PRIMARY CARE
OF THE
NEWBORN

PRIMARY CARE OF THE NEWBORN

a Mosby handbook

HENRY M. SEIDEL, MD
Professor Emeritus of Pediatrics,
The Johns Hopkins University School of Medicine;
Attending Physician, Department of Pediatrics,
The Johns Hopkins Hospital,
Baltimore, Maryland

BERYL J. ROSENSTEIN, MD
Professor of Pediatrics,
The Johns Hopkins University School of Medicine;
Attending Physician, Department of Pediatrics,
The Johns Hopkins Hospital,
Baltimore, Maryland

AMBADAS PATHAK, MD
Assistant Professor of Pediatrics,
The Johns Hopkins University School of Medicine;
Clinical Associate Professor of Pediatrics,
University of Maryland School of Medicine;
Distinguished Emeritus Staff,
Department of Pediatrics,
Greater Baltimore Medical Center,
Baltimore, Maryland

THIRD EDITION

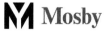 Mosby

A Harcourt Health Sciences Company

St. Louis   London   Philadelphia   Sydney   Toronto

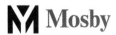

M Mosby

A Harcourt Health Sciences Company

Editor: Elizabeth M. Fathman
Project Manager: Carol Sullivan Weis
Senior Production Editor: Karen M. Rehwinkel
Designer: Mark A. Oberkrom

Mosby, Inc.
A Harcourt Health Sciences Company
11830 Westline Industrial Drive
St. Louis, Missouri 63146

Printed in the United States of America

ISBN 0-323-01111-X

01   02   03   04   05   TG/FF   9   8   7   6   5   4   3   2

Contributors

Max M. April, MD, FAAP, FACS
Co-Director of Pediatric Otolaryngology,
Department of Otolaryngology,
Lenox Hill Hospital,
New York, New York

James F. Casella, MD
Rainey Professor of Pediatric Hematology,
Department of Pediatrics, Division of Hematology,
The Johns Hopkins University School of Medicine;
Chief, Pediatric Hematology,
The Johns Hopkins Hospital,
Baltimore, Maryland

Bernard A. Cohen, MD
Associate Professor of Pediatrics and Dermatology,
The Johns Hopkins University School of Medicine;
Director of Pediatric Dermatology,
The Johns Hopkins Children's Center,
Baltimore, Maryland

Marvin Cornblath, MD
Lecturer, Department of Pediatrics,
The Johns Hopkins University School of Medicine,
Baltimore, Maryland

John P. Gearhart, MD
Professor of Pediatric Urology and Pediatrics,
The Johns Hopkins University School of Medicine;
Director of Pediatric Urology,
The Johns Hopkins Hospital,
Baltimore, Maryland

Ada Hamosh, MD, MPH
Assistant Professor of Pediatrics, Institute of Genetic Medicine,
The Johns Hopkins University School of Medicine;
Attending Physician, The Johns Hopkins Hospital,
Baltimore, Maryland

Rebecca N. Ichord, MD
Assistant Professor, Department of Neurology and Pediatrics,
The Johns Hopkins University School of Medicine,
Baltimore, Maryland

Timothy R.B. Johnson, MD
Bates Professor of Diseases of Women and Children;
Chair, Department of Obstetrics and Gynecology,
University of Michigan,
Ann Arbor, Michigan

Jean S. Kan, MD
Professor of Pediatrics, Division of Pediatric Cardiology,
The Johns Hopkins University School of Medicine;
Co-Director, Division of Pediatric Cardiology,
The Johns Hopkins Hospital,
Baltimore, Maryland

Gregory J. Kato, MD
Associate Professor of Pediatrics and Oncology,
Department of Pediatrics, Division of Hematology,
The Johns Hopkins University School of Medicine;
Attending Physician, Department of Pediatrics,
The Johns Hopkins Hospital,
Baltimore, Maryland

Janet S. Kinney, MD
Staff Neonatologist, Department of Neonatology,
Baylor University Medical Center,
Dallas, Texas

Carlton K.K. Lee, PharmD, MPH
Assistant Professor, Department of Pediatrics,
The Johns Hopkins University School of Medicine;
Clinical Coordinator, Pediatrics,
Department of Pharmacy,
The Johns Hopkins Hospital,
Baltimore, Maryland

Robert M. Naclerio, MD
Professor and Chief,
Section of Otolaryngology-Head and Neck Surgery,
The University of Chicago,
Chicago, Illinois

Catherine A. Neill, MD, FRCP
Professor Emeritus,
Department of Pediatrics,
The Johns Hopkins University School of Medicine;
Pediatric Cardiologist Emeritus,
Department of Pediatrics,
The Johns Hopkins Hospital,
Baltimore, Maryland

Ambadas Pathak, MD
Assistant Professor of Pediatrics,
The Johns Hopkins University School of Medicine;
Clinical Associate Professor of Pediatrics,
University of Maryland School of Medicine;
Distinguished Emeritus Staff,
Department of Pediatrics,
Greater Baltimore Medical Center,
Baltimore, Maryland

Michael X. Repka, MD
Professor, Department of Ophthalmology;
Associate Professor, Department of Pediatrics,
The Johns Hopkins University School of Medicine;
Attending Physician, Department of Ophthalmology,
The Johns Hopkins Hospital,
Baltimore, Maryland

Beryl J. Rosenstein, MD
Professor, Department of Pediatrics,
The Johns Hopkins University School of Medicine;
Attending Physician, Department of Pediatrics,
The Johns Hopkins Hospital,
Baltimore, Maryland

Jose M. Saavedra, MD
Attending Physician, Department of Pediatrics,
Division of Gastroenterology and Nutrition,
The Johns Hopkins Hospital,
Baltimore, Maryland

Henry M. Seidel, MD
Professor Emeritus of Pediatrics,
The Johns Hopkins University School of Medicine;
Attending Physician, Department of Pediatrics,
The Johns Hopkins Hospital,
Baltimore, Maryland

Patricia H. Smouse, MSN, CPNP
Assistant in Pediatrics, Department of Pediatrics,
The Johns Hopkins University School of Medicine,
Baltimore, Maryland

Paul D. Sponseller, MD
Professor, Department of Orthopedic Surgery,
The Johns Hopkins University School of Medicine;
Head, Division of Pediatric Orthopedics,
The Johns Hopkins Hospital,
Baltimore, Maryland

Mark C. Steinhoff, MD
Professor of International Health, Department of Pediatrics,
The Johns Hopkins University School of Medicine;
Attending Physician, Department of Pediatrics,
The Johns Hopkins Hospital,
Baltimore, Maryland

Kristyne M. Stone, MS
Genetic Counselor, Department of Gynecology and Obstetrics,
The Johns Hopkins University School of Medicine,
The Johns Hopkins Hospital,
Baltimore, Maryland

Timothy Townsend, MD
Associate Professor, Department of Pediatrics
The Johns Hopkins University School of Medicine;
Attending Physician, Department of Pediatrics,
The Johns Hopkins Hospital,
Baltimore, Maryland

Judith W. Vogelhut, RN, BS, CPNP, IBCLC
Nurse Coordinator, Breastfeeding Center,
Department of General Pediatrics and Adolescent Medicine,
The Johns Hopkins University School of Medicine,
The Johns Hopkins Hospital,
Baltimore, Maryland

Jean S. Wheeler, BSN, CPNP
Assistant in Pediatrics, Department of Pediatrics,
The Johns Hopkins University School of Medicine,
Baltimore, Maryland

Siew-Jyu Wong, MD
Instructor, Department of Pediatrics,
The Johns Hopkins University School of Medicine;
Former Director of Newborn Nurseries,
Greater Baltimore Medical Center,
Baltimore, Maryland

To our children and grandchildren, who are also our teachers; to the nurse practitioners and residents with whom we have worked.

Preface

The Nelson 2 Nursery in The Johns Hopkins Hospital and the New-born Nursery at the Greater Baltimore Medical Center are the facilities in which the editors of this volume have had the privilege of caring for newborn infants. Each of us has been long accustomed to carrying *The Harriet Lane Handbook,* one of us for almost 50 years, and each of us has believed that there is still room in our pockets for a companion volume devoted solely to the care of the newborn in the first hours and days of life, the newborn who is *not* a resident in an intensive care nursery.

The need for information—the kind and amount that can stimulate initial thoughts and insights and ease the way to a needed course of immediate action—is a constant in the service of our patients. With *Primary Care of the Newborn* in its third edition, it continues to be our hope that this compact volume can achieve that end for practitioners young and old and for their patients.

Henry M. Seidel
Beryl J. Rosenstein
Ambadas Pathak

Acknowledgments

We owe a great deal to many men and women who have helped make the third edition of this handbook a reality. Many of our colleagues have reviewed individual sections, and others have made numerous contributions in many ways. They include Nancy Barnett, MD; Francine Cheese; George Dover, MD; Edward E. Lawson, MD; Angella J. Olden, MS, RN; Linda Packham; Radha Pathak, MD; and Diann L. Snyder, RN, MS.

We wish, too, to include those teachers, mentors, and colleagues who have contributed so much to our experience in the care of babies: Harry Gordon and Alexander Schaffer long ago and, today, Billy Andrews, Mary Ellen Avery, Jeffrey Maisels, and Nicholas Nelson.

Those who do not write books or contribute to their development have not had the pleasant opportunity to learn about and get to know those whose job it is to ensure a positive outcome and who work quietly and effectively behind the scenes. For us, Liz Fathman, Paige Mosher Wilke, Peggy Perel, Carol Sullivan Weis, and Karen Rehwinkel epitomize these professionals in the best possible way. We thank them for making our task easy and our relationship with them a pleasure.

Contents

PRIMARY CARE
OF THE
NEWBORN

1

Prenatal Visit

HENRY M. SEIDEL

I. GENERAL

Prenatal visits are invaluable, particularly during a first pregnancy, when practitioner and patient are strangers. These visits provide an opportunity to learn much about each other (e.g., history relevant to the pregnancy, practice habits of the practitioner) and to begin to build the foundation of trust and mutual respect essential in continuity care and in moments of great stress, such as in cases of congenital defect in the neonate. During the visits there is much to discuss, ideally with both mother and father so that full information and necessary education facilitate active family participation in decision making and initiate counseling about the experience of living with an infant. A partnership is formed with the goal of serving the parents and baby.

N.B.: If there has not been opportunity for a prenatal visit, everything discussed in this chapter is relevant to the time of first introduction to the baby and family (see Chapter 5). Also, in lieu of this basic visit if it is not possible, a brief "get to know you" visit may at least ease future interactions. At the least, a telephone call can acquaint the parents with the rudiments of the practitioner's office practices.

II. TIMING

By early in the third trimester much of the *history* of the pregnancy is available and parents have time to seek other resources if they are dissatisfied with the practitioner for any reason.

III. DETAILS OF THE HISTORY
A. Family.
1. Consanguineous marriage.
2. Development of a chart of genetic lineage when indicated.
3. Particular disease concerns: Questions regarding heritable and contagious illness; effect of major illness in parents or in others in family of the expected child.

4. Status of siblings.
5. Specific topics, at the least, that should be addressed include the following:
   a. Allergy.
   b. Blood dyscrasia.
   c. Cardiovascular conditions (e.g., congenital disorders, rheumatic fever).
   d. Pulmonary conditions.
   e. Renal conditions.
   f. Contagion (e.g., tuberculosis, syphilis, hepatitis, herpes, acquired immunodeficiency syndrome [AIDS], rubella, and much more).

B. Pregnancy.

1. Previous pregnancies; results.
2. Intercurrent illness.
   a. Infection of any kind (e.g., hepatitis, tuberculosis, sexually transmitted disease, herpes).
   b. Vaginal bleeding.
   c. Toxemia (pretoxic states).
3. Chronic illness (e.g., lupus erythematosus, diabetes, thyroid disease).
4. Weight gain (excessive or insufficient).
5. Time and intensity of fetal movement.
6. Care of animals (e.g., cats and the possibility of toxoplasmosis).
7. Drugs.
   a. Prescribed (e.g., anticonvulsants, anticoagulants).
   b. Over-the-counter (OTC).
   c. Illicit (in some areas, illicit drug use is virtually an epidemic).
   d. Tobacco and/or alcohol intake.

C. Prenatal screening.

1. Amniocentesis.
2. Sonography.
3. Chorionic villus sampling (CVS).
4. Rh sensitization and setup.
5. Maternal and paternal blood type.
6. Serologic studies for sexually transmitted disease (rapid plasma reagin [RPR] for syphilis; hepatitis B surface antigen, and human immunodeficiency virus [HIV] status).
7. Tuberculin test.
8. Alpha-fetoprotein.
9. Radiographs.
10. Serologic studies for cytomegalovirus (CMV) or toxoplasmosis.

D. Social.

1. Family constellation.
   a. Members of household.
   b. Intergenerational relationships: Grandparents, aunts and uncles, close family friends.
   c. Sources of child care: Relatives, paid helpers.
   d. Sources of income.
   e. Attitudes on discipline.

2. Physical setting.
3. Religious preferences (e.g., question of blood transfusion, mandate for circumcision).
4. Ethnic preferences, background.

IV. ANTICIPATORY GUIDANCE
A. Feeding options. Mother's preference; father's support.
B. Rooming in and the meaning of bonding.
C. Circumcision, yes or no?
D. Necessary home furnishings and equipment; type of diapers.
E. The first ride home. Appropriate automobile restraints.
F. Preparing siblings for the baby's arrival.
G. Practitioner's practice rules, preferences, and style.
1. Call arrangements.
2. Appointment schedules.
3. Fees and billing.
4. Hospital affiliations.
H. Open-ended discussion.
1. Explore potential of expressed or unexpressed concerns (e.g., What do I do when I want to "flush the baby down the toilet?").
2. Handouts.

N.B.: Though clearly more than enough for an hour's conversation, this visit is essential to the development of sound, ongoing relationships; no one appropriate approach or style is best. There is lots of room for individual variation in length, frequency, and content of discussion; content may be shared with first postpartum visit.

V. ADOLESCENT PREGNANCY
A. The teenager is, of course, subject to all the pleasures and problems of pregnancy and delivery. In addition, as with all patients, the practitioner should be aware of the particular circumstance and characteristics of the adolescent, including the following:
1. Level of education.
2. Communication skills.
3. Family structure.
4. Relationship with putative father.
B. The practitioner should also:
1. Adjust his or her language and style of presentation to the needs of the patient without limiting the range of issues for discussion. The information does not have to be communicated in one session.
2. Involve family if at all possible.
3. Involve father of the child if at all possible.

N.B.: Be sure to discuss and provide for follow-up contraception.

VI. CULTURAL CONSIDERATIONS
The prenatal interview and *any* ensuing interactions require insight into the culture of the family and an understanding of what it is that differentiates individuals and groups if all patient needs are to be appropriately served (see Appendix J). Any individual may and

most often does belong to more than one group or subgroup. These multiple classifications can be the result of any combination of ethnic origin, religion, gender, social network, occupation, or profession.

A. Some guidelines to cultural understanding.

1. Respect individuals as unique, with culture as one determinant.
2. Respect the unfamiliar.
3. Identify and examine personal cultural beliefs. Acute self-understanding engenders ability to put into context and constrain personal likes and dislikes.
4. Recognize that different cultural groups have varying practices that attempt to promote health and cure illness. If the cultural view is "scientific" in that a precise cause can be determined for every problem, the family is more apt to be comfortable with Western approaches to care. A more naturalistic or "holistic" approach views life as part of a greater whole that must be in harmony. If the balance is disturbed, illness can result, and the goal then is to retrieve balance or harmony. Aspects of these concepts are evident among many persons of Hispanic, Native American, Asian, and Arab cultures, and they are increasingly evident in the United States today. There are also beliefs in the "supernatural," forces for good and evil that determine individual fate. In such a context, illness may be thought to be a punishment for wrongdoing.
5. Be willing to modify care in keeping with the patient's cultural background.
6. Appreciate that each person's cultural values are often deep set and possibly difficult or undesirable to change.
7. Do not confuse the physical and the cultural or allow the physical to symbolize the cultural. This does not deny the interdependence of the physical with the cultural. Skin color, for example, precedes most of the experience of life and the subsequent obvious interweaving of color with cultural experience.
8. Do not assume homogeneity in any group. The stereotype is to be rejected. People within groups can and do respond differently to the same stimuli.
9. The health care worker and the newborn's caretaker must understand one another fully and clearly. Ask if not sure. Do not make assumptions without validation from the family.

B. Family relationships.

Family structure and the social organizations to which a family belongs (e.g., churches, clubs, and schools) are among the many imprinting and constraining cultural forces, particularly with the shift toward dual-income families, single-parent families, an increasing number of teenage pregnancies, the prevalence of divorce, and the increasing involvement of fathers in child care.

N.B.: One type of behavior may predict another type (e.g., mothers who take advantage of appropriate prenatal care will generally provide appropriate infant care regardless of educational level, marital status, family relationships, or illicit drug use).

C. Questions that can provide cultural insights.
1. Health beliefs and practices.
   a. How does the family define health and illness?
   b. What is the attitude toward preventive health measures?
   c. Are there health topics that may be particularly sensitive or that are considered taboo?
   d. What are the attitudes toward pain, handicapping conditions, chronic disease, death, and dying?
2. Religious influences and special rituals.
   a. Is the family adherent to a religion? To what degree?
   b. Are there special religious practices or beliefs that may affect health care?
   c. What events, rituals, and ceremonies are considered important within the life cycle, such as birth and baptism?
3. Language and communication.
   a. What language is spoken in the home?
   b. How well is English understood, both spoken and written?
   c. Are there special behaviors for demonstrating respect or disrespect?
4. Parenting styles and role of family.
   a. Who makes the decisions in the family?
   b. What is the composition of the family and the number of generations involved? Which relatives compose the family unit?
   c. What is the role of and attitude toward children in the family?
   d. Are there special beliefs and practices surrounding conception, pregnancy, childbirth, lactation, and child rearing?

VII. ETHICAL CONSIDERATIONS
The ethical context to the relationship with the newborn and the family has been better defined in recent years. Ethics does not provide answers; rather, it offers a disciplined approach to understanding and to determining ultimate behavior. Given a problem (e.g., a perceived necessary violation of confidentiality), several concepts must be considered.

A. Autonomy. The need for self-determination. With a newborn, parents, family, and other significant persons must be included and the boundaries of their autonomy clearly set. The core question is, Who shall speak for the baby?

B. Beneficence. Beneficence is the mandate to do good for the patient. There is always a concern that the need to do good may be too eagerly pursued and may result in a paternalism that might smother the family's autonomy.

C. Nonmaleficence. Nonmaleficence is the mandate to do no harm to the patient; *primum non nocere.*

D. Utilitarianism. Utilitarianism is the practical need to consider the allocation of resources for the greater good of the larger community (distributive justice).

E. Fairness and justice. Fairness and justice enable recognition of the often precarious balance between the competing interests of the individual and the community.

F. Deontologic imperatives. Deontologic imperatives are the duties of care providers established by tradition and in a cultural context.

These principles often come into conflict (e.g., the use of limited resources in situations thought to be futile, the difficulties in end-of-life decisions). Consideration of each with the baby in mind can, however, lead to helpful outcomes. Respect for all involved and flexibility in attitudes are key ingredients in the search for answers. Another unfortunate danger, the initiation of inappropriate social contact (e.g., gift giving, sexual favors), can be readily avoided in a relationship that facilitates limit setting.

BIBLIOGRAPHY

Charney E: Counseling of parents around the birth of a baby, *Pediatr Rev* 4:167, 1982.

Committee on Bioethics: Appropriate boundaries in the pediatrician-family-patient relationship, *Pediatrics* 104:334, 1999.

Committee on Psychosocial Aspects of Child and Family Health: The prenatal visit, *Pediatrics* 97:141, 1996.

VanderHeide A, VanderMaas PJ, VanderWal G, et al: The role of parents in end-of-life decisions in neonatology: physicians views and practices, *Pediatrics* 101:413, 1998.

Wessel MA: The prenatal pediatric visit, *Pediatrics* 32:926, 1963.

2

High-Risk Pregnancy

TIMOTHY R.B. JOHNSON

I. DEFINITION OF HIGH-RISK PREGNANCY

A. **Varies depending on patient population.**

B. **The most common high-risk conditions** include age >35, age <17, postterm pregnancy, associated medical complications, previous preterm labor, multiple pregnancy, and socioeconomic problems. Some maternal medical problems can be associated with specific neonatal conditions (Box 2-1).

C. **Risk assessment is useful.** An attempt is made to identify the 20% of patients that account for 60% or more of perinatal morbidity and mortality.

D. **Various risk assessment scores** have been developed for perinatal morbidity and mortality. Generally, risk is assessed at registration, in middle to late pregnancy, and again in labor. Obstetric preconception assessment is recommended, analogous to a prenatal visit. Risk assessment has been developed for preterm labor and includes historical assessment and home uterine activity monitoring.

E. **The term *high-risk pregnancy* can have medicolegal implications.** As with the term *asphyxia,* the term *high-risk pregnancy* must be used carefully. Depending on the degree of risk, referral to perinatal specialists or neonatal specialists prenatally is indicated.

F. **Group B streptococcus screening** and treatment protocols exist; the pediatrician should be aware of what protocols are in use (Figs. 2-1 and 2-2).

G. **Human immunodeficiency virus (HIV).** Zidovudine (AZT) and retroviral therapy have been shown to decrease vertical transmission of HIV. Therapy should follow the most current recommendation. Cesarean section is recommended for delivery (Table 2-1).

II. PRENATAL RECORD

A. **One advantage of prenatal care is the identification of risk factors.** Many risk factors are associated with a commonly derived medical obstetric history. Major factors include the following:

BOX 2-1
Neonatal Complications of Maternal Disease

DIABETES MELLITUS
Congenital malformation (especially caudal regression)
Macrosomia
Birth trauma
Intrauterine growth retardation (IUGR)
Fetal death
Cardiomyopathy
Hypoglycemia
Respiratory distress syndrome
Hyperbilirubinemia
Polycythemia
Hypocalcemia
Hypomagnesemia

TOXEMIA/PREECLAMPSIA
IUGR
Magnesium sulfate exposure
Acidosis/decreased fetal reserve

BLOOD DISORDERS
Rh and atypical antibodies/ABO incompatibility
Hyperbilirubinemia and kernicterus
Alloimmune thrombocytopenia
Fetal thrombocytopenia
Isoimmune thrombocytopenia*
? Neonatal thrombocytopenia

---

*Many other specific conditions can cause similar or associated fetal complications (myasthenia gravis/neonatal myasthenia, lupus/neonatal lupus syndrome, myotonic dystrophy).

1. Previous history of preterm labor, illicit drug use, alcohol consumption, smoking, low socioeconomic status, and problematic genetic background.
2. Previous history of stillbirth or miscarriage.
3. Associated medical complications, such as hypertension or diabetes.
B. Laboratory studies (Fig. 2-3) can identify risk and should include the following:
1. Blood type, Rh status, and antibody status.
2. Syphilis serology.
3. Hematocrit.
4. Hepatitis B screen.
5. HIV test.
6. Gonococcus culture.

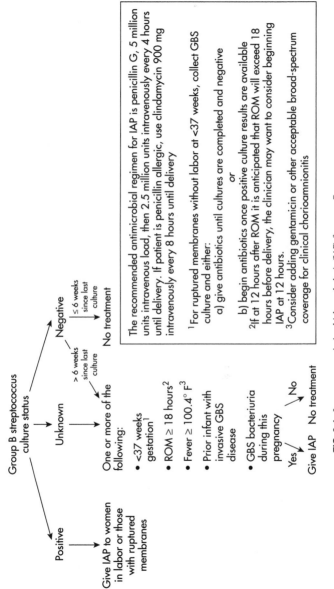

Group B streptococcus culture status

Positive → Give IAP to women in labor or those with ruptured membranes

Unknown

Negative
- > 6 weeks since last culture
- ≤ 6 weeks since last culture → No treatment

One or more of the following:
- <37 weeks gestation[1]
- ROM ≥ 18 hours[2]
- Fever ≥ 100.4° F[3]
- Prior infant with invasive GBS disease
- GBS bacteriuria during this pregnancy

Yes → Give IAP
No → No treatment

The recommended antimicrobial regimen for IAP is penicillin G, 5 million units intravenous load, then 2.5 million units intravenously every 4 hours until delivery. If patient is penicillin allergic, use clindamycin 900 mg intravenously every 8 hours until delivery

[1] For ruptured membranes without labor at <37 weeks, collect GBS culture and either:
   a) give antibiotics until cultures are completed and negative

   or

   b) begin antibiotics once positive culture results are available

[2] If at 12 hours after ROM it is anticipated that ROM will exceed 18 hours before delivery, the clinician may want to consider beginning IAP at 12 hours.

[3] Consider adding gentamicin or other acceptable broad-spectrum coverage for clinical chorioamnionitis

FIG. 2-1. Intrapartum antimicrobial prophylaxis (IAP) for group-B streptococcus.

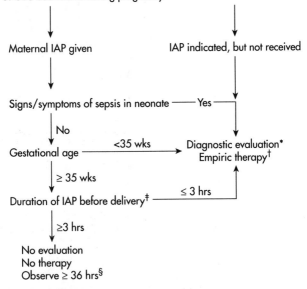

Indications for IAP

A. Positive maternal rectovaginal culture for GBS during pregnancy
   (unless cesarean section is performed on a woman not in labor
   with intact membranes)

or

B. GBS status unknown within 6 weeks of delivery, *and*
1. <37 weeks gestational age (unless delivered for pure maternal
   indications [e.g., preeclampsia]), *or*
2. ROM ≥ 18 hours, *or*
3. Maternal temperature ≥ 100.4° F (38° C), *or*
4. Prior infant with GBS disease, *or*
5. GBS bacteriuria during pregnancy

Maternal IAP given   IAP indicated, but not received

Signs/symptoms of sepsis in neonate —— Yes

No

Gestational age ——— <35 wks ——→ Diagnostic evaluation*
                                    Empiric therapy†
≥ 35 wks
                        ≤ 3 hrs
Duration of IAP before delivery‡ ———

≥3 hrs

No evaluation
No therapy
Observe ≥ 36 hrs§

---

*Blood culture, urine antigen for GBS (if IAP received), lumbar
 puncture if symptoms and sufficiently stable or at discretion of
 physician. Chest radiograph if cardiopulmonary signs; complete
 blood cell (CBC) and differential at discretion of physician.
†Duration of therapy is institution specific, may discontinue if count
 and antigen level and chest radiograph are negative after 36
 hours and patient is well.
‡Penicillin or other antibiotics are effective against GBS.
§No discharge before 36 hours.

FIG. 2-2. Guidelines for management of the neonate born to a mother who is a candidate for IAP.

TABLE 2-1
Pediatric AIDS Clinical Trials Group 076 AZT Regimen

Time of AZT administration	Regimen
Antepartum	Oral administration of 100 mg AZT five times daily, initiated at 14-34 weeks gestation and continued throughout the pregnancy*
Intrapartum	During labor, intravenous administration of AZT in a 1-hour initial dose of 2 mg/kg body weight, followed by a continuous infusion of 1 mg/kg body weight/hour until delivery†
Postpartum	Oral administration of AZT to the newborn (AZT syrup) at 2 mg/kg body weight/dose every 6 hours for the first 6 weeks of life, beginning at 8-12 hours after birth NOTE: Intravenous dosage for infants who cannot tolerate oral intake is 1.5 mg/kg body weight every 6 hours

From Centers for Disease Control and Prevention: *MMWR* 47(RR-2):2, 1998.
AZT, Zidovudine.
*AZT is generally part of a triple antiviral therapy regimen.
†From American College of Obstetricians and Gynecologists: *Scheduled cesarean delivery and the prevention of vertical transmission of HIV infection,* ACOG Committee opinion #219, August 1999.

C. The prenatal record should clearly indicate high-risk conditions that have been identified and should detail the management plan. Example: "Partner of intravenous (IV) drug user—HIV infection. Plan: Screening for HIV status."

III. RISK-SCORING FORMS

A. Various risk-scoring forms have been developed, both freestanding and associated with the prenatal record. Example: The Hollister record (Hollister Inc., Libertyville, Ill.), a computer-based record; genetic risk-scoring systems; preterm labor risk-scoring systems.

B. There is no well-defined prenatal record that is used throughout the United States. Generally used forms include those of the American College of Obstetricians and Gynecologists (Fig. 2-4), the Hollister record, and various other forms. The prenatal and hospital obstetric forms contain much important risk-assessment information for appropriate newborn care.

	Preconception or 1st visit	6-8*	14-16	24-28	32	36	38	39	40	41
						Weeks				
History										
Medical, including genetic	X									
Psychosocial	X									
Update medical & psychosocial		X	X	X	X	X	X	X	X	X
Physical examination										
General	X									
Blood pressure	X	X	X	X	X	X	X	X	X	X
Height	X									
Weight	X	X	X	X	X	X	X	X	X	X
Height & weight profile	X									
Pelvic examinatin & pelvimetry	X	X								
Breast examination	X	X								
Fundal height			X	X	X	X	X	X	X	X
Fetal position & heart rate			X	X	X	X	X	X	X	X
Cevical examination	X									
Laboratory tests										
Hemoglobin or hematocrit	X	X		X		X				
Rh factor	X									
Pap smear	X									
Diabetic screen				X						
MSAFP			X							
Urine										
Dipstick (protein, sugar)	X	X	X	X	X	X	X	X	X	X
Culture		X								
Infections										
Rubella titer	X									
Syphilis test	X			X						
Gonococcal culture	X	X				X				
Hepatitis B	X									
HIV (offered)	X	X								
Illicit drug screen (offered)	X									
Genetic screen	X									

*If preconception care has preceded.

FIG. 2-3. Medical components of prenatal care. Note that screens for syphilis, hepatitis B, HIV, and illicit drugs may need to be repeated at delivery in high-risk situations.

Patient Addressograph

DATE _____

NAME _____
 LAST   FIRST   MIDDLE

ID # _____ HOSPITAL OF DELIVERY _____

NEWBORN'S PHYSICIAN _____ REFERRED BY _____

FINAL EDD_____		PRIMARY PROVIDER/GROUP _____

BIRTH DATE		AGE	RACE	MARITAL STATUS	ADDRESS:		
MONTH DAY YEAR				S M W D SEP			
OCCUPATION				EDUCATION	ZIP:	PHONE:	(H)	(O)
☐ HOMEMAKER				(LAST GRADE COMPLETED)	INSURANCE CARRIER/MEDICAID #		
☐ OUTSIDE WORK							
☐ STUDENT	Type of Work						
HUSBAND/FATHER OF BABY:			PHONE:		EMERGENCY CONTACT:		PHONE:

TOTAL PREG	FULL TERM	PREMATURE	AB. INDUCED	AB. SPONTANEOUS	ECTOPICS	MULTIPLE BIRTHS	LIVING

MENSTRUAL HISTORY

LMP ☐ DEFINITE ☐ APPROXIMATE (MONTH KNOWN)   MENSES MONTHLY ☐ YES ☐ NO   FREQUENCY: Q _____ DAYS   MENARCHE _____ (AGE ONSET)
  ☐ UNKNOWN ☐ NORMAL AMOUNT/DURATION   PRIOR MENSES _____ DATE   ON BCP AT CONCEPT. ☐ YES ☐ NO   hCG + ____ / ____ / ____
  ☐ FINAL _____

PAST PREGNANCIES (LAST SIX)

DATE MONTH / YEAR	GA WEEKS	LENGTH OF LABOR	BIRTH WEIGHT	SEX M/F	TYPE DELIVERY	ANES.	PLACE OF DELIVERY	PRETERM LABOR YES / NO	COMMENTS / COMPLICATIONS

PAST MEDICAL HISTORY

	O Neg + Pos.	DETAIL POSITIVE REMARKS INCLUDE DATE & TREATMENT		O Neg + Pos.	DETAIL POSITIVE REMARKS INCLUDE DATE & TREATMENT
1. DIABETES			16. D (Rh) SENSITIZED		
2. HYPERTENSION			17. PULMONARY (TB, ASTHMA)		
3. HEART DISEASE			18. ALLERGIES (DRUGS)		
4. AUTOIMMUNE DISORDER			19. BREAST		
5. KIDNEY DISEASE / UTI			20. GYN SURGERY		
6. NEUROLOGIC/EPILEPSY					
7. PSYCHIATRIC			21. OPERATIONS / HOSPITALIZATIONS (YEAR & REASON)		
8. HEPATITIS / LIVER DISEASE					
9. VARICOSITIES / PHLEBITIS					
10. THYROID DYSFUNCTION			22. ANESTHETIC COMPLICATIONS		
11. TRAUMA/DOMESTIC VIOLENCE			23. HISTORY OF ABNORMAL PAP		
12. HISTORY OF BLOOD TRANSFUS			24. UTERINE ANOMALY/DES		
	AMT./DAY PREPREG	AMT./DAY PREG	#YEARS USE	25. INFERTILITY		
13. TOBACCO				26. RELEVANT FAMILY HISTORY		
14. ALCOHOL						
15. STREET DRUGS				27. OTHER		

COMMENTS: _____

The American College of Obstetricians and Gynecologists, 409 12th Street, SW, PO Box 96920, Washington, DC 20090-6920   Copyright © 1997 (Version 4)

ACOG ANTEPARTUM RECORD (FORM A)

FIG. 2-4. American College of Obstetricians and Gynecologists (ACOG) antepartum record. (Copyright 1997, ACOG.)   *Continued*

Patient Addressograph

SYMPTOMS SINCE LMP

GENETIC SCREENING/TERATOLOGY COUNSELING
INCLUDES PATIENT, BABY'S FATHER, OR ANYONE IN EITHER FAMILY WITH:

	YES	NO		YES	NO
1. PATIENT'S AGE ≥ 35 YEARS			12. MENTAL RETARDATION/AUTISM		
2. THALASSEMIA (ITALIAN, GREEK, MEDITERRANEAN, OR ASIAN BACKGROUND); MCV < 80			IF YES, WAS PERSON TESTED FOR FRAGILE X?		
3. NEURAL TUBE DEFECT (MENINGOMYELOCELE, SPINA BIFIDA, OR ANENCEPHALY)			13. OTHER INHERITED GENETIC OR CHROMOSOMAL DISORDER		
4. CONGENITAL HEART DEFECT			14. MATERNAL METABOLIC DISORDER (EG. INSULIN-DEPENDENT DIABETES, PKU)		
5. DOWN SYNDROME			15. PATIENT OR BABY'S FATHER HAD A CHILD WITH BIRTH DEFECTS NOT LISTED ABOVE		
6. TAY-SACHS (EG. JEWISH, CAJUN, FRENCH CANADIAN)			16. RECURRENT PREGNANCY LOSS, OR A STILLBIRTH		
7. SICKLE CELL DISEASE OR TRAIT (AFRICAN)			17. MEDICATIONS/STREET DRUGS/ALCOHOL SINCE LAST MENSTRUAL PERIOD		
8. HEMOPHILIA			IF YES, AGENT(S):		
9. MUSCULAR DYSTROPHY			18. ANY OTHER		
10. CYSTIC FIBROSIS					
11. HUNTINGTON CHOREA					

COMMENTS/COUNSELING: _____

_____

INFECTION HISTORY	YES	NO		YES	NO
1. HIGH RISK HEPATITIS B/IMMUNIZED?			4. RASH OR VIRAL ILLNESS SINCE LAST MENSTRUAL PERIOD		
2. LIVE WITH SOMEONE WITH TB OR EXPOSED TO TB			5. HISTORY OF STD, GC, CHLAMYDIA, HPV, SYPHILIS		
3. PATIENT OR PARTNER HAS HISTORY OF GENITAL HERPES			6. OTHER (SEE COMMENTS)		

COMMENTS: _____

_____ INTERVIEWER'S SIGNATURE _____

INITIAL PHYSICAL EXAMINATION

DATE ____ / ____ / ____   PREPREGNANCY WEIGHT _____   HEIGHT _____   BP_____

1. HEENT	☐ NORMAL	☐ ABNORMAL	12. VULVA	☐ NORMAL	☐ CONDYLOMA	☐ LESIONS
2. FUNDI	☐ NORMAL	☐ ABNORMAL	13. VAGINA	☐ NORMAL	☐ INFLAMMATION	☐ DISCHARGE
3. TEETH	☐ NORMAL	☐ ABNORMAL	14. CERVIX	☐ NORMAL	☐ INFLAMMATION	☐ LESIONS
4. THYROID	☐ NORMAL	☐ ABNORMAL	15. UTERUS SIZE	_____ WEEKS		☐ FIBROIDS
5. BREASTS	☐ NORMAL	☐ ABNORMAL	16. ADNEXA	☐ NORMAL	☐ MASS	
6. LUNGS	☐ NORMAL	☐ ABNORMAL	17. RECTUM	☐ NORMAL	☐ ABNORMAL	
7. HEART	☐ NORMAL	☐ ABNORMAL	18. DIAGONAL CONJUGATE	☐ REACHED	☐ NO	_____ CM
8. ABDOMEN	☐ NORMAL	☐ ABNORMAL	19. SPINES	☐ AVERAGE	☐ PROMINENT	☐ BLUNT
9. EXTREMITIES	☐ NORMAL	☐ ABNORMAL	20. SACRUM	☐ CONCAVE	☐ STRAIGHT	☐ ANTERIOR
10. SKIN	☐ NORMAL	☐ ABNORMAL	21. SUBPUBIC ARCH	☐ NORMAL	☐ WIDE	☐ NARROW
11. LYMPH NODES	☐ NORMAL	☐ ABNORMAL	22. GYNECOID PELVIC TYPE	☐ YES	☐ NO	

COMMENTS (Number and explain abnormals): _____

_____ EXAM BY _____

ACOG ANTEPARTUM RECORD (FORM B)

FIG. 2-4, cont'd. American College of Obstetricians and Gynecologists (ACOG) antepartum record. (Copyright 1997, ACOG.)

NAME _____
| LAST | FIRST | MIDDLE |

DRUG ALLERGY:

RELIGIOUS/CULTURAL CONSIDERATIONS _____ | ANESTHESIA CONSULT PLANNED ☐ YES ☐ NO

PROBLEMS/PLANS	MEDICATION LIST:	Start date	Stop date
1.	1.		
2.	2.		
3.	3.		
4.	4.		
5.	5.		
6.	6.		

EDD CONFIRMATION

INITIAL EDD:

LMP ___/___/___ = EDD ___/___/___
INITIAL EXAM ___/___/___ = ___WKS = EDD ___/___/___
ULTRASOUND ___/___/___ = ___WKS = EDD ___/___/___
INITIAL EDD ___/___/___ INITIALED BY _____

18-20-WEEK EDD UPDATE:

QUICKENING ___/___/___ +22 WKS = ___/___/___
FUNDAL HT. AT UMBIL. ___/___/___ +20 WKS = ___/___/___
FHT W/FETOSCOPE ___/___/___ +20 WKS = ___/___/___
ULTRASOUND ___/___/___ = ___WKS = ___/___/___
FINAL EDD ___/___/___ INITIALED BY _____

VISIT DATE (YEAR)	WEEKS GEST. (BEST EST.)	FUNDAL HEIGHT (CM)	PRESENTATION	FHR	FETAL MOVEMENT	PRETERM LABOR SIGNS/SYMPTOMS (+ PRESENT, O ABSENT)	CERVIX EXAM (DIL/EFF/STA)	BLOOD PRESSURE	EDEMA	WEIGHT	URINE (GLUCOSE/ALBUMIN)	NEXT APPOINTMENT	PROVIDER (INITIALS)	COMMENTS:

PROBLEMS: _____

COMMENTS: _____

ACOG ANTEPARTUM RECORD (FORM C)

FIG. 2-4, cont'd. For legend see opposite page. *Continued*

LABORATORY AND EDUCATION

Patient Addressograph

INITIAL LABS	DATE	RESULT	REVIEWED
BLOOD TYPE	/ /	A B AB O	
D (Rh) TYPE	/ /		
ANTIBODY SCREEN	/ /		
HCT/HGB	/ /	_____ % _____ g/dl.	
PAP TEST	/ /	NORMAL / ABNORMAL / ____	
RUBELLA	/ /		
VDRL	/ /		
URINE CULTURE/SCREEN	/ /		
HBsAg	/ /		
HIV COUNSELING/TESTING	/ /	☐ POS. ☐ NEG. ☐ DECLINED	
OPTIONAL LABS	**DATE**	**RESULT**	
HGB ELECTROPHORESIS	/ /	AA AS SS AC SC AF TA₂	
PPD	/ /		
CHLAMYDIA	/ /		
GC	/ /		
TAY-SACHS	/ /		
OTHER			
8–18-WEEK LABS (WHEN INDICATED/ELECTED)	**DATE**	**RESULT**	
ULTRASOUND	/ /		
MSAFP/MULTIPLE MARKERS	/ /		
AMNIO/CVS	/ /		
KARYOTYPE	/ /	46, XX OR 46, XY / OTHER____	
AMNIOTIC FLUID (AFP)	/ /	NORMAL____ ABNORMAL____	
24–28-WEEK LABS (WHEN INDICATED)	**DATE**	**RESULT**	
HCT/HGB	/ /	_____ % _____ g/dl.	
DIABETES SCREEN	/ /	1 HOUR_____	
GTT (IF SCREEN ABNORMAL)	/ /	____FBS ____1 HOUR	
		____2 HOUR ____3 HOUR	
D (Rh) ANTIBODY SCREEN	/ /		
D IMMUNE GLOBULIN (RhlG) GIVEN (28 WKS)	/ /	SIGNATURE_____	
32–36-WEEK LABS (WHEN INDICATED)	**DATE**	**RESULT**	
HCT/HGB (RECOMMENDED)	/ /	_____ % _____ g/dl.	
ULTRASOUND	/ /		
VDRL	/ /		
GC	/ /		
CHLAMYDIA	/ /		
GROUP B STREP (35-37 WKS)	/ /		

COMMENTS/ADDITIONAL LABS

PLANS/EDUCATION (COUNSELED ☐)

☐ ANESTHESIA PLANS _____
☐ TOXOPLASMOSIS PRECAUTIONS (CATS/RAW MEAT) _____
☐ CHILDBIRTH CLASSES _____
☐ PHYSICAL/SEXUAL ACTIVITY _____
☐ LABOR SIGNS _____
☐ NUTRITION COUNSELING _____
☐ BREAST OR BOTTLE FEEDING _____
☐ NEWBORN CAR SEAT _____
☐ POSTPARTUM BIRTH CONTROL _____
☐ ENVIRONMENTAL/WORK HAZARDS _____

☐ TUBAL STERILIZATION _____
☐ VBAC COUNSELING _____
☐ CIRCUMCISION _____
☐ TRAVEL _____
☐ LIFESTYLE, TOBACCO, ALCOHOL _____
REQUESTS _____

TUBAL STERILIZATION	DATE	INITIALS
CONSENT SIGNED	____/____/____	

PROVIDER SIGNATURE (AS REQUIRED) _____

AA201   12345/10967

ACOG ANTEPARTUM RECORD (FORM D)

FIG. 2-4, cont'd. For legend see page 14.

FIG. 2-4, cont'd. For legend see page 14.

BIBLIOGRAPHY

American College of Obstetricians and Gynecologists: *Scheduled cesarean delivery and the prevention of vertical transmission of HIV infection,* ACOG Committee opinion #219, August 1999.

Creasy RK, Gummer BA, Liggins GC: System for predicting spontaneous preterm birth, *Obstet Gynecol* 55:692, 1980.

Gabbe SG, Niebyl JR, Simpson JL (editors): *Obstetrics: normal and problem pregnancies,* ed 3, New York, 1996, Churchill-Livingstone.

3

Perinatal Monitoring

TIMOTHY R.B. JOHNSON

I. GENETIC SCREENING AND PRENATAL DIAGNOSIS

A. Alpha-fetoprotein (AFP). An AFP test is a maternal blood screening test that can detect elevated AFP levels in the amniotic fluid, which can be an indication of anomaly (neural tube defect, ventral wall defect, congenital nephrosis, twins, death, inaccurate dates); low values increase the risk of chromosomal abnormalities.

B. Triple test. The triple test combines the AFP, human chorionic gonadotropin (HCG), and estriol values to more precisely identify the risk of fetal chromosomal anomalies.

C. Genetic probes are available for many disorders (e.g., cystic fibrosis [CF], sickle cell). Prenatal genetic centers have access to the most current tests, are reliable, and offer counseling. Chorionic villus sampling (CVS) can be performed from 11 to 14 weeks gestation; amniocentesis can be performed from 15 to 20 weeks. Karyotype or fluorescence in situ hybridization (FISH) techniques are available.

II. ULTRASOUND

Most pregnant women undergo one or more ultrasound survey examinations during which measurements can be made to assess gestational age. The most accurate measurements are those obtained before 28 weeks. At least two measurements (e.g., biparietal diameter and femur length) are used. Late intrauterine growth retardation (IUGR) can be recognized by ultrasound. Targeted ultrasound scans (formally called *level II*) direct attention to suspicious areas of fetal development. Ultrasound screening for fetal anomalies using recognized high-risk findings (e.g., nuchal thickening and short femur in Down syndrome) is used in some screening protocols.

III. ASSESSMENT OF THE HIGH-RISK NEONATE (FETAL ASSESSMENT)

A. Fetal movement counting. Fetal movement counting can begin as early as 28 weeks; the mother is asked to count fetal movements on a daily basis. Although randomized clinical trials have not documented efficacy of routine fetal movement counting, it is often used in high-risk pregnancies and can be used routinely.

B. **A sharp diminution of fetal movement** or no fetal movement in a 24-hour period is an alarm for further evaluation of the fetus.

IV. NONSTRESS TESTING

The nonstress test (NST) uses the electronic fetal monitor to assess fetal well-being.

A. **Evidence of fetal well-being** during an NST consists of two fetal heart rate accelerations of 20 beats per minute lasting for 20 seconds. Generally, this test is done twice weekly.

B. **The sensitivity of the NST is fair and the specificity is poor.** The incidence of stillbirth within 1 week of a reassuring test result is approximately 3:1000. More frequent testing (two to three times per week) may increase the sensitivity of the test.

C. **The positive (nonreassuring, nonreactive) test result** can lead to further testing or delivery, depending on clinical circumstances.

V. CONTRACTION STRESS TESTS

The contraction stress test consists of similarly derived electronic fetal heart rate strips and the induction of contractions either by intravenous oxytocin or nipple stimulation to see whether decelerations of the heart rate occur.

A. **A positive test result is one in which there are late decelerations after contractions, or variable decelerations,** which can be indications of cord compression or oligohydramnios. The incidence of death within 1 week of a reassuring test result is 0.6:1000.

B. **A positive test result can lead to further testing or delivery,** although care must be taken because of a high rate of false-positive test results.

VI. BIOPHYSICAL PROFILE

The biophysical profile includes electronic fetal heart rate testing (NST) and ultrasound examination to evaluate fetal movement, breathing, and tone and to measure amniotic fluid volume. Two points are assigned for each reassuring result. Testing is generally done on a weekly basis or more often. Test scores <4 generally indicate need for delivery.

A. **A high score of 10 is associated with a good outcome.** Some add placental grading (with a "mature" placenta suggesting adverse outcome) to their scoring system.

B. **Scores of <4 are associated with increased perinatal risk.**

C. **The incidence of death within 1 week of a reassuring test result is approximately 0.5:1000.** The positive predictive value is high at about 80%.

VII. OLIGOHYDRAMNIOS/POLYHYDRAMNIOS/ AMNIOTIC FLUID INDEX

Oligohydramnios and polyhydramnios can be clinically diagnosed using ultrasound techniques. The amniotic fluid index (AFI) (Figs. 3-1 and 3-2) is the most widely used technique and combines measurements of the deepest vertical pocket in each of four quadrants to give an aggregate AFI score. Values <5 = oligohydramnios; >18 = poly-

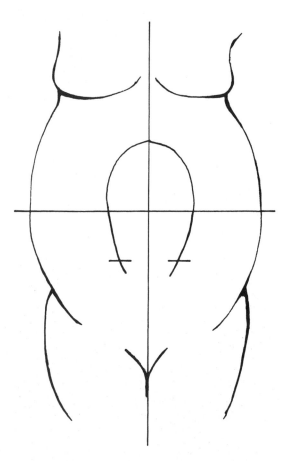

FIG. 3-1. Amniotic fluid index. Quadrant boundaries for amniotic fluid index after 20 weeks.

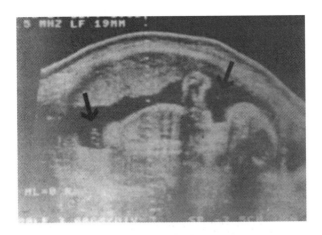

FIG. 3-2. Amniotic fluid *(arrow)* is easily identified sonographically.

hydramnios. The AFI has recently been combined with the NST in a two-test strategy known as the *modified biophysical profile.* Evidence of oligohydramnios should lead to a search for congenital anomalies such as renal agenesis and other conditions associated with oligohydramnios. In cases of polyhydramnios, consider tracheoesophageal (TE) fistula, anencephaly, hydranencephaly, and neural tube defects.

VIII. DOPPLER

Umbilical arterial Doppler studies and other Doppler studies that assess placental function and uteroplacental blood flow can be used. These studies are occasionally useful in cases associated with hypertensive disease and IUGR. Monitoring too early and therapy with aspirin may delay appreciation of such problems, although work on this topic is still investigational. At present, routine Doppler study is not indicated and the modality is useful only as an adjunct in the evaluation of high-risk pregnancy and only in the aforementioned cases. A systolic/diastolic (S/D) ratio of 3 or greater, as measured by continuous or pulsed Doppler and displayed on a spectrum analyzer, is associated with increased placental resistance and increased perinatal mortality and morbidity.

IX. ELECTRONIC FETAL MONITORING

Intrapartum monitoring generally consists of electronic fetal monitoring (EFM), which measures heart rate and uterine contractions. Internal modes consist of a scalp electrode, which has a minimal risk of infection, or an intrauterine pressure catheter, which is associated with risk of chorioamnionitis. External devices use Doppler and tocodynamometry.

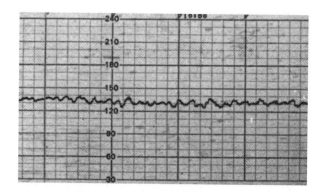

FIG. 3-3. Normal heart rate and variability.

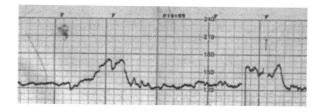

FIG. 3-4. Normal rate variability and fetal heart rate accelerations.

A. Fetal heart rate. The areas assessed include the following:
1. Baseline rate, the normal rate being 120 to 160 beats per minute (Fig. 3-3).
2. Baseline variability; decrease in beat-to-beat variability is an ominous sign.
3. Periodic changes. The presence of accelerations (Fig. 3-4) is reassuring (see NST, p. 19); the presence of decelerations (Fig. 3-5) or late decelerations suggests uteroplacental insufficiency; variable decelerations suggest cord compression. Variable decelerations are unusual in the absence of ruptured membranes or oligohydramnios.
B. EFM is sensitive but has low specificity and is therefore often backed up with scalp pH sampling. Randomized controlled trials have not proven that EFM improves perinatal outcome or has any effect on long-term neurodevelopment (e.g., cerebral palsy), even in preterm infants.
C. Risks of scalp electrode placement include scalp abscess. With internal monitoring, there is an increasing risk of ascending infection because the membranes are ruptured.

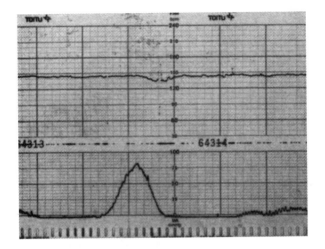

FIG. 3-5. Decreased beat-to-beat variability and late deceleration of fetal heart rate after contraction.

D. **Scalp pH sampling value of >7.25 is normal;** 7.2 to 7.25 is borderline; <7.2 indicates acidosis.

E. **Occasionally, methods are used to stimulate fetal reactivity in labor.** These include pinching the scalp, scratching the scalp, scalp blood sampling, and vibroacoustic stimulation to induce fetal heart-rate accelerations.

X. LUNG MATURITY

Pulmonary maturity is a major predictor of good neonatal outcome and usually can be assessed by amniotic fluid characteristics.

A. **A lecithin/sphingomyelin (L/S) ratio >2 generally suggests maturity.** When phosphatidylglycerol (PG) is present, there is a very low risk of respiratory distress syndrome. The PG level is seldom mature at <36 weeks of gestation.

B. **The Shake test is a foam stability test.** It is more rapid than the L/S ratio and it has comparable sensitivity and specificity to the L/S.

C. **Rapid foam stability tests are clinically available that also assess fetal lung maturity.** Rapid tests of L/S can be performed on amniotic fluid obtained transabdominally in sterile fashion, by vaginal collection of fluid, or from gastric aspirate from the newborn.

XI. PRETERM LABOR/PREMATURE RUPTURE OF MEMBRANES

Prematurity is a major cause of infant morbidity and mortality. Preterm labor is diagnosed by regular uterine contractions associated with cervical change. Cervical change without contractions is termed *cervical incompetence* and generally occurs before 20 weeks.

A. Preterm labor, when diagnosed, is generally treated aggressively with betamimetics, magnesium sulfate, or indomethacin. Potential side effects of each include the following:

1. Betamimetics: Fetal tachycardia.
2. Magnesium sulfate: Pharmacologic impact on the fetus.
3. Indomethacin: Premature closure of the ductus, decreased amniotic fluid.

B. Premature rupture of membranes is a common cause of prematurity. There is an association with vaginal infection and cervical infection, although the exact mechanisms and etiologic organisms are unknown. Premature rupture of membranes is managed by various protocols, including the following:

1. Patients are often hospitalized until delivery occurs.
2. Patients may be discharged if risk of ascending infection is found to be low.
3. Antibiotic coverage for prevention of group B streptococcus and corticosteroids should be considered. Antibiotic treatment for a short course also appears to improve fetal outcome. Broad-spectrum antibiotics are reserved for clinical evidence of infection.
4. Preterm labor and premature ruptured membranes not associated with evidence of chorioamnionitis can be treated with tocolytic therapy and other agents. Culture for pathogens can be useful; infection with group B streptococci and *Neisseria gonorrhoeae* should be eradicated.

XII. FEVER

Fever in the obstetric patient must be evaluated in a rigorous fashion. Common causes include the following:

A. Pyelonephritis.

B. Viral syndrome.

C. Chorioamnionitis. Often associated with fever, leukocytosis, maternal/fetal tachycardia, purulent vaginal discharge, or premature rupture of membranes. The diagnosis of chorioamnionitis is often clinical, with positive evidence from Gram's stains if *organisms* (but not leukocytes) are present; a positive leukocyte esterase test is often useful.

XIII. APGAR SCORE

The Apgar score was developed to identify those infants needing resuscitation.

A. Apgar scoring is generally performed at 1 minute and 5 minutes after birth, although if the score is depressed at 5 minutes, the test should be repeated at 10 minutes.

B. The Apgar score (Table 3-1) depends on gestational age. Many premature infants have decreased Apgar scores purely representative of low gestational age.

C. The Apgar score is not predictive of long-term neurologic outcome or development of cerebral palsy and is not a

TABLE 3-1
Apgar Score

Sign	0	1	2
Heart rate	Absent	Under 100 beats/min	Over 100 beats/min
Respiratory effort	Absent	Slow (irregular)	Good crying
Muscle tone	Limp	Some flexion of extremities	Active motion
Reflex irritability	No response	Grimace	Cough or sneeze
Color	Blue, pale	Pink body, blue extremities	All pink

good indicator of perinatal asphyxia. The diagnosis of perinatal asphyxia should be restricted to those infants with a low 10-minute Apgar score, early neonatal seizures, and early hypotonia.

BIBLIOGRAPHY

American Academy of Pediatrics: Use and abuse of the Apgar score, *Pediatrics* 78:1148, 1986.
Gabbe SG, Niebyl JR, Simpson JL (editors): *Obstetrics: normal and problem pregnancies,* ed 3, New York, 1996, Churchill-Livingstone.

4

Neonatal Resuscitation

Siew-Jyu Wong

Every hospital (level 1, 2, or 3) with delivery services should have skilled personnel immediately available for neonatal resuscitation, and appropriate equipment should be present at all deliveries. Although the percentage of anticipated high-risk deliveries has been increasing steadily, there are still unavoidable, unanticipated high-risk deliveries that require the presence of skilled personnel in house at all times. Such personnel include trained registered nurses, neonatal nurse practitioners, respiratory therapists, physician assistants, and physicians skilled in neonatal resuscitation.

There are numerous causes of an unanticipated compromise of the newborn at delivery. Examples include precipitous delivery; prenatally undiagnosed congenital malformations, such as bilateral choanal atresia or congenital diaphragmatic hernia; and cord accidents, such as short cord, rupture of cord, true knot, tight nuchal cord, or prolapsed cord.

I. CONDITIONS COMMONLY ASSOCIATED WITH ANTICIPATED MODERATE-RISK AND HIGH-RISK DELIVERIES

A. **Prematurity** (<37 weeks).
B. **Cesarean section** (except for elective repeat cesarean section).
C. **Pregnancy-induced hypertension.**
D. **Multiple gestation.**
E. **Intrauterine growth retardation (IUGR).**
F. **Oligohydramnios or polyhydramnios.**
G. **Significant vaginal bleeding.**
H. **Postterm gestation.**
I. **Meconium staining.**
J. **Abnormal fetal monitoring pattern.**
K. **Administration of narcotics within 4 hours of delivery.**
L. **Abnormal presentation.**
M. **Maternal diabetes.**
N. **In utero drug or alcohol exposure.**
O. **Rh sensitization.**
P. **Prolonged labor, rupture of membranes (ROM)** >24 hr or maternal fever/chorioamnionitis.

N.B.: The American Academy of Pediatrics (AAP) and the American Heart Association (AHA) have developed an excellent neonatal resuscitation program, referred to as the *NRP*. Encourage your hospital to provide training programs for **all** personnel involved in the care of the pregnant mother and the newborn. Details of resuscitation as outlined in the aforementioned program include the following:

1. Resuscitation supplies and equipment list.
2. Overview of resuscitation in the delivery room. This is an easy-to-follow algorithm to determine the specific intervention needed.
3. Medications for neonatal resuscitation. This is a comprehensive and updated list of indicated medications.

II. NEONATAL RESUSCITATION SUPPLIES AND EQUIPMENT
A. Suction equipment.
1. Bulb syringe.
2. DeLee mucus trap with a 10F catheter or mechanical suction.
3. Suction catheters: 3F, 6F, 8F, and 10F.
4. An 8F feeding tube and 20-ml syringe.
5. Meconium aspirator.

B. Bag-and-mask equipment.
1. Infant resuscitation bag with a pressure-release valve or pressure manometer; the bag must be capable of delivering 90% to 100% oxygen.
2. Face masks: Newborn and premature sizes (cushioned-rim masks preferred).
3. Oxygen with flowmeter and tubing.

C. Intubation equipment.
1. Laryngoscope with straight blades, No. 0 (premature)* and No. 1 (newborn).
2. Extra bulbs and batteries for laryngoscope.
3. Endotracheal tubes, sizes 2.5, 3.0, 3.5, and 4.0 mm.
4. Stylet.
5. Scissors.
6. Tape and/or other securing device for endotracheal tube.
7. Alcohol sponges.
8. CO_2 detector (optional).
9. Laryngeal mask airway (optional).

D. Medications.
1. Epinephrine 1:10,000, 3-ml or 10-ml ampules.
2. Naloxone hydrochloride (1 mg/ml).
3. Isotonic crystalloid for volume expansion, 100 or 250 ml.
   a. Normal saline.
   b. Ringer's lactate.
4. Sodium bicarbonate 4.2% (5 mEq/10 ml), 10-ml ampules.
5. Dextrose 10%, 250 ml.
6. Normal saline, 30 ml for flushes.

---

*Laryngoscopic blade No. 00 is available for extremely-low-birth-weight (ELBW) infants.

E. Miscellaneous.
1. Radiant warmer.*
2. Stethoscope.
3. Warm linens.
4. Clock.
5. Oropharyngeal airways (0, 00, and 000 sizes or 30-, 40-, and 50-mm lengths).
6. Monitors: Cardiotachometer with electrocardiograph (ECG) oscilloscope (desirable). Pulse oximeter.
7. Adhesive tape, ½-inch or ¾-inch width.
8. Syringes, 1, 3, 5, 10, 20, and 50 ml.
9. Needles, 25, 21, and 18 gauge.
10. Alcohol, povidone-iodine sponges.
11. Gloves (sterile and nonsterile) and other appropriate personal blood and body fluid protection equipment.
12. Umbilical artery catheterization tray.
13. Umbilical tape.
14. Umbilical catheters, 3½F and 5F.
15. Three-way stopcocks.
16. A 5F feeding tube.

III. OVERVIEW OF RESUSCITATION IN THE DELIVERY ROOM (Fig. 4-1)

IV. MEDICATION FOR NEONATAL RESUSCITATION (Table 4-1)

V. SPECIAL PROBLEMS
A. **Meconium.** All infants who have meconium-stained fluid should undergo thorough oral, nasal, and pharyngeal suctioning at the delivery of the head. If the infant is not vigorous at birth, with depressed respirations, low tone and/or a heart rate <100 beats per minute, tracheal suctioning should be done immediately after delivery.
B. **Diaphragmatic hernia.** If diagnosed prenatally or suspected in a non-IUGR newborn with scaphoid abdomen and respiratory distress, do not use face-mask ventilation; proceed immediately to tracheal intubation to provide intermittent positive-pressure breathing (IPPB).
C. **Airway obstruction (e.g., bilateral choanal atresia, neck masses).** Proceed immediately to endotracheal intubation.
D. **Extremely-low-birth-weight (ELBW) infants** who require resuscitation should have early tracheal intubation; administration of surfactant should be done after stabilization. Premature infants have fragile germinal matrix and immature cerebrovascular autoregulation that may be further impaired by asphyxia, so volume expanders (normal saline) and sodium bicarbonate, which is hyperosmolar, should be given slowly.

---

*Polyethylene occlusive skin wrapping for <28 weeks gestation to decrease heat loss; it is very difficult to keep these neonates warm because of very little body fat and high surface area for conductive, evaporative, and radiation heat loss.

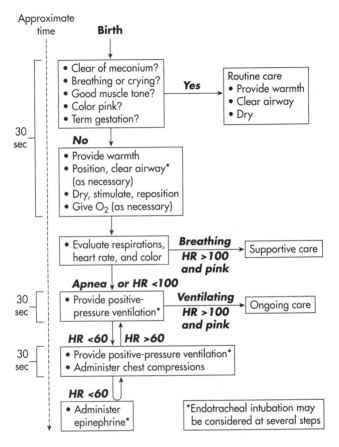

Approximate time

Birth

- Clear of meconium?
- Breathing or crying?
- Good muscle tone?
- Color pink?
- Term gestation?

Yes →

Routine care
- Provide warmth
- Clear airway
- Dry

30 sec

No ↓

- Provide warmth
- Position, clear airway* (as necessary)
- Dry, stimulate, reposition
- Give O$_2$ (as necessary)

↓

- Evaluate respirations, heart rate, and color

Breathing HR >100 and pink → Supportive care

Apnea ↓ **or HR <100**

30 sec

- Provide positive-pressure ventilation*

Ventilating HR >100 and pink → Ongoing care

HR <60 ↓ **HR >60** ↑

30 sec

- Provide positive-pressure ventilation*
- Administer chest compressions

HR <60 ↓

- Administer epinephrine*

*Endotracheal intubation may be considered at several steps

FIG. 4-1 Algorithm for resuscitation of the newly born infant. *HR*, Heart rate. Modified from Kattwinkel J (editor): *Textbook of neonatal resuscitation*, ed 4, Chicago, 2000, American Heart Association and American Academy of Pediatrics.

E. **Infants with severe malformations.** Resuscitate first if there is no prior prenatal discussion with parents. If resuscitation is successful, establish diagnosis, to be followed by compassionate supportive discussion with parents regarding management and continuation of life support.

TABLE 4-1
Medication for Neonatal Resuscitation

Drug	Indication	Concentration and dose	Route	Precaution
Epinephrine	Heart rate <60 after 30 sec of **adequate** ventilation and chest compression	1:10,000; 0.1-0.3 ml/kg every 3-5 min	Endotracheal Intravenous Intraosseous	Do not give intraarterially
Volume expanders (normal saline or Ringer's lactate)	*Hypovolemia suspected:* Shocked infant with history of blood loss, such as maternal vaginal bleeding, or infant who has not responded to other resuscitative measures	10 ml/kg slowly over 5-10 min; may repeat the dose after clinical assessment and observation of response	Intravenous Intraosseous	Give slowly over 5-10 min and observe response before repeating dose

| Sodium bicarbonate | Insufficient data for recommendation; if using, give only during prolonged cardiac arrest unresponsive to other resuscitative measures | 0.5 mEq/ml; 1-2 mEq/kg very slowly over 2 min | Intravenous Intraosseous | Give very slowly over at least 2 min; do not give intraarterially |
| Naloxone | Respiratory depression with history of maternal narcotic administration within 4 hours of delivery | 1 mg/ml; 0.1 mg/kg | Endotracheal Intravenous Subcutaneous or intramuscular if circulation is good | Do not give to infants whose mothers have or are suspected of recent narcotic drug abuse; provide ventilatory support before and during administration until adequate response is observed; continue to observe for hypopnea or apnea because repeat dosing might be necessary |

F. Extremely immature infants. Prepartum discussions with high-risk parents regarding prognosis and resuscitation should be done on an ongoing basis if possible. In case of uncertainty, after a rapid assessment of the infant after birth, resuscitative options include noninitiation of efforts, initiation and discontinuation, initiation and trial of therapy. All will include parental involvement and support of family.

G. Pleural effusion and pneumothoraces. Hydropic newborns may need thoracentesis and paracentesis at birth and transfusion for severe anemia. Pneumothoraces at birth associated with pulmonary hypoplasia may complicate resuscitation and require thoracentesis.

H. Severe hypovolemia. Hypovolemia should be suspected in a newborn not responding to adequate ventilation. History of labor and delivery events may help in establishing the diagnosis, and volume replacement with normal saline should be provided.

VI. SPECIAL PRECAUTIONS

A. Avoid using excessive pressure in resuscitation.

B. Be gentle with suctioning.

C. Always make sure adequate ventilation is established. Medication is **not** a substitute for ventilation.

D. Continue monitoring and support in a special unit until transition to a normal postnatal life is established. Watch blood pressure and perfusion, respirations, and oxygen saturation. Check blood glucose. Guidelines should be established for the continuing care of this newborn as to whether the care should be in the "normal newborn unit" or in the "special care unit."

E. Discontinuation of resuscitative effort may be appropriate if there is no spontaneous circulation after 15 minutes.

The following are controversial issues regarding newborn resuscitation addressed in September 1999 at the Evidence Evaluation (E2) conference and the recommendations made were discussed in February 2000 by the Emergency Cardiovascular Care (ECC) Committee (publication anticipated in 2000 by the Neonatal Program Resuscitation Steering Committee, American Academy of Pediatrics and American Heart Association):

1. Tracheal suctioning when meconium-stained amniotic fluid is present.
2. Room air versus 100% oxygen for resuscitation.
3. Cerebral hypothermia after perinatal asphyxia.
4. Fluids for volume replacement.
5. Discontinuation and noninitiation of resuscitation in the delivery room.

BIBLIOGRAPHY

Goldsmith JP, Spitzer AR: Controversies in neonatal pulmonary care, *Clin Perinatal* 25(1):39-45, 203-214, 228, 229, 1998.

Jain L, Keenan W: Resuscitation of the fetus and newborn, *Clin Perinatal* 26(3):641-656, 731, 1999.

Kattwinkel J (editor): *Textbook of neonatal resuscitation,* ed 4, Chicago, 2000, American Heart Association and American Academy of Pediatrics.

Taeusch HW, Ballard RA: *Avery's diseases of the newborn,* ed 7, Philadelphia, 1998, WB Saunders.

5

Physical Examination
of the Newborn

HENRY M. SEIDEL

Ideally, the full-term newborn should be examined at least two and preferably three times between birth and discharge: in the delivery room immediately at birth (in the event of a high-risk pregnancy or delivery), in the nursery within 12 hours at most, and at discharge. On one of the latter two occasions, it is important to examine the infant in the presence of the mother and if possible the father. This is a marvelous means for education, for observing their interaction with the baby, and for reinforcing the physician's ongoing relationship with the parents. Some examiners prefer to do the first nursery physical alone in case there are unanticipated findings. A premature, sick, or congenitally defective infant's particular needs may mandate changes in approach. The short hospital stay imposed by the demands of managed care unfortunately tends to compress these steps. The guidelines for perinatal care acknowledge this by suggesting that one examination no later than 24 hours after birth and within 24 hours before discharge from the hospital will be satisfactory. This recommendation confronts the reality of medicine today, but it is without universal agreement.

N.B.: If there has not been opportunity for a prenatal visit, everything discussed in Chapter 1 is relevant to the time of first introduction to baby and family. No physical examination is complete without a thorough, well-understood family, maternal, and fetal history. Given a healthy infant after an uncomplicated delivery, there are transitional stages that set the context of examination.

I. THE CONTEXT OF THE EXAMINATIONS: PATTERNS OF ACTIVITY
A. First 15 to 30 minutes.
1. Immediate tachycardia to 160 to 180 beats per minute, with a gradual drop to 100 to 120 beats per minute.

2. Irregular respirations, tachypnea to 60 to 80 respirations per minute, brief moments of apnea.
3. Moist-sounding lung fields, transient grunting and retraction.
4. Awake, moving, alert, easily startled, crying, transient tremors.

B. Next 60 to 90 minutes.

1. Sleepy or sleeping, somewhat unresponsive.
2. Heart rate 100 to 120 beats per minute, transient tachycardia.
3. Respiratory rate 50 to 60 respirations per minute, transient tachypnea.
4. Usually, passage of meconium.

C. The next 10 minutes to several hours. Again, awake, alert, easily startled, crying, easily stimulated, and reactive.

D. At last, behaving like a baby. "Over" being born, eager for feeding and the world, and eager at times for sleep.

II. DELIVERY-ROOM EXAMINATION

Remember that inspection is at least as important as touching and listening. The baby should be nude and under a warmer, and the Apgar 1-minute score (see Table 3-1) should be determined. Immediate concerns include assessment of pulmonary, cardiovascular, and central nervous system (CNS) function. If a pediatrician is not called to the delivery room, these observations become the responsibility of those in attendance, and the nursery examination should then be performed as soon as possible. The list of observations noted can be altered depending on the particular circumstance. The full list is probably achievable only in an ideal world (Box 5-1).

N.B.: Whenever you observe something that violates your sense of the expected–the "normal"–pay attention. It may be a clue to something obvious or something obscure, one of many hidden anomalies or infrequently detected syndromes.

A. Particular attention should be given to the following:

1. Apgar scores at 1 and 5 minutes: A 5-minute score >8 is reassuring; a 1-minute score <7 suggests the possibility of CNS difficulty; a score of <4 reflects a need for resuscitation.
2. Placenta: Look for infarction, separation at margin, velamentous insertion of vessels, meconium staining, foul odor.
3. Umbilical cord: The cord should have two arteries and one vein; only one artery (<1:100 births) suggests associated congenital defects. The cord should be examined early before drying obscures findings. The average cord length at term is 50 to 60 cm (a shortened cord may be associated with in utero hypotonia).
4. Perinatal events: Consider the possibility of birth trauma (e.g., shoulder dystocia, evidence of asphyxia, cord around neck) (Table 5-1).
5. Obvious and unexpected abnormalities (e.g., meningomyelocele, club feet, cleft lip, nevi, hemangiomas).
6. Weight: If baby weighs >4 kg, think of maternal diabetes and baby's potential for hypoglycemia.
7. Using a small catheter, probe the nares (for suction and to judge patency) and, if indicated, the stomach (for aspiration and to judge

BOX 5-1
Delivery Room Assessment

A. GENERAL

1. Whole
   a. Proportions
   b. Symmetry
   c. Facies
   d. Gestational age (approximate)
2. Skin: color, subcutaneous tissue, and imperfections (bands and birthmarks)
3. Neuromuscular
   a. Movements
   b. Responses
   c. Tone (flexor)

B. HEAD AND NECK

1. Head
   a. Shape
   b. Circumference
   c. Molding
   d. Swellings
   e. Depressions
   f. Occipital overhang
2. Fontanelles, sutures
   a. Size
   b. Tension
   3. Eyes
   a. Size
   b. Separation
   c. Cataracts
   d. Colobomas
4. Ears
   a. Placement
   b. Complexity
   c. Preauricular tags or sinuses
5. Mouth
   a. Symmetry
   b. Size
   c. Clefts
6. Neck
   a. Swellings
   b. Fistula

From Nelson NM: Neonatal adaptations. In Hoekelman RA, et al, editors: *Primary pediatric care,* St Louis, 1992, Mosby.   *Continued*

BOX 5-1
Delivery Room Assessment—cont'd

C. LUNGS AND RESPIRATION
1. Retraction
2. Grunt
3. Air entry (breath sounds)

D. HEART AND CIRCULATION
1. Rate
2. Rhythm
3. Murmurs
4. Sounds

E. ABDOMEN
1. Musculature
2. Bowel sounds
3. Cord vessels
4. Distention
5. Scaphoid shape
6. Masses

F. GENITALIA AND ANUS
1. Placement
2. Testes
3. Labia
4. Phallus

G. EXTREMITIES
1. Bands
2. Digits (number and overlapping)

H. SPINE
1. Symmetry
2. Scoliosis
3. Sinuses

---

esophageal continuity); excessive stomach contents, as little as 30 ml, suggest intestinal obstruction.

8. Possible voiding or passage of meconium: Note vigor of urinary stream and ensure patency of relevant orifices. (Catheter in rectum is not routine; it can help ensure patency if there is a question.)

N.B.: Atresia higher up in the rectum can sometimes be difficult to detect. The baby must ultimately have a stool.

9. Mouth: Cleft palate.

TABLE 5-1
Obstetric Situations in Which Delivery Trauma May Occur

Type of injury	Normal vertex	Cesarean	Premature	Precipitate	Breech extraction	Large infant	High midforceps
HEMORRHAGE							
Cerebral							
Subdural							X
Subarachnoid				X	X	X	X
Intraventricular			X				
Abdominal							
Liver					X	X	
Spleen					X	X	
Adrenal gland					X	X	
Cutaneous, presenting part	X				X		
Conjunctival	X						

From Nelson NM: Neonatal adaptations. In Hoekelman RA, et al (editors): *Primary pediatric care*, St. Louis, 1992, Mosby.   *Continued*

TABLE 5-1
Obstetric Situations in Which Delivery Trauma May Occur—cont'd

Type of injury	Normal vertex	Cesarean	Premature	Precipitate	Breech extraction	Large infant	High midforceps
						DIFFICULTY	
FRACTURE OR DISLOCATION							
Clavicle						X	
Humerus					X		
Femur					X		
Skull							X
NERVE INJURY							
Brachial plexus						X	
Spinal cord					X		
Facial	X						
LACERATION		X					

From Nelson NM: Neonatal adaptations. In Hoekelman RA, et al (editors): *Primary pediatric care*, St. Louis, 1992, Mosby.

10. Color: Generalized cyanosis turns to pink as respirations are established.
    a. Persistent generalized central cyanosis: Cardiac abnormality, pulmonary compromise, sepsis.
    b. Pallor: Asphyxiation, anemia, acute blood loss.
    c. Meconium staining: Asphyxiation, other causes of fetal distress; stained fingernails suggest prolonged distress.
11. Respiratory pattern: Tachypnea; grunts; flaring alae nasi; intercostal retractions of more than momentary duration, particularly after suctioning; stridor; presence or absence of abnormal breath sounds of any sort.
12. Cardiac auscultation: Grossly apparent murmurs, quality of heart sounds, arrhythmia.
13. Pulses: Strength, palpability. Do not forget to assess the femoral pulses.
14. Abdomen: Prominence (masses), concave (diaphragmatic hernia), auscultation (presence or absence of borborygmi).
15. Genitalia: Rule out ambiguity, undescended testes, hypospadias.
16. Reactivity: Compatible with expected neuromuscular behavior for the first few minutes of life.
B. In addition, measure weight and assess gestational age. It is vital to assess the appropriateness of growth and development to gestational age. The date of the last menstrual period (LMP) is a helpful indicator even if flawed by the irregularities of memory, contraception, and previous pregnancies. The sonographic record can also help, completing the triad of LMP, sonogram, and physical examination (PE). The key designations are *AGA,* appropriate for gestational age; *SGA,* small for gestational age; and *LGA,* large for gestational age.
1. Birth weight and length alone are insufficient for determining gestational age, although the infant can be placed in an appropriate percentile for these measures using standardized charts. Using a variety of physical and neuromuscular characteristics, there are standardized criteria necessary for making a more accurate assessment of gestational age (Fig. 5-1).
2. Vascularity of the anterior capsule of the lens can be an additional guide. Direct ophthalmoscopy during the second day of life can indicate the degree of vascularity from major involvement of the entire capsule before 28 weeks of gestational age to only peripheral fringe involvement, if that, after 34 weeks. This is most helpful in the very premature baby (Fig. 5-1).
3. SGA: Weight below the 10th percentile for gestational age may be related to a variety of factors, including the following:
    a. Maternal.
        (1) Chronic disease (e.g., cardiovascular, renal, diabetes, hemoglobinopathies).
        (2) Habits (e.g., drugs [legal and illegal], cigarettes, diet preferences).
        (3) Obstetric (e.g., placental infarct, separation, velamentous vessel insertion).

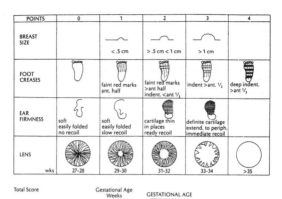

POINTS	0	1	2	3	4
BREAST SIZE		< .5 cm	> .5 cm < 1 cm	> 1 cm	
FOOT CREASES		faint red marks ant. half	faint red marks >ant half indent. <ant ⅓	indent >ant. ⅓	deep indent. >ant ⅓
EAR FIRMNESS	soft easily folded no recoil	soft easily folded slow recoil	cartilage thin in places ready recoil	definite cartilage extend. to periph. immediate recoil	
LENS wks	27–28	29–30	31–32	33–34	>35

Total Score	Gestational Age Weeks
1	28
2	29
3	29½
4	30½
5	31

GESTATIONAL AGE

For scores >5: Score + 26 = weeks gestational age (example: score = 6 (+ 26) = 32 weeks gestational age).

BREAST SIZE—measured by picking up the breast tissue between finger and thumb.
0 = no breast tissue palpable.
1 = breast tissue palpable on one or both sides, neither being more than 0.5cm in diameter.
2 = breast tissue palpable on both sides, one or both being 0.5 to 1cm in diameter.
3 = breast tissue palpable on both sides, one or both being more than 1 cm in diameter.
PLANTAR SKIN CREASES—assessed by noting the creases which persist when the skin of the sole is stretched from toes to heel.
0 = no skin creases present.
1 = skin creases are faint red marks over the anterior half of the sole.
2 = creases are definite red marks over more than the anterior half of the sole, and indentation is present over no more than the anterior third.
3 = as (2) but the indentation is present over more than the anterior third of the sole.
4 = deep indentations present > ant ⅓ of sole
EAR FIRMNESS—tested by palpation and folding of the upper pinna between finger and thumb.
0 = pinna feels soft, and is easily folded into bizzare positions without springing back into position spontaneously.
1 = pinna feels soft along the edge and is easily folded, but returns slowly to the correct position spontaneously.
2 = cartilage can be felt to the edge of the pinna, though it is thin in places, and the pinna springs back readily after being folded.
3 = pinna firm, with definite cartilage extending to the periphery, and springs back into position immediately after being folded.
LENS—tested by examination of the anterior vascular capsule of the lens².
0 = vessels completely covering the lens.
1 = small area of clearing, the diameter of which is less than one fourth that of the lens.
2 = larger area of clearing, the diameter of which is one fourth of one half that of the lens.
3 = small loops at the periphery with diameter of the area of clearing more than one half that of the lens.
4 = lens completely clear or having only an occasional strand or faint loop.

Adapted from personal communication of Palmor C from data of:
1. Narayanan I, et al. Pediatrics 69(1):27, 1982
2. Hittner HM et al. J Pediatr 91:456, 1977

FIG. 5-1. Rapid assessment of gestational age. (From Nelson NM: Neonatal adaptations. In Hoekelman RA, Friedman SB, Nelson NM, et al (editors): *Primary pediatric care,* St. Louis, 1992, Mosby.)

b. Neonate.
   (1) Severe congenital anomalies.
   (2) Congenital infection.
   (3) Inborn errors of metabolism.
   (4) Twin-to-twin competitions (e.g., for blood).
The clinical picture, diagnostic and management decisions, and prognosis depend on the clinical circumstance.

N.B.: Mortality and morbidity are increased when birth weight for an infant born at term is equal to or below the 3rd percentile relative to gestational age.

4. LGA (weight beyond the 90th percentile for gestational age, or weighing >4000 g) may be related to a variety of factors, including the following:
   a. Maternal: Chronic disease, most commonly diabetes.
   b. Parental (e.g., body habitus, race, gestational weight gain).
   c. Neonate: Congenital growth disorders.
      (1) Beckwith-Wiedemann syndrome (e.g., macrosomia, macroglossia, omphalocele, occasional hypoglycemia).
      (2) Sotos syndrome (e.g., big head, big hands, hypertelorism, big jaw).
   d. A compelling obstetric concern pits baby size against pelvic outlet; judgment often must be made before delivery with examination, sonogram, and pelvic measurements to guide management and mode of delivery.

III. NURSERY EXAMINATION

A. First steps. Best done within 12 hours of delivery. The purpose is assessment of the baby's stability after the rush of perinatal and immediate postnatal events and of continuing respiratory, cardiovascular, and neurologic competence. At the start the baby should be nude, warmed, and offered a pacifier (or gloved finger). The strength and eagerness of sucking gives a first, important message about "competence." Begin gently with inspection, proceeding to auscultation, gentle and then deep palpation, and finally the more stimulating experiences of abduction of the hips, examination of the mouth, and elicitation of Moro's and other neurologic reflexes. If the baby is particularly reactive and crying, note the intensity and pitch—how shrill or how stridulous the cry may be.

B. The setting. Most examiners want parental presence at this point. Watching the mother hold and react to the baby offers clues to her feelings, from warmth and tenderness to tension, and much between. The father's behavior indicates his approach and attitudes toward mother and baby, ranging from wholehearted to tentative or noninvolvement. The length of stay is probably too brief these days to count on a third (discharge) examination for this opportunity.

C. The conclusion. Minute attention is then given to each aspect of the full examination. Adopt a comfortable sequence and style; remember that a fixed routine, whatever it might be, helps prevent missed observations, and in the long run, no specific sequence, so long as it is inclusive, offers better outcomes. Be ready, however, to be flexible given the demands of the baby's condition. Among the myriad of possible findings on both history and physical examination, the information in Tables 5-2 to 5-11 suggests the range of those that require parental reassurance at most to those suggesting

TABLE 5-2
Levels of Surveillance of the Newborn Based on the Obstetric History

History	Normal	Alert	Alarm
		LEVEL OF SURVEILLANCE	
Pregnancy surveillance	Registered during first trimester	Unregistered during second trimester	Unregistered and in labor
Genetic disease	None known	In family	In sibling of fetus
Uterine volume		Polyhydramnios	Oligohydramnios
Fetal movement		Increased	Decreased
Biochemical		Decreased estriol levels	
Biophysical		Positive oxytocin challenge test	Uterine ultrasound abnormality
Maternal disease		Diabetes and hypertension	Active tuberculosis
Rupture of membranes		<36 weeks	
Labor	36-42 weeks	<36, >42 weeks	<34 weeks
Delivery			
Vaginal		"Difficult" breech	
Cesarean	Elective (repeat)	Elective (initial)	Emergency
Fetus	Apgar 8-10	Apgar 4-7, visible congenital anomaly	Asphyxia (Apgar <4) and hydrops fetalis

From Nelson NM: Neonatal adaptations. In Hoekelman RA, et al (editors): *Primary pediatric care,* St. Louis, 1992, Mosby.

genuine alarm. There may be disagreement about some of the listings (e.g., rupture of the membranes at <36 weeks might alarm some and alert others, yawning might alert some to drug exposure, and polydactyly might alert rather than alarm others).

IV. GENERALIZATIONS
A. Skin. Inspection should be followed by gentle palpation of affected areas to judge the feel of the skin and to discover associated underlying findings.
1. Acrocyanosis is common, particularly if the baby is insufficiently warmed; mottling is also common, particularly peripherally.
2. Vernix caseosa—cheesy, greasy, and white—covers large areas of skin, more so in premature infants.
3. Lanugo, fine hair investing much of the body, is common, particularly in premature infants; it disappears after several weeks. Scalp hair,

TABLE 5-3
**Levels of Surveillance of the Newborn Based
on Vital Functions**

	LEVEL OF SURVEILLANCE		
Vital function	Normal	Alert	Alarm
Respiration	Paradoxic	Periodic tachypnea or retractions	Apnea, bradycardia, grunting, or gasping
Circulation	Acrocyanosis and heart rate 110-165 beats/min	Tachycardia, or cardiac murmur	Central cyanosis, hypertension, bradycardia, hypotension, enlarged heart, or pallor
Metabolism	Body temperature of 95.9° to 99.5° F (36.5° to 37.5° C)	Hyperthermia	Hypothermia
Digestion	Drooling or "transitional" stools	Spitting	Vomiting or diarrhea
Excretion		No voiding (>24 hr) and no stooling (>24 hr)	Dribbling stream
Behavior	Alert, responsive, reactive, startle, or sneeze	Hyperactive, jittery, or yawning	Coma or convulsions

From Nelson NM: Neonatal adaptations. In Hoekelman RA, et al (editors): *Primary pediatric care,* St. Louis, 1992, Mosby.

ordinarily dark at birth, usually falls out in several weeks and often changes color.
4. The longer the fingernail, the more mature the baby.
5. Breaks in skin, or sinuses, defects, and tags are surface clues to underlying cysts and masses, particularly those that are preauricular, along the sternocleidomastoid area, and midline from the nose over the head and down to the coccyx.
6. The fatter the baby, the lesser the redness.
7. Color: Pallor, plethora, cyanosis, and clinically apparent jaundice suggest a variety of illnesses described more completely in sections devoted to hematology, cardiovascular, respiratory, and gastrointestinal disease.

TABLE 5-4
Levels of Surveillance of the Newborn Based on Examination of the Skin and Its Appendages

Characteristic	LEVEL OF SURVEILLANCE		
	Normal	Alert	Alarm
Color (age of occurrence)			
Cyanosis	Acrocyanosis (<12 hr)	Central (<1 hr)	Central (>1 hr)
Jaundice	>24 hr	18-24 hr	<18 hr
Pallor			<3 min
Epidermis	Dermatoglyphics	Excoriations	Sloughing
Hair	Lanugo	Lumbosacral tuft and scalp defect	
Texture	Soft and moist	Dry and scaling	Thickened and crusting
Vascular pattern	Harlequin, mottling (cold)	Persistent mottling	
Cysts	Milia and Epstein pearls		
Papules	Acne and miliaria		
Desquamation	Delicate scaling (>2 days)	Peeling (<2 days)	Denuded sheets (anytime)
Hemangiomas	Telangiectatic (forehead, lids, lips, and nape)	Telangiectatic (trigeminal) and angiomatous (few)	Angiomatous (multiple)
Hemorrhage	Petechiae (head or upper body)	Petechiae (elsewhere)	Ecchymoses and purpura
Macules	Mongolian spots	Café au lait spots (<6 spots)	Café au lait spots (>5 spots) and "mountain ash" leaf
Pustules	Erythema toxicum		Large and dermal
Vesicles			Any
Nodules		Subcutaneous fat necrosis	Sclerema

From Nelson NM: Neonatal adaptations. In Hoekelman RA, et al (editors): *Primary pediatric care,* St. Louis, 1992, Mosby.

TABLE 5-5

Levels of Surveillance of the Newborn Based on the Head and Neck Examination

	LEVEL OF SURVEILLANCE		
Location	Normal	Alert	Alarm
Skull	Caput succeda-neum molding, or occipital overhang	Cephalhematoma, craniotabes, large fontanel, or forceps mark	Craniosynostosis, transillumination, or bruit
Facies		Hypoplasia or palsy	
Eyes		Mongoloid slant	Aniridia and enlarged cornea
Nose		Nasal obstruction	
Mouth		High-arched palate or macroglossia	Cleft palate and/or lip or micrognathia
Ears		"Simple" structure or low set	
Neck	Rotation ± 90°	Dimple or webbing	

From Nelson NM: Neonatal adaptations. In Hoekelman RA, et al (editors): *Primary pediatric care,* St. Louis, 1992, Mosby.

8. Jaundice is common—perhaps half of all neonates are jaundiced; the earlier the onset, the more acute the problem. Intensity can be measured by descent on the body—the lower and the more peripheral the appearance of jaundice, the higher the bilirubin level. Use daylight preferably for making the judgment; applying pressure with a finger on the infant's forehead or other area, which empties the capillary bed, provides the best opportunity to pick up the color change. Clinically apparent jaundice indicates a bilirubin level of >6 mg/dl.
9. Melanin is not always fully apparent at birth. It often takes a while to appear, and pigmentation below the nails and on the scrotum or vulva provides an early clue to later skin color.
10. A variety of spots, blotches, plugs, and growths are common; the presence of vesicles is always of concern (e.g., may indicate herpes).
11. Yellow-green meconium staining of vernix or fingernails suggests possible fetal distress.

B. Head and neck.
1. Caput succedaneum is more common than cephalhematoma; caput can cross suture lines, but a cephalhematoma is limited by them. Differentiation at first examination may be difficult.
2. A subgaleal hemorrhage is not common and crosses suture lines.
3. Molding is common and appropriate in vaginal deliveries but is not

TABLE 5-6
Levels of Surveillance of the Newborn Based on the Chest Examination

	LEVEL OF SURVEILLANCE		
Characteristic	Normal	Alert	Alarm
Respiration		Paradoxic, periodic, or retractions	Apnea, expiratory grunt, or flaring alae nares
Auscultation		Decreased air entry	Bowel sounds
Chest roentgenogram		Enlarged heart	Oligemia or plethora
Cardiac			
Impulse	Tapping	Heaving, lifting	
Pulses	Full	Decreased	Absent (femoral) and lag (cardiac-radial)
Rate and rhythm	110-165, sinus arrhythmia	Sinus bradycardia	Persistent sinus tachycardia
Sounds	"Tic-toc"	S_2 widely split	S_2 fixed split
Murmurs	Systolic (<24 hr)	Systolic (>24 hr)	Diastolic
Electrocardiograph (QRS)			
Vector	+35° to +180°		0 to −90°; −90° to −180°
Amplitude			
V_1	Rs	Rs	rS
V_6	qrS	qRs	qRs

From Nelson NM: Neonatal adaptations. In Hoekelman RA, et al (editors): *Primary pediatric care,* St. Louis, 1992, Mosby.

    so in cesarean. The molding will often obscure the fontanelle, but the head returns to its expected shape in a few days.

4. Intracranial bruits will not be heard unless they are listened for.
5. Hydrocephaly may not be found unless the skull is transilluminated.
6. Low-set or "funny-looking" ears: Look for other anomalies, particularly renal, and hearing loss; ears are often floppy and may be folded on themselves.
7. Dimples in the neck or about the ears: Look for cysts; dimples in this area occur in 1:100 infants and most often are no problem.
8. Nose may be distorted and flat after delivery; it should recover to the expected shape in a few days.

TABLE 5-7
Levels of Surveillance of the Newborn Based on Examination of the Abdomen

	LEVEL OF SURVEILLANCE		
Characteristic	Normal	Alert	Alarm
Shape	Cylindric	Scaphoid	Distended
Muscular wall	Diastasis recti		Absent
Umbilicus	Amniotic navel or cutaneous navel	Exudation or leakage, granuloma, hernia, inflammation, or less than three cord vessels	Gastroschisis, omphalitis, or omphalocele
Liver	Smooth edge		Enlarged
Spleen	Nonpalpable	Palpable	Enlarged
Kidneys	Lobulated or palpable (lower poles)	Horseshoe	Enlarged

From Nelson NM: Neonatal adaptations. In Hoekelman RA, et al (editors): *Primary pediatric care,* St. Louis, 1992, Mosby.

TABLE 5-8
Levels of Surveillance of the Newborn Based on Examination of the Perineum

	LEVEL OF SURVEILLANCE		
Location	Normal	Alert	Alarm
Anus		Coccygeal dimple	Imperforate, fistula, patulous
Female			
Clitoris		Enlarged, hooded	
Vulva	Bloody secretion, edema, gaping labia, or hymenal tags		Hydrometrocolpos
Male			
Gonad	Edema, hydrocele	Bifid scrotum, cryptorchidism, inguinal hernia	
Phallus	Phimosis	Chordee, hypospadias	Microphallus

From Nelson NM: Neonatal adaptations. In Hoekelman RA, et al (editors): *Primary pediatric care,* St. Louis, 1992, Mosby.

TABLE 5-9
Levels of Surveillance of the Newborn Based on Examination of the Musculoskeletal System

	LEVEL OF SURVEILLANCE		
Characteristic	Normal	Alert	Alarm
Fetal posture	Flexor, position of comfort	Frank breech	Extensor
Hand	Webbing	Cortical thumb, overlapping fingers, short, incurved little finger	Polydactyly, syndactyly
Foot	Dorsiflex 90°, plantar flex 90°, abduct or adduct forefoot 45°, invert or evert ankle 45°	Decreased range of motion	Fixed
Extremities	Tibial bowing		Constriction bands, amputations
Neck	Rotate ±90°		
Joints		Reluctance to use	Subluxation (hips), contracture

From Nelson NM: Neonatal adaptations. In Hoekelman RA, et al (editors): *Primary pediatric care,* St. Louis, 1992, Mosby.

9. A large, potentially obstructive tongue suggests concern (e.g., hypothyroidism); watch the baby feed to be sure that it is not a problem.
10. An apparent tongue tie is common; time, use, and stretching almost always take care of it.
11. Teeth at birth are unusual; 1:10 are extra, usually unrooted teeth and may need removal by a dentist; 9:10 are prematurely erupted and should be left in unless extremely loose. Natal teeth may be a clue to a variety of syndromes.
12. Extremely wide sutures and a huge fontanelle deserve sonographic study; rarely, absence of the corpus callosum (e.g., as seen in Aicardi syndrome) may be found.

C. Chest.
1. Paradoxic respirations may or may not be a problem; retractions or grunting intensify the concern.
2. Bowel sounds in the chest usually mean trouble (e.g., diaphragmatic hernia).
3. Swollen breasts in a boy or girl—the result of passively transferred maternal hormones—are ordinarily no problem and will subside.

TABLE 5-10
Levels of Surveillance of the Newborn Based on Examination of the Nervous System

Characteristic	Normal	Alert	Alarm
		LEVEL OF SURVEILLANCE	
State	*Awake:* crying, active, quiet alert *Asleep:* active, indeterminate, quiet	Hyperalert, lethargic	Stupor, coma
Motor			
Posture	Flexor, symmetric	Extensor, asymmetric	Obligatory, decerebrate
Tone	Obtuse popliteal angle	Limp in upright suspension	Limp in ventral suspension
Movement	All extremities, nonrepetitive, random, symmetric	Jitteriness, tremor	Seizures
Reflexes	Deep tendon, grasp, Moro, placing and stepping, sucking, tonic neck	Asymmetric, do not habituate	Absent
Sensory	Pinprick response slow (2-3 sec)	Pinprick response equivocal	No response

From Nelson NM: Neonatal adaptations. In Hoekelman RA, et al (editors): *Primary pediatric care,* St. Louis, 1992, Mosby.

4. A chest radiograph should be a quick resort if physical examination is worrisome.
5. Diminished peripheral pulses are a concern (e.g., coarctation of the aorta, increased cardiac impulses equally, left ventricular hypertrophy); an echocardiogram and cardiology consult should be a quick resort if findings are worrisome.

D. Abdomen.
1. A draining umbilicus should *not* be ignored.
2. Triple dye confuses an umbilical examination.
3. Only one cord artery mandates concern about a congenital anomaly, particularly renal.
4. Enlargement of the liver cannot be judged by palpation alone; percuss the upper border.
5. Many physicians believe newborn kidneys are easy to palpate; others, equally adept, dispute this. The sonogram is a valuable tool for this or other worrisome abdominal findings.

TABLE 5-11
**Levels of Surveillance of the Newborn Based
on Examination of the Cranial Nerves**

| Cranial nerves | LEVEL OF SURVEILLANCE | | |
	Normal	Alert	Alarm
Forebrain: 2	Fix and follow (visual-evoked potential)	Equivocal (arc <60 degrees)	No response
Midbrain: 3, 4, 6, and 8	Pupillary response, doll's eye response	Unequal, disconjugate, nystagmus	Absent, fixed position
Hindbrain:			
8	Crib-O-Gram (auditory-evoked potentials)	Diminished	No response
5, 7, and 12	Sucking	Weak	Unequal
9 and 10	Swallowing	Uncoordinated	
11	Sternocleidomastoid muscles	Weak	

From Nelson NM: Neonatal adaptations. In Hoekelman RA, et al (editors): *Primary pediatric care,* St. Louis, 1992, Mosby.

E. Perineum. Be careful: assigning the wrong sex in the presence of ambiguous genitalia confuses the infant's and the family's life, sometimes irreparably.

N.B.: Babies have been shown to void prenatally on ultrasonography. Postnatally, most have voided by 12 hours, almost all by 24. Be sure; an obstruction or absent kidneys can occur. Swollen labia and hymenal tags are common and will shrink, usually within a month.

F. Musculoskeletal system.

1. Gently press on the infant's soles; the fetal position and quiet can often be restored.
2. Worry about persistent extension of the extremities, particularly in the full-term (and even in the premature) infant.
3. Syndactyly and polydactyly should alert a practitioner to the possibility of other anomalies; a second toe longer than the great toe is not unusual among those from around the Mediterranean Sea. Clinodactyly might indicate other anomalies.
4. "Fisting" (clenching) might mean neurologic difficulty, but not always.
5. Do *not* miss dislocated hips (dysplasia).
6. Any persistent rigidity or resistance to passive motion should be a source of concern.

G. Nervous system.
1. Newborns are sensate individuals aware of their environment.
2. Early depression suggests asphyxia, sepsis, trauma, or drugs; later depression (once feeding is well established) suggests an inborn error of metabolism.
3. Extension and asymmetry in posture are causes for concern, particularly when persistent.
4. Floppiness is hard to judge; this often calls for a second observer for confirmation.
5. Real seizures are hard to define; degrees of cortical inhibition are hard to define; jitteriness is common; if a finger gently applied to a shaking limb quiets it, it is probably not a seizure.

V. NEONATAL BEHAVIORAL AND DEVELOPMENTAL ASSESSMENT

The newborn period represents a moment in a developmental process already 9 months along and moving forward rapidly, abetted by an already well-developed CNS housed in a not nearly so mature body. The infant is from the start an interactive being with a sophisticated sensory apparatus and a much more compromised motor ability. Genetic and environmental factors contribute to the potentiation (or constraint) of these abilities. An undesirable outcome can sometimes be traced to a single risk factor, but most often the hazards are multiple and individual causes are obscured. It is necessary to evaluate the newborn's behavioral developmental status and to anticipate (and perhaps forestall) risk.

N.B.: A single assessment is but a "snapshot"; a sequence of assessments is usually needed to get the full story.

A. Prenatal and perinatal risk factors.
1. Maternal.
   a. Anatomic.
      (1) Structural malformations of uterus and birth canal.
      (2) Inadequate pelvic outlet.
   b. Disease.
      (1) Infection (e.g., genitourinary tract): Viral (e.g., rubella, herpes, severe flu), bacterial (e.g., group B streptococcus, tuberculosis), sexually transmitted infection.
      (2) Mild to severe anemia from any cause (e.g., sickle cell anemia).
      (3) Chronic systemic disease (e.g., renal, cardiovascular, pulmonary).
      (4) Metabolic abnormality (e.g., diabetes, thyroid).
   c. Variables of pregnancy.
      (1) Maternal age: Increasing risk with decreasing or increasing age (e.g., ages .20 and .35 years).
      (2) Birth weight: Increasing risk if underweight or overweight.
      (3) Gestational age: Increasing risk with younger age.
      (4) Birth status: Increasing risk with diminished Apgar score, especially if prolonged.

N.B.: Diagnosis of asphyxia should never be based solely on Apgar scores at 1 and 5 minutes.

        (5) Complications.
            (a) Eclampsia, milder toxemia.
            (b) Abnormal fetal position.
            (c) Polyhydramnios.
            (d) History of prematurity, spontaneous and elective abortion, cesarean section, multiparity, prior fetal anomaly.
    d. Habit factors.
        (1) Alcohol.
        (2) Smoking.
        (3) Drugs (prescribed, over the counter, or illicit).
        (4) Adequacy of prenatal care.
  2. Other gestational influences: Malnutrition for any reason (e.g., underweight for length); baby *may* be neurologically compromised. Ponderal index = weight (g)/(length [cm])^3 × 100: malnutrition indicated by a score of 2 or less.

B. Perinatal risk factors. Complications of delivery include the following:

  1. Premature rupture of membranes.
  2. Evidence of fetal distress (e.g., bradycardia, tachycardia).
  3. Sluggish labor.
  4. Inappropriate anesthesia: The heavier the medication, the greater the likelihood of compromise.

N.B.: An effort has been made to score these factors. At the moment, I suggest being alert to the potential risks; scoring is not as yet a necessarily fruitful clinometric step.

C. Clinometric assessment of a newborn's development and behavioral state has been attempted in a variety of ways. I suggest the following as best suited to the need.

N.B.: These scales measure a point in time; they are best used in a sequence, or confusion may result. Remember that a score will vary if taken during the "alert period" right after delivery or during the subsequent "depressed period" and then the "recovery."

  1. Apgar score: Already in universal use.
  2. Brazelton behavioral scale, or neonatal behavioral assessment scale (NBAS) (Box 5-2). This scale takes advantage of the full-term neonate's ability to react and participate in the environment (e.g., selecting the human face over inanimate objects for intense gazing, responding to variations in speech, and to cuddling in the fetal position). The findings vary with the baby's level of sleep or alertness and the age in hours; the most fruitful observations are made when the infant is quiet but alert. Notably, an infant's neurologic and organizational competency is better judged by the Brazelton behavioral scale performed by someone experienced with it and a competent neurologic examination (Box 5-3) than by the neurologic examination alone.
  3. Neuromuscular competency: Neuromuscular assessment (Box 5-3) can complement the NBAS observations in judging the effect of known risk factors for an individual neonate.

BOX 5-2
Brazelton Behavioral Scale

Environmental interactions
Alertness
Consolability
Cuddliness
Orientation
Stress responses
Skin color lability
Startle reaction
Tremulousness
Motor processes
Activity
Defensive reactions
Hand-to-mouth movement
Maturity
Reflex
Tone
Physiologic state
Habituating to stimuli
Self-quieting

From Nelson NM: Neonatal adaptations. In Hoekelman RA, et al (editors): *Primary pediatric care,* St. Louis, 1992, Mosby.

BOX 5-3
Techniques for Assessment of Neuromuscular Maturity

POSTURE
With the infant supine and quiet, score as follows:
    Arms and legs extended = 0
    Slight or moderate flexion of hips and knees = 1
    Moderate to strong flexion of hips and knees = 2
    Legs flexed and abducted, arms slightly flexed = 3
    Full flexion of arms and legs = 4

POPLITEAL ANGLE
With the infant supine and the pelvis flat on the examining surface, the leg is flexed on the thigh and the thigh is fully flexed with the use of one hand. With the other hand the leg is then extended, and the angle attained is scored as in Fig. 5-1.

Modified from Amiel-Tison C: *Arch Dis Child* 43:89, 1968; and Dubowitz LMS, et al: Clinical assessment of gestational age in the newborn infant, *J Pediatr* 77:1, 1970.
Continued

BOX 5-3
**Techniques for Assessment of Neuromuscular
Maturity—cont'd**

SQUARE WINDOW

Flex the hand to the wrist; exert pressure sufficient to get as much flexion as possible. The angle between the hypothenar eminence and the anterior aspect of the forearm is measured and scored according to Fig. 5-1. Do not rotate the wrist.

ARM RECOIL

With the infant supine, fully flex the forearm for 5 seconds, then fully extend by pulling the hands and releasing. Score the reaction according to the following:

   Remains extended or random movements = 0
   Incomplete or partial flexion = 1
   Brisk return to full flexion = 2

SCARF SIGN

With the infant supine, take the infant's hand and draw it across the neck and as far across the opposite shoulder as possible. Assistance to the elbow is permissible by lifting it across the body. Score according to the location of the elbow:

   Elbow reaches beyond the opposite anterior axillary line = 0
   Elbow reaches to the opposite anterior axillary line = 1
   Elbow is between opposite anterior axillary line and midline of thorax = 2
   Elbow is at midline of thorax = 3
   Elbow does not reach midline of thorax = 4

HEEL-TO-EAR MANEUVER

With the infant supine, hold the infant's foot with one hand and move it as near to the head as possible without forcing it. Keep the pelvis flat on the examining surface. Score as in Fig. 5-1.

VI. NEONATAL PAIN ASSESSMENT

Newborns have pain and react to it. Behavioral changes can be assessed. These include the following:

A. Facial expression.
B. Crying.
C. Bodily activity.
D. Wakefulness.
E. Consolability.
F. Sociability.

Scoring systems can help in judging severity of pain (Table 5-12).
N.B.: The potential of pain in the newborn should never be ignored.

TABLE 15-12
Infant Pain Score

Indicator	0	Behavior Scale 1	Behavior Scale 2	Score*
Sleep during preceding hour	None	Short naps (5-10 min)	Longer naps	
Facial expression: brow bulge, open mouth, chin quiver, stretch mouth horizontal, nasolabial furrow, eye squeeze	Marked	Less marked	Calm	
Quality of cry	Screaming, pain, high pitched	Modulated, infant can be distracted	No cry	
Spontaneous motor activity	Thrashing, incessant agitation	Moderate	Normal	
Excitability and responsiveness to stimulation	Tremulous, clonic movement, spontaneous Moro's reflex	Excessive reactivity to any stimulation	Quiet	
Flexion of fingers and toes	Pronounced and constant	Less marked, intermittent	Absent	
Sucking	Absent or disorganized	Intermittent (3 or 4), stops with crying	Strong, rhythmic, pacifies	
Overall tone	Strong, hypertonicity	Moderate hypertonicity	Normal	
Consolability	None after 2 minutes of comforting	Quiet after 1 minute of effort	Quiet within 1 minute	
Sociability (eye contact) in response to voice, smile, or face	Absent	Difficult to obtain	Easy and prolonged	
			Total:	

From Strauss SG, Lynn AM, Spear RM: *Contemp Pediatr* 19:80, 1995.
*0 = Severe pain, 20 = comfort.

VII. DISCHARGE EXAMINATION

The compression of time spent in the hospital often precludes separate first, nursery, and discharge examinations. Regardless, the effort should be made if at all possible, for the baby's sake, for parental education or reassurance, for the family dynamic, and for reinforcement of the continuity relationship with the practitioner (see Chapter 28).

BIBLIOGRAPHY

American Academy of Pediatrics and American College of Obstetricians and Gynecologists: *Guidelines for prenatal care,* ed 4, Elk Grove Village, Ill and Washington DC, 1997, AAP and ACOG.

Amiel-Tison C: Neurological evaluation of the maturity of newborn infants, *Arch Dis Child* 43:89, 1968.

Ballard JL, Novak KK, Driver M: A simplified score for assessment of fetal maturation of newly born infants, *J Pediatr* 95:769, 1979.

Dubowitz LMS, Dubowitz V, Goldberg C: Clinical assessment of gestational age in the newborn infant, *J Pediatr* 77:1, 1970.

Eisen LN, Field TN, Bandstra ES, et al: Perinatal cocaine effects on neonatal stress behavior and performance on the Brazelton scale, *Pediatrics* 88:477, 1991.

Hittner HM, Hirsch NJ, Rudolph AJ: Assessment of gestational age by examination of the anterior capsule of the lens, *J Pediatr* 94:455, 1977.

McIntire DD, Bloom SL, Casey BM, Leveno KG: Birth weight in relation to morbidity and mortality among newborn infants, *New Engl J Med* 340:1234, 1999.

Naeye RL: Umbilical cord length: clinical significance, *J Pediatr* 107:278, 1985.

Nelson NM: Neonatal adaptations. In Hoekelman RA, Friedman SB, Nelson NM, et al (editors): *Primary pediatric care,* St. Louis, 1992, Mosby.

Oh W, Merenstein G: Fourth edition of the Guidelines for Perinatal Care: summary of changes, *Pediatrics* 100:1021, 1997.

Sanders M, Allen M, Alexander GR, et al: Gestational age assessment in pre-term neonates weighing less than 1500 grams, *Pediatrics* 88:542, 1991.

Strauss SG, Lynn AM, Spear RM: Progress in pain control for very young infants, *Contemp Pediatr* 12:80, 1995.

6

Transitional Period: The First 6 Hours of Adaptation From Intrauterine to Extrauterine Life

Patricia H. Smouse

I. TRANSITIONAL PERIOD
A. Complex process of physiologic adjustments.
1. Changes in function of organ systems.
   a. Onset of respiration.
   b. Change from fetal to neonatal circulation.
   c. Change of hepatic and renal function.
   d. Clearance of meconium from bowel.
2. Reorganization of metabolic processes.
B. Patterns of activity (see pp 33-34).
1. Normal transition (Fig. 6-1).
   a. Period of reactivity: Initial 15 minutes of life.
      (1) Spontaneous startle reactions.
      (2) Tremors.
      (3) Crying.
      (4) Increased motor activity.
      (5) Excellent time for initial feeding and bonding.
   b. Second stage: Next 60 to 90 minutes of life.
      (1) Marked decrease in motor activity.
      (2) Neurologic component of maturation assessments examination may be affected by marked hypotonia.
   c. Second period of reactivity: Lasts 10 minutes to several hours.

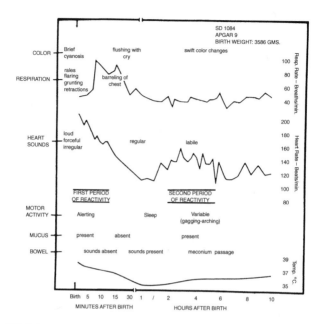

FIG. 6-1. A summary of the physical findings noted during the first 10 hours of extrauterine life in a representative infant with high Apgar score delivered under spinal anesthesia without prior medications. (From Desmond MM, Rudolf AJ, Phitaksphraiwan P: *Pediatr Clin North Am* 13:656, 1966.)

2. Abnormal transition: Although variability may be seen in aforementioned stages, certain findings require further evaluation, work-up, and possibly treatment.
   a. Respiratory: Rule out pneumonia, respiratory distress syndrome, transient tachypnea of the newborn, sepsis, pneumothorax, congenital heart disease, polycythemia.
      (1) Respiratory rate >100 or >70 after the first 8 hours (placing infant in prone position may cause mild respiratory distress).
      (2) Respirations accompanied by grunting, flaring, retractions after first 2 hours of life.
      (3) Central cyanosis after first 5 minutes.
   b. Neurologic: Rule out sepsis, maternal drug abuse, maternal medication administration during labor or pregnancy (including magnesium sulfate), neuromuscular disorder, chromosomal anomaly, hypoglycemia, polycythemia.
      (1) Inability of a term infant to suck.
      (2) Extreme or persistent jitteriness or hypertonia.
      (3) Extreme or persistent hypotonia.

C. Temperature homeostasis.

1. Importance of heat balance.
   a. Decrease metabolic and oxygen requirements.
   b. Essential for stabilization after delivery.
2. Monitoring temperature in the newborn.
   a. Rectal temperature should be checked within first hour of life (normal is 36.5° to 37.5° C).
   b. Axillary temperature should be monitored thereafter (normal is 36.5° to 37.4° C).
   c. If axillary temperature is subsequently abnormal, rectal temperature should be taken to confirm temperature instability.
   d. Infant should be maintained, until stable, under a radiant warmer with the servo control mode set at 36.5° to 37.0° C.
   e. An abnormal body tempeture may not be an indicator of thermal stress but of the inability of the baby to adequately compensate.
3. Hypothermia.
   a. Etiology.
      (1) Large amounts of evaporative heat loss.
      (2) Increased surface area/body mass ratio.
      (3) Decreased subcutaneous tissue.
      (4) Sepsis.
   b. Risk situations.
      (1) Premature and small for gestational age (SGA) infants.
      (2) Air conditioned labor and recovery rooms.
      (3) Inadequate or delayed drying and warming after delivery.
   c. Neonatal response.
      (1) Nonshivering thermogenesis.
      (2) Hypoxemia.
      (3) Metabolic acidosis.
      (4) Depletion of glycogen stores.
      (5) Reduction of blood glucose levels.
      (6) Increased oxygen consumption.
   d. Prevention and treatment.
      (1) Rapid drying with prewarmed towels immediately after birth.
      (2) Covering the head with a cap.
      (3) Placing under radiant warmer set to maintain rectal temperature between 36.5° and 37.0° C.
      (4) Skin-to-skin contact with the mother may be substituted if infant and mother are stable.
      (5) After initial stability is determined, the infant may be bathed and then closely monitored for temperature instability for another hour.
      (6) Normal newborns may then be dressed, swaddled, and placed in an open bassinet.
      (7) Premature (<37 weeks), SGA, and unstable infants should be maintained undressed in an isolette set at neutral thermal environment.

4. Hyperthermia.
   a. Etiology.
      (1) Impaired ability to sweat in response to environmental temperatures.
      (2) Sepsis.
      (3) Maternal fever at delivery.
      (4) Overbundling or overwarming.
   b. Risk situations.
      (1) Maternal fever.
      (2) Prolonged resuscitation under warmer.
      (3) Lack of proper probe placement while infant is under radiant warmer or in isolette.
   c. Neonatal response.
      (1) Hypernatremia.
      (2) Volume depletion.
      (3) Increased metabolic demands.
      (4) Apnea.
   d. Prevention and treatment.
      (1) Tape the thermometer probe securely to the anterior abdominal wall with the infant in the supine position.
      (2) Treat hyperthermia (skin temperature = 37.5° to 39.0° C) by undressing the neonate and exposing to room temperature.

II. ASSESSMENT OF THE NEWBORN

A. Gestational age assessment. Used to anticipate needs, clinical course, and outcome of premature, postmature, SGA, and large for gestational age (LGA) infants.
1. Performed on every neonate soon after birth.
2. Scoring systems.
   a. Dubowitz (Table 6-1, Fig. 6-2).
      (1) Detailed scoring system that combines external physical characteristics and neurologic findings.
      (2) Ideally performed between 12 to 24 hours of life.
   b. Ballard (Fig. 6-3).
      (1) An abbreviated version of the Dubowitz examination that retains the neurologic criteria that do not require the infant to be alert and vigorous.
      (2) Accuracy ±2 weeks.
   c. Rapid assessment (Table 6-2, Fig. 6-4).
3. Determine relationship of gestational age to birth weight by plotting on a birth weight–gestational age chart appropriate to the population.

B. SGA infant. Weight <10th percentile for estimated gestational age.
1. Associated with a higher morbidity and mortality rate than for a premature infant of comparable weight.
2. Symmetric growth retardation versus asymmetric growth retardation.
   a. Symmetric growth retardation.
      (1) Proportionately small infant (head, weight, and length <10th percentile).
      (2) Represents slow growth rate beginning early in the pregnancy.

TABLE 6-1
Scoring System for External Criteria

External sign	SCORE*				
	0	1	2	3	4
Edema	Obvious edema of hands and feet; pitting over tibia	No obvious edema of hands and feet; pitting over tibia	No edema		
Skin texture	Thin, gelatinous	Thin and smooth	Smooth; medium thickness; rash or superficial peeling	Slight thickening; superficial cracking and peeling, especially of hands and feet	Thick and parchment-like; superficial or deep cracking
Skin color	Dark red	Uniformly pink	Pale pink; variable over body	Pale; only pink over ears, lips, palms, or soles	
Skin opacity (trunk)	Numerous veins and venules clearly seen, especially over abdomen	Veins and tributaries seen	A few large vessels clearly seen over abdomen	A few large vessels seen indistinctly over abdomen	No blood vessels seen

From Farr V, Mitchell RG, Nelligan GA, et al: *Develop Med Child Neurol* 8:507, 1966.
*If score differs on two sides, take the mean.

Continued

TABLE 6-1
Scoring System for External Criteria—cont'd

External sign	0	1	2	3	4
			Score*		
Lanugo (over back)	No lanugo	Abundant; long and thick over whole back	Hair thinning, especially over lower back	Small amount of lanugo and bald areas	At least half of back devoid of lanugo
Plantar creases	No skin creases	Faint red marks over anterior half of sole	Definite red marks over more than half of anterior; indentations over less than one third of anterior half of sole	Indentations over more than one third of anterior half of sole	Definite deep indentations over more than one third of anterior half of sole
Nipple formation	Nipple barely visible; no areola	Nipple well defined; areola smooth and flat, diameter <0.75 cm	Areola stippled, edge not raised, diameter <0.75 cm	Areola stippled, edge raised, diameter >0.75 cm	
Breast size	No breast tissue palpable	Breast tissue on one or both sides, <0.5 cm diameter	Breast tissue both sides; one or both 0.5-1.0 cm	Breast tissue both sides; one or both >1 cm	

Ear form	Pinna flat and shapeless, little or no incurving of edge	Incurving of part of edge of pinna	Partial incurving whole of upper pinna	Well-defined incurving whole of upper pinna
Ear firmness	Pinna soft, easily folded, no recoil	Pinna soft, easily folded, slow recoil	Cartilage to edge of pinna, but soft in places, ready recoil	Pinna firm, cartilage to edge; instant recoil
Genitals Male	Neither testis in scrotum	At least one testis high in scrotum	At least one testis right down	
Female (with hips half abducted)	Labia majora widely separated, labia minora protruding	Labia majora almost cover labia minora	Labia majora completely cover labia minora	

From Farr V, Mitchell RG, Nelligan GA, et al: *Develop Med Child Neurol* 8:507, 1966.
*If score differs on two sides, take the mean.

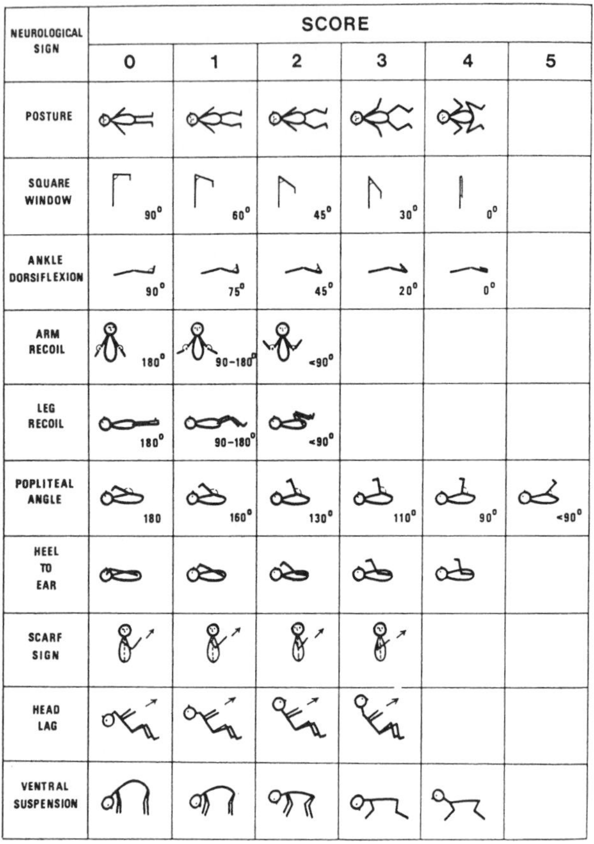

NEUROLOGICAL SIGN	SCORE					
	0	1	2	3	4	5
POSTURE						
SQUARE WINDOW	90°	60°	45°	30°	0°	
ANKLE DORSIFLEXION	90°	75°	45°	20°	0°	
ARM RECOIL	180°	90–180°	<90°			
LEG RECOIL	180°	90–180°	<90°			
POPLITEAL ANGLE	180	160°	130°	110°	90°	<90°
HEEL TO EAR						
SCARF SIGN						
HEAD LAG						
VENTRAL SUSPENSION						

FIG. 6-2. Scoring system for neurologic criteria. (From Dubowitz LMS, et al: *J Pediatr* 77:1, 1970.)

   (3) More likely to represent severe genetic constraints on growth, a dysmorphic syndrome, or congenital infection (e.g., TORCH syndrome).
  b. Asymmetric growth retardation.
   (1) Greatest reductions are in weight and length with relative sparing of the head circumference.
   (2) Newborn appears wasted and malnourished.
   (3) Usually the result of an extrinsic influence on the fetus later in gestation when growth is usually rapid.

Neuromuscular Maturity

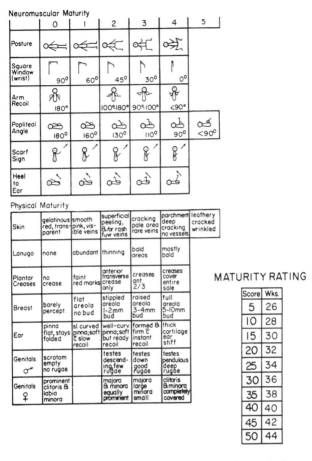

Physical Maturity

MATURITY RATING

Score	Wks.
5	26
10	28
15	30
20	32
25	34
30	36
35	38
40	40
45	42
50	44

FIG. 6-3. Scoring system for simplified clinical assessment of maturation in newborn infants. (From Ballard JL, et al: *J Pediatr* 95:769, 1979.)

    (4) Seen with multiple-gestation pregnancies, pregnancy-induced hypertension, placental insufficiency, in utero drug exposure (including tobacco).

3. Clinical problems associated with SGA.
    a. Asphyxia and intrauterine distress.
    b. Respiratory distress.
    c. Persistent fetal circulation.

TABLE 6-2
Estimation of Gestational Age

Evaluation	APPROXIMATE WEEK OF GESTATION WHEN FINDINGS APPEAR							
	24	28	30	32	34	36	38	40	
Head circumference in cm ± 2 SD	Clinical	23-28.3	25-30.4	26.8-32.4	28.6-34	30.5-35.5	32-36.5	33-37	Based on 300 single live births—all Caucasian
Sole creases		Anterior transverse crease only →				Occasional creases anterior two thirds →		Sole covered with creases →	If small, may represent fetal malnutrition
Breast nodule diameter		Not palpable—absent →				2 mm →	4 mm →	7 mm →	
Scalp hair		Fine and fuzzy / Hard to distinguish individual strands →						Appears as individual strands →	Thick and silky →
Earlobe		Pliable—no cartilage →					Some cartilage →		Stiffened by thick cartilage →
Testes and scrotum		Testes in lower canal / Scrotum small—few rugae →					Intermediate →		Testes pendulous, scrotum full, extensive rugae →

(Clinical)

From Behrman RE, et al: *Adv Pediatr* 17:13-55, 1970.

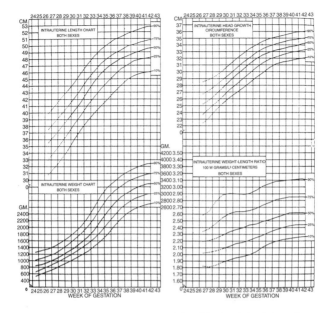

FIG. 6-4. Percentiles of intrauterine growth in weight, length, head circumference, and weight/length ratio. (From Lubchenco LO, et al: *Pediatrics* 37:403, 1966.)

    d. Hypoglycemia.
    e. Hypothermia.
    f. Polycythemia.
    g. Congenital malformations.
C. LGA infant. Weight >90th percentile for estimated gestational age.
  1. Etiology.
    a. Infants of diabetic mothers (except mothers with advanced disease).
    b. Genetic predisposition (large parents).
    c. Beckwith-Wiedemann syndrome.
  2. Clinical problems associated with LGA.
    a. Birth injuries.
      (1) Fractured clavicle.
      (2) Brachial plexus injury.
      (3) Facial palsy.
    b. Hypoglycemia.
    c. Polycythemia.

III. INITIAL MANAGEMENT
A. Monitoring. Avoid separation of mother and newborn whenever possible.

1. Vital signs.
   a. Temperature, pulse, and respirations every 15 minutes for first hour or until stable.
   b. Measurement of temperature, pulse, and respirations should continue every hour for 4 hours, then every 8 hours if stable.
   c. Note changes in respiratory status, color, tone, mucus production, meconium passage (see Appendix G), first void (see Table G-1).
2. Screening tests.
   a. Hematocrit/hemoglobin.
      (1) Normal range for a hematocrit level in a full-term neonate is 45% to 65%.
      (2) Normal range for a hemoglobin level in a full-term neonate is 15 to 22 g/dl.
      (3) If obtaining a heel-stick measurement and infant is stable, obtain blood at about 4 hours of age when peripheral blood flow is improved (capillary hemoglobin exceeds venous level by about 3.6 g in the first week of life).
      (4) Indications for testing: Perinatal asphyxia, respiratory distress, pallor, plethora, twins, infant of diabetic mother, SGA, uncontrolled delivery.
   b. Blood glucose.
      (1) Normal range is 40 to 130 mg/dl.
      (2) Indications for screening: SGA, LGA, prematurity, infant of diabetic mother, twins, perinatal asphyxia, poor feeding, plethora.
   c. Blood type and Coombs' test should be considered under the following circumstances:
      (1) If mother is Rh negative, to determine the need for maternal Rhogam administration.
      (2) If mother is O+, to rule out AB incompatibility; this is especially important in conjunction with early discharge policy.
      (3) If the maternal blood type is unknown, to rule out Rh incompatibility.
   d. Rapid plasma reagin (RPR) or serologic test for syphilis (STS).
      (1) Screening before hospital discharge is generally preferable, particularly when prenatal care has been inadequate or screen was not performed on mother at delivery.
      (2) Most accurate screen for congenital syphilis is serial testing of mother prenatally and again at delivery.
      (3) Cord blood and neonatal serum may not be as sensitive as maternal serum.
   e. Human immunodeficiency virus (HIV).
      (1) Ideally performed prenatally on mother.
      (2) Should be performed on a baby to be placed for adoption whose maternal status is unknown.
      (3) Should be performed on infant of high-risk mother who was not screened or who refused screening.

B. Prophylaxis.

1. Eye prophylaxis.
   a. Purpose is prevention of neonatal gonococcal infection.

    b. Current recommendation is routine administration of one of the following to all newborns within the first hour of life (refer to Appendix I for proper instillation technique).

      (1) Erythromycin, 0.5% ophthalmic ointment or drops in single-dose tubes or ampules instilled in each eye.

      (2) 1% silver nitrate solution in single-dose ampule (associated with high incidence of chemical conjunctivitis).

      (3) Tetracycline, 1% ophthalmic ointment or drops in single-dose ampule.

N.B.: All of the aforementioned agents are equally effective in the prevention of gonococcal infection but do *not* prevent chlamydial eye infection.

    c. Infant born to mother with known gonococcal infection.

      (1) When prophylaxis is administered correctly infant should be adequately protected.

      (2) Current recommendation, however, is to administer a single dose of ceftriaxone, 125 mg intravenously or intramuscularly; for low-birth-weight infants, the dose is 25 to 50 mg/kg.

2. Vitamin K_1 administration.

    a. Purpose of prophylaxis: To prevent hemorrhagic disease of the newborn.

      (1) Infants develop vitamin-K deficiency by day 2 to 3 of life if supplement is not given at birth.

      (2) Maternal drugs that interfere with vitamin-K synthesis: Phenytoin (Dilantin), phenobarbital, salicylates.

      (3) One recommended policy is to double the dose of vitamin K_1 for infants of mothers on anticonvulsant therapy.

    b. Standard recommended dose: Single intramuscular dose of 0.5 to 1.0 mg phytonadione (vitamin K_1) in the anterolateral thigh to all newborns within 1 hour of birth.

3. Hepatitis B vaccine and hepatitis B immunoglobulin (see Chapter 20 and Table 20-3).

C. Initial feeding.

1. Timing.

    a. After establishing respiratory stability, temperature homeostasis, and absence of neurologic dysfunction (usually between 1 and 6 hours of life).

    b. Benefits of early feeding.

      (1) Maintain normal metabolism during transition to extrauterine life.

      (2) Decrease incidence of hyperbilirubinemia in breast-fed infants.

      (3) Decrease incidence of hypoglycemia.

      (4) Decrease incidence of dehydration.

      (5) Early onset of breast-feeding may contribute to breast-feeding success.

2. What to feed.

    a. Breast milk.

    b. Standard infant formula with iron.

3. Technique.
   a. Breast-feed or bottle-feed.
      (1) Stable respiratory status.
      (2) >34 weeks, or 32 to 34 weeks with good suck-swallow coordination.
   b. Gavage.
      (1) Poor suck-swallow coordination.
      (2) Severe SGA.
      (3) <32 weeks.
      (4) Respiratory rate 60-80/minute (gavage not indicated if respiration rate >80/minute).
4. Frequency/amount of feeds.
   a. Healthy full-term infant.
      (1) Breast-fed infants should nurse on demand (avoid rigid feeding schedules; frequent feedings, 8 to 12 feedings per day, should be encouraged to help establish maternal milk supply, prevent engorgement, and decrease neonatal jaundice).
      (2) Formula-fed infants usually feed on demand every 3 to 5 hours and should progress rapidly from about 30 ml every feed to full feeds (120 kcal/kg per day) by 3 to 5 days of life.
   b. Infants <2500 grams require more careful consideration of fluid and caloric requirements based on weight (Table 6-3).

D. Skin care.
1. Bathing.
   a. After stabilization.
   b. Nonmedicated soap may be used to remove blood and meconium.
   c. Vernix caseosa need not be removed.
   d. Cleanse skin abrasions carefully with an antiseptic such as Betadine.
2. Cord care.
   a. No single procedure is recommended to prevent colonization or subsequent infection.
   b. Currently acceptable method is initial application of triple dye or antibiotic ointment followed by regular application of alcohol with every diaper change.

E. Indications for isolette use.
1. Temperature regulation of the preterm or cold-stressed infant.
2. Reverse isolation for infant.
3. Facilitate observation of the high-risk or unstable infant.
4. Kangaroo Mother Care (KMC): Safe alternative to isolette for small, stable infants.
   a. Mothers are used as "incubators" and main source of food and stimulation.
   b. Babies are kept 24 hours a day in strict upright position, skin-skin contact, firmly attached to mother's chest.
   c. Strict criteria recommended for feedings, evaluation, timing of hospital discharge, and length of KMC.
   d. Advantages include mother-infant bonding and reduction in number of hospital days without compromising growth of infant.

TABLE 6-3
Infant Feeding Guidelines

Feeding	BIRTH WEIGHT (GESTATIONAL AGE)		
	1500-2000 g (≥32, ≤36 weeks)	2000-2500 g (>36 weeks)	>2500 g (>36 weeks)
Route	Gavage through a nasogastric tube; may attempt bottle if >1600 g, >34 weeks, and neurologically intact	Breast or bottle if neurologically intact	Breast or bottle if neurologically intact
Type	Breast milk or premature formula; for infants 1800 g, regular formula may be considered (controversial)	Breast milk or regular formula	Breast milk or regular formula
Initial	Sterile water, 2.5 ml/kg; if tolerated, begin formula	Sterile water, 2.5 ml/kg; if tolerated begin breast milk or formula	Sterile water, 2.5 ml/kg; if tolerated, begin breast milk or formula
Subsequent	2.5 ml/kg every 3 hr and advance as tolerated	Advance as tolerated	Advance as tolerated

Modified from Gomella GM: *Neonatology management, procedures, on-call problems, diseases, and drugs,* ed 4, Norwalk, Conn, 1999, Appleton and Lange.

BIBLIOGRAPHY

American Academy of Pediatrics: Peter G (editor): *1997 Redbook: report of the Committee on Infectious Diseases,* ed 24, Elk Grove Village, Ill, 1997, American Academy of Pediatrics.

Ballard JL, Novak KK, Driver M: A simplified score for assessment of fetal maturation of newly born infants, *J Pediatr* 95:769, 1979.

Behrman RE, Fisher D, Paton JB, et al: In utero disease and the newborn infant, *Adv Pediatr* 17:13-55, 1970.

Charpak N, Ruiz-Pelacz JR: Kangaroo mother versus traditional care for new infants ≤ 2000 grams: a randomized, controlled trial, *Pediatrics* 100:682, 1997.

Cheng TL, Partridge JC: Effect of bundling and high environmental temperature on neonatal body temperature, *Pediatrics* 92:238, 1993.

Chhabra RS, Brion LP, Castro M, et al: Comparison of maternal sera, cord blood, and neonatal sera for detecting presumptive congenital syphilis: relationship with maternal treatment, *Pediatrics* 91:88, 1993.

Desmond MM, Rudolph AJ, Phitaksphraiwan P: The transitional nursery: a mechanism for preventive medicine in the newborn, *Pediatr Clin North Am* 13:656, 1966.

Donn SM: *The Michigan manual,* Mount Kisco, NY, 1992, Futura.

Dubowitz LMS, Dubowitz V, Goldberg C: Clinical assessment of gestational age in the newborn infant, *J Pediatr* 77:1, 1970.

Gomella GM: *Neonatology: management, procedures, on-call problems, diseases and drugs,* Norwalk, Conn, 1999, Appleton & Lange.

Klaus MH, Fanaroff AA: *Care of the high-risk neonate,* Philadelphia, 1993, WB Saunders.

Lubchenco LO, Hansman C, Boyd E: Intrauterine growth in length and head circumference as estimated from live births at gestational ages 26 to 42 weeks, *Pediatrics* 37:403, 1966.

7

The Head

BERYL J. ROSENSTEIN

I. EVALUATION

A. Attention should be paid to the size and configuration of the head. Look for ridging or separation of sutures, size of the fontanels, skull defects, asymmetry, and softening. Head size, measured by maximum occipitofrontal head circumference, and the size of the fontanels should be compared with appropriate standards. Serial head circumference measurements are more important than any single value.

N.B.: Occipitofrontal circumference may not be a valid measure in a newborn with an abnormally shaped head (e.g., craniosynostosis).

B. Examination should include the following:

1. Percussion: A hollow or "cracked-pot" sound will be heard over dilated ventricles.
2. Auscultation: A bruit can be heard with vascular lesions.
3. Transillumination: Will be positive with subdural hematoma, cortical atrophy, porencephaly, hydranencephaly.

C. In a patient with a large or asymmetric head, it is important to look for evidence of increased intracranial pressure, which may include the following:

1. Distention of scalp veins.
2. Separation of cranial sutures (especially squamosal).
3. Enlargement and distention of fontanels.
4. Sixth-nerve palsy, rarely seen in the newborn period.
5. "Setting sun" eye findings.
6. Vomiting, irritability, lethargy.

N.B.: Because of open sutures, however, signs of increased intracranial pressure such as papilledema are rarely seen in the newborn period.

D. Diagnostic procedures that may be helpful include skull radiographs, ultrasound, computed tomography (CT) with and without contrast medium, magnetic resonance imaging (MRI), cerebral angiography (rarely), and radionuclide bone scans.

II. FONTANELS
A. Size.
1. At birth the anterior fontanel is highly variable in size and shape. Mean size (average of length plus width) is 2.5 6 1.5 cm. It is rare for the posterior fontanel to be larger than 0.5 cm. The anterior fontanel tends to enlarge during the first postnatal month.
2. In otherwise normal infants, there is no correlation between the size of the anterior fontanel and the time of closure and head circumference.

B. Large anterior fontanel.
1. A nonbulging, large anterior fontanel may be seen in the following disorders:
   a. Achondroplasia.
   b. Apert syndrome.
   c. Cleidocranial dysostosis.
   d. Hypophosphatasia.
   e. Osteogenesis imperfecta.
   f. Pyknodysostosis (osteopetrosis, cranial and digital anomalies, dwarfism, frontal and occipital bossing).
   g. Kenny syndrome.
   h. Down syndrome.
   i. Trisomy 13 and 18.
   j. Hypothyroidism.
   k. Rubella syndrome.
   l. Russell-Silver syndrome.
   m. Intrauterine malnutrition.
   n. Hydrocephalus.
2. A large anterior fontanel with widened sutures (>1 cm) may be seen in normal infants.
3. A large anterior fontanel may be associated with poor calcification of the cranium or delayed closure of the anterior fontanel, but normal head growth.

C. Small anterior fontanel.
1. A small or closed anterior fontanel does not always correlate with small head circumference.
2. With a cranium of normal size and shape and without ridging along sutures, a small anterior fontanel is usually of no significance.
3. A small anterior fontanel may be a normal variant or may be secondary to one of the following disorders:
   a. Primary microcephaly.
   b. Craniosynostosis (sagittal or coronal sutures).
   c. Hyperthyroidism.
   d. A wormian bone in the anterior fontanel.

D. Third fontanel.
1. A third fontanel is not a true fontanel, but is a bony defect of variable size situated along the sagittal suture, 2 cm anterior to the posterior fontanel. It ranges in size from 0.7 to 3.5 cm.
2. A third fontanel is present in approximately 6% of neonates and occurs more often in preterm than full-term infants.

3. A large third fontanel (>13 mm) is associated with minor congenital anomalies and is a common finding in infants with Down's syndrome.

III. SKULL SOFTENING

Skull softening may be seen in a variety of conditions, including the following:

A. Cleidocranial dysostosis. Complete or partial absence of the clavicles; large head with defective ossification.

B. Craniotabes.
1. Reduction in bone mineralization of the skull.
2. Most often occurs in the occipital and parietal bones along the lambdoidal sutures.
3. Usually of no clinical significance.

C. Lacunar skull.
1. Defects in the inner table of the cranial vault.
2. Skull radiograph shows decreased densities described as "soap bubble" rarefactions.
3. May be associated with spina bifida or other central nervous system (CNS) abnormalities.

D. Osteogenesis imperfecta.

E. Multiple wormian bones. Small multiple bones that occur within sutures.

IV. LARGE HEAD

A large head is defined as an occipitofrontal circumference greater than three standard deviations above the mean or above the 98th percentile. Differential diagnosis includes the following:

A. Birth trauma. A large head may be secondary to cephalhematoma, subgaleal effusion, or caput succedaneum. These are usually obvious on physical examination and resolve spontaneously over days to weeks.

B. Benign familial macrocephaly.
1. The absolute head circumference is large, but serial measurements demonstrate a proportionate rate of growth; sutures and fontanels are normal; neurologic examination is normal.
2. This condition is often familial and inherited as an autosomal dominant trait. Determination of the head circumference of other family members (physical examination, photographs, hat size) may be helpful. Diagnosis may be suggested by prenatal ultrasound in association with appropriate family history.
3. May rarely be associated with underlying CNS structural or storage disease (megalocephaly), such as the following:
   a. Retardation, hypotonia, convulsions.
   b. Achondroplasia (may be associated with mildly to moderately dilated ventricles).
   c. Cerebral gigantism (Sotos syndrome).
   d. Beckwith-Wiedemann syndrome.
4. A normal CT scan is the definitive diagnostic test.

C. Hydrocephalus.

1. Hydrocephalus is the most common cause of head enlargement in the newborn period (0.39 to 0.87 cases per 1000 births); congenital cases are more common than acquired (3:1).
2. Etiology.
   a. Congenital.
      (1) Aqueductal stenosis is the most common cause.
      (2) Dandy-Walker syndrome: Cystic dilation of the fourth ventricle, with defective development of the cerebellum. Associated malformations include capillary angioma, cardiac malformations, ophthalmic anomalies, agenesis of the corpus callosum, and occipital meningocele.
      (3) Arnold-Chiari malformation: Downward displacement of the cerebellar tonsils through the foramen magnum; downward displacement of the cervical cord; often seen with meningomyelocele.
      (4) Vein of Galen malformation: Dilated vein compresses aqueduct; a bruit can be heard over the vertex; cardiac failure.
      (5) Choroid plexus papilloma: Overproduction of cerebrospinal fluid (CSF).
      (6) Holoprosencephaly.
      (7) Hydranencephaly.
   b. Acquired.
      (1) Posthemorrhagic; usually secondary to intraventricular bleed or temporal lobe hematoma.
      (2) Inflammatory or postinflammatory; secondary to meningitis.
      (3) Toxoplasmosis.
   c. Syndromic.
      (1) Trisomies.
      (2) Craniosynostosis.
      (3) VACTERL association.
      (4) Smith-Lemli-Opitz.
      (5) Hunter-Hurler.
3. Clinical manifestations.
   a. There may be obvious head enlargement at birth or gradual enlargement; this may be the only manifestation in the newborn period.
   b. Anorexia, vomiting, lethargy, hyperirritability.
   c. Signs of increased intracranial pressure (rare in the newborn).
   d. "Cracked-pot" sign on percussion over dilated ventricle.
4. Diagnosis.
   a. Confirmed by CT studies with and without contrast medium.
   b. MRI may help define anatomic abnormalities.
   c. Ultrasound useful for serial assessment of ventricular size.
   d. Cerebral angiography may be helpful in delineation of vascular lesions.
   e. Transillumination is usually negative unless cerebral mantle is <1 cm.

f. Antenatal diagnosis can be made by ultrasound. If the fetus has progressive hydrocephalus and the biparietal diameter is >100 mm, delivery should be by elective cesarean section.

N.B.: Fetal hydrocephalus occurs in 1 of 2000 pregnancies. Polyhydramnios occurs in about 30% of the pregnancies and is frequently the only sign of hydrocephalus. The presence of additional malformations is a poor prognostic sign. Prenatal cytogenetic studies are indicated, especially when there are associated abnormalities. The overall outcome is not good. Prenatal shunting procedures have shown no improvement over that expected from the natural history.

  5. Treatment.
- a. Direct operative procedure (e.g., removal of congenital cyst).
- b. Ventricular shunting procedure.
- c. The role of acetazolamide and furosemide in neonatal posthemorrhagic ventricular dilation remains highly controversial.
- d. Prognosis depends on the underlying etiology.

D. Subdural collections.

1. Etiology.
   - a. Hematoma secondary to birth trauma or bleeding disorder.
   - b. Hygroma secondary to traumatic laceration of piarachnoid.
   - c. Effusion secondary to meningitis.
2. Clinical features.
   - a. Head enlargement with boxlike configuration and biparietal bossing.
   - b. Signs of increased intracranial pressure.
   - c. Positive transillumination.
   - d. Retinal hemorrhages with traumatic hematoma.
3. Diagnosis is by CT scan or ultrasound.
4. Treatment may include evacuation of blood and subdural shunting.
5. Prognosis depends on the following:
   - a. Nature and severity of the underlying problem.
   - b. Size, location, and duration of the lesion.
   - c. Success or failure of interventions.

E. Intracranial cysts and tumors.

1. Tumors are exceedingly rare.
2. Hydranencephaly.
   - a. Absence of cerebral hemispheres with intact dura, skull, and scalp.
   - b. Large head, spasticity, seizures, lack of eye fusion.
   - c. Diagnosis is by ultrasound or CT scan; on transillumination, islands of preserved cortical tissue are seen as small opacities.
3. Porencephaly.
   - a. Abnormal CSF cavities within the cerebral hemispheres.
   - b. Seizures, focal neurologic deficit, hydrocephalus, overlying cranial defects.
   - c. Diagnosis is by ultrasound or CT scan; transillumination is locally positive.
   - d. Treatment includes surgical removal or shunting of the cyst.

4. Miscellaneous.
    a. Neurofibromatosis.
    b. Bannayan syndrome (lipomatosis, angiomatosis, macrocephaly).

V. SMALL HEAD
A. A small head is defined as an occipitofrontal circumference greater than three standard deviations below the mean or less than the 3rd percentile.
1. It is always secondary to delayed brain growth and development.
2. Although microcephaly is significantly correlated with low IQ scores, the relationship is not absolute.

B. Etiology.
1. Intrauterine infection (rubella, cytomegalovirus [CMV], toxoplasmosis).
2. Chromosomal abnormalities: Trisomies 13, 18, 21; deletion syndromes (4, 5, 13).
3. Familial.
    a. Autosomal recessive, dominant, or X-linked.
    b. Furrowed brow, backward sloping of the forehead, and small cranial volume.
4. In utero drug exposure (e.g., cocaine, alcohol).
5. Intrauterine growth retardation (IUGR) secondary to malnutrition, hypertension, placental insufficiency.
6. Poorly controlled maternal phenylketonuria; aminoacidurias.
7. Component of a variety of syndromes, including the following:
    a. Rubinstein-Taybi.
    b. Smith-Lemli-Opitz.
    c. de Lange.
    d. Prader-Willi.
8. Perinatal infection (e.g., herpes simplex).
9. Intrapartum or neonatal hypoxic-ischemic insults.

C. Diagnosis. Based on physical examination, serologic studies, family history, skull radiographs, neuroimaging studies, amino acid screening, and chromosome analysis.

D. There is no specific therapy; prognosis depends on the underlying etiology.

VI. ABNORMAL HEAD CONFIGURATION
A. Frontal bossing. May be seen in achondroplasia, osteopetrosis, GM_1 gangliosidosis, and I-cell disease (lysosomal storage disease).

B. Molding.
1. Molding is a common finding secondary to the fetal head passing through the birth canal.
2. Molding usually consists of lengthening in the occipitofrontal diameter, flattening of the forehead, narrowing of the biparietal diameter, and protuberance of the occiput.
3. The configuration steadily improves over a period of several days.

C. Craniosynostosis.

1. Premature closure of one or more of the cranial sutures. Because this usually occurs prenatally, a diagnosis can be made in the neonatal period. Affects approximately 1 in 2000 children. A single suture is involved in 80% of cases; multiple sutures are involved in 20%. There may be an increased incidence with breech positioning and with twins.

2. At birth the cranial bones tend to override one another. Within hours to days the bones no longer override, definite sutures are established, and the edges of the flat bones are separated by fibrous tissue.

3. Growth normally occurs perpendicular to the line of the suture but is inhibited by the premature closure of the suture. The skull is forced to grow parallel to the fused suture, but additional growth abnormalities can occur throughout the calvarium. In infants with nonsyndromic craniosynostosis, there is no reduction in intracranial volume.

4. The final configuration of the head depends on the sutures involved. The deformity is greatest in the axial direction of the affected suture. Closure of one of the paired sutures results in flattening of the skull on that side.

5. Single-suture synostosis usually results only in cosmetic defect and does not impair brain growth; hydrocephalus is a rare event in cases of nonsyndromic craniosynostosis and never occurs in cases of single-suture synostosis other than by coincidence; in contrast, it is a relatively frequent finding in cases of syndromic craniosynostosis.

6. Etiology.
   a. Often unknown.
   b. May be secondary to developmental, mechanical, teratogenic (fetal hydantoin syndrome), metabolic, or genetic factors; a number of mutations in the fibroblast growth factor receptor family of genes have been identified.
   c. Is not related to abnormalities of brain growth, but may occur in association with CNS malformations.
   d. May occur as an isolated defect or (when multiple sutures are involved) as a component of a syndrome (e.g., Apert, Crouzon, Pfeiffer, Saethre-Chotzen).

7. Diagnosis.
   a. Physical findings: Irregular or asymmetric skull; detection of an area where overriding sutures cannot be felt; inability to move the cranial bones in relation to one another; palpation of a bony ridge along the suture line; hypertelorism; difference in level or position of the eyes and ears.
   b. Careful fundoscopic examination is needed to rule out optic atrophy, papilledema.

N.B.: An open anterior fontanel does not rule out craniosynostosis.

   c. Skull radiographs.
   d. Three-dimensional CT is useful in cases of complicated suture pathology, when the diagnosis is in question, to evaluate under-

lying brain abnormalities, and to rule out increased intracranial pressure.

e. Ear, nose, and throat (ENT); ophthalmology; and genetics consultations are often indicated.

8. Specific defects.

a. Sagittal.

(1) Sagittal defects are the most common type of defect seen (50% of cases); they occur in males more often than females (4:1); they may be familial and are rarely associated with other abnormalities.

(2) Scaphocephaly, or "boat shaped"; increased anteroposterior length and decreased cranial width; neurologic examination and development are normal. The suture is usually ridged and quite long.

(3) Plain-film radiographs confirm the diagnosis.

(4) The head may assume a more normal shape over time without treatment.

N.B.: Some cases occur in premature infants laid with their heads turned to the side ("NICUcephaly").

b. Coronal.

(1) Coronal defects occur in females more often than males; unilateral and bilateral types occur with equal frequency; there is a familial incidence in 8% of cases.

(2) Unilateral synostosis leads to flattening of the forehead on the side of the involved suture and contralateral forehead bossing (anterior plagiocephaly); there may be associated abnormalities in binocular eye movement.

(3) Bilateral synostosis causes brachycephaly—a short head with expansion of the vertex and lateral aspects of the skull. It may be associated with retardation, developmental abnormalities, proptosis, and strabismus.

c. Metopic.

(1) Trigonocephaly: Bullet-shaped configuration of the forehead with a prominent ridge in the midforehead region (frontal keel), narrow forehead, close-set eyes. A palpable and often visible ridge is present along part or all of the suture.

(2) Plain-film radiographs confirm the diagnosis.

(3) May be associated with related anomalies of the limbs/digits, cleft palate, coloboma, genitourinary and cardiac anomalies, and holoprosencephaly; 5% of cases are familial.

(4) May be associated with mental retardation, which is most likely related to associated CNS abnormalities.

d. Lambdoid.

(1) True lambdoid synostosis is relatively rare (2% to 4% of all cases of craniosynostosis); occurs in males more often than females.

(2) Presents as flattening of the occipital bone with compensatory bossing of the ipsilateral frontal region. In severe cases, the head may be shaped like a parallelogram.

(3) Diagnosis is based on perisutural ridging of the suture and radiologic evidence of bony fusion.

(4) In later infancy, it needs to be differentiated from positional (deformational) flattening, seen with increased frequency after the recent recommendation for supine sleeping position.

(5) Most children with true lambdoid synostosis benefit from surgical correction.

e. Multiple synostoses.

(1) Oxycephaly: The skull expands toward the vertex, resulting in a pointed, tower-shaped head.

(2) May be associated with increased intracranial pressure, mental retardation, and neurologic complications.

(3) Early surgery is almost always indicated.

9. Treatment.

a. Indications for treatment are cosmetic only, except when multiple sutures are involved or there is evidence of increased intracranial pressure or interference with binocular vision.

b. Optimum timing of surgery is 3 to 6 months of age; the only indication for surgical intervention in the neonatal period is to relieve intracranial pressure, which occurs in only a small percentage of affected children.

VII. ENCEPHALOCELE/MENINGOCELE

A. An encephalocele represents the protrusion of a portion of the brain and meninges through a skull defect. If only the meninges herniate, the lesion develops into a meningocele. The incidence is 1:5000 births; 75% occur in the occipital area, 25% in the frontal area. They are often associated with other congenital defects or associated CNS abnormalities. Hydrocephalus is a common problem in patients with large occipital encephaloceles.

B. An encephalocele causes a soft, fluctuant, balloonlike mass that protrudes from the cranium. It may pulsate and may be covered by erythematous translucent or opaque material, or by normal skin; it may vary in size from 1 cm to two to three times the infant's head circumference.

C. Diagnosis.

1. Plain-film radiographs show the associated skull defect.
2. Transillumination may be helpful.
3. CT, MRI, and ultrasound can provide information on associated cerebral anomalies.
4. In many cases, the presence of a large convexity encephalocele is diagnosed prenatally based on an elevated alpha-fetoprotein level or abnormalities seen on in utero ultrasonograms.

D. Treatment. Whenever possible, surgical repair early in life should be performed.

E. Prognosis.

1. The size of the sac is not a reliable predictor of functional outcome.
2. Meningoceles have a substantially better prognosis than encephaloceles.

3. The finding of substantial brain tissue in the sac or association with an underlying syndrome (e.g., Meckel syndrome) is a poor prognostic sign.

VIII. CONGENITAL SCALP DEFECT (APLASIA CUTIS CONGENITA)

A. Localized area of congenital absence of skin. This condition usually occurs at the vertex; at birth it may appear ulcerated and crusted and may appear to be infected. Over time the area epithelializes but remains devoid of hair. The underlying skull is usually intact, but the lesion may extend to the dura or meninges.

B. Etiology.

1. A congenital scalp defect may be inherited as autosomal dominant (sometimes in association with limb abnormalities) or may occur sporadically; a detailed family history is important.
2. The defect may be isolated or may occur with other cerebral or extracranial anomalies, such as those associated with the following:
   a. Johanson-Blizzard syndrome (mental retardation, congenital deafness, hypothyroidism).
   b. Chromosome 4 deletion.
   c. Cleft lip or palate; tracheoesophageal fistula; renal and cardiac anomalies.
   d. Trisomy 13.
   e. Epidermal nevus syndrome.

C. Treatment. Treatment is usually conservative, but plastic surgical repair may be indicated in selected cases.

IX. NATAL TEETH

A. Clinical features.

1. Natal teeth are defined as teeth present at the time of birth; neonatal teeth, which are less common, erupt from birth to 30 days of age.
2. Natal teeth may be fully erupted or partially covered by gingival tissue; they are almost always the lower central incisors and often occur in pairs. Most represent premature eruption of deciduous teeth, but occasionally they represent supernumerary teeth.
3. Incidence is 1:2000 to 1:4000 births; natal teeth may occur as early as 26 weeks gestation.
4. Most natal teeth occur as isolated events, but there is a positive family history in 15% to 25% of cases (may be autosomal dominant). There is an increased incidence in cases involving cleft lip and palate. Natal teeth may also be seen with several syndromes (e.g., Ellis-van Creveld [chondroectodermal dysplasia], Hallermann-Streiff [oculomandibulofacial syndrome], Jadassohn-Lewandowsky [pachyonychia congenita], Pfeiffer and Teebi [hypertelorism]).
5. Complications include the following:
   a. Discomfort during feeding.
   b. Trauma to the mother's nipple during feeding.
   c. Ulceration of the adjacent lip or tongue.

   d. Aspiration of a loose tooth (always mentioned but rarely documented).
B. Management.
1. Dental radiography is always indicated to differentiate premature eruption of deciduous teeth from supernumerary teeth and to provide information about tooth root development and the relationship of the tooth to adjacent teeth.
2. Extraction is indicated if the tooth is supernumerary or very loose; this is best done by a dentist, who must be alert to the possibility of excessive bleeding.
3. If the tooth is not causing any difficulty it should be left in place.
   a. Early mobility often resolves within a month.
   b. Early extraction may lead to overcrowding of the permanent teeth or loss of the permanent tooth bud.

BIBLIOGRAPHY

Brann AW Jr, Schwartz JF: Developmental anomalies and neuromuscular disorders. In Fanaroff AA, Martin RJ (editors): *Neonatal-perinatal medicine*, ed 4, St. Louis, 1987, Mosby.

Chemke J, Robinson A: The third fontanelle, *J Pediatr* 75:617, 1969.

Cohen MM Jr: Sutural biology and the correlates of craniosynostosis, *Am J Med Genet* 47:581, 1993.

Duc G, Largo RH: Anterior fontanel: size and closure in term and preterm infants, *Pediatrics* 78:904, 1986.

Frieden IJ: Aplasia cutis congenital: a clinical review and proposal for classification, *J Am Acad Dermatol* 14:646, 1986.

Jacobson RI: Congenital structural defects. In Swaiman KF (editor): *Pediatric neurology: principles and practice*, St. Louis, 1989, Mosby.

Leung AKC: Natal teeth, *Am J Dis Child* 140:249, 1986.

Menkes JH: Malformation of the central nervous system. In Taeusch HW, Ballard RA, Avery ME (editors): *Schaffer and Avery's diseases of the newborn*, ed 6, Philadelphia, 1991, WB Saunders.

Popich GA, Smith DW: Fontanels: range of normal size, *J Pediatr* 130:386, 1972.

Shilito J Jr, Matson DD: Craniosynostosis: a review of 519 surgical patients, *Pediatrics* 41:829, 1986.

Tan KL: Wide sutures and large fontanels in the newborn, *Am J Dis Child* 130:386, 1976.

8

Otolaryngology

MAX M. APRIL AND ROBERT M. NACLERIO

I. AIRWAY OBSTRUCTION

A. Stridor.

1. Harsh sound produced by turbulent airflow through a partial obstruction. *Stridor* is a description, not a disease entity. Symptoms associated with the site of airway obstruction are listed in Table 8-1. There are three types of stridor:
   a. Inspiratory.
   b. Expiratory.
   c. Biphasic.
2. Stridor may be associated with abnormalities of feeding (nasal, oropharyngeal, supraglottic) or crying (glottic).
3. If there is stridor with severe airway compromise the first step in treatment is establishment of a stable airway with endotracheal intubation.

B. Nasal obstruction.

1. Choanal atresia.
   a. Newborn infants are obligate nasal breathers.
      (1) Bilateral atresia is recognized at birth (respiratory distress) when the infant has paradoxic cyanosis (cyanotic with mouth closed but not with crying).
      (2) Unilateral atresia is usually not recognized clinically until the infant is older, when the unilateral nasal obstruction is complicated by purulent rhinorrhea.
   b. Incidence is 1:8000 births.
   c. Unilateral to bilateral ratio is 2:1.
   d. 90% of nasal obstructions involve the bony plates; 10% are membranous.
   e. Up to 50% of infants with choanal atresia have associated anomalies (CHARGE association: *c*oloboma, *h*eart disease, *a*tresia choanae, *r*etarded central nervous system [CNS], *g*enital hypoplasia, *e*ar anomalies).
   f. Diagnosis: Diagnosis is suspected when a 6F catheter cannot be passed through the nasal airway (make sure catheter is seen in

TABLE 8-1
Symptoms Associated With Site of Airway Obstruction*

Site of obstruction	Inspiratory stridor	Expiratory stridor	Feeding problems	Abnormal cry
Nose	++		++	+
Oropharynx	++		++	
Supraglottis	++		++	++
Glottis/subglottis	++	++	+	++
Trachea		++		

*+, Mild symptoms; ++, moderate to severe symptoms.

    mouth, not curled in nose); diagnosis can be confirmed by computed tomography (CT) scan.
    g. Treatment: Establish an oral airway using a McGovern nipple (a large nipple modified with its end cut off and ties attached to secure it in place, acting like an oral airway).
    h. Surgical repair (transnasal [endoscopic] versus transpalatal) may be required. A tracheotomy should be performed for obstruction related to CHARGE association.
  2. Congenital nasal masses (intranasal or extranasal) can be caused by the following:
    a. Encephalocele: Herniation of brain.
      (1) An encephalocele is compressible and pulsates.
      (2) An encephalocele enlarges with crying.
    b. Glioma: Glial tissue that has lost a CNS connection (80% of cases) or has an intracranial extension (20%). Gliomas are noncompressible and nonpulsatile.
    c. Dermoid: Contains ectodermal and mesodermal elements; often contains hair follicles in a dimple.
    d. Diagnosis: CT scan or magnetic resonance imaging (MRI).
    e. Treatment: Surgical excision.
  3. Nasal septal dislocation.
    a. Related to passage through birth canal.
    b. Incidence is 1% to 3% of newborns (higher in primiparas).
    c. Diagnosis: External nose twisted, with poor tip and dorsal support on vertical pressure (compression test).
    d. Treatment: Reduction (mechanical repositioning by otolaryngologist) with local anesthesia in nursery.
  4. Craniofacial anomalies.
    a. Crouzon disease (craniofacial dysostosis): Craniostenosis, midface hypoplasia, and bulging eyes.
    b. Apert syndrome (acrocephalosyndactyly): Crouzon disease with syndactyly.
C. Oropharyngeal obstruction.
  1. Macroglossia.
    a. Down syndrome.
    b. Hypothyroidism.

    c. Beckwith-Wiedemann syndrome (exomphalos, macroglossia, gigantism), often with visceromegaly.

  2. Glossoptosis: Pierre Robin sequence (micrognathia, cleft palate).

D. Supraglottic larynx.

1. Laryngomalacia.
   a. Laryngomalacia is the most common congenital anomaly.
   b. Inspiratory stridor is present; it is worse when the infant is supine, excited, or feeding.
   c. Stridor may improve when the infant is prone or resting.
   d. The infant has a normal cry, and cyanosis is absent.
   e. Diagnosis: Confirmed by fiberoptic laryngoscopy.
   f. Treatment: Usually self-limited (12 to 24 months); rarely, laser excision of the aryepiglottic fold or a portion of the epiglottis is needed for failure to thrive infants or those in extreme distress (1% to 4%).

2. Laryngeal cleft.
   a. A laryngeal cleft causes respiratory distress during feeding.
   b. Diagnosis: Confirmed by barium swallow and endoscopy.
   c. Treatment: Surgical repair.

3. Laryngocele.
   a. A laryngocele is a cystic lesion in the larynx.
   b. It presents in the newborn as stridor or airway obstruction.
   c. Diagnosis: Confirmed by endoscopy with or without plain-film radiographs.
   d. Treatment: Endoscopic marsupialization.

E. Glottic obstruction.

1. Web-type obstruction.
   a. Poor cry is an indication.
   b. Airway symptoms depend on size of obstruction.
   c. Diagnosis: Confirmed by endoscopy.
   d. Treatment: Endoscopic division, with possible intraluminal stent placement.

2. Vocal cord paralysis: Second most common anomaly.
   a. Bilateral.
      (1) Causes acute respiratory distress.
      (2) Infant may have normal cry.
      (3) Seen in Arnold-Chiari malformation, hydrocephalus, and meningocele.
      (4) Diagnosis: Confirmed by fiberoptic nasolaryngoscopy.
      (5) Treatment: Tracheotomy is needed in 50% of cases. If CNS-related problem is treated, many infants do not need tracheotomy.
   b. Unilateral.
      (1) Infants with unilateral vocal cord paralysis are often asymptomatic.
      (2) Indications are a hoarse cry, possible aspiration.
      (3) Diagnosis: Confirmed by fiberoptic nasolaryngoscopy.
      (4) Treatment: Observation.

3. Atresia.
   a. Rare.
   b. Incompatible with life unless tracheoesophageal fistula is also present.

F. Subglottic obstruction.
1. Congenital subglottic stenosis.
   a. Congenital subglottic stenosis usually causes recurrent croup or stridor after a few months.
   b. Diagnosis: Endoscopy reveals a lumen <3.5 mm in diameter.
   c. Treatment: Depends on extent of obstruction; it may respond to endoscopic treatment or the patient may need tracheotomy with subsequent laryngotracheal reconstruction.
2. Subglottic hemangioma.
   a. A subglottic hemangioma usually appears as stridor at 1 to 6 months of age but can appear in neonates.
   b. 50% have associated skin hemangiomata.
   c. Diagnosis: Endoscopy.
   d. Treatment: CO_2 laser, steroids, tracheotomy, interferon-α.

G. Tracheobronchial obstruction. The following entities are associated with varied signs and symptoms ranging from mild expiratory stridor and no distress to tachypnea and acute distress necessitating immediate intervention.
1. Stenosis.
   a. Diagnosis: Endoscopy, fluoroscopy.
   b. Treatment is based on severity of the stenosis (i.e., endoscopic versus open surgical management).
2. Tracheomalacia.
   a. Indication is collapse of the lower airway.
   b. Diagnosis: Confirmed by endoscopy or fluoroscopy.
   c. Treatment: Condition often improves with time, but tracheotomy may be necessary.
3. Vascular ring.
   a. Double aortic arch.
   b. Right aortic arch.
   c. Innominate artery compression.
   d. Pulmonary artery sling.
   e. Diagnosis: Confirmed by endoscopy, barium swallow, or MRI.
   f. Treatment depends on severity of the obstruction; may need open thoracic repair.
4. Tracheoesophageal fistula (TEF). Presentation may be immediate, with first feed not tolerated (see a and b below), or more subtle, with recurrent aspiration (see c below).
   a. Proximal esophagus blind pouch with distal TEF (87% of cases).
   b. Isolated esophageal atresia (8%).
   c. H type (4%).
   d. Diagnosis: Confirmed by barium swallow and/or inability to pass a nasogastric tube into the stomach.
   e. Treatment: Surgical repair.

H. External compression. See section on neck masses later in this chapter.

II. CLEFT LIP AND PALATE
A. Incidence.
1. Cleft lip and palate is the second most common and significant congenital deformity, occurring in 1:1000 births (club foot is the most common).
2. The highest incidence occurs in Native Americans, followed by whites and then blacks.
3. 50% of cases involve both cleft lip and palate; 25% cleft palate only; 20% cleft lip only; 5% cleft lip and alveolus.

B. Manifestations.
1. Diagnosis is obvious on examination.
2. Most affected newborns have associated middle ear effusions.
3. Feeding difficulties: A longer nipple and compressible bottle are required, with more frequent burping.
4. Bifid uvula: 10% to 20% of cases are associated with a submucosal cleft palate.

C. Surgical repair.
1. Cleft palate.
   a. Early repair (10 to 12 months) is better for speech.
   b. Late repair (24 to 30 months) is better for facial growth.
2. Cleft lip. Early repair (within the first year) is best.

III. EAR
A. External ear.
Conditions that affect the external ear include the following:
1. Congenital aural atresia.
   a. Incidence is 1:10,000 to 1:20,000 births.
   b. Unilateral.
      (1) Twice as common as bilateral.
      (2) Diagnosis: Auditory brainstem response (ABR) to document sensorineural hearing and contralateral hearing.
      (3) Treatment: Separate procedures for auricle and middle ear.
   c. Bilateral.
      (1) Use of a bone-conducting hearing aid should begin at 6 months of age.
      (2) Surgical repair should be done at age 4 to 5 years.
2. Microtia: Various degrees of hypoplasia of external ear with or without middle ear involvement.
3. Positional: Malformations and positional aberrations of the pinna suggest a variety of genetic defects. If it is rotated or low set, this is especially so; associated anomalies are apt to be severe (e.g., renal agenesis, CNS defects).

B. Middle ear.
Otitis media: Rare in neonate.
1. Causes sepsis, fever, or both.
2. May involve gram-negative organisms in neonatal period.
3. Diagnosis: Tympanocentesis for diagnosis and culture.

4. Treatment: Intravenous antibiotics if gram-negative infection or infant <4 weeks old.

C. Hearing loss.

1. Incidence of severe hearing loss at birth is 1:1000.
2. Incidence of severe hearing loss in neonatal intensive care unit (NICU) is 1:60.
3. There is a high risk for hearing loss with the following conditions:
   a. Family history of congenital hearing loss.
   b. Birth weight <1500 g.
   c. 5-minute Apgar score <5.
   d. TORCH group of infections.
   e. Severe hyperbilirubinemia.
      (1) >22 mg/dl in infant weighing >2000 g.
      (2) >17 mg/dl in infant weighing <2000 g.
   f. Intraventricular hemorrhage.
   g. Bacterial meningitis/neonatal sepsis.
   h. External ear deformities.

N.B.: Recent reports on the subject of universal newborn screening recommend that every infant have evoked otoacoustic emissions (EOAE) or ABR testing before 3 months of age.

IV. FACIAL PARALYSIS

A. Birth trauma.

1. May be related to large size, forceps delivery, or pressure through birth canal.
2. Diagnosis: Associated ecchymosis, synkinesis (contraction of unexpected facial muscles with voluntary movement).
3. Treatment: Observation; most recover spontaneously.
4. If not resolved after 14 days, serial electromyography should be performed.

B. Möbius syndrome.

1. Usually associated with bilateral abducens nerve paralysis.
2. May also involve cranial nerves 3, 4, 7, 10, 12.
3. May include micrognathia, club foot, and/or absence of the pectoralis muscle.
4. No treatment is available.

C. Goldenhar syndrome.

1. Oculoauriculovertebral dysplasia.
2. Hemifacial microsomia: Faulty development of first and second branchial arches.
3. Can have reconstructive surgery when older.

D. Agenesis of depressor anguli oris muscle.

1. Unilateral; asymmetry is prominent when baby cries.
2. Associated with cardiovascular, skeletal, and genitourinary abnormalities.

V. NECK MASSES

A. Lymphatic malformations/cystic hygroma.

1. Soft, diffuse, painless.
2. Cystic; transilluminates; often multiloculated.

3. Often in posterior triangle of neck.
4. Can involve mucosal surfaces.
5. Does not regress.
6. Diagnosis by MRI or CT.
7. Treatment: Surgical excision.

B. Hemangioma/vascular malformations.

1. Associated skin hemangiomata in 50% of cases.
2. Usually reddish-blue, soft; often involves overlying skin.
3. Rapid growth first 6 months.
4. Most regress by 5 years of age.
5. Treatment: Observation; surgical excision is warranted if spontaneous bleeding, airway distress, or coagulopathy occurs.

C. Thyroglossal duct cyst.

1. Tract from tongue base to thyroid gland.
2. Painless, midline mass with normal overlying skin.
3. Most often between hyoid bone and thyroid.
4. Moves with deglutition and tongue protrusion.
5. Diagnosis by ultrasound; thyroid scan also used to discover functioning thyroid tissue other than cyst.
6. Treatment: Surgical excision (Sistrunk procedure).

D. Teratoma.

1. All three germ layers are involved (ectoderm, mesoderm, endoderm).
2. Solid mass.
3. Plain-film radiographs reveal calcification in 50% of cases.
4. Treatment: Surgical excision.

E. Sternocleidomastoid (SCM) tumor of infancy.

1. Also known as *fibromatosis coli.*
2. Torticollis is associated with a firm, nontender nodule under the SCM muscle.
3. Occurs between 7 and 28 days of life.
4. Treatment: Massage, passive stretching, and positioning.
5. Be alert for associated congenital hip deformity.

F. Branchial cleft anomalies.

1. Cyst: No internal or external opening; may present in adolescence or adulthood.
2. Sinus tract: External opening.
3. Fistula: Internal and external opening.
4. May involve first, second, or third branchial arches.
5. Fistulas and sinus tracts that occur at birth have an external opening (pit) along lower anterior border of SCM muscle.
6. Treatment is surgical excision when the child is older.

BIBLIOGRAPHY

Cotton RT: The problem of pediatric laryngotracheal stenosis, *Laryngoscope* 101(suppl 56):1, 1991.

Evans JNG: Management of the cleft larynx and tracheoesophageal clefts, *Ann Otol Rhinol Laryngol* 94:627, 1985.

Holinger LD: Etiology of stridor in the neonate, infant and child, *Ann Otol Rhinol Laryngol* 89:397, 1980.

Morgan DW, Baily CM: Current management of choanal atresia, *Int J Pediatr Otorhinolaryngol* 19:1, 1990.

National Institutes of Health: Early identification of hearing impairment in infants and young children, *NIH Consensus Statement* 11(1):1, 1993.

Paradise JL: Universal newborn hearing screening: should we leap before we look? *Pediatrics* 103:670, 1999.

Thomsen JR, Koltai PJ: Sternomastoid tumor of infancy, *Ann Otol Rhinol Laryngol* 98:955, 1989.

VanSon JAM, Julsrud PR, Hagler DJ, et al: Surgical treatment of vascular ring, *Mayo Clin Proc* 68:1056, 1993.

9

Ophthalmology

MICHAEL X. REPKA

I. GENERAL CONSIDERATIONS
A. Few infants will have any significant abnormality detectable on examination.
B. Subconjunctival hemorrhage is not unusual and ordinarily resolves spontaneously.
C. The examination requires a penlight to test for a pupillary response and to examine the anterior segment, including the conjunctiva, sclera, cornea, anterior chamber, and iris. Direct ophthalmoscopy is necessary to examine the clarity of the media, specifically looking at the quality of the red reflex.

N.B.: Disruptions in the red reflex are always abnormal and may represent a corneal opacity, cataract, vitreous hemorrhage, or retinal detachment.

D. The visual acuity of the full-term neonate is approximately 20/800, adequate to fixate a high-contrast target.
E. The ocular motor system is well established at birth. Eye movements may be tested with a doll's-head maneuver, such as by spinning the infant around the examiner. The eyes will deviate in the direction opposite to the spin. However, alignment need not be normal until 6 to 8 weeks after birth. During the neonatal period, esotropic (turning in) and, more frequently, exotropic (turning out) deviations of the eyes are common.
F. Nearly any problem identified will require consultation, preferably with an ophthalmologist experienced with the ocular examination of an infant.

II. CATARACT
A. Diagnosis.
1. The diagnosis of cataract is best made while examining the red reflex with a direct ophthalmoscope; an opacity in the red reflex is most often the result of a lens anomaly.
2. A cataract may be unilateral (more common) or bilateral.

3. A cataract may range in severity from an insignificant dotlike opacity that is not going to impair visual development through a completely white lens that completely obscures the red reflex.
4. The morphology of the cataract is rarely helpful in establishing an etiology. Help with its description should be sought.
B. Evaluation. Items to be considered in the evaluation of a cataract include the following:
1. History.
   a. A history and eye examination of the infant's parents should be obtained for evidence of autosomal dominant cataracts.
   b. Maternal drug exposure: Substances to look for include naphthalene, phenothiazines, steroids, vitamin D, and antimetabolites.
   c. Maternal infection: The TORCH group of infections should be considered.
2. Physical examination: Look for dysmorphic features that might suggest specific syndromes (e.g., trisomy 21 or Hallermann-Streiff [oculomandibulofacial dyscephalia, or "parrot nose"; bilateral cataracts, often with microphthalmia, microcornea, or glaucoma; hypotrichosis; and dwarfism are possible; all cases are sporadic]).
3. Laboratory evaluation.
   a. Laboratory tests should be performed when there is no history of familial infantile or juvenile cataract and the cataracts are bilateral.
   b. Tests should be used selectively based on the clinical findings. Most patients will require few or no tests.
   c. Blood tests should be done to determine levels of the following:
      (1) Glucose.
      (2) Calcium.
      (3) Amino acids.
      (4) TORCH titers, rapid plasma reagin (RPR).
   d. Urine tests should be done to determine the presence or levels of the following:
      (1) Amino acids.
      (2) Reducing substances.
      (3) Blood and protein screens.
      (4) Lipid bodies.
      (5) Copper.
   e. Specialized tests can determine the presence or levels of the following:
      (1) Red blood cell (RBC) galactose 1-phosphate uridyltransferase.
      (2) RBC glucose-6-phosphatase activity.
      (3) RBC galactokinase activity.
      (4) White blood cell (WBC) α-mannosidase activity.
      (5) Plasma phytanic acid.
C. Differential diagnosis.
1. Autosomal dominant conditions are the most common cause of cataracts in otherwise healthy children.
2. Cataracts may develop after intrauterine infection with rubella, rubeola, varicella, herpes simplex virus (HSV), cytomegalovirus (CMV), or toxoplasmosis.

3. Chromosomal abnormalities: Trisomies 13, 15, 18, or 21; Turner syndrome.
4. Prematurity.
5. Cataracts can be associated with other ocular malformations or with metabolic disorders such as the following:
   a. Galactosemia: Cataracts associated with galactosemia can occasionally be reversed with the institution of dietary management.
   b. Hypoparathyroidism and pseudohypoparathyroidism.
   c. Diabetes mellitus.
   d. Refsum disease.
   e. Lowe oculocerebrorenal syndrome.
   f. Hypoglycemia.
   g. Mannosidosis.
   h. Hereditary hemorrhagic nephritis (Alport syndrome).
6. Systemic syndromes.
   a. Hallermann-Streiff.
   b. Congenital stippled epiphysis (Conradi syndrome).
   c. Smith-Lemli-Opitz (ears slanted or low set; ptosis; micrognathia; syndactyly of second and third toes; cryptorchidism; significant hypospadias).
7. Associated with dermatologic disorders or craniofacial dysostosis.

III. CONGENITAL DEFECTS
A. Aniridia.
1. Incidence is 1:75,000.
2. Autosomal dominant.
   a. Chromosome 2.
   b. Nystagmus, poor vision, cataracts, glaucoma.
3. Sporadic.
   a. 25% develop Wilms tumor. These patients have chromosome 11p13 deletion.
   b. Associated with genitourinary anomalies and mental retardation.
B. Albinism.
1. Incidence is 1:20,000.
2. Autosomal recessive, autosomal dominant, X-linked.
3. Variable visual loss, nystagmus, high refractive error.
C. Microphthalmos and cryptic eye.
1. The reduction in the size of an eye may vary from a nearly imperceptible difference to no formed eye visible in the orbit. In the latter instance the orbit usually contains a cystic structure, which may cause the lower lid to bulge forward and the floor of the orbit to be pushed into the maxillary sinus. This structure is readily detected with imaging. Anophthalmos is extremely rare.
2. Usually unilateral.
3. 40% of affected children have other, nonocular anomalies.
4. Evaluation.
   a. Ophthalmologic and pediatric examination.
   b. Orbital transillumination.
   c. Consider ultrasound and neuroimaging.

5. Management.
    a. Highly individualized. Includes serial aspiration or resection.
    b. Lids need progressive enlargement by the use of progressively larger prostheses or orbital expanders.
6. Prognosis: Generally poor; vision is directly related to the degree of malformation.

D. Coloboma.
1. Pathogenesis: Failure of fusion of the embryonic fissure.
2. A coloboma variably affects the retina, optic nerve, iris, and choroid.
3. Types of coloboma include the following:
    a. Isolated: Sporadic or autosomal dominant.
    b. Part of a malformation syndrome.
        (1) CHARGE association.
            (a) Coloboma (80%).
            (b) Heart anomalies.
            (c) Choanal atresia.
            (d) Retardation.
            (e) Genital anomalies.
            (f) Ear anomalies.
        (2) Aicardi syndrome: Infantile spasms, abnormal corpus callosum, and mental retardation.
    c. Associated with chromosomal abnormalities.
        (1) Trisomies 13 and 22.
        (2) Wolf-Hirschhorn (4p): Mental retardation, short stature, microcephaly, cardiac septal defects, and cleft lip or palate.
        (3) Cat's eye syndrome (22+).
4. Visual prognosis depends on the extent of ocular involvement. Macular or optic nerve involvement causes permanently reduced visual acuity.

IV. CLOUDY CORNEA
A. A wide variety of abnormalities may be responsible for producing a corneal opacity at birth. Careful, rapid therapy is needed to preserve vision.
B. Differential diagnosis.
1. Birth trauma, often associated with a forceps delivery.
2. Infantile glaucoma (see below).
3. Infection: Rubella, HSV.
4. Corneal drying (exposure keratopathy).
5. Metabolic conditions; occasionally seen at birth but more often in childhood.
    a. Mucopolysaccharidosis I-H and I-S.
    b. Mucolipidosis IV.
6. Corneal anomalies.
    a. Replacement by dermoid tissue; most commonly a fleshy mass at the limbus.
    b. Sclerocornea.
    c. Corneal endothelial absence or abnormality.

C. Evaluation.
1. Emergent determination of intraocular pressure. May require general anesthesia or sedation.
2. Ophthalmologic examination to define diagnosis and assist in selection of therapy.
3. Echography of posterior segment.

D. Management.
1. Reduce elevated intraocular pressure.
2. Corneal transplant for bilateral corneal opacities, when not produced by glaucoma, within the first 10 weeks of life. The treatment of unilateral opacities must be individualized because the ultimate prognosis for vision in such a disadvantaged eye is extremely poor.

V. CONJUNCTIVITIS

A. Conjunctivitis during the first month of life is termed *ophthalmia neonatorum.* The incidence is about 2% but ranges from 0.5% to 12%.

B. Prophylaxis.
1. Erythromycin 0.5% ointment.
2. Tetracycline 1% ointment.
3. Silver nitrate 1% drops.
4. All three agents are effective against *Neisseria gonorrhea.*
5. None is highly effective against chlamydia.
6. 2.5% povidone-iodine solution is equally as effective as antimicrobials and is less expensive and less toxic.

C. Differential diagnosis.
1. Chemical-related secondary to use of silver nitrate drops.
2. Chlamydia; may represent 50% of cases.
3. Bacterial.
   a. *N. gonorrhea:* Most dangerous because of the possibility of rapid corneal perforation.
   b. *Staphylococcus aureus* and *Staphylococcus epidermidis.*
   c. *Streptococcus pneumoniae* and *Streptococcus viridans.*
   d. Haemophilus species.
4. HSV.

D. Evaluation.
1. Chemical conjunctivitis appears in the first 24 to 48 hours.
2. Always rule out *N. gonorrhea* and determine if the isolated strain is penicillinase producing. Make certain topical prophylaxis was given.
3. HSV usually appears later, often in the second week after delivery.
4. Microscopic evaluation and cultures are nearly always necessary.
   a. Giemsa and Gram's stains.
   b. Direct fluorescent antibody, enzyme immunoassay, or DNA probes are diagnostic tests for chlamydia.
   c. Chocolate agar in CO_2; reduced blood agar; thioglycolate broth.
   d. Viral cultures as indicated.

E. Therapy.
1. Preliminary therapy is based on clinical presentation and stains of the conjunctival scrapings.

2. *N. gonorrhea:* ceftriaxone 25 to 50 mg/kg per day intravenously or intramuscularly for 7 days; for hyperbilirubinemic infants, especially those who are premature, cefotaxime 50 to 100 mg/kg per day intravenously or intramuscularly in two divided doses.

3. Chlamydia: Erythromycin syrup, 50 mg/kg per day orally in four divided doses for 14 days. Topical therapy is ineffective. Alternative treatment: Azithromycin 20 mg/kg orally daily for 3 days.

4. HSV: Trifluridine 1% every 2 hours for 7 days; should be given with ophthalmologic consultation; ophthalmologic examination is necessary because this treatment will control only epithelial disease.

F. Public health referral and treatment is necessary for mother and all sexual partners.

VI. INFANTILE GLAUCOMA

A. The presentation in infants is entirely different from that in older children and adults. The onset may seem to be nearly instantaneous; symptoms and signs develop over just a few hours.

B. Incidence is 1:10,000.

C. Signs and symptoms.

1. Cloudy cornea is the most common presentation in the neonate.
2. Photophobia.
3. Corneal enlargement (buphthalmos): A horizontal diameter of 9.5 mm is normal.
4. Increased intraocular pressure (IOP) is needed to prove the diagnosis; it is sometimes appreciable on gentle palpation of the eye.
5. Optic nerve cupping and atrophy.
6. Poor vision is a late sign.

D. Evaluation.

1. The pressure should be measured with a tonometer in the office using topical anesthesia, or on occasion, in a facility with anesthesia. General anesthesia and sedation should be avoided because they lower the pressure. Most clinicians attempt to determine the IOP in the office without medication in infants and with ketamine sedation in the operating room.
2. Measure horizontal corneal diameter; >10.5 mm, or progressive enlargement in the infant is a reliable sign of uncontrolled pressure.

E. Differential diagnosis.

1. Primary congenital open-angle glaucoma.
   a. Usually occurs between 3 and 9 months but may occur in the neonate.
   b. Autosomal recessive with incomplete penetrance.
2. Secondary.
   a. Sturge-Weber syndrome.
   b. Lowe syndrome (oculocerebrorenal).
   c. Neurofibromatosis type 1.
   d. Anterior segment malformation syndromes.
   e. Trauma.
   f. Rubella.

F. Therapy.

1. The choice of therapy is governed by the optic nerve appearance, the IOP, and the corneal diameter.
2. Medical therapy is intended as a temporary measure.
   a. Topical β-blockers may produce systemic drug levels and adverse reactions (e.g., wheezing, bradycardia) in the neonate.
   b. Carbonic anhydrase inhibitors: topical and/or acetazolamide 15 mg/kg per day orally divided into two to four doses.
3. Surgery: The objective is long-term control of the glaucoma. Multiple procedures are often needed.

VII. LEUKOCORIA
A. Leukocoria always requires ophthalmologic evaluation.
B. Differential diagnosis.

1. Cataract.
2. Persistent hyperplastic primary vitreous; usually unilateral, with microphthalmos.
3. Cloudy cornea.
4. Retinal detachment, including retinopathy of prematurity.
5. Vitreous hemorrhage: Think of "shaken baby" syndrome.
6. Retinal coloboma.
7. Vitreous inflammation: Toxoplasmosis.
8. Retinoblastoma, toxocariasis: Rare in the neonate but common in toddlers.

BIBLIOGRAPHY

American Academy of Pediatrics Committee on Infectious Diseases: *1997 Redbook: report of the Committee on Infectious Diseases,* ed 24, Elk Grove Village, Ill, 1997, American Academy of Pediatrics.

Birch EE, Stager DR: Prevalence of good visual acuity following surgery for unilateral congenital cataract, *Arch Ophthalmol* 106:40, 1988.

Crawford JS, Morin JD (editors): *The eye in childhood,* New York, 1983, Grune & Stratton.

Isenberg ST, Apt L, Wood M: A controlled trial of povidone-iodine as prophylaxis against ophthalmia neonatorum, *N Engl J Med* 332:562, 1995.

Katzman GH: Pathophysiology of neonates: subconjunctival hemorrhage, *Clin Pediatr* 31:149, 1992.

Laga M, Plummer FA, Piot P, et al: Prophylaxis of gonococcal and chlamydial ophthalmia neonatorum: a comparison of silver nitrate and tetracycline, *N Engl J Med,* 318:653, 1988.

Merin S, Crawford JS: The etiology of congenital cataracts, *Can J Ophthalmol* 6:178, 1971.

Nelson LB, Calhoun JH, Harley RD: *Pediatric ophthalmology,* Philadelphia, 1991, WB Saunders.

Nixon RB, Helveston EM, Miller KK, et al: Incidence of strabismus in neonates, *Am J Ophthalmol* 100:798, 1985.

Rapoza PA, Quinn TC, Kiessling LA, et al: Epidemiology of neonatal conjunctivitis, *Ophthalmology* 93:456, 1986.

10

Cardiology

JEAN S. KAN AND CATHERINE A. NEILL

Cardiac problems in the newborn form a spectrum of severity, ranging from profound cyanosis or heart failure needing immediate attention to a soft, localized cardiac murmur heard in a healthy infant. Some acute problems arise as the ductus closes shortly after birth in infants with "duct-dependent" lesions of the right or left side of the heart. Rather than remembering a long list of rare defects, the primary care provider needs to know the signs of immediate or impending cardiac difficulty and have a swift and organized approach to diagnosis and management. The following tools of diagnosis may be useful:

I. FIVE TOOLS OF DIAGNOSIS
1. Physical examination, physical examination, physical examination: (not *every* infant with a heart murmur needs an echocardiogram!).
2. Electrocardiogram (ECG): Left axis deviation (abnormal superior vector) is always abnormal and may indicate complete atrioventricular (AV) canal, tricuspid atresia, or other rarer defects. An ECG examination is also essential in arrhythmias.
3. Radiography: A chest radiograph can show distinctive cardiac contour in tetralogy of Fallot (TOF) (e.g., pulmonary venous congestion is seen in early left heart failure), or with obstructed pulmonary veins.
4. A hyperoxia test is needed if central cyanosis is suspected. Pulse oximetry measurement in both extremities may prove valuable before discharge if there is any question of left heart obstruction.
5. An echocardiogram and cardiac consultation are mandatory if a serious problem is clinically suspected.

II. RECOGNITION OF A CARDIAC PROBLEM: FIVE METHODS OF PRESENTATION
Cyanosis, heart failure/cardiovascular collapse, or arrhythmia are the usual urgent signs of cardiac disorder. Additionally, the infant may have a syndrome that includes a heart defect, or may present with an isolated murmur.

A. Cyanosis.

1. Causes and consequences: Central cyanosis is always a source of concern because it may be a sign of severe cardiac, respiratory, or neurologic compromise. Peripheral cyanosis (acrocyanosis) is a frequent benign finding in normal infants. Once clinical evaluation and a hyperoxia test have confirmed that cyanosis is from cardiac causes (i.e., the result of a fixed cardiac right-to-left shunt), urgent cardiac evaluation is needed. Profound cyanosis and hypoxia (e.g., an arterial PO_2 of 50 mmHg or less) can lead to acidosis and irreversible organ damage.

   a. Severe cyanosis and hypoxia:
      (1) Transposition (d-TGA).
      (2) Pulmonary atresia with the following:
         (a) Large ventricular septal defect (e.g., TOF) with outflow atresia.
         (b) Intact ventricular septum, hypoplastic right ventricle.
         (c) Tricuspid atresia.
         (d) Other, including Ebstein anomaly, single ventricle, or double outlet ventricle.

   b. Milder cyanosis (PO_2 80-90).
      (1) TOF with pulmonary stenosis but no atresia.
      (2) Admixture defects, including truncus arteriosus, single or double outlet ventricle, and total anomalous pulmonary venous return (TAPVR) with obstruction.

   The old mnemonic of the **6 Ts** can be helpful: **T**ransposition, **T**etralogy of Fallot, **T**ricuspid or pulmonary atresia with hypoplastic or single ventricle, **T**runcus arteriosus, **T**otal anomalous pulmonary venous return, and **T**ransitional circulation (also known as *persistent fetal circulation* [PFC] or *persistent pulmonary hypertension of the newborn* [PPHN]).

2. Diagnosis. Once central cyanosis is recognized, the likely cause must be rapidly determined. Although physical, radiographic, and ECG findings can provide leads to diagnosis, immediate echocardiography is essential. If transitional circulation is severe, inhaled nitric oxide, high-frequency ventilation, or extracorporeal membrane oxygenation (ECMO) may be needed. For the other five diagnoses, transfer to a tertiary cardiac center with facilities for neonatal cardiac surgery is urgent. For infants with the first three diagnoses (transposition, TOF, or hypoplastic right ventricle), especially when the PO_2 remains less than 100 mm Hg, prostaglandin E_1 infusion during transfer is usually recommended to keep the ductus patent and to maintain PO_2 above critical levels. Key echocardiographic findings include the following:

   a. In transposition, the posterior artery, arising from the left ventricle, is seen to bifurcate soon after it leaves the heart, showing that the pulmonary artery and not the aorta arises from the left ventricle.

   b. In TOF with extreme pulmonic stenosis, the aorta overrides a large ventricular septal defect and the pulmonary arteries are small.

   c. In tricuspid or pulmonary atresia, the right ventricle is small or hypoplastic and the pulmonary arteries are small. Doppler study will often show that flow to the lungs takes place entirely through the patent ductus, rather than from the right ventricle.

3. Treatment.
  a. Transposition: Arterial switch procedure is the treatment of choice, usually without prior cardiac catheterization. Some centers still perform a Rashkind atrial septostomy before arterial switch. The switch procedure is now almost universally preferred to atrial types of operation such as the Mustard procedure. In full-term infants without additional anomalies, a 1-year survival rate of 90% or greater is expected.
  b. Tetralogy: Primary open repair is performed, usually in the first 6 months of life. A 1-year survival rate of 90% or greater can be expected in full-term infants without other major defects. However, if there is outflow atresia or severely hypoplastic pulmonary arteries, an aortopulmonary shunt (Blalock-Taussig procedure or variant) may precede open repair. (The role of interventional cardiac catheterization in "rehabilitating" diminutive pulmonary arteries is being evaluated at a few large centers.) Outflow atresia, low birth weight, and major extracardiac defects are unfavorable risk factors.
  c. Tricuspid atresia with hypoplastic right ventricle: An arterial (Blalock-Taussig) shunt procedure is performed, sometimes with atrial septostomy. A Fontan operation (anastomosis of the systemic veins to the pulmonary artery) is necessary by around 2 years of age. An intermediate operation, known as a *bilateral Glenn procedure,* is now often done at around 6 months of age.
    (1) In a hypoplastic right ventricle resulting from pulmonary atresia with intact septum, a shunt is used to enlarge the right ventricle; several operations may be needed.
    (2) Interventional cardiac catheterization may supplement surgery.
  d. Total anomalous pulmonary venous return can usually be corrected in the newborn period using cardiopulmonary bypass and deep hypothermia. In small premature infants surgery may be delayed for a few weeks.
  e. Truncus arteriosus is repaired with patch closure of the ventricular septal defect and a homograft to join the right and left pulmonary arteries to the right ventricle. These infants need close monitoring after repair because many have hypocalcemia and other evidence of DiGeorge syndrome. Transfusion should be with irradiated blood because of probable immune deficiency.
  f. Transitional circulation may respond to inhaled nitric oxide and ventilatory and pressor support; ECMO is needed for severely affected infants.

B. Heart failure/cardiovascular collapse.

1. Causes and types: Persistent tachypnea, often associated with feeding difficulty, is the earliest and most important sign of impending heart failure in the neonate. Rarely, heart failure presents in the perinatal period, either in utero associated with fetal nonimmune hydrops, or immediately after delivery. Consider severe valvar insufficiency, arrhythmia, or a primary myocardial disorder if any of the following are present:
  a. Arteriovenous fistula (cerebral [vein of Galen], hepatic, other).

    b. Ebstein or other anomaly of the tricuspid valve.

    c. Tetralogy with absent pulmonary valve (pulmonary valvar insufficiency).

    d. Complex defects such as unbalanced atrioventricular canal with atrioventricular valve regurgitation.

    e. Myocardial disease, myocarditis, cardiomyopathy.

    f. Prolonged or recurrent arrhythmias, usually atrial tachycardia or flutter (occasionally after in utero cocaine exposure); rarely, bradyarrhythmia from complete heart block.

2. Depending on the degree of failure, diuretics and digitalization may be needed before any surgery. Prognosis is guarded because severe tricuspid regurgitation and cardiomegaly in utero may have led to pleural effusion and resulting lung hypoplasia. For critical myocardial disease, cardiac biopsy and emergency treatment with immunoglobulin may follow referral to a tertiary cardiac center.

3. Unlike infants with cyanosis or perinatal heart failure, these infants may appear normal at birth. However, if there is an obstructive defect involving the left side of the heart, normal systemic blood flow depends on persistent patency of the ductus arteriosus. As the duct closes, there is the sudden onset of poor perfusion, mottling, feeding difficulty, and metabolic acidosis. Onset may be a day or two after birth or later in the first month; murmurs may be faint or absent. Differential diagnosis includes sepsis and inherited metabolic disorders.

    a. Left heart flow defects with duct dependency.

       (1) Coarctation of the aorta (isolated or with an accompanying ventricular septal defect or complex defect [e.g., single ventricle]).

       (2) Interrupted aortic arch, usually with a large ventricular septal defect.

       (3) Aortic valve stenosis, critical.

       (4) Hypoplastic left heart syndrome (HLHS) with aortic or mitral valve atresia and hypoplastic left ventricle.

    b. Diagnosis: Clinical clues to diagnosis include tachypnea, right ventricular heave, pulse and blood pressure discrepancy between arm and leg on examination, cardiomegaly and pulmonary venous congestion on chest radiographs, and a high index of suspicion. Echocardiography and Doppler study can usually localize the site of obstruction, the size of the left ventricle, and any added defects.

    c. Treatment: Prostaglandin E_1 infusion, stabilization of acidosis, and early surgery. Prostaglandin infusion should be started at the first clinical suspicion of pending cardiovascular collapse while arrangements are being made for echocardiography and transfer to a tertiary cardiac center.

       (1) Coarctation repair has an excellent outcome; if late restenosis occurs, balloon angioplasty has replaced repeat surgery.

       (2) Interrupted aortic arch can usually be treated by primary repair, involving primary anastomosis of the separated ends of the aortic arch and patch closure of the ventricular defect. There is about a 20% chance of accompanying DiGeorge syn-

drome, with hypocalcemia and immune deficiency. The calcium level must be monitored, and blood products given should be irradiated. Restenosis of the area of arch repair is common and often responds to balloon angioplasty.

(3) Aortic valve stenosis is now treated by valve dilation. This can be done surgically by inserting a surgical dilator from the left ventricle or by catheter balloon valvuloplasty in the catheterization laboratory.

(4) Hypoplastic left heart syndrome was once uniformly fatal. There are now two surgical options. One is the Norwood procedure, which involves two or three staged operations in the first 3 years of life. The other is cardiac transplantation. Prostaglandin infusion and maintenance of normal perfusion and metabolism are carried out while the family is reviewing the options of surgery. (Compassionate care without surgery is still the choice of some families, but rapid improvements in surgical outcome now make this a rare option.)

d. Another cause of heart failure that develops after birth is left-to-right shunts, including a large ventricular septal defect (VSD), a persistent ductus arteriosus (PDA), and atrioventricular (AV) canal defects.

(1) Treatment: Reduce fluid intake to maintenance, induce diuresis, and plan for early surgery.

(2) PDA in a premature infant is the most common of these problems: in premature infants closure may be induced by indomethacin, but in term infants this is ineffective.

(3) For the other defects, primary open repair is the treatment of choice, but pulmonary artery banding is still occasionally done for large VSDs in the muscular part of the ventricular septum, in complex AV canal defects, or in low-birth-weight infants. Prognosis after primary open repair is good, with less than 10% mortality at 1 year after surgery.

C. Cardiac arrhythmias. Arrhythmias may occur in utero or in the neonatal period.

1. Premature contractions, whether atrial (PACs) or ventricular (PVCs), are usually benign variants.

2. Tachyarrhythmia.

a. Supraventricular tachycardia (SVT). Although the heart rate is labile in normal newborns, a rate above 230 beats per minute is virtually never the result of sinus tachycardia. SVT is usually re-entry in type; rarely, it can be the result of an ectopic atrial focus.

b. Atrial flutter.

c. Ventricular tachycardia (extremely rare).

3. Bradyarrhythmia: Apnea-bradycardia (a major problem in premature infants, rare in full-term infants); heart block, second or third degree.

4. Diagnosis: Arrhythmias are often detected on clinical examination or on monitoring, but a 12-lead ECG is needed for full evaluation. Because arrhythmias are of more concern if the heart is structurally abnormal, an echocardiogram is advisable. Holter monitoring may be

recommended for sustained arrhythmia, for persistent or multifocal PVCs, or when the nature of the arrhythmia is in doubt.

5. Treatment.

    a. Supraventricular tachycardia or atrial flutter can lead to heart failure within 24 hours of onset, occasionally even sooner.

        (1) Vagal maneuvers: A cold wet washcloth applied to the face will stimulate the "diving reflex" and is the first treatment. Continuous electrocardiographic monitoring should be done. After this or any other therapy, once the tachycardia is broken, a 12-lead ECG is needed to determine if Wolff- Parkinson-White (pre-excitation) syndrome is present.

        (2) Adenosine

        (3) Digitalization, beta blockers, or an esmolol drip are other medical methods of treatment; verapamil should not be used. Reentry tachycardias usually respond rapidly to vagal maneuvers or adenosine, but with an ectopic atrial focus more than one medication may be needed.

        (4) Electroconversion is the treatment of choice if the patient is unstable, or if there is evidence of heart failure or hypotension. Transesophageal pacing is an excellent alternative if equipment and expertise are available.

        (5) Cardiac consultation is needed for long-term management.

    b. Heart block in infants with heart defects is often poorly tolerated; cardiac pacing is almost invariably indicated. Infants with structurally normal hearts and complete heart block usually have a mother with lupus erythematosus or with Ro antibodies. Pacing is rarely needed unless the ventricular rate is below 50 beats per minute, or the infant is symptomatic.

D. Cardiac syndromes. Recent advances in molecular biology and genetics are revolutionizing our understanding of the interrelationship between heart defects, syndromes, and genetic disorders. In the Baltimore-Washington Infant Study (BWIS), in which all live-born infants with heart defects were registered over a 9-year period, over 25% were found to have extracardiac anomalies. The biologic basis of many of these associations is being rapidly clarified. In the newborn period the syndrome may be obvious and lead to immediate evaluation for a heart defect; Down syndrome is a good example because the incidence of heart defects is high (around 50%) and about two thirds of the defects are severe (complete AV cana), often without a significant murmur. By contrast, sometimes recognition of a heart defect such as interrupted aortic arch may lead to evaluation for hypocalcemia and to FISH studies because of the high likelihood of 22q11 microdeletions. Table 10-1 includes a few important syndromes and their related heart defects.

With improving fetal ultrasound and other studies, more syndromes are being identified in utero. Nevertheless, some young parents still encounter the tragic dilemma presented by a newborn with multiple handicaps and shortened life expectancy, as in trisomies 13 or 18. The primary

TABLE 10-1
Syndrome-Related Heart Defects

Syndrome	Heart defects
Trisomies	
Trisomy 21 (Down)	Complete AV canal; VSD; TOF; other
Trisomy 18	Polyvalvar thickening; VSD; TOF with pulmonary atresia
Trisomy 13	VSD, other
XO: Turner	Coarctation, other left heart defects
22q11 microdeletions	TOF (severe forms) with pulmonary atresia, absent pulmonary valve
DiGeorge, velocardiofacial, CHARGE, other	Right aortic arch; interrupted aortic arch; truncus arteriosus; other, including VSD, TOF
VACTERL	VSD, TOF, coarctation, other
Ivemark/heterotaxy	
Asplenia	Complete AV canal with d-TGA and pulmonary atresia; TAPVR obstructed
Polysplenia	VSD with pulmonary stenosis; interrupted IVC, partial anomalous pulmonary venous return
Noonan	Pulmonary valve stenosis with dysplasia; hypertrophic cardiomyopathy
Marfan	Dilated ascending aorta, pulmonary artery; mitral regurgitation
Williams	Supravalvar aortic/pulmonary stenosis

physician can help the family and others on the health care team discuss and resolve the ethical issues involved.

E. Cardiac murmurs without symptoms.

1. Murmurs getting fainter from birth until 1 week of age usually are due to transient tricuspid regurgitation, to a closing patent ductus arteriosus, or to peripheral pulmonic stenosis (frequent in premature infants).
2. Causes of murmurs that persist for several days or appear soon after birth include the following:
   a. Ventricular septal defect.
   b. Tetralogy of Fallot.
   c. Aortic stenosis.
   d. Pulmonary stenosis, valvar or peripheral.
   e. Atrioventricular canal defects.
   f. Patent ductus arteriosus.

Every infant with a "cardiac murmur without symptoms" should be carefully checked for signs of cardiovascular compromise or cyanosis. In a newborn with TOF, clinical cyanosis may be present only on crying; even an infant with transposition and a large VSD may appear only minimally cyanotic, particularly if anemia or dark pigmentation of the skin make evaluation more difficult. Pulse oximetry and a hyperoxia test will resolve doubts and should be used frequently now that discharge is occurring very early.

3. Although cardiac murmurs are less specific in the newborn than in childhood, their location and timing are similar.

   a. In general, a loud murmur heard at birth and that persists more likely indicates outflow stenosis (pulmonary or aortic valve stenosis or infundibular stenosis in TOF) than a small VSD.

   b. An ejection murmur, beginning after the first heart sound, indicates outflow stenosis. If it is loudest at the lower left sternal border, the primary care physician should suspect TOF with infundibular stenosis. If the murmur is maximal in the pulmonary area and radiating to the lung fields, pulmonary stenosis should be considered. If there is an ejection click, valvar stenosis is possible; no click could indicate peripheral stenosis. The murmur of aortic stenosis is accompanied by a click and radiates to the neck.

   c. An echocardiogram is always indicated if outflow stenosis is suspected. The only exception is a soft murmur that radiates to the lung fields, compatible with mild peripheral pulmonary stenosis.

4. Small ventricular septal defect.

   a. The murmur is usually not heard in the first few hours after birth; it is localized to the lower left sternal border and often stops before the second heart sound. The signs and symptoms listed previously are absent.

   b. Because of the high rate of spontaneous closure of such defects (40% in the first year of life) neonatal cardiac evaluation and echocardiography are not always needed.

5. Other murmurs.

   a. The murmur of patent ductus is heard best in the pulmonary area and peaks at the second heart sound; it is often abbreviated, not truly "continuous."

   b. Complete AV canal may have confusing murmurs, but the diagnosis can be suspected in an infant with tachypnea, a right ventricular heave, and an apical murmur. All such infants require cardiac evaluation, particularly those with Down's syndrome.

   c. A soft pulmonary ejection murmur may also indicate an atrial septal defect (ASD) or left-to-right shunt through a PFO. An echocardiogram is rarely indicated. If a high-caliber study is done, an accurate prognosis of the likelihood of early spontaneous closure can be given.

III. GOING HOME

A. Five Clinical Pearls to Rule Out Significant Heart Disease.

There are a few cardiac problems, such as ASD or hypertrophic cardiomyopathy, that can be detected only rarely in the neonate, and in which later diagnosis and surgical repair in childhood carries no risk to the infant. However, an occasional newborn is discharged from the hospital with a "normal" cardiovascular examination, only to return a few days later with obvious cyanosis or heart failure with cardiovascular collapse. The five points below are illustrated in Fig. 10-1 and are helpful on discharge physical or on the first well-baby follow-up examination to exclude any ductus-dependent or other critical heart defect needing treatment in infancy.

1. Precordial impulse: The RV impulse is markedly accentuated in almost all critical heart defects.
2. Second heart sound: If loud, single, or readily palpable, a second heart sound may indicate elevated pulmonary artery pressure. This is normal immediately after birth, but not by 48 hours or later, when the pulmonary vascular resistance has fallen.
3. Cyanosis, perfusion: The examiner should check again for central cyanosis, cyanosis on crying, or inadequate perfusion. Pulse oximetry above and below the ductus (right arm and leg) may be useful when in doubt.

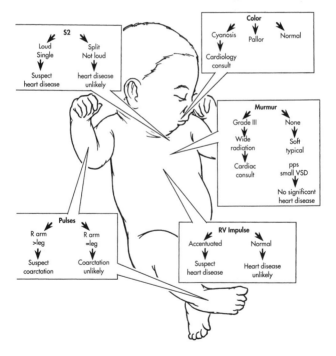

FIG. 10-1. Going home: Cardiac clues on discharge physical or first well-baby visit.

4. Upper and lower extremity pulses: The examiner should check again for coarctation, with diminished pulsatile flow and pressure in legs.
5. Murmur: The examiner should analyze for atypical qualities. If a murmur is not characteristic of peripheral pulmonic stenosis, small VSD, or other benign murmurs of early infancy, further evaluation should be done.

In conclusion, the primary care provider plays a pivotal role in the care of infants with heart problems, just as he or she does in those born with normal hearts. This role includes early diagnosis, optimal referral, and acting as ombudsman in coordination of long-term care.

BIBLIOGRAPHY

Ferencz C, Rubin JD, Lofredo CA, Magee CA: *Epidemiology of congenital heart disease: the Baltimore-Washington Infant Study, 1981-1989,* Mount Kisco, NY, 1993, Futura.

Flanagan MF, Yeager SB, Weindling SN: Cardiac disease. In Avery GB, Fletcher MA, MacDonald MG (editors): *Neonatology: pathophysiology and management of the newborn,* Philadelphia, 1999, Lippincott, Williams and Wilkins.

Fost N: Bioethics of the mother, fetus and newborn. In Fanaroff AA, Martin RJ (editors): *Neonatal-perinatal medicine,* ed 6, St. Louis, 1997, Mosby.

Gillette PC, Garson A: *Pediatric cardiac arrhythmias,* Philadelphia, 1999, WB Saunders.

Payne RM, Johnson MC, Grant JW, Strauss AW: Toward a molecular understanding of congenital heart disease (Review), *Circulation* 91:494-504, 1995.

Snider AR, Serwer GA, Ritter SB: *Echocardiography in pediatric heart disease,* ed 2, St. Louis, 1997, Mosby.

11

Pulmonary System

SIEW-JYU WONG

Fetal breathing movements can be observed by about 11 weeks of gestation. Movements increase with gestational age but diminish sharply within 3 days of labor. These movements can be stimulated by smoking and hypercapnia and depressed by hypoxia and barbiturates. Lung liquid is reabsorbed to some extent during labor. The first breath is taken about 9 seconds after delivery. Once the first breath is taken and the lungs inflate, there is a major stimulus to the release of lung surfactant into the alveolar space.

I. APNEA: CESSATION OF AIR EXCHANGE
A. Types.
1. Central apnea: No respiratory effort for 15 seconds; may be associated with hypoxemia and bradycardia.
2. Obstructive apnea: Resulting from airway obstruction; may be positional, functional (caused by poor tone of pharyngeal dilator [e.g., in prematurity], reflex spasms [e.g., in reaction to regurgitation of milk], or incoordination of pharyngeal muscles during feeding), or structural (see Chapter 8).
3. Mixed apnea: A combination of central and obstructive types.
B. Causes.
1. At delivery (see Chapter 4).
2. In the nursery, causes for central and mixed apnea include the following:
   a. Maternal drugs (e.g., sedatives, analgesics, magnesium).
   b. Metabolic imbalance (e.g., hypoglycemia, acidosis, alkalosis, hyperammonemia, electrolyte imbalance).
   c. Infection (e.g., sepsis, meningitis, necrotizing enterocolitis [NEC]).
   d. Temperature instability.
   e. Hematologic disorders (e.g., anemia or polycythemia).
   f. Seizures, especially if apnea is accompanied by tachycardia rather than bradycardia.
   g. Hypoxia: In premature and small for gestational age (SGA) infants with delayed autonomic system maturation, hypoxia triggers hypopneic response rather than hyperpneic response.

   h. Cardiovascular system (CVS) disorders (e.g., shock, patent ductus arteriosus [PDA]), with decreased blood flow to central nervous system (CNS).
   i. CNS disorders (e.g., immature CNS), congenital malformations of the CNS, chromosomal anomalies such as trisomies 13 or 18, intracranial hemorrhage, or intraventricular hemorrhage.
   j. Gastrointestinal disorders (e.g., gastroesophageal reflux and swallowing difficulties).

C. Diagnosis and management.

1. History: An obstetric history should be taken to look for risk factors that could affect the pulmonary system, such as a difficult delivery, maternal fever or chorioamnionitis, drug abuse, drugs administered to the mother before and (if breast-feeding) after birth, resuscitation of the infant needed at birth, or a low Apgar score. Umbilical cord pH levels, gestational age, and events associated with apnea (e.g., drastic temperature changes, feeding, seizure activity) should also be noted.

2. Physical examination: During the physical examination, the practitioner should note the infant's temperature and the presence of either fever or hypothermia. He or she should also note the presence of dysmorphic features and malformation, skin color and perfusion, blood pressure, irritability or lethargy, tone and activity, the state of the anterior fontanel, the presence (if any) of milk in nasal and nasopharyngeal passages, the quality of respiratory effort, and the presence of any murmur, petechiae, or hepatosplenomegaly. Gestational age should also be noted.

3. Laboratory evaluation (if the cause is not obvious) should be considered to assess the following: glucose and electrolyte (Ca^{++}, Mg^{++} pH, NH_3) levels, complete blood cell count (CBC) and differential, blood gases, gastric pH levels, and the possibility of sepsis. Other studies may be indicated, such as chest radiographs, a spinal tap, ultrasound of the head, electroencephalogram, or a pneumogram with an esophageal pH probe.

N.B.: Subarachnoid hemorrhage is not uncommon; if no cause is found, computed tomography (CT) of the head should be considered to rule out this condition because ultrasound will not detect it.

II. RESPIRATORY DISTRESS

Respiratory distress is indicated by the following signs, either singly or in combination: cyanosis, tachypnea, retractions, grunting, and nasal flaring. It may initially be related to nonrespiratory events.

A. Causes of respiratory distress.

1. Sepsis.
2. Hematologic (polycythemia).
3. Cardiac (cyanotic and noncyanotic heart disease).
4. Shock.
5. Metabolic (acidosis, hypoglycemia, hyperammonemia).
6. Respiratory.

B. Respiratory-related causes.

1. Airway problems: At times prenatal ultrasound might detect potential airway problems such as tumors, vascular malformations, and encephaloceles in or around the nose, mouth, pharynx, or neck that cause airway obstruction. Certain congenital syndromes with craniofacial anomalies are associated with airway problems. Examples of lesions that may cause airway problems include the following:

   a. Nasal obstruction: Choanal atresia/stenosis, atresia seen in CHARGE association.

   b. Pharyngeal obstruction (e.g., glossoptosis with micrognathia and central cleft palate in Pierre Robin sequence [NOTE: Laryngeal mask airway (LMA) is helpful in managing this]). Pharyngeal masses such as encephaloceles and polyps may also cause obstruction.

   c. Vocal cord disorders: These may be functional, as seen in Arnold-Chiari malformation, or structural, as in laryngomalacia or a laryngeal web.

   d. Subglottic lesions: Laryngotracheal edema may be caused by intubation related to the presence of meconium, or hemangiomas, tracheomalacia, stenosis, or atresia.

   e. Paratracheal lesions (e.g., goiter, superior mediastinal masses, cystic hygromas, or vascular ring). Esophageal atresia with or without tracheoesophageal fistula (TEF) may cause aspiration into the lungs.

2. Poor respiratory muscle effort.

   a. Diaphragmatic paralysis.

      (1) Diaphragmatic paralysis may result from phrenic nerve injury and is usually associated with difficult delivery, shoulder dystocia, brachial plexus injury, and clavicular fracture, singly or together.

      (2) Chest radiographs may show unilateral elevation of the paralyzed hemidiaphragm.

      (3) Ultrasound may show absence of movement or paradoxic movement of the paralyzed leaf.

      (4) Other causes include phrenic nerve compression by tumors such as neuroblastoma, and iatrogenic injury during insertion of chest tubes.

   b. Myopathies, muscular dystrophies, and myasthenia.

3. Parenchymal causes.

   a. Transient tachypnea of the newborn (TTN).

      (1) TTN is a diagnosis of exclusion. There is an increased incidence of TTN in cesarean section deliveries (especially if they are not preceded by labor and are before 39 completed weeks of gestation), in infants who are male, in macrosomic infants, and in infants whose mothers have asthma.

      (2) TTN usually involves tachypnea with minimal evidence of respiratory distress, with or without O_2 requirement.

      (3) Chest radiographs show fluid in fissures (sometimes minimal), pleural effusion, and streaky parenchymal changes with hyperinflation.

    (4) O$_2$ needs are short term; tachypnea may last longer. Follow-up chest radiographs show rapid clearing of fluid, usually within 24 hours. TTN might be complicated by pulmonary hypertension.

  b. Respiratory distress syndrome (RDS).

    (1) RDS occurs characteristically in preterm infants and is related to surfactant deficiency. There is an increased risk of RDS with decreasing gestational age, maternal diabetes, white male infants, acute asphyxia, second twin, and family history of RDS. PDA complicates recovery from RDS. In older gestational age infants, pulmonary hypertension might complicate management. RDS might occur in "term infants." If the infant is not following a typical course with response to surfactant and with improvement over time, certain cardiac lesions such as total anomalous pulmonary venous return [TAPVR] should be considered, and genetic surfactant protein-B deficiency should be considered.

    (2) Prevention of RDS is primary. Early prenatal care allows identification of an at-risk woman and education for all pregnant women to get them to be sensitive to the possibility of premature labor. This allows early detection of labor, improves the effectiveness of tocolysis, and permits the use of betamethasone to hasten lung maturity. Prenatal betamethasone also has been shown to decrease intraventricular hemorrhage [IVH] and periventricular leukomalacia [PVL] in very-low-birth-weight (VLBW) infants. However, multiple (i.e., more than two) courses of prenatal steroids might be deleterious.

    (3) Prompt and appropriate resuscitation at delivery decreases asphyxia-related surfactant destruction.

    (4) Shortly after birth, the preterm infant with RDS will start to show signs of respiratory distress, with tachypnea, retractions, grunting, and cyanosis. Chest radiographs in mild cases may show minimal underexpansion, progressing in 24 to 48 hours to the typical ground-glass reticulogranular appearance with air bronchogram. In moderate cases, RDS may start out with typical reticulogranular appearance with air bronchogram; in severe cases there is blurring of heart, diaphragm, and rib-cage borders because of marked atelectasis ("total whiteout").

    (5) Management includes the following:

      (a) Respiratory support in the form of early institution of nasal continuous positive airway pressure [NCPAP] might avoid the need for intubation and assisted ventilation, especially in the bigger infants.

      (b) Infection and pneumonia should be ruled out; antibiotics should be used as needed; other immature organ systems should be supported.

      (c) Exogenous surfactant should be administered to infants with RDS who require endotracheal intubation for mechanical ventilatory support. Exogenous surfactant used prophylactically in very small infants at delivery has been shown to decrease the severity of RDS in the short term.

The availability of exogenous surfactant is associated with decreased national neonatal and infant mortality.

(d) Persistent pulmonary hypertension of the newborn (PPHN) is a complication of RDS, especially in infants of older gestational age.

(e) Acute complications of barotrauma, such as pulmonary interstitial emphysema [PIE], pneumothoraces, and pneumopericardium, are constantly considered with any deterioration.

(f) Pneumonias such as those caused by group B streptococcus and ureaplasma urealyticum should be considered when there is early appearance of PIE.

(6) Adult respiratory distress syndrome (ARDS) has been described in full-term infants and is characterized by shock, asphyxia, and aspiration.

c. Meconium aspiration syndrome (MAS).

(1) The incidence of meconium-stained amniotic fluid depends on infant maturity; it is rare at <37 weeks. An associated risk of asphyxia mandates the presence of skilled personnel at delivery.

(2) Management should be preventive. At delivery of the head at the perineum or at the uterine incision in cesarean section, the obstetrician should clear the infant's airway by DeLee suctioning. If thick and particulate meconium is present, the infant should receive tracheal suctioning.

(3) MAS can occur in utero. With severe stress the fetus may pass meconium; deep fetal gasping causes the aspiration of meconium-mixed amniotic fluid into the lungs.

(4) Diagnosis is by history, the presence of respiratory distress, and subsequent chest radiograph.

(5) Management of MAS is complex, involving management for asphyxia-related effects on the CNS, CVS, and renal and gastrointestinal systems, and pulmonary support. Particular attention is needed to avoid further stress (e.g., hypoxia, hypercapnia, cold stress, hypoglycemia, noise, discomfort, and metabolic imbalance) to avoid or prevent worsening of PPHN. Pneumomediastinum and pneumothorax are common; antibiotics are usually given. High-frequency ventilation without or with nitric oxide [NO], or extracorporeal membrane oxygenation (ECMO) may be lifesaving.

d. Pneumonia.

(1) Risk factors for pneumonia include premature labor, premature rupture of membranes, prolonged rupture of membranes, maternal chorioamnionitis, maternal fever, asphyxia, difficult delivery, and tracheoesophageal fistula.

(2) Onset is usually early, with signs of respiratory distress, apnea, hypotension, shock, and secondary PPHN.

(3) Chest radiographs may show patchy or streaky infiltrates, but findings may be indistinguishable from those of RDS. Hence

in infants with RDS, pneumonia should be ruled out if antibiotics are not given.

(4) Workup includes cultures of blood, tracheal aspirate, urine, and cerebrospinal fluid (CSF); lumbar puncture (LP) should be postponed if infant is unstable; CSF and urine can be sent for rapid antigen detection.

(5) Mortality remains high. Ampicillin and gentamicin remain the drugs of choice to cover group B streptococci, *Haemophilus, Pneumococcus, Listeria, Escherichia coli,* and other gram-negative organisms. The Centers for Disease Control and Prevention (CDC), American College of Obstetricians and Gynecologists (ACOG), and the American Academy of Pediatrics (AAP) have established guidelines for intrapartum antibiotic prophylaxis.

(6) Congenital syphilis should be considered, especially in at-risk situations.

(7) Septic shock, PPHN, leukopenia, thrombocytopenia, and disseminated intravascular coagulation (DIC) complicate management. Intravenous immunoglobulin (IVIG), monoclonal antibodies, white blood cell (WBC) transfusion, and granulocyte-colony stimulating factor (G-CSF) have been used. High-frequency ventilation, without or with NO, and ECMO may be helpful when conventional ventilation fails.

e. PPHN could be primary or secondary. Secondary PPHN is defined as PPHN associated with parenchymal problems as mentioned above, cardiac lesions, or hypoplastic lungs. Hypoplastic lungs can occur with constraints on lung development during the critical period (<28 weeks gestation), such as oligohydramnios caused by prolonged, premature, or very preterm rupture of membranes, or poor renal function; intrathoracic, large, space-occupying lesions in early gestation, such as congenital diaphragmatic hernia (CDH), pleural effusions, and congenital cysts. In primary PPHN, there is no pulmonary cause. In the prenatal and intrapartum history there might be suggestions of fetal hypoxemia, distress, or conditions causing premature closure of the PDA, such as indomethacin use. An echocardiogram will provide definitive diagnosis and rule out congenital cardiac lesions as the cause of the cyanosis, although preductal and postductal O_2 saturation and PAO_2 will be of some help. PPHN could be fatal. The goal is to relax the pulmonary vasculature, keep the infant well oxygenated, avoid handling and stimulation, provide sedation and analgesia, give sodium bicarbonate to keep base deficit to zero, and provide pressure support as needed to keep systemic blood pressure higher than pulmonary pressure without causing systemic hypertension. Various pharmaceutical pulmonary vasodilators, such as tolazoline, magnesium, and prostaglandins, have been tried. In most cases, assisted ventilation is needed; in severe cases, high-frequency ventilation, without or with NO, is necessary, and, finally, ECMO is used to tide the infant over the critical period. Infants born at very high altitudes who are not genetically adapted might develop pulmonary hypertension after the first few days of life.

4. Space-occupying lesions.
   a. Diaphragmatic hernia (DH).
      (1) When DH is diagnosed by prenatal ultrasound, the mother should be transferred for delivery to a tertiary center with pediatric surgery capabilities. However, not all cases are anticipated prenatally.
      (2) DH is one of the causes of unanticipated newborn resuscitation in a supposedly low-risk pregnancy (and hence a reason for immediate availability of trained, skilled personnel in all hospitals with delivery services).
      (3) After uneventful labor and delivery, the infant may deteriorate rapidly after the first gasp; DH should be suspected when an appropriate or large-for-gestational-age newborn whose delivery is not frank breech has a scaphoid abdomen and develops acute respiratory distress.
      (4) These infants should be given only endotracheal intermittent positive pressure breathing (IPPB) because ventilation by face mask will distend the herniated gastrointestinal contents and worsen the respiratory status.
      (5) Pneumothoraces are common because of bilateral hypoplastic lungs. Thoracentesis may be needed in the delivery room.
      (6) Accompanying PPHN complicates management. High-frequency ventilation, with or without NO, or ECMO may help.
      (7) DH is sometimes associated with trisomies 13 or 18 and Rubinstein-Tabyi syndrome.
      (8) Surgery is definitive treatment.
   b. Pneumothorax and pneumomediastinum.
      (1) Spontaneous pneumothorax occurs in 1% to 2% of live births. Spontaneous symptomatic pneumothorax, however, occurs in 1:1500 live births and may be associated with single umbilical artery and renal malformations. Symptomatic infants are noted to be tachypneic, with minimal retractions, grunting, and nasal flaring. They may be cyanotic in room air. On auscultation, there is diminished air entry on the affected side, muffled heart sounds, and shifting of the cardiac impulse. Transillumination may not be positive in a full-size newborn. A chest radiograph is diagnostic. Treatment is supportive, with spontaneous resolution. Thoracentesis is indicated only in cases of tension pneumothorax.
      (2) Most pneumothoraces are not spontaneous and are associated with iatrogenic hyperinflation during newborn resuscitation, or with RDS, MAS, or hypoplastic lungs. Thoracentesis and thoracostomy are frequently needed in those with severe and persistent respiratory distress.
   c. Chylothorax, pleural effusion (e.g., in fetal hydrops).

    d. Other causes: Tumors, enteric or bronchial cysts, cystic adenomatoid malformation of the lungs, or congenital lobar emphysema.

III. ABNORMALITIES IN GAS EXCHANGE

Gas exchange in the alveolar-capillary unit depends on ventilation, membrane thickness and area, perfusion, ventilation-perfusion mismatch, venous gas tension, and inspired gas tension.

A. Ventilation. Ventilation is the movement of gas by convection, bulk flow, and molecular diffusion through the conducting airways into the alveoli, where gas exchange takes place, resulting in the elimination of CO_2 and the uptake of O_2 into the pulmonary capillary blood.

B. Minute ventilation = (Tidal volume − Physiologic dead space) × Respiratory rate.

1. Hypoventilation: Inadequate gas exchange leading to increased PA_{CO_2} and end-tidal P_{CO_2}.
   a. Causes.
      (1) Poor respiratory effort caused by central depression, phrenic nerve injury, or respiratory muscle weakness in myopathies, myasthenia, dystrophies, or fatigue.
      (2) Airway obstruction (see Chapter 8).
      (3) Restrictive causes from within (e.g., RDS, pulmonary interstitial emphysema (PIE), hypoplastic lungs, or pneumonia) or from without (e.g., pneumothorax, tumors, or pleural effusion).
   b. Effects: Moderate increase in P_{CO_2} increases respiratory drive, with increase in respiratory rate and depth, heart rate, stroke volume, cardiac output, systolic blood pressure, pulse pressure with systemic vasodilation, and intrapulmonary vasoconstriction. Worsens PPHN.
   c. Acute rise of P_{CO_2} causes CO_2 narcosis, respiratory depression, decreased myocardial contractility, hypotension, and shock.
2. Hyperventilation: Excessive ventilation resulting in hypocapnia and decreased end-tidal P_{CO_2}.
   a. Causes.
      (1) Compensatory for metabolic acidosis.
      (2) Response to mild-to-moderate hypoxemia.
      (3) Local limited atelectasis stimulating stretch receptors.
      (4) Iatrogenic.
   b. Effects: Marked hypocapnia with alkalosis decreases ionized calcium and potassium, increases nerve and muscle excitability, decreases cerebral blood flow, and shifts the oxygen hemoglobin dissociation curve to the left with decreased O_2 release at tissue level. Systemic vasoconstriction and decreased tissue perfusion coupled with decreased O_2 release may result in tissue hypoxia. Cerebral vasoconstriction might contribute to the development of periventricular leukomalacia [PVL] in the susceptible preterm infant.

C. Membrane thickness and area. Increased membrane thickness and decreased area retard the rate of gas exchange. Causes include the following:

1. Fluid in alveolar and interstitial space (seen in retained lung fluid), inflammation, or congestive heart failure.
2. Air, as in interstitial emphysema.
3. Hypoplastic lungs and atelectatic lungs with decreased area for gas exchange.

D. Perfusion. Reduced pulmonary capillary blood flow is seen in PPHN (either primarily or associated with various pulmonary disorders), polycythemia with its attendant hyperviscosity, and certain cyanotic congenital heart diseases (e.g., severe pulmonic stenosis, pulmonary atresia, and Tetralogy of Fallot [TOF]). In both cases, the right-to-left shunt through the PDA and patent foramen into the systemic circulation decreases the O_2 saturation. After tissue extraction, the O_2 saturation in the mixed venous return is even lower, and when this blood is returned to the lungs the severe hypoxemia causes further pulmonary vasoconstriction, thereby setting off a vicious cycle of increased pulmonary vascular resistance, decreased pulmonary flow, increasing shunt, and increased systemic hypoxemia, which increases pulmonary vascular resistance.

E. Ventilation-perfusion (V/Q) mismatch. Wasted perfusion occurs in atelectatic alveoli, causing low V/Q. Wasted ventilation occurs in overventilated alveoli, causing high V/Q.

F. Venous gas tension. In cyanotic states, shock, and severe anemia, the mixed venous Po_2 may be extremely low. This blood is then returned to the alveolar-capillary unit. With equilibration after gas exchange, the resulting Po_2 may still be low. It is therefore important to recognize the presence of these factors and rectify if possible. Causes of poor tissue perfusion with resulting increased tissue extraction and low venous Po_2 include the following:

1. Hypovolemia: Hypovolemia can be caused by massive fetomaternal transfusion, twin-to-twin transfusion, fetoplacental transfusion with cord compression, placental abruption, placenta previa, vasa previa, incision into the anterior placenta at cesarean section, position of newborn at delivery and timing of cord clamping, massive internal hemorrhage (e.g., hepatic, intracranial, adrenal, subaponeurotic).
2. Cardiogenic shock: Causes of cardiogenic shock include myocardial depression in severe asphyxia and some congenital heart disease (e.g., hypoplastic heart, cardiac arrhythmia, myocarditis, and myopathies).
3. Sepsis.

IV. INDICATIONS FOR CARDIORESPIRATORY MONITORING

A. <35 completed weeks of gestation.
B. Infants with observed episodes or history of episodes of apnea, tachypnea, bradycardia, or tachycardia.
C. Infants receiving O_2.
D. Infants with a history of sudden infant death syndrome in siblings.

BIBLIOGRAPHY

Centers for Disease Control and Prevention: Prevention of perinatal group B streptococcal disease: a public health perspective, *MMWR* 45[RR-7]:1-24, 1996.

Donn SM, Faix RG: *Neonatal emergencies,* New York, 1991, Futura.

Goldsmith JP, Karotkin EH: *Assisted ventilation of the neonate,* ed 3, Philadelphia, 1996,
WB Saunders.

Goldsmith JP, Spitzer AR: Controversies in neonatal pulmonary care, *Clin Perinatol*
25(1):1-248, 1998.

Jain L, Keenan W: Resuscitation of the fetus and newborn, *Clin Perinatol* 26(3):549-
792, 1999.

Thibeault DW, Gregory GA: *Neonatal pulmonary care,* ed 2, Norwalk, Conn, 1986,
Appleton-Century-Crofts.

12

Gastroenterology

Jose M. Saavedra

I. GASTROINTESTINAL (GI) DISTURBANCES
A. Vomiting/regurgitation.
1. General comments.
   a. *Vomiting* is the forceful expulsion of GI contents. It is an integrated reflex response involving contraction of the respiratory, abdominal, and GI muscles. *Regurgitation* is a more passive, effortless phenomenon, most likely representing the ultimate degree of gastroesophageal (GE) reflux. The differentiation is not always obvious.
   b. Regurgitation of the first few feedings in a newborn is common.
   c. 80% of infants under 3 months of age regurgitate formula at least once a day.
2. Persistent regurgitation without other signs or symptoms usually represents "uncomplicated" GE reflux (see GE reflux, p. 126).
   a. Hematemesis may represent a benign or serious conditions (see GI bleeding, p. 121).
   b. Bilious vomiting often indicates obstruction and a potential surgical emergency.
3. Etiology of vomiting.
   a. Usually not bilious.
      (1) Overfeeding.
      (2) Milk/formula protein sensitivity.
      (3) Sepsis, urinary tract infection, meningitis.
      (4) Necrotizing enterocolitis (NEC).
      (5) Central nervous system (CNS) lesion.
      (6) Pyloric stenosis.
      (7) Metabolic abnormalities (hypercalcemia, galactosemia, aminoacidopathies).
      (8) Electrolyte imbalance.
      (9) Drugs (digoxin, anticonvulsants).
      (10) Hirschsprung disease.
      (11) Lactobezoars.
   b. Usually bilious.
      (1) Congenital anomalies such as malrotation (with or without volvulus).

        (2) Atresia.
        (3) Stenosis.
        (4) Webs.
        (5) Aberrant superior mesenteric artery (SMA).
        (6) Annular pancreas.
        (7) Preduodenal portal vein.
        (8) Persistent omphalomesenteric duct (see Intestinal obstruction, p. 124).
        (9) Intestinal dysmotility (pseudoobstruction).
        (10) Visceral myopathies.

4. Diagnosis and management.
   a. Review feeding and medication history, look for signs of infection, obtain serum electrolytes.
   b. Plain-film abdominal radiograph with upright or cross-table lateral view (looking for specific pattern of obstruction or free air).
   c. Gentle passage of gastric tube for decompression if GI obstruction is suspected.
   d. Bilious vomiting and hematemesis should prompt surgical consultation.
   e. Upper GI series to rule out obstruction and anomalies and evaluate GI motility (usually unnecessary if complete obstruction is suspected). Abdominal ultrasound if pyloric stenosis is suspected.
   f. Neurologic evaluation and CNS imaging (looking for CNS congenital anomalies, malformation).

B. Diarrhea.

1. General comments.
   a. Stool frequency among breast-fed infants can range from once every several days to 12 times per day. Frequency in formula-fed infants fluctuates less and is usually between one and seven stools per day.
   b. Stool output of >10 g/kg per day suggests diarrhea, although this is not necessarily a practical definition.
   c. Changes in daily stool volume may be more helpful to diagnosis and are usually not subtle if the etiology is infectious.
   d. Stools of breast-fed infants can normally be loose and acidic and contain reducing sugars.

2. Etiology of diarrhea.
   a. GI infections in order of frequency: viral, enteropathogenic *Escherichia coli* (EPEC), *Salmonella, Pseudomonas, Klebsiella, Enterobacter, Proteus, Staphylococcus aureus, Campylobacter fetus,* and *Shigella.* Viral infections in infants under 2 months of age are usually asymptomatic. After 3 months of age, rotavirus becomes the most common infectious cause of diarrhea in infants.
   b. Sepsis.
   c. Overfeeding.
   d. Antibiotics.
   e. Milk protein allergy.
   f. NEC.

g. Malabsorption syndromes: These can be postinfectious in nature, or can be caused by cystic fibrosis, human immunodeficiency virus (HIV), or other congenital malabsorptive conditions (rare: Shwachman syndrome, congenital lactase deficiency, microvillus inclusion disease, glucose-galactose malabsorption, congenital sucrase-isomaltase deficiency).

h. Cholestasis (biliary atresia, Alagille syndrome).

i. Familial chloridorrhea.

j. Bowel resection (short bowel syndrome, blind loop syndrome).

k. Hirschsprung disease (enterocolitis).

l. Intestinal obstruction (diarrhea may be an initial symptom).

m. Metabolic: Galactosemia, tyrosinemia, enterokinase deficiency.

n. Maternal ulcerative colitis.

3. Diagnosis and management.

a. Review family, feeding, and medication history. Assess hydration status and treat fluid and electrolyte imbalances. Obtain stool specimen for culture and assessment of leukocytes and blood; assess serum for electrolyte levels and liver profile.

b. Obtain abdominal radiographs to assess gas distribution pattern and to seek evidence of obstruction, free air, or intestinal pneumatosis.

c. In a "sick-looking" infant, blood culture and systemic antibiotics (ampicillin and gentamicin) may be necessary if etiology appears infectious or NEC is suspected.

d. If diarrhea persists more than 2 weeks (chronic), investigate for malabsorption of carbohydrate (stool pH <5.5, reducing sugars present) or fat (72-hour stool collection). Consider use of lactose-free or medium-chain triglyceride–containing formula. Pancreatic function tests, stool electrolyte levels, intestinal biopsy (for inflammatory, infectious, or malabsorptive conditions), or rectal suction biopsy (for Hirschsprung's disease) may be necessary for definitive diagnosis.

C. Bleeding.

1. General comments.

a. Hematemesis usually indicates bleeding above the ligament of Treitz.

b. Grossly bloody stools usually indicate lower GI bleeding.

c. Swallowed maternal blood during delivery or breast-feeding can explain up to 30% of neonatal "GI bleeding."

2. Etiology of bleeding.

a. Most common causes of upper GI bleeding.

(1) Disseminated intravascular coagulation (DIC) after infection, shock, anoxia, etc.

(2) Gastritis and gastroduodenal ulcers after severe perinatal stress or sepsis.

(3) Pyloric stenosis.

(4) Hemorrhagic disease of the newborn.

(5) Coagulopathy (hemophilia rarely causes bleeding in newborns).

b. Most common causes of lower GI bleeding.

      (1) Anal fissures (most common cause of hematochezia in apparently well infants).

      (2) NEC (most frequent cause of GI bleeding in premature infants).

      (3) Acute enterocolitis (infectious: *Salmonella, Shigella,* EPEC, *Clostridium difficile*).

      (4) Volvulus.

      (5) Intussusception.

      (6) Meckel's diverticulum.

      (7) Hirschsprung disease (enterocolitis).

      (8) GI duplications.

      (9) Milk/formula protein sensitivity.

      (10) Polyps, hemangiomas (rare).

      (11) Rectal injury (e.g., from thermometer).

3. Diagnosis and management.

   a. Hemoccult testing of vomitus or stool will confirm presence of blood.

   b. The Apt test will differentiate maternal from infant's blood. Examine mother's nipples; pumping of breast may be helpful.

   c. Passage of nasogastric or orogastric tube and gastric lavage with saline may confirm upper GI bleeding. Never use cold saline.

   d. Check to see if vitamin K was given. Check for petechiae and other bleeding sites.

   e. Perform meticulous examination of the anal canal for anal fissures.

   f. Obtain stool sample for culture and to examine for leukocytes and *C. difficile* toxin.

   g. Obtain abdominal radiographs for evidence of obstruction, intestinal pneumatosis; upper GI series for evidence of obstruction, and congenital anomalies; obtain ultrasound examination if pyloric stenosis is suspected.

   h. Blood transfusion may be necessary. Supportive care and management of underlying condition are required.

   i. Antacids and H_2 blockers may be useful in suspected or confirmed gastritis or ulcers.

   j. Upper or lower GI endoscopy and biopsy may be indicated for definitive diagnosis.

D. Delayed passage of meconium/constipation.

1. General comments.

   a. Approximately 70% of neonates pass meconium within 12 hours, 95% within 24 hours, and >99% within 48 hours.

   b. Failure to pass meconium in the first 24 hours should raise suspicion and warrants close observation and possible workup.

   c. Passage of meconium does not rule out intestinal obstruction.

   d. 97% of infants have between one and nine bowel movements daily in the first week.

   e. 93% of infants have between one and seven bowel movements daily between 2 and 20 weeks of age. The variability is greater in breast-fed infants.

f. Consistency (hard, dry stools) and difficulty with passage (excessive straining, irritability, crying) are more important in determining the need for intervention in an infant with infrequent stools.

2. Etiology.
   a. Delayed passage of meconium.
      (1) Intestinal obstruction.
      (2) Spinal defects (meningocele, sacral agenesis, diastematomyelia).
      (3) Maternal drugs (opiates, ganglionic blocking agents, magnesium sulfate).
      (4) Meconium ileus.
      (5) Meconium plug syndrome.
      (6) Ileus (electrolyte imbalance, sepsis).
   b. Infrequent passage of stools.
      (1) Hypothyroidism.
      (2) Spinal defects (meningocele, sacral agenesis, diastematomyelia).
      (3) Hypotonia (Down syndrome).
      (4) Drugs (antihistamines, opiates, phenothiazines).
      (5) Hirschsprung disease.
      (6) Idiopathic ("functional" constipation).

3. Diagnosis and management.
   a. Perineal and rectal examination are essential.
   b. Abdominal radiographs for evidence of obstruction; an unprepped barium enema may be used to look for a "transition zone" if Hirschsprung disease is suspected.
   c. Prolonged jaundice, lethargy, and low body temperature should prompt thyroid function studies.
   d. A sweat test or screening for cystic fibrosis gene mutations is indicated in suspected or confirmed meconium ileus.
   e. Anorectal manometry, rectal suction biopsy, or both are necessary to confirm Hirschsprung disease.
   f. In the absence of a primary condition, stool softening can be achieved by adding corn syrup or malt soup extract (1 to 2 teaspoons three times daily) to the infant's formula.
   g. Clinical or radiologic signs of intestinal obstruction and frequent or severe episodes of fecal impaction require a GI and surgical consultation.

E. Abdominal distention.

1. General comments.
   a. Distention may indicate the following:
      (1) Increased intraluminal air (usually a result of intestinal obstruction).
      (2) Pneumoperitoneum (free intraabdominal air, usually the result of a perforation).
      (3) Ascites.
   b. Intraluminal air can usually be distinguished from free air on a plain-film radiograph. Cross-table lateral and upright radiographs are helpful.

2. Etiology.
   a. Increased intraluminal gas (see Intestinal obstruction, below); also seen with severe aerophagia (e.g., with pain, discomfort, or stress or after mask ventilation [bagging]).
   b. Pneumoperitoneum.
      (1) Spontaneous gastric perforation.
      (2) Perforated Meckel's diverticulum.
      (3) Perforated appendix.
      (4) Bowel perforation secondary to NEC, volvulus.
      (5) Pulmonary air leaks can also dissect into the peritoneal cavity.
   c. Ascites (may be identified prenatally by ultrasound).
      (1) Urinary tract anomalies.
      (2) Peritonitis.
      (3) Lymphatic (thoracic duct) obstruction.
      (4) Hepatic or portal vein obstruction.
      (5) Congenital infections.
      (6) Hemolytic disease of the newborn.
      (7) Cardiac or renal anomalies.
3. Diagnosis and management: See the section on intestinal obstruction or specific conditions later in this chapter.

N.B.: When suspected, most of these conditions require GI and surgical consultation.

F. Intestinal obstruction.

1. General comments.
   a. Vomiting (particularly if bilious), abdominal distention, and constipation are the cardinal signs, and *they constitute a potential surgical emergency.* Not all are always present. Vomiting predominates in proximal obstruction, distention in distal obstruction.
   b. Polyhydramnios is most commonly caused by congenital GI obstruction.
   c. Early pooling of secretions before starting feedings and scaphoid abdomen are also indicators of possible GI obstruction (esophageal atresia without tracheoesophageal fistula).
2. Etiology.
   a. Mechanical.
      (1) Congenital.
         (a) Atresia.
         (b) Stenosis.
         (c) Pyloric stenosis.
         (d) Meconium ileus.
         (e) Imperforate anus.
         (f) Malrotation, with or without volvulus.
         (g) Annular pancreas.
         (h) Incarcerated hernia.
         (i) Hirschsprung disease.
         (j) Aberrant superior mesenteric artery (SMA)
         (k) Preduodenal portal vein.
         (l) Intestinal duplications.

(m) Persistent omphalomesenteric duct (peritoneal bands).
(2) Acquired.
    (a) Intussusception.
    (b) NEC.
    (c) Meconium plug syndrome.
    (d) Peritoneal adhesions (after meconium peritonitis).
    (e) Mesenteric artery thrombosis.
b. Functional.
    (1) Ileus (electrolyte imbalance, hypermagnesemia, NEC, sepsis, asphyxia).
    (2) Maternal drugs (opiates, ganglionic blocking agents, magnesium sulfate).
    (3) Hypothyroidism.
    (4) Adrenal insufficiency.
3. Diagnosis and management.
  a. After obtaining a history (maternal, medications, procedures), assess the patient's vital signs and hydration status. Examinations (including rectal) should be done to look for distention, masses, bleeding sites, somatic anomalies. *If obstruction is suspected, act quickly.*
  b. Hold all oral or tube feedings.
  c. Decompress the stomach with a nasogastric or orogastric tube.
  d. Establish intravenous access and correct fluid and electrolyte deficits.
  e. Begin antibiotic therapy if sepsis is suspected.
  f. Obtain emergency surgical consultation.
  g. Radiologic studies and findings:
    (1) Plain-film abdominal radiographs are most helpful initially. In the newborn, gas is usually present in the stomach at 1 hour of life, in the cecum by 3 hours, and in the rectosigmoid by 8 to 10 hours. The progression is slower in premature newborns.
    (2) Absence of air may indicate esophageal atresia without tracheoesophageal fistula.
    (3) Mechanical causes (e.g., atresia, stenosis, Hirschsprung disease) usually result in marked distention with many air fluid levels proximal to the obstruction and little or no gas beyond.
    (4) Functional causes (e.g., electrolyte imbalance, sepsis, drugs) usually show diffuse distention with few air fluid levels.
    (5) Upper GI contrast studies are usually unnecessary and generally contraindicated in apparent complete obstruction. Contrast enema can help in diagnosing malrotation and Hirschsprung disease; it can also be therapeutic in meconium ileus, meconium plug syndrome, and intussusception (see specific conditions later in this chapter).
  h. Ultrasound can help with prenatal diagnosis (e.g., polyhydramnios, echogenic bowel, ascites, duodenal atresia). It is useful postnatally if pyloric stenosis is suspected.

II. SPECIFIC GASTROINTESTINAL CONDITIONS
A. GE reflux.
1. General comments.
   a. Regurgitation secondary to GE reflux is normal in the great majority of infants. When severe or persistent, look for signs of intestinal obstruction.
   b. Complicated reflux refers to GE reflux accompanied by failure to thrive (poor weight gain), esophagitis (pain or discomfort with regurgitation, upper GI bleeding), or cardiorespiratory symptoms (apnea, reactive airway disease, bradycardia, aspiration).
   c. Xanthines used for managing newborn apnea, and manipulation of the infant (such an with chest physiotherapy) can exacerbate reflux episodes.
2. Diagnosis and management of GE reflux.
   a. In complicated GE reflux, an upper GI series should be obtained to rule out a partial obstruction. Esophageal pH monitoring studies are rarely necessary if regurgitation is obvious; pH monitoring may be helpful in documenting severity of GE reflux, subclinical reflux, and correlation with cardiorespiratory complications (e.g., apnea, bradycardia). Upper endoscopy may be necessary to rule out esophagitis when symptoms are irritability and GI blood loss.
   b. Treatment.
      (1) The infant should be put in the prone position, if possible with the head elevated (avoid the supine or semiseated position).
      (2) Small, frequent feedings are best.
      (3) Formula can be thickened with 1 tablespoon of dry rice cereal per ounce.
      (4) Pharmacologic therapy (e.g., metoclopramide, H_2 blockers) should be reserved for complicated reflux once obstruction has been ruled out.
      (5) Continuous nasogastric feedings may alleviate the complications of reflux.
      (6) Surgery (fundoplication) may be indicated in complicated reflux refractory to other therapy.
B. Pyloric stenosis.
1. General comments.
   a. Pyloric stenosis is defined as hypertrophy of the pyloric circular muscle and is of unknown etiology.
   b. It usually occurs between the third and fifth weeks of life but has been observed from birth to the twelfth week. It is more common in first-born boys.
   c. Signs and symptoms include persistent and progressive worsening of vomiting, usually projectile, occasionally bloody, never bilious. Failure to thrive and jaundice may be associated findings.
   d. Palpation of a pyloric tumor ("olive") in the epigastrium just to the right of midline, if definite, is diagnostic.
   e. Electrolyte profile shows hypochloremic metabolic alkalosis.

2. Diagnosis and management.
   a. When pyloric stenosis is suspected, ultrasound confirms the presence of a pyloric tumor and narrow pyloric channel.
   b. Radiographs (usually unnecessary) show gastric distention with little or no air in small bowel and a string sign on contrast study.
   c. Treatment includes hydration and correction of metabolic alkalosis and surgical pyloromyotomy.

C. Necrotizing enterocolitis (NEC).

1. General comments.
   a. The etiology of NEC is unclear, but several risk factors have been identified.
      (1) The primary risk factor is prematurity; however, up to 20% of affected infants are full term. Other risk factors include small for gestational age, maternal hemorrhage and preeclampsia, cyanotic heart disease, polycythemia, in utero cocaine exposure, umbilical catheters, exchange transfusions, and asphyxia.
      (2) Precipitating factors include enteral feeding (up to 10 times more common in enteral-fed versus nonenteral-fed infants), ischemia, bacteria (e.g., altered bowel flora or mucosal barrier). Breast milk and low-volume early feedings ("gut priming") may be protective.
   b. NEC most commonly involves the terminal ileum and colon but can occur throughout.
   c. Signs and symptoms of NEC include lethargy, abdominal distention, bloody stools, ileus, vomiting, ascites, apnea, shock, DIC, perforation. Progression can be gradual (several days) to fulminant (several hours).
2. Diagnosis and management.
   a. Diagnosis: The clinical picture and radiologic findings show distended loops, air fluid levels, pneumatosis intestinalis (intramural air), intrahepatic air, and ascites. Free air indicates perforation.
   b. Treatment is mostly supportive. The infant should receive nothing by mouth; a nasogastric tube can be used for decompression. Hypotension, anemia, and thrombocytopenia should be treated. Antibiotics should be given as needed. Serial abdominal radiographs should be taken to monitor the infant's course.
   c. Surgery is indicated for perforation, peritonitis, and acidosis unresponsive to medical management.
   d. Prognosis: The mortality rate for infants with NEC is 20% to 40%. Up to 10% will go on to develop a second episode. Strictures, lymphangiectasis, malabsorption, and short bowel syndrome are late complications in up to 25% of survivors.

D. Milk/formula protein sensitivity (allergy).

1. General comments.
   a. GI protein sensitivity can manifest as an enteropathy or enterocolitis, usually in reaction to cow's milk–based formula, but it is also associated with soy and other allergens.

b. Enterocolitis causes acute blood-streaked diarrheal stools, usually between 5 days and 3 weeks of age. The infant may be irritable, but otherwise has no other findings. Enterocolitis has also been described in breast-fed infants. Proctoscopy and biopsy confirm proctocolitis.

c. Enteropathy is characterized by prolonged diarrhea with protein loss and occult blood, emesis, and failure to thrive. It usually occurs at 2 to 3 months of age.

2. Management consists of removing the offending protein from the infant's or the mother's diet. Protein hydrolysate formulas are useful for this purpose.

E. Esophageal atresia and tracheoesophageal (TE) fistula.

1. General comments.

   a. Esophageal atresia with distal TE fistula is the most common form (85%); TE fistula without atresia, known as "H type" occurs in 5% of cases.

   b. Esophageal atresia with a TE fistula proximal to the atretic segment is very rare.

2. Diagnosis and management.

   a. In esophageal atresia, polyhydramnios occurs in one third of the cases. Immediate vomiting with feedings, large amounts of secretions, and respiratory distress are present.

   b. Abdominal distension occurs if there is a distal fistula. A gasless abdomen indicates no fistula or an obliterated fistula.

   c. A soft 5F to 8F feeding tube that can't be advanced or that coils (visualized by radiograph) confirms atresia.

   d. When atresia is apparent, the infant should be placed in the upright position, with constant secretion aspiration by catheter inserted into the esophageal pouch, until surgical correction is done.

   e. H-type fistulas do not often present with symptoms perinatally. Chronic respiratory problems or recurrent pneumonias over months or years are suggestive.

F. Intestinal atresia (complete obstruction of the lumen).

1. Esophageal.

   a. General comments.

      (1) Polyhydramnios occurs in 30% to 50% of cases; 85% are accompanied by distal TE fistula; up to 40% are accompanied by other anomalies (e.g., imperforate anus, malrotation, cardiovascular anomalies, VACTERL syndrome).

      (2) Signs and symptoms include a large amount of oral secretions, brisk regurgitation of feedings, abdominal distention (if TE fistula is present, see above), respiratory distress, and resistance on passage of nasogastric tube.

      (3) Radiographic findings include the absence of air in the bowel if there is no TE communication.

   b. Diagnosis and management.

      (1) If esophageal atresia is suspected, a soft 5F to 8F feeding tube can be carefully passed until resistance is met. A plain-film radiograph after injection of a small amount of air will con-

firm diagnosis. The use of contrast material is usually unnecessary.

(2) A sump tube should be passed and connected to suction. Intravenous hydration should be started promptly.

(3) Endotracheal intubation may be necessary.

(4) Obtain immediate surgical consultation.

2. Duodenal.

a. General comments.

(1) Polyhydramnios is frequently associated with duodenal atresia. Obstruction is usually distal to the bile duct. Approximately 30% of infants with atresia will have Down syndrome; 50% may have other GI anomalies (e.g., annular pancreas, malrotation, esophageal atresia, and small bowel and anorectal anomalies).

(2) Signs and symptoms include bile-stained vomitus in the first few hours, delayed passage of meconium, upper abdominal distention (may be absent), visible abdominal peristalsis, and occasionally jaundice.

b. Diagnosis and management.

(1) Radiographic findings show a "double bubble" sign (dilated stomach and duodenum) with no air beyond (see Intestinal obstruction, p. 124-125).

(2) Gastric decompression and surgical correction are indicated.

3. Small bowel.

a. General comments.

(1) Jejunal and ileal atresias are more common and have fewer (7%) associated anomalies than duodenal atresias. Only 1% are associated with Down syndrome. Approximately 15% of cases may present as meconium ileus, or occasionally as meconium peritonitis.

(2) Signs and symptoms include delayed passage of a small amount of meconium. Vomiting and distention occur within 48 to 72 hours. Jaundice may be present.

b. Diagnosis and management.

(1) Radiographic findings show dilated loops and air fluid levels. Calcifications will be present if there was meconium peritonitis.

(2) A contrast enema should be done to rule out Hirschsprung disease and meconium ileus.

(3) Gastric decompression and surgical correction are indicated (see Intestinal obstruction, p. 124-125).

G. GI duplications.

1. General comments.

a. GI duplications are cystic or tubular malformations lined by intestinal mucosa, with smooth muscle and sharing of a common blood supply with the adjacent gut.

b. They can occur at any level. Tubular duplications frequently communicate with the adjacent lumen.

c. Duplications can enlarge, obstruct, bleed, or lead to volvulus or intussusception. Some may go unrecognized until adulthood.

2. Diagnosis and management.
  a. Duplications should be suspected in cases involving unexplained obstruction, bleeding, mass, perforation, volvulus, or intussusception.
  b. Ultrasound and computed tomography can help diagnose cystic duplications. A Meckel's scan may be positive if the duplication contains ectopic gastric mucosa.
  c. Duplications should be surgically removed (see the sections on GI bleeding and GI obstruction earlier in this chapter).

H. Malrotation/volvulus.
1. General comments.
  a. Malrotation results from an arrest in the normal counterclockwise rotation of the bowel about the axis of the superior mesenteric artery during gestation.
  b. Volvulus of the midgut at the level of the resulting narrow mesenteric stalk causes obstruction and strangulation. This constitutes an extreme surgical emergency.
  c. Signs and symptoms: Typically, the infant appears and feeds well and has normal stools. There is sudden onset of bilious vomiting, with or without distention, and passage of blood-tinged stools. Signs of cardiovascular collapse and sepsis may rapidly ensue.
2. Diagnosis and management.
  a. See management of intestinal obstruction, p. 124-125.
  b. Plain-film radiographs show dilated small bowel.
  c. After stabilization, contrast enema can be done, which will reveal the cecum in the right upper quadrant. Upper GI contrast study (by nasogastric tube) will show absence of the normal duodenal loop and the ligament of Treitz to the left of the midline.
  d. Emergency surgery is indicated to relieve volvulus. Resection of nonviable bowel may be required and may lead to short bowel syndrome.

I. Meconium ileus.
1. General comments.
  a. Meconium ileus is obstruction of distal small bowel and proximal colon caused by inspissated meconium. It is almost always (98%) associated with cystic fibrosis and may present as echogenic fetal bowel on prenatal ultrasound.
  b. Meconium ileus accounts for up to 32% of neonatal small-bowel obstructions.
  c. Signs and symptoms include failure to pass meconium, even after digital examination; abdominal distention in the first 12 to 24 hours; and bilious vomiting within 48 hours after birth. Abdominal examination may indicate hard, palpable, freely movable masses.
  d. Up to 30% of cases are associated with volvulus, atresia, peritonitis, or pseudocysts.
2. Diagnosis and management.
  a. Radiographic findings may suggest meconium peritonitis (e.g., abdominal calcifications on plain-film radiographs). If perforation has not occurred, the small bowel will appear distended, thick-walled, granular, and with tiny air bubbles mixed with meconium.

An enema with soluble contrast material will show an empty and narrow distal colon (microcolon) and may be therapeutic.
b. A sweat test (difficult in neonates) or identification of cystic fibrosis gene mutations is confirmatory.
c. Treatment: See Intestinal obstruction, p. 124-125. Once perforation and atresia are excluded, enemas with isoosmolar contrast material or acetylcysteine may relieve the obstruction. If unsuccessful, surgical decompression, often with an enterostomy, is necessary.

J. Meconium plug syndrome.

1. General comments.
   a. Meconium plug syndrome involves obstruction of the colon, usually distal, with meconium or mucus. Also called *small left hemicolon syndrome* or *functionally immature colon.*
   b. Meconium plug syndrome is usually seen in premature infants, infants of diabetic mothers, or acutely ill neonates. It may be an early manifestation of cystic fibrosis or Hirschsprung disease.
   c. Signs and symptoms include failure to pass or difficulty passing stools, evidence of intestinal obstruction, and normal rectal examination, which may be enough to stimulate passage of the plug and relieve obstruction.
2. Diagnosis and management.
   a. Rectal stimulation with digital examination or glycerine suppository.
   b. Soluble-contrast enema may demonstrate a narrowed distal colon and may be therapeutic.
   c. Normal stooling pattern should resume by 48 hours after decompression. If not, consider Hirschsprung disease.

K. Meckel's diverticulum.

1. General comments.
   a. Meckel's diverticulum is a remnant of the omphalomesenteric duct, which arises from the ileum proximal to the ileocecal valve. More than 50% contain ectopic gastric or pancreatic tissue. Meckel's diverticula are present in 1% to 3% of the general population.
   b. Signs and symptoms include bleeding, usually painless, resulting from peptic ulceration. It may also present as intussusception.
2. Diagnosis can be made by technetium scan. Administration of an H_2 blocker 48 to 72 hours before the procedure will increase sensitivity of the scan.
3. Treatment is surgical excision.

L. Anal fissure.

1. General comments.
   a. An anal fissure is a slitlike tear in the anal canal, usually caused by passage of large, hard stools. Pain and irritability may be elicited with bowel movements.
   b. Bright-red blood can be seen on the surface of stools or occasionally isolated after defecation.
2. Diagnosis and management.
   a. Examination in the knee-chest position, parting the buttocks to visualize the anal canal to the mucocutaneous junction, is all that is necessary.

b. Management includes a stool softener such as malt soup extract, 1 to 2 teaspoons three times daily, and thorough cleansing of the perianal area with water after bowel movements.

M. Hirschsprung disease.

1. General comments.
   a. Hirschsprung disease is defined as congenital absence of ganglion cells of the bowel (usually distally).
   b. Most cases occur in full-term infants.
   c. Only 15% of cases are diagnosed in the first month of life, 80% by 1 year. Between 3% and 10% of infants with Down syndrome have Hirschsprung disease.
   d. Signs and symptoms: 94% of infants with Hirschsprung disease do not pass meconium in the first 24 hours. Constipation, abdominal distention, and empty rectum on digital examination (especially in long-segment disease) with rapid passage of stools after examination are suggestive.
   e. Explosive stools, poor feeding, hematochezia, fever, and shock characterize enterocolitis, which can be fatal.
2. Diagnosis and management.
   a. If the clinical picture is consistent, anal manometry and rectal suction biopsy with acetylcholinesterase staining can be highly suggestive or diagnostic. A "transition zone" on an unprepped contrast enema is less likely to be seen in a neonate. Lower endoscopy can confirm ileocolitis.
   b. Treatment of ileocolitis includes restoration of fluid and electrolyte balance, evacuation of the colon with a rectal tube, and administration of antibiotics.
   c. Full-thickness surgical biopsy and resection of the affected segment are confirmatory and therapeutic.

N. Anorectal anomalies.

1. General comments.
   a. Anorectal anomalies are generally classified as "high"/rectal or "low"/anal depending on occurrence above or below the puborectalis levator sling.
   b. More than 50% (especially high malformation) are associated with other anomalies (e.g. vertebral, genitourinary, other intestinal).
   c. Low anomalies include anal stenosis, imperforate anal membrane, and anal agenesis (the most common of low anomalies). Anal agenesis usually is accompanied by a fistulous tract to the vulva or perineum.
   d. High anomalies include rectal atresia (obstructing membrane above levator) and rectal agenesis (most common of all anorectal lesions, commonly accompanied by rectourethral or rectovaginal fistula).
2. Diagnosis and management.
   a. Diagnosis is made by inspection and by the infant's failure to pass meconium normally.
   b. Surgical correction is required, either by anoplasty or a diverting colostomy, depending on the case.

BIBLIOGRAPHY

Berseth CL: Gastrointestinal and nutritional conditions. In Taeusch HW, Ballard RA, Avery ME (editors): *Avery's diseases of the newborn,* Philadelphia, 1998, WB Saunders.

Brown RL: Care of the surgical intensive care nursery graduate: the primary pediatrician's perspective, *Pediatr Clin North Am* 45(6): 1327-1352, 1998.

Grand RJ, Watkins JB, Torte FM: Development of the human gastrointestinal tract, *Gastroenterology* 70:790, 1976.

Jona JZ: Advances in neonatal surgery, *Pediatr Clin North Am* 45(3): 605-617, 1998.

La Gamma EF, Browne LE: Feeding practices for infants weighing less than 1500 g at birth and the pathogenesis of necrotizing enterocolitis, *Clin Perinatol* 21:271, 1994.

Neu J: Necrotizing enterocolitis: the search for unifying pathogenic theory leading to prevention, *Pediatr Clin North Am,* 43:409, 1996.

13

Genitourinary System

JOHN P. GEARHART

I. SPECIMEN COLLECTION METHODS FOR URINALYSIS AND CULTURE

A. Clean catch. A polyethylene bag should be attached with adhesive to the perineum and over the genitalia.

1. Cleanse area with povidone-iodine 10% (Betadine soaks) three times.
2. Rinse thoroughly with sterile water.
3. Attach bag and wait.
4. Retrieve as soon as possible after voiding, within 1 hour if findings are to be reliable.

B. Suprapubic bladder aspiration. A palpably distended bladder is preferable. Infant's diaper should be dry, with no indication of voiding in the previous 60 minutes.

1. To prevent voiding during procedure, exert gentle anterior rectal pressure in girls, penile pressure in boys.
2. Place infant in supine, frog-leg position.
3. Cleanse area three times with povidone-iodine 10% and 70% alcohol.
4. Puncture site should be midline, 1 to 2 cm above symphysis pubis.
5. Use a syringe with a 22-gauge 1-inch needle. Insert 10 to 20 degrees to perpendicular, aimed a bit to caudad.
6. Apply gentle suction as needle is introduced until urine spurts into syringe. Advance needle no more than 1 inch (2.5 cm).
7. Aspirate urine gently.

N.B.: Bladder aspiration is to be avoided in the event of demonstrated or possible anatomic urinary tract anomalies.

C. Catheterization.

1. Cleanse area as for clean catch.
2. Use well-lubricated, sterile no. 3 or no. 5 pediatric feeding tube.

N.B.: Catheterization is to be avoided unless there is concern about the reliability of previous cultures and the need for culture is great, or in the event of clinical improvement and continued bacterial growth in voided culture.

II. VOIDING PATTERNS

Oliguria, anuria, or a poor urinary stream may be an indication of a urologic emergency. Voiding will have occurred in two thirds of all neonates within 12 hours of birth and in at least 90% during the first 24 hours. Failure to void within the first 24 hours should cause concern.

A. Delayed voiding with a palpably distended bladder suggests possible lower urinary tract obstruction (e.g., posterior urethral valves or other structural abnormalities).

B. Neurogenic bladder. Distention may be the sole, subtle clue to a neurologic defect.

C. Anuria with or without Potter facies suggests renal agenesis.

D. Oliguria, hematuria, or both suggest a vascular catastrophe, such as the following:
1. Renal vein thrombosis.
2. Renal artery thrombosis.
3. Renal cortical necrosis.

E. A weak or sputtering urinary stream requires careful examination of the penis during voiding. Possible causes and their signs include the following:
1. Posterior urethral valves: stream weak, dribbling, or absent.
2. Urethral diverticula, often secondary to anterior urethral valves (rare): stream weak, dribbling.
3. Megalourethra with inadequate corpora spongiosum: urethra dilates and fills under increased pressure of voiding.

III. CLUES TO POSSIBLE PRESENCE OF UROLOGIC DISORDER

A. History: maternal, prenatal (prenatal ultrasound performed?), and perinatal.
1. Past maternal history of fetal wastage.
2. Chromosomal abnormalities (e.g., trisomies).
3. Oligohydramnios.
   a. Severe obstructive uropathy.
   b. Eagle-Barrett (prune-belly) syndrome.
   c. Renal agenesis.
4. Polyhydramnios: neonatal ovarian cysts.
5. Maternal bleeding during pregnancy, particularly first trimester.
6. Maternal illness during pregnancy (e.g., diabetes, rubella).
7. Maternal age >35 years.
8. Maternal cocaine use.
9. Toxemia of pregnancy. Therapy with magnesium sulfate during labor may cause neuromuscular blockade with generalized hypotonia and bladder distention.
10. Perinatal asphyxia.
    a. Renal cortical necrosis.
    b. Renal tubular necrosis.
    c. Renal vein thrombosis.

B. Single umbilical artery. Approximately 0.9% of all babies have a single umbilical artery. There is ongoing controversy regarding the urologic significance. The mortality rate is almost four times that of neonates in general; of those who die, 28% have genitourinary (GU) malformation, roughly the same percentage as in those with two arteries.

N.B.: Nevertheless, a sonogram is indicated in babies born with a single umbilical artery.

C. Physical examination findings. The following physical findings provide the most common clues to uropathy:

1. Potter facies (large, low-set, flabby ears; widely spaced eyes).
   a. Renal agenesis.
   b. Eagle-Barrett (prune-belly) syndrome.
   c. Bilateral multicystic kidneys.
2. External ear deformity.
3. Widely spaced nipples; supernumerary nipples in white babies.
4. Deficiency of abdominal musculature.
   a. Eagle-Barrett syndrome.
   b. Cryptorchidism.
5. Palpable, enlarged kidneys at first examination.
6. Abnormalities of genitalia.
7. Abnormalities of anus.
8. Sacral dermal sinus.
9. Obvious meningomyelocele; absence of sacral segments.
10. Cardiac anomalies (associated renal defects in as high as 12% of cases).
11. Imperforate anus (reported incidence of renal defect as high as 38%, particularly with high rectal atresia).
12. Tracheoesophageal fistula.
13. Polydactyly and associated anomalies of the extremities.
    a. Renal agenesis.
    b. Urethral duplication.

N.B.: Renal defects are associated with a number of congenital anomalies; the presence of any significant anomaly or a constellation of several minor anomalies suggests a search for renal disease, including studying voiding patterns, urinalysis, and sonography.

IV. CIRCUMCISION

The controversy surrounding newborn circumcision continues to evolve. Recent studies suggest that a decreased incidence of urinary tract infection and bacteremia is a possible benefit of circumcision; however, most of these early investigations have not been confirmed. If there is any abnormality of the penis or scrotum, circumcision should be deferred until a pediatric urologic consultation is obtained.

A. Foreskin.

1. Without intervention, the foreskin should separate and become freely mobile by 4 to 7 years of age.

N.B.: The newborn's foreskin should never be forcibly retracted; additional adhesions joining foreskin to glans readily develop, with phimosis the common result.

2. Cleanliness requires attention only to what can be seen—again, there should be no forced retraction of the foreskin.

B. Complications of circumcision.

1. Bleeding.
    a. Most often, local pressure will suffice to stanch bleeding; if not, sponges with 1:200,000 epinephrine should be held to the area for 10 to 15 minutes.
    b. A urologic consultation should be requested if bleeding persists. (**Do not cauterize** without a consultation!)
2. Infection (rare).
    a. Warm soaks to penis.
    b. Broad-spectrum antibiotic coverage (e.g., ampicillin and gentamicin) can be given pending culture results.

N.B.: Proceed slowly. Not everything that looks infected is infected. This is a raw, healing surface. It is not necessary to delay discharge after circumcision until the infant has voided.

3. Inappropriate operative result.
    a. Insufficient removal of skin. If repair is necessary, simple revision can be done when the child is older. Most often, growth solves the problem. Advise restraint and the passage of time.
    b. Excessive removal of skin (common cause of litigation).
        (1) Allow healing (if excess skin removal is noted at time of circumcision; if noted later, immediate urologic consultation is required).
        (2) If penis is displaced downward or otherwise distorted, mobilization of available skin and grafting may be necessary for both functional and cosmetic purposes.
    c. Injury to urethra (rare, requires immediate urologic consultation).
    d. Tourniquet injury to penis from constricting gauze (rare, requires immediate urologic consultation).

V. HYPOSPADIAS

Hypospadias is common, occurring in 8:1000 live male births. It is five times more common with in vitro pregnancy. Less severe forms predominate, making up approximately 87% of the total. In 10% the urethral meatus is on the proximal penile shaft; in 3% the meatus is in the penoscrotal or perineal region.

A. Associated anomalies.

1. Undescended testes (10%).
2. Upper urinary tract malformation. Ordinarily uncommon; potential increases to 45% in the presence of the following:
    a. Imperforate anus.
    b. Cardiac malformation.
    c. Myelomeningocele.

N.B.: Renal ultrasonography and urologic consultation are essential in this event.

B. Therapeutic considerations.

1. Repair as early as possible in the first year (current practice).
    a. Extent of abnormality guides decision on exact timing.
    b. Separation anxiety diminished.

    c. Technical management simplified.

    d. Simpler malformations may be repaired on outpatient basis (soft silastic urethral stents are facilitative).

    e. Complex malformations, such as penoscrotal or perineal hypospadias, require hospitalization and an experienced pediatric urologist.

2. In the event of association with undescended testis, consider workup for intersex anomaly.

3. Appropriate attention should be given to associated anomalies.

VI. EPISPADIAS

Epispadias may occur alone (1:112,000 births) or in combination with exstrophy (1:30,000 births). Incontinence is a common problem. Surgical correction is generally deferred to about 1 year of age.

VII. THE UNDESCENDED TESTIS

Cryptorchidism is one of the most common disorders seen in the newborn. In some premature babies, birth may occur before the onset of normal testicular descent during the last trimester of gestation. Only 3% of full-term males examined at birth have a true undescended testis; almost 30% of premature males have undescended testis. The lower the birth weight, the greater the incidence of cryptorchidism. The cryptorchid state is usually easily determined at birth when the scrotum is relatively large, minimal subcutaneous fat exists, and the cremasteric reflex is absent. The incidence of cryptorchidism at 1 year of age is 0.8%. In 10% of patients with cryptorchidism the defect is bilateral, and in less than 3% one or both of the testes are absent.

A. Localization of a nonpalpable testis. Possible locations of an undescended testis, given careful physical examination, include the following:

1. Inguinal region, obscured by abundant subcutaneous fat, small size, or both.

2. Intraabdominal, inside a hernial sac just proximal to the internal ring, and thus not palpable.

3. Intraabdominal, not associated with a hernial sac.

4. Congenital absence.

B. Management.

1. In the immediate newborn period, watchful waiting and parental education are keys to management of the undescended testis.

2. With associated hypospadias, consider an intersex abnormality.

3. By 1 year of age, for the fewer than 1% that have not yet descended, consult with a pediatric urologist.

    a. Sonography is helpful only if the testis is in the inguinal canal.

    b. Magnetic resonance imaging (MRI) and computed tomography (CT) are of doubtful value for intraabdominal study.

    c. Surgery ultimately is necessary in any event (unless the testis is definitely absent).

C. Potential therapeutic approaches.

1. Hormonal stimulation (gonadotropin-releasing hormone or human chorionic gonadotropin).

   a. Use of these hormones is controversial; success in achieving full descent is relatively infrequent.

   b. Hormone stimulation is often helpful if the cryptorchidism is unilateral; it enables some descent to make the testis palpable before corrective surgery.

   c. In the event of bilateral cryptorchidism, a trial of hormonal stimulation is justified despite the low success rate.

2. Surgery for localizing the testis and placing it in the scrotum is usually done after the first birthday because descent is unlikely after 1 year.

   a. Laparoscopy is helpful to localize the testis and even to help with bringing the testis down.

   b. Histologic changes in a cryptorchid testis apparent at 24 to 30 months suggest the need for earlier surgery.

   c. Long-term fertility is uncertain in any event. Recent studies suggest 80% to 85% fertility in unilateral and just over 50% in bilateral cases. Further studies are necessary to validate the benefit of earlier surgery.

VIII. PRENATAL HYDRONEPHROSIS

Prenatal evaluation of the genitourinary tract with ultrasonography has become common. In some countries (e.g., England and Belgium), all pregnant women are evaluated at 16 weeks and 19 weeks in the search for malformations of the major fetal organ systems. In the United States, however, routine ultrasonography is not as prevalent. It formerly was limited to those with problem pregnancies or a history of an infant born with a major malformation. However, this procedure is becoming more widespread. Diagnosis and management should be guided by the following principles and steps:

A. The majority of upper and lower urinary tract anomalies are easily demonstrated by 19 weeks of gestation.

B. By 22 weeks the entire tract is visible and easily studied.

C. If a major genitourinary problem (e.g., hydronephrosis) is discovered, ultrasound examination should be repeated and followed during pregnancy and again just after birth, to confirm or rule out the problem. If an associated condition (e.g., oligohydramnios) is also present, weekly ultrasound examination to follow progress and to guide clinical decision making is justified.

N.B.: Hydronephrosis can be seen on one examination and be completely resolved on the next. Even the fetal bladder can be seen to empty and refill on ultrasonographic examination.

D. If a major genitourinary problem persists on postnatal examination, voiding cystourethrograms and appropriate upper-tract studies (e.g., diuretic renograms) can differentiate reflux from anatomic obstructive lesions of the upper or lower tract.

E. If an obstructive lesion is found, prompt surgery within a few weeks of birth is usually (but not always) indicated, with excellent expectation of normal renal growth and stable renal function.

F. On the relatively infrequent occasion when the exact nature of the lesion is not clearly shown, follow-up with ultrasonography or diuretic renal scans (with the guidance of the pediatric urologist) is justified until the nature of the lesion becomes apparent.

IX. ABDOMINAL MASSES COMMON TO THE URINARY TRACT

A. Differential diagnosis. The discovery of an abdominal mass on the first physical examination is a relatively common clinical finding. Many conditions must be considered in the differential diagnosis.

1. Hydronephrosis.
   a. Ureteropelvic junction (UPJ) obstruction. This is the most common cause of abdominal mass; 20% to 30% are bilateral, with slightly more than half occurring in males.
   b. If bilateral, be certain that bladder outlet obstruction is not also present. This is, however, less common than the UPJ lesion.
   c. Surgical repair usually provides an excellent result.

2. A multicystic dysplastic kidney is a common cause of abdominal mass. It is usually unilateral; cysts are usually few in number, large and variable in size, and loosely bound together.
   a. If the condition is bilateral, it is frequently associated with Potter facies.
   b. The mass often feels lobulated.
   c. The kidney is nonfunctional on renal scanning or excretory urography.
   d. Nuclear renal scan, not ultrasonography, is used to evaluate function in the contralateral kidney.
   e. Lesions generally regress during infancy and early childhood.
   f. Surgery, usually nephrectomy, is not indicated if ultrasonography indicates regression.

3. Renal vein thrombosis is relatively less common and is usually unilateral.
   a. Risk factors.
      (1) Trauma.
      (2) Dehydration.
      (3) Infection.
      (4) Maternal diabetes.
      (5) Polycythemia.
   b. Clinical picture.
      (1) Firm, enlarging kidney.
      (2) Gross hematuria (caused by hemorrhagic renal infarction).
      (3) Anemia (possible, secondary to hemolysis or hematuria).
   c. Treatment.
      (1) Watchful waiting.
      (2) Nephrectomy usually is not necessary.

4. Adrenal hemorrhage is also not uncommon.
    a. Risk factors.
        (1) Prolonged labor.
        (2) Difficult, traumatic delivery.
        (3) Vigorous resuscitative effort.
        (4) Excessive abdominal compression for any reason.
        (5) Sepsis.
        (6) Urinary tract infection.
    b. Clinical picture.
        (1) An abdominal mass, although not always readily evident, is usually located in the flank.
        (2) Anemia, pallor.
        (3) Lethargy, even shock.
        (4) Jaundice.
        (5) Hematuria, usually microscopic.
        (6) Renal scanning indicates the kidney is displaced downward and outwardly rotated.
        (7) Demonstrable infection in urinary tract or elsewhere.
    c. Differential diagnosis.
        (1) Renal vein thrombosis: usually gross hematuria.
        (2) Hydronephrosis in the upper pole of a duplicated collecting system.
        (3) Renal hemorrhage; may not be differentiated before surgery.
    d. Treatment.
        (1) Fluid replacement and maintenance.
        (2) Electrolyte repair.
        (3) Steroid therapy, possible.

N.B.: Rarely, there is progression to bilateral involvement.

        (4) Blood transfusion should be used cautiously and only if anemia is profound.
        (5) Antibiotics are appropriate treatment for demonstrated infection.

5. Mesoblastic nephroma. The most common renal tumor in childhood is Wilms tumor. Those discovered in neonates are most often not true Wilms tumors but mesoblastic nephromas. Clinical management is identical for either.
    a. Tumor may not at first be palpable on physical examination.
    b. Ultrasonography or renal scans performed for other reasons may define the lesion even before a physical examination is performed.
    c. Metastatic spread to lungs or bone may be demonstrated.
    d. Treatment: nephrectomy.

6. Neuroblastoma is also a common abdominal tumor of childhood. One third to one half of these tumors are found in the first year of life.
    a. Neuroblastomas are often palpable.
    b. Plain-film abdominal radiographs may reveal calcification in up to 60% of cases.
    c. CT scans best define the extent of disease before surgery.
    d. Radionuclide bone scans or radiographic bone survey may reveal skeletal metastases.

e. Vanillylmandelic acid (VMA) and homovanillic acid (HVA): one or both levels can be elevated in up to 90% of cases.

f. Metastases to bone marrow, bone, and liver are most common.

g. Treatment options include surgery, chemotherapy, or radiation; requires consultation with a urologist, oncologist, or radiation therapist.

7. Hydrometrocolpos is rare. It is the result of fluid distention of the vagina and uterus secondary to vaginal obstruction and excessive secretion of cervical glands.

a. Associated anatomic anomalies include the following:

(1) Vaginal atresia (the most common anomaly).

(2) Imperforate hymen.

(3) Imperforate anus.

(4) Cloacal anomaly.

(5) Ambiguous genitalia.

b. Diagnosis is based on physical examination and ultrasonography; retrograde genitography will be needed to demonstrate the level and cause of obstruction.

c. Treatment is usually surgical.

8. Polycystic kidneys. Condition is autosomal recessive (infantile).

a. Affects both kidneys.

b. Shows no gender preference.

c. Symptoms include palpable masses and renal failure.

d. On ultrasound, cysts are too small to see and renal size is enlarged.

e. Management includes control of hypertension, congestive heart failure, renal failure, and hepatic failure.

f. Survivors face dialysis and renal transplantation.

9. Distended bladder. 90% of newborns void during the first 24 hours of life and essentially all void by 48 hours of life unless there is a problem such as the following:

a. Posterior urethral valves.

b. Neurogenic bladder.

c. Pelvic/vaginal rhabdomyosarcoma (rare).

d. Ureterocele obstructing the bladder outlet.

B. Diagnostic approach after physical examination.

1. Ultrasound of abdomen and pelvis to determine if lesion is solid or cystic.

2. Voiding pattern.

3. Urinalysis to look for hematuria (gross or microscopic), proteinuria, or evidence of infection.

4. A follow-up examination, if necessary and as appropriate, should be scheduled with a pediatric urologist. Additional studies include the following:

a. Renal diuretic scan.

b. CT scan.

c. MRI.

d. Excretory urography.

e. Retrograde genitography.

f. Urine culture.

g. A variety of other studies related to associated findings.

X. AMBIGUOUS GENITALIA SHOULD BE CONSIDERED AN EMERGENCY!!!

A. Congenital adrenal hyperplasia is a common cause of ambiguous genitalia. Unrecognized, the salt-losing type of adrenal hyperplasia carries a high mortality rate. Immediate evaluation and monitoring are indicated. Serum electrolytes and blood and urine steroid studies are also indicated (see p. 363).

B. Gender identification must be made as soon as possible. Social and emotional imperatives are on a par with anatomic and physiologic considerations.

1. Karyotyping should be performed.
2. Retrograde genitography, performed by a pediatric urologist in the radiology department, should determine the takeoff of the vagina and urethra from the urogenital sinus.

N.B.: Hypospadias associated with undescended testes should be thoroughly evaluated to avoid erroneous assignment of gender.

C. Parental counseling and education should be provided. Choose words carefully until the situation is clarified by the appropriate workup. Samples include the following:

1. Ambiguous genitalia = incomplete forming.
2. Phallus = penis, clitoris.
3. Gonads = testes, ovaries.

XI. VAGINAL DISCHARGE AND VAGINAL BLEEDING

A. Most newborn girls have a thick, often profuse vaginal discharge as a result of prenatal stimulation by maternal hormones. The discharge may be blood tinged. This is a self-limited condition requiring explanation but no intervention.

B. Causes of concern.

1. Discharge may be from an ectopic ureter inserting into the vagina. A clear and persistent discharge may be urine.
   a. Urinalysis is recommended.
   b. Upper-tract imaging can be used to search for possible duplication of the urinary tract with ectopia.
2. Bleeding from the vagina is not common and may be caused by the following:
   a. A prolapsed ectopic ureterocele descending through the bladder neck and exiting through the urethral meatus; a discolored mass may be seen.
   b. Rhabdomyosarcoma of the vagina. This bleeds easily; a friable, discolored mass can be visualized.
   c. Urethral prolapse.

N.B.: Each of these conditions mandates immediate pediatric urologic consultation.

XII. VULVAR ABNORMALITY

A. Clitoris. Hypertrophy (e.g., as the only sign of the adrenogenital syndrome.

B. Imperforate hymen. May be associated with hydrocolpos or hematocolpos.

C. Aberrant location of urethral meatus. It should be just ventral to the vaginal introitus. An aberrant location indicates a possible urogenital sinus anomaly.

D. Prolapsed ureterocele. May present as a perineal mass; may be confused with hydrocolpos.

E. Poorly defined urethral and vaginal orifices. This suggests the possibility of a urogenital sinus or cloacal outlet anomaly.

    a. Careful examination of anal competence is required.

    b. May be associated with an abdominal mass.

XIII. INGUINAL HERNIA AND HYDROCELE IN THE NEWBORN

A. Inguinal hernia. In clinical practice, the majority of infantile inguinal hernias appear during the first year, with the diagnosis commonly made in the first month after birth; new cases are less frequent as childhood advances. The overall incidence in the pediatric population is from 1% to 4%. In premature infants weighing <2000 g at birth the incidence rises to >15%. The condition affects boys nine times more frequently than it does girls.

1. In recent years controversy has arisen with regard to the desirability of routine bilateral exploration in cases of apparent unilateral inguinal hernia. Clinically undiagnosed hernias on the contralateral side have been reported to occur as often as 60% of the time. However, other studies have shown that only 15% of patients developed a clinical hernia later on in childhood on the contralateral, unexplored side. Thus it may be reasonably argued that routine operation on the second side in the younger child may be unnecessary in up to 85% of cases. When additional consideration is given to the close association of the spermatic vessels and vas deferens to the patent processus vaginalis, it will be appreciated that routine exploration is not without risk in the young infant. Indeed, there is an incidence of testicular atrophy of approximately 0.5% after infantile hernia repair.

2. Usual presentation: Many infantile inguinal hernias appear during the first month of life and a majority within the first 3 months of life; they are usually detected by the parent after discharge and present as a bulge in the groin after a period of crying or straining during a bowel movement. The swelling is generally absent in the morning and more noticeable in the latter part of the day. Sometimes the hernia is not clinically apparent to the clinician but the child's parent is convinced of its presence, especially during periods of infant distress.

3. Features of physical examination.

    a. Roll the spermatic cord gently over the pubic tubercle; the affected side is more readily palpated and bulkier than the more delicate structure on the contralateral side.

    b. Inspect the scrotum. Are both testes fully descended? Up to 6% of congenital inguinal hernias are associated with incomplete testicular descent.

    c. If, in a girl, a gonad is palpable in the hernial sac at the time of surgery, one must be certain that this is an ovary and not a testis.

N.B.: A phenotypic female with a testis may have androgen insensitivity syndrome.

   B. Hydrocele. A hydrocele is a collection of fluid between the parietal and visceral layers of the tunica vaginalis. Hydroceles usually occur during infancy but can appear even into adulthood. During infancy it is believed that a patent processus vaginalis contributes to the collection of peritoneal fluid in the tunica vaginalis. A hydrocele is common after birth, occurring in about 6% of full-term males. It causes a transilluminating, painless, oval scrotal swelling that may extend along the spermatic cord. Because a hydrocele at birth almost universally occurs secondary to a patent processus vaginalis, therapy should be delayed until after the processus closes, which may occur spontaneously within the first year of life. The patent processus vaginalis also explains why the size of an infant hydrocele may vary from time to time.

N.B.: Occasionally, an inguinal hernia may be suspected in a patient with a hydrocele. Careful follow-up will be needed in the first few months of life to make sure that one is dealing with a true infant hydrocele and not an inguinal hernia. There can be an association if the hydrocele persists after 1 year of life or continues to increase in size; surgical therapy will then be required.

XIV. HEMATURIA

Microscopic or gross hematuria in the neonate should be considered an emergency; gross hematuria is rare. All causes require immediate and accurate diagnosis and include the following:

A. Renal artery thrombosis is potentially lethal. There has been a recent increase in incidence.
1. It is commonly associated with umbilical artery catheterization.
2. The clinical presentation, in whole or in part, includes the following:
   a. Hypertension/congestive heart failure.
   b. Hematuria.
   c. Proteinuria.
   d. Azotemia.
   e. Duskiness of lower extremities after placement of umbilical artery catheter.
   f. Nonopacification of involved kidney on nuclear renal scanning.
3. Management.
   a. Treatment of hypertension if present.
   b. Nephrectomy should be performed only if blood pressure elevation is severe and difficult to control medically.

B. Renal vein thrombosis (see p. 140); potentially lethal.

C. Renal cortical necrosis; potentially lethal.
1. Associated with the following:
   a. Hypoxia/intrauterine distress.
   b. Dehydration.
   c. Sepsis.
   d. Blood loss.
   e. Birth trauma.
2. Clinical presentation not unlike bilateral renal vein thrombosis.
   a. Enlarged kidneys.

   b. Thrombocytopenia.
   c. Anemia.
   d. Azotemia.
   e. Hematuria.
   3. Diagnosis. Renal nuclear scanning can differentiate from renal vein thrombosis.
   4. Management is supportive and includes management of renal failure.
   C. Obstructive uropathy (see pp. 140-142), particularly after difficult, traumatic delivery.
   D. Renal tumor (see pp. 140-142), particularly after difficult, traumatic delivery.

XV. URACHUS (PERSISTENT BAND OR LUMEN)
   A. Presentation.
   1. Inversion of umbilicus, apparent pain on voiding (persistent band).
   2. Draining urine at umbilicus (patent lumen). A potential of infection exists if sinuses or cysts form, involving the entire tract from umbilicus to bladder.
   B. Diagnosis.
   1. Ultrasound of bladder and infraumbilical abdominal wall.
   2. Methylene blue, instilled at umbilicus, voided in urine.
   3. Carmine red dye, orally, discharged at umbilicus in the rare event of associated enteric fistula.
   C. Management. Surgical excision.

XVI. EXSTROPHY OF BLADDER (About 1 in 30,000 Births)
N.B.: Prompt referral to an experienced pediatric urologist is mandatory.

BIBLIOGRAPHY

American Academy of Pediatrics Task Force on Circumcision: Circumcision policy statement, *Pediatrics* 103:686, 1999.

American College of Obstetricians and Gynecologists: *Ultrasound in pregnancy,* Technical Bulletin 116, Washington, DC, 1988, ACOG.

Elder JS, Duckett JW: Management of the fetus and neonate with hydronephrosis detected by prenatal ultrasonography, *Pediatr Ann* 17:19, 1988.

Hadlock FP, Deter RL, Carpenter R, et al: Sonography of fetal urinary tract anomalies, *Am J Radiol* 137:261, 1981.

Lawson TL, Foley WD, Berland LL, et al: Ultrasonic evaluations of fetal kidneys, *Radiology* 138:153, 1988.

Mussels M, Gaudoy CL, Bason WM: Renal anomalies in the newborn found by deep palpation, *Pediatrics* 47:97, 1971.

Perlmutter DF, Lawrence JH, Krauss AN, Auld PAM: Voiding after neonatal circumcision, *Pediatrics* 96:1111, 1995.

Pinto KJ, Noe HN, Jenkins GR: Management of neonatal testicular torsion, *J Urol* 158:1196, 1997.

Silver RI, Roriguez RI, Chang TS, Gearhart JP: In vitro fertilization is associated with an increased risk of hypospadias, *J Urol* 161:1954, 1999.

Stephens FD: *Congenital malformations of the urinary tract,* New York, 1983, Praeger.

14

The Nervous System

REBECCA N. ICHORD

I. HYDROCEPHALUS
A. Fetal ventriculomegaly.
1. Definition. Enlarged ventricular diameter with enlarged head circumference for gestational age.
2. Causes. Fetal ventriculomegaly is isolated in <20% of cases and occurs with other anomalies in >80% of cases. Common causes include the following:
   a. Developmental anomalies associated with fetal ventriculomegaly include neural tube defects (NTDs), aqueductal stenosis, Dandy-Walker malformation (DWM), multiple congenital anomalies, encephalocele, and holoprosencephaly.
   b. Acquired in utero insults include porencephaly, infection (e.g., toxoplasmosis, cytomegalovirus [CMV]), hydranencephaly, and in utero intracranial hemorrhage.
   c. Idiopathic communicating hydrocephalus.
3. Detection can be made by fetal ultrasound of the choroid plexus: ventricular disproportion at 12 to 22 weeks gestation and an increased ratio of lateral ventricle width to hemisphere width after 22 weeks.
4. Natural history. The majority of these cases that are detected early do not survive to term; among survivors, the outcome is determined by the same factors as in hydrocephalus diagnosed postnatally.
   a. Death, or survival with major handicap, if associated with major anomalies or congenital infection.
   b. Variable intact survival with need for postnatal shunt. Majority of cases of isolated nonsyndromic hydrocephalus have normal intelligence if the condition is managed aggressively and is free of complications.
5. Evaluation. The aim of an evaluation is to prenatally define associated anomalies or the cause of the ventriculomegaly. Examinations include the following:
   a. Detailed fetal ultrasound for central nervous system (CNS) and non-CNS anomalies or NTDs; further morphologic evaluation of the fetus can sometimes be obtained using magnetic resonance imaging (MRI).

    b. Fetal karyotype and gender determination if the pedigree shows an X-linked pattern.

    c. Pedigree and indicated examination of family members.

    d. Serology for toxoplasmosis, CMV.

    e. Assessment of alpha-fetoprotein (AFP) levels.

6. Management. There is little consensus concerning the role of in utero cerebrospinal fluid (CSF) diversion procedures or mode of delivery.

    a. If prenatal study shows nonviable anomalies, major anomalies, or poor prognosis, consider nonintervention or pregnancy termination with appropriate family consultation and counseling.

    b. If there are no major anomalies or the prognosis is reasonable, weekly fetal ultrasound and assessment of lung maturity should be done. If there is progressive or severe ventriculomegaly, the fetus should be delivered by cesarean section as early as it is safe to do so.

    c. In utero ventricular tap should be performed only in extreme circumstances if early delivery is not feasible.

    d. In utero shunting has unproven value and a high complication rate.

    e. Provide prenatal counseling to family of possibility of inaccurate diagnosis based on fetal ultrasound. Verify abnormality postnatally with computed tomography (CT) or MRI.

B. Congenital hydrocephalus.

1. Definition. Congenital hydrocephalus is ventriculomegaly with macrocephaly (head circumference greater than two standard deviations above the mean for gestational age) or excessive head growth in the first months of life.

2. Incidence. 0.5 to 3:1000 live births; about one third of cases occur among premature infants, two thirds occur in term infants.

3. Causes include the following:

    a. Posthemorrhagic. Congenital hydrocephalus can be caused by intraventricular hemorrhage (IVH) usually related to germinal matrix hemorrhage occuring prenatally; subdural hemorrhage, which is often associated with trauma; parenchymal hemorrhage or subarachnoid hemorrhage, which may be associated with vascular malformations or coagulopathy; spontaneous choroid plexus hemorrhage is a possible cause in term infants with isolated intraventricular hemorrhage without coagulopathy.

    b. Postinfectious. Bacterial meningitis, lymphocytic choriomeningitis.

    c. Tumor. Choroid plexus papilloma usually produces severe hydrocephalus and has unfavorable outcome; hamartoma may also cause hydrocephalus.

    d. Vascular. Vein of Galen malformation, venous sinus thrombosis.

    e. Genetic and syndromic. NTDs (e.g., myelomeningocele, encephalocele); aqueductal stenosis may be idiopathic (70%) or genetic (30%). Of genetic causes of aqueductal stenosis, some are autosomal recessive, and some are X-linked related to multiple genetic defects in the L1 neural cell adhesion molecule (LCAM); other malformation syndromes with hydrocephalus include Joubert syndrome, DWM, Walker-Warburg syndrome, holoprosencephaly, and VACTERL (an acronym for *v*ertebral, *a*nal, *c*ardiac, *t*racheal, *e*sophageal, *r*enal, and *l*imb; used to designate a pattern of congenital anomalies) with hydrocephalus.

4. Clinical signs and symptoms (in increasing order of gravity). Excessive head growth, suture diastasis, bulging fontanel, irritability, vomiting, sixth nerve palsy, downward gaze preference, posturing or hypertonia, lethargy, apnea/bradycardia. Cushing's triad (hypertension, irregular respiration, and bradycardia) and papilledema are rare.

5. Natural history. There is a high mortality rate if untreated; developmental handicap depends on the cause, other anomalies, and occurrence of shunt complications. The majority of cases require revisions for shunt malfunction (40% to 50%) or infection (10%), mostly in the first year. Most survivors (>60%) have normal intelligence regardless of initial cortical mantle thickness.
   a. Aqueductal stenosis and myelomeningocele. More than 90% of affected children have normal IQ; there is a high risk of learning disability. A majority (60% to 80%) need a shunt by the age of 6 months.
   b. Dandy-Walker or other major CNS malformations. The majority of cases have subnormal IQ and variable motor deficits. Almost all need a shunt.
   c. Posthemorrhagic, postinfectious. These cases occur mostly after higher-grade IVH (30% to 50% of grades 3 and 4); a majority of survivors have major handicap, especially if <28 weeks gestation at birth; about half need a shunt.

6. Evaluation should include the following:
   a. Clinical examination for associated anomalies.
   b. Neuroimaging. A baseline head ultrasound should be obtained if frequent ventricular monitoring is anticipated; a head CT should be done for etiologic and preoperative definition; a head MRI should be done if there is suspicion of a brainstem or posterior fossa abnormality, tumor, neuronal migration defect, or vascular malformation.
   c. Consider lumbar puncture (LP) if communicating hydrocephalus is shown on neuroimaging and if CSF pressure or protein content will influence the surgical decision. Normal full-term newborn opening pressure is <10 cm H_2O.
   d. Transcranial Doppler (TCD). Assessment of resistive index (RI) can provide a serial noninvasive measure of intracranial compliance. Large intersubject variance of RI limits conclusions about absolute values of intracranial pressure; however, RI is a sensitive indicator of changes in intracranial compliance over time within an individual infant. Combined with data on head circumference, clinical symptoms, and static imaging, TCD can assist with decisions on if and when to perform ventricular drainage or permanent shunting.
   e. Family pedigree and examination of indicated family members.

f. Additional studies to establish cause, as indicated by clinical findings and neuroimaging, include karyotype, TORCH serology, and eye examination for chorioretinitis.

7. Management. Treatment of obstructive hydrocephalus in NTDs, aqueductal stenosis, and other syndromic cases is straightforward and involves shunt placement within the first month. Shunt infection rates increase in NTDs when closure of the primary defect is delayed more than 36 hours. Treatment for posthemorrhagic hydrocephalus is more variable and controversial. The aim is to diminish operative risk and postoperative complications and to avoid shunting, if possible, while minimizing the neurologic sequelae of elevated intracranial pressure. Efficacy of all treatments for posthemorrhagic hydrocephalus in premature infants in improving neurodevelopmental outcome is uncertain. Clinical monitoring of the medically managed infant should continue for 6 to 12 months postnatally to detect late-onset or recurrence after discontinuation of medical therapy.

a. Nonsurgical treatment is indicated if the patient is medically unstable, too small for surgery, or if ventriculomegaly is borderline in severity and not accompanied by symptomatic intracranial hypertension.

(1) Diuretics are most useful in the treatment of posthemorrhagic hydrocephalus, in which their use can delay or prevent the need for permanent shunt placement. Furosemide (1 to 2 mg/kg per day) and acetazolamide (25 mg/kg per day divided into three daily doses, increasing up to 100 mg/kg per day if needed) are used. Patients should be monitored and treated for electrolyte and acid-base abnormalities. Monitoring for hypercalciuria can be done to prevent nephrocalcinosis. Some centers use acetazolamide alone to reduce the incidence of nephrocalcinosis.

(2) CSF diversion procedures.

(a) Serial LP can be used only in communicating hydrocephalus. Indications are controversial; some advocate it within 3 days of diagnosis of grades 3 or 4 IVH; others reserve it for symptomatic or rapidly progressive posthemorrhagic hydrocephalus, or if diuretics are ineffective and the patient is not a surgical candidate. Frequency and duration of taps and volume of CSF removed are individualized. Pretap and posttap ultrasound or TCD have been suggested to monitor efficacy of LP in individual infants. Complications include infection. Serial LP may delay but not prevent the need for a shunt.

(b) Ventricular drainage via direct tap, indwelling drain, or reservoir. Useful in cases of noncommunicating hydrocephalus, or when diuretics or serial LPs fail and symptoms of intracranial pressure elevation dictate decompression. Complications include infection, obstruction, and hemorrhage. Many centers favor use of subcutaneous reservoirs over indwelling drains because of a lower complication rate. External diversion procedures are commonly favored over medical treatment in babies with severe progressive hydrocephalus after grade 3 or 4 hemorrhage who are too small (<2 kg) or too ill to readily tolerate a permanent shunt placement. Typical schedules of CSF removal involve twice daily to every other day taps, removing 2 to 10 ml at a time. Treatment schedules are individualized according to head growth, symptoms, ultrasound parameters, and direct measurement of opening and closing pressures. Devices can be kept in place for a prolonged period (2 to 3 months), with variable infection rates (8% to 30%). Most (60% to 80%) ultimately require replacement with a permanent shunt.

   (c) Intraventricular thrombolytics. Small series using intraventricular urokinase or rtPA have been reported. Although these therapies can achieve clot lysis, they have shown variable ability to improve outcomes in terms of ease of controlling ventriculomegaly or the need for a permanent shunt; complications include new hemorrhage.

  b. Surgical treatment applies when the underlying disorder is unlikely to resolve spontaneously, ventricular enlargement is progressive or symptomatic, and operative risk factors are optimal. A ventriculoperitoneal route is preferred over a ventriculoatrial one.

II. NEURAL TUBE DEFECTS
A. Spinal defects.

1. Myelomeningocele (spina bifida cystica).
    a. Definition. Failure of posterior neural tube closure with defects in meninges, bone, and skin, resulting in maldevelopment, injury, and dysfunction of neural elements.
    b. Incidence. 0.5 to 2:1000 live births in United States; 1 to 6:1000 live births in United Kingdom.
    c. Pathogenesis. Folic acid deficiency plays a significant role, leading public health policy makers to recommend folate supplementation by all pregnant women (400 μg/day) and women of childbearing age (4000 μg/day). This intervention is believed capable of preventing 50% to 70% of cases of NTDs. Genetic factors also play a role. Inheritance is multifactorial, unless it is syndromic. Recurrence risk is 5% if there is a single affected first-degree relative (sibling, parent), 10% if there are two affected first-degree relatives, 2% if there is an affected second-degree relative, and 1% if there is an affected third-degree relative.
    d. Clinical features.
        (1) Frequency by level affected. Above the thoracolumbar junction: 5%; at the thoracolumbar junction: 45%; at the lumbar level: 20%; at the lumbosacral junction: 20%; and at the sacral area: 10%.
        (2) Neurologic examination. The head circumference is usually normal or small before back repair. There are frequent (25% to 30%) lower brainstem signs (e.g., suck-swallow dysfunction, stri-

dor, apnea). Motor and sensory deficits vary according to level and are often asymmetric; there is often sensorimotor dissociation (Table 14-1).

(3) Associated features. An Arnold-Chiari anomaly is seen in all cases. Hydrocephalus is found in 90% of cases with lumbar lesions and 60% with lesions at other sites. Bladder incontinence is common, with increased risk for urinary tract infection. Foot and spine deformities are seen.

e. Outcome. Cognitive studies show normal IQ if spinal defects are nonsyndromic and there are no major shunt complications. There is a high prevalence of higher cortical dysfunction and a need for special education resources. Motor and bowel/bladder functional outcomes depend on the level of the lesion (Table 14-2) and may decline in childhood or adolescence because of tethered cord syndrome. Diagnosis of lesion level and of motor prognosis can be accurately determined by prenatal ultrasound. Sudden death during sleep accounts for 10% of mortality, and may be related to sleep-disordered breathing.

f. Management. A high incidence of latex allergy has led some centers to institute latex prophylaxis measures at birth.

TABLE 14-1
Motor and Sensory Findings in Myelomeningocele

Spinal cord level	Motor function	Sensory function	Reflex
L1-2	Hip flexion	Inguinal to anterior upper thigh	
L3-4	Knee extension	Anterior lower thigh and knee to medial lower leg	Knee
L5-S1	Ankle flexion, knee extension	Lateral lower leg and medial foot to sole of foot	Ankle
S1-2	Ankle extension, hip extension	Sole of foot, posterior leg and thigh	
S3-4	Bowel and bladder sphincters	Perineum and buttocks	Anal wink

TABLE 14-2
Functional Prognosis in Myelomeningocele With Optimal Aggressive Management

Level	Prognosis
Above L3	Mostly wheelchair bound
L4-S1	Partial ambulation with assistive devices
Below S1	Ambulate without assistance

(1) Mode of delivery. There is no broad consensus; data are inconclusive concerning the benefit of a prelabor cesarean section.

(2) A preoperative neurologic evaluation should look for associated conditions and clinically define motor and sensory levels. Preoperative ultrasound or CT examinations of the head can be used to define intracranial anatomy. An MRI of the head should be done if the infant is symptomatic from lower brainstem compression (Arnold-Chiari).

(3) Chiari malformation. Consider MRI of the head during the neonatal period in all patients with a Chiari malformation. Obtain sleep study and feeding and swallowing evaluations early in the treatment course if there are any feeding problems, apnea, stridor, disordered breathing during sleep, or signs of lower cranial nerve dysfunction on examination. Consider posterior decompression if there are any significant signs or symptoms of lower brainstem dysfunction or cervicomedullary compression. Evaluation and intervention of neonates with symptomatic Chiari anomalies should proceed rapidly because of the high risk of rapid and irreversible progression of brainstem dysfunction.

(4) Urinary tract management. Monitor voiding patterns and postvoiding residuals; obtain a urology consultation. Upper and lower tract imaging should be done in the first month.

(5) Back repair should be performed within 48 hours of birth, if possible; preoperative antibiotics should be used if a CSF leak is present; postoperative antibiotic use is at the discretion of the surgeon.

(6) Hydrocephalus. Monitor daily for head circumference, signs of increased intracranial pressure, and back wound healing. Shunt when dictated by progressive symptoms.

(7) Psychosocial issues. Provide informative and supportive family counseling throughout.

2. Occult dysraphism (spina bifida occulta).
   a. Definition. Incomplete bony fusion of vertebral elements with intact skin/meningeal elements, with or without neural involvement.
   b. Clinical findings in the neonate. Overlies the lumbosacral spine. May cause CNS infection, root entrapment, tethered cord, spine deformity, or, rarely, hydrocephalus or Arnold-Chiari.
      (1) Skin, subcutaneous. Simple midline dimples have low risk (<1%) of underlying spinal dysraphism; high-risk (>40% have associated spinal defects) cutaneous lesions include large dimples (>5 mm), high (>2.5 cm above anus) or raised lesions with complex pigmentation, hair, or hemangioma.
      (2) Vertebrae, cord. Incomplete fusion, meningocele, lipomyelomeningocele, syringomyelia, diastematomyelia.
      (3) Neurologic findings create a variable picture. Some are symptomatic as newborns, others develop upper motor neuron signs or sphincter dysfunction in infancy, and still others remain clinically silent. There are rare isolated lumbosacral root syndromes and progressive paraparesis in adolescence.

    c. Management. Spinal ultrasound of the neonate can be used to screen suspicious lesions; MRI of the spine is needed for comprehensive definition of abnormalities. This should be followed by a careful neurologic examination for upper motor neuron signs (e.g., spasticity, hyperreflexia, clonus), urinary tract and orthopedic evaluation, neurosurgical consultation, and prenatal and genetic counseling. Early surgery is recommended for lipomeningocele, dermoid sinus or cyst, diastematomyelia, or symptomatic tethered cord (as indicated by bladder dysfunction or upper motor neuron findings on examination).

B. Cranial defects.

1. Anencephaly is the complete failure of anterior neural tube closure. There is a 100% rate of stillborn or neonatal mortality. Most cases are detectable by fetal ultrasound or maternal AFP screening. Autopsy and karyotype can rule out syndromes. Family and genetic counseling are needed.

2. Encephalocele is partial failure of anterior neural tube closure.
   a. 75% are occipital, 15% are frontoethmoid, and 10% are located in other sites.
   b. Clinical features include microcephaly if there is extensive brain herniation, or associated neuronal migration disorder. There is an infection risk if the skin is broken. Neurologic deficits depend on the site (rare in frontal lesions) and extent of brain herniation; one third have spinal defects. There is high prenatal and perinatal mortality for large occipital defects. Outcome is related to site (posterior lesions have worse outcome than frontal) and severity of lesion and presence of associated anomalies. A majority have associated major malformations.
   c. Genetics. Encephaloceles may be syndromic (e.g., Meckel syndrome); most are multifactorial. The recurrence risk is the same as with myelomeningocele.
   d. Management. Defer invasive management pending full evaluation of the defects and family consultation and counseling. The route of delivery is debatable; consider cesarean section if aggressive therapy is planned. Evaluation includes measurement of head circumference, complete physical examination, karyotype if associated anomalies or syndrome are suspected, neuroimaging to define ventricular size and extent of malformation (MRI is most informative). Surgical treatment involves aggressive surgery for frontal lesions, or palliative surgery for occipital lesions. Hydrocephalus should be monitored and treated (occurs in 70% of occipital lesions, 10% of frontal lesions).

III. INTRACRANIAL HEMORRHAGE

A. Premature infants.
Types of intracranial hemorrhage in premature infants cover a broad spectrum, including periventricular hemorrhage (PVH) and periventricular white matter (PVL) injuries (Table 14-3).

1. Incidence. Most centers report declining incidence in the 1990s; the incidence increases with decreasing gestational age; babies <1500 g at birth have PVH in 14% to 47% of cases; 5% to 16% have PVL.

TABLE 14-3
Spectrum of Periventricular Injuries in Prematurity

Pathologic lesion	Radiologic correlate by ultrasound
Subependymal hemorrhage	Grade 1 PVH
Intraventricular hemorrhage without ventriculomegaly	Grade 2 PVH
Intraventricular hemorrhage with ventriculomegaly	Grade 3 PVH
Periventricular white matter hemorrhage, usually with IVH	Grade 4 PVH
Periventricular or subcortical white matter ischemic changes	
Transient edema, ischemia	Transient echodensities
Noncystic gliosis, calcification	Prolonged flare, >2 wk
Cystic necrosis	Cystic PVL
Posthemorrhage ventriculomegaly	Ventricular dilation

PVH, Periventricular or intraventricular hemorrhage; *PVL,* periventricular white matter injuries.

2. Pathogenesis. The pathogenesis for intracranial hemorrhage includes ischemia to watershed regions, hemorrhage during reperfusion into ischemic regions, and a histologically immature vascular bed. Risk factors include prolonged hypotension, decreasing gestational age, difficult vaginal delivery, chorioamnionitis, outborn status, respiratory distress syndrome (RDS), fluctuating blood pressure, coagulopathy, and patent ductus arteriosus.

3. Clinical features. Intracranial hemorrhage is often clinically silent, but clinical features may include lethargy, bulging fontanel, apnea/bradycardia, posturing, seizures, tone abnormalities, eye movement abnormalities, or falling hematocrit. Most occur in the first 4 days of life.

4. Management begins with maternal transport. In the newborn, avoid hypotension, hypercarbia, and wide blood pressure fluctuations; correct coagulopathies (see pp. 150-151). Serial ultrasound studies of the head should be performed to assess periventricular lesions; CT or MRI scans should be done with peripheral parenchymal or posterior fossa/brainstem lesions. See the section on posthemorrhagic hydrocephalus on p. 148.

5. Outcome. There is high mortality in grade 4 PVH (30% to 50%); with grade 1 or 2 PVH, there is no increased risk of major handicap; with grade 3 PVH, there is a moderately increased risk of major handicap (10% to 20%). The majority of infants with grade 4 PVH have a major handicap. In PVL, the risk of major handicap variably increases with increasing extent of lesions; motor handicaps predominate.

6. Promising preventive interventions undergoing clinical trial include the use of antenatal phenobarbital, antenatal steroids, postnatal indomethacin, and antenatal magnesium.

B. Full-term infants.

1. Types of hemorrhage include intraventricular, subarachnoid, subdural, and parenchymal.
2. Causes include trauma, arteriovenous malformation, hemorrhage into an infarct, or coagulopathy.
3. Clinical features depend on the cause, location, and severity. They may include acute global encephalopathy, isolated focal seizures, signs of increased intracranial pressure, subacute focal motor deficits, or craniofacial trauma. Significant intraventricular or subarachnoid blood causes chemical meningitis. There is a risk of acute or subacute onset of hydrocephalus.
4. Evaluation includes ultrasound of the head for initial screen and serial ventricular monitoring, MRI of the head for cause, cerebral angiography if arteriovenous malformation is suspected. Rule out coagulopathy, including inherited hypercoagulable states.
5. Management includes hemodynamic/respiratory support, anticonvulsants as needed, decompression of symptomatic hydrocephalus, correction of coagulopathy, and surgery as indicated for symptomatic subdural and amenable arteriovenous malformations. Family counseling and rehabilitation are also required.
6. Outcome may be good if there is no diffuse hypoxic-ischemic injury and if hydrocephalus is aggressively treated.

IV. SEIZURES

A. Clinical features. *Seizure types* refer to individual ictal events of any cause; *seizure syndromes* refer to recognizable patterns of recurrent seizures.

1. Clinical seizure types include paroxysmal involuntary behavior caused by hypersynchronous CNS activity; these are distinguished from reflexes and dystonia, which are more likely stimulus sensitive and suppressible by restraint or repositioning.
   a. Tonic. Focal or generalized sustained posturing of limbs or trunk.
   b. Clonic. Focal or multifocal rhythmic (1 to 3 per second) jerking movements.
   c. Myoclonic. Focal or multifocal, generalized, fleeting, nonrhythmic spasms (predominantly flexors).
   d. Subtle, fragmentary. Tonic or jerking eye movements, oral-buccal-lingual movements, limb automatisms, apneic spells, autonomic paroxysms.
   e. Status epilepticus. The criteria for diagnosis are controversial in neonates; some have suggested to treat seizures as status if during a 2- to 4-hour continuous electroencephalogram (EEG) recording, more than 30% of the record consists of electrographic or electroclinical seizures.
2. Seizure syndromes.
   a. Benign familial neonatal convulsions are isolated clonic seizures, beginning day 2 to 3. Findings include a normal neurologic examination, minimally abnormal EEG, and a positive family history. Most resolve within months.

  b. With myoclonic encephalopathy, the onset is in the first week; multifocal myoclonic seizures progress to mixed intractable seizures and global neurologic dysfunction. There is burst suppression on EEG. Seizures may be the result of inborn errors of metabolism; rule out nonketotic hyperglycemia.

  c. Pyridoxine deficiency/dependency. A careful history may suggest intrauterine seizures. These seizures are extremely resistant to standard anticonvulsants and are diagnosed by therapeutic trial of intravenous pyridoxine with EEG monitoring.

3. Seizure syndromes must be differentiated from tremors, jitteriness, stimulus-provoked clonus, decerebrate posturing from intracranial pressure (ICP) elevation, normal stretching, and sleep myoclonus.

4. EEG. Electrographic seizures without clinical events are common in the neonatal intensive care unit (NICU) population; EEG results correlate more likely with focal and multifocal clonic, focal tonic, or generalized myoclonic seizures.

B. Causes. Frequency varies among centers and populations.

1. Hypoxic-ischemic encephalopathy (30% to 60%).

2. Vascular (20% to 30%). Intracranial hemorrhage, thromboembolic infarction, venous occlusive infarct.

3. Infection (5% to 10%). Congenital (TORCH), acquired viral encephalitis, bacterial meningitis.

4. Metabolic. Transient disturbances involving Ca^{++}, Na^+, Mg^{++}, or glucose, or inborn errors of metabolism that include hyperglycinemia, amino and organic acidopathies, peroxisomal disorders, oxidative metabolism defects, sulfite oxidase deficiency, pyridoxine deficiency/dependency, mitochondrial disorders, or glucose transporter defect.

5. Drugs, toxins. Drug withdrawal (especially heroin and methadone), maternal cocaine use, xanthines, lidocaine.

6. Trauma. Contusions, hemorrhage.

7. Genetic and malformation syndromes. Phakomatoses (tuberous sclerosis, incontinentia pigmenti), major CNS malformations (e.g., holoprosencephaly), migration defects (e.g., lissencephaly), chromosomal disorders (uncommon in trisomy 21).

C. Evaluation. Examinations are sequential, depending on known causative factors.

1. Carefully document the nature of events and time course.

2. Screen all infants for Na^+, Ca^{++}, Mg^{++}, and glucose levels; acid-base status; hematologic and clotting profiles; and oxygenation.

3. A detailed examination should be conducted for focal deficits, global encephalopathy, signs of intracranial hypertension, cranial trauma, and genetic/congenital syndromes.

4. Neuroimaging. If there is no benign correctable metabolic disturbance, obtain screening sonograms of the head. Include a Doppler examination for sagittal sinus thrombosis if available. Better definition of abnormalities can be obtained by CT or MRI scans if stroke, diffuse ischemia, or extraaxial hemorrhage is suspected; MRI should be done if venous sinus thrombosis is suspected. Studies may need to

be repeated at 7 to 10 days if abnormalities are poorly defined on the first examination.

5. LP should be done in all infants, especially if infection is suspected and to define subarachnoid hemorrhage (SAH) not well visualized by imaging.

6. Use of EEG is controversial. The severity and duration of background abnormalities are very important for characterizing the severity of global acute brain injury. Prolonged EEG with simultaneous real-time clinical observation is helpful to distinguish clinical nonepileptic events from epileptic events and to monitor frequency of electrographic seizures and their response to anticonvulsant drugs.

7. Metabolic studies. If cause is undetermined by other studies, consider determining levels of serum ammonium, plasma amino acids, urine organic acids, blood lactate and pyruvate, plasma long-chain fatty acids, plasma uric acid, and urinary sulfites. Careful attention should be paid to CSF glucose levels; measure CSF glycine if plasma glycine level is equivocally elevated.

D. Management. There are no definitive controlled prospective clinical studies showing whether aggressive anticonvulsant therapy alters long-term functional outcome or incidence of late-onset epilepsy. Standards of treatment are widely variable and are determined by consensus among neonatologists and neurologists within a given center.

1. General. Correct fluid/chemical imbalances; maintain adequate ventilation, oxygenation, and perfusion; maintain normoglycemia and normothermia; avoid syndrome of inappropriate antidiuretic hormone (SIADH).

2. Anticonvulsants. Efficacy of standard anticonvulsants is poor. One third of cases are controlled with a loading dose of phenobarbital or phenytoin, and two thirds are controlled with combined phenobarbital and phenytoin. Severity of seizures and resistance to anticonvulsants are directly related to severity of underlying brain disorder; they usually remit spontaneously over hours or days.

a. Whom to treat. Infants with recurring clinical seizures with an adverse hemodynamic or respiratory impact on the infant (e.g., ictal apnea); infants with frequent (multiple/hour) clinical or electrographic seizures associated with severe acute brain injury (e.g., hemorrhage or ischemia) in whom it is desirable to minimize secondary brain metabolic stress arising from frequent seizures.

b. Drugs. Phenobarbital (first line), phenytoin (second line), or benzodiazepines (short term). See Table 14-4 for dosage guidelines. The general strategy is to give a full loading dose of the first drug (phenobarbital most commonly), followed by repeat boluses of one fourth of the loading dose at time intervals of 1 to 24 hours, titrating to achieve the desired level of seizure control. If seizure activity fails to improve significantly after loading dose of the first drug, then give the loading dose of the second drug (phenytoin, most commonly). Benzodiazepines are useful for short-term control while awaiting infusion or equilibration of longer-acting anticonvulsants. Monitor continuously for arrhythmia, hypotension,

TABLE 14-4
Anticonvulsant Drugs in Newborns

Drug	Dose	Comment
Phenobarbital	*Loading:* 15-20 mg/kg intravenously *Maintenance:* 3-6 mg/kg/day intravenously or orally once daily	Monitor for respiratory, cardiac depression; aim for blood levels of 20-50 mg/L
Phenytoin (or phosphenytoin)	*Loading:* 15-20 mg/kg intravenously *Maintenance:* 5-10 mg/kg/day intravenously, or 5-40 mg/kg/day orally, divided twice a day	Monitor for cardiac toxicity; ensure patency of intravenous line to avoid serious burns; absorption by oral route is poor
Diazepam	0.3 mg/kg/dose intravenously 0.5 mg/kg/dose rectally	Short acting; monitor for hypotension, respiratory depression
Lorazepam	0.05 mg/kg/dose intravenously	Short acting; monitor for hypotension, respiratory depression; may provoke myoclonus
Midazolam infusion for status epilepticus	0.15 mg/kg starting dose, then 0.1 mg/kg/hr, increasing every 1-2 hrs to 0.4 mg/kg/hr	Monitor for hypotension, respiratory depression; use with EEG monitoring; taper over 2-6 hrs after achieving 12-24 hrs of clinical and EEG control of seizures

and respiratory depression during drug infusion. Ensure patency of intravenous line, especially when giving phenytoin. Obtain post-loading blood levels to help guide subsequent dosing. "Minimal therapeutic" levels are defined by achieving desired control of seizure activity, and "maximal therapeutic" levels are defined by presence of hemodynamic depression or failure to further augment seizure control with added dosing of the same drug. Midazolam infusion has been recommended for neonatal status epilepticus resistant to standard anticonvulsants, and it should be used with continuous EEG monitoring.

c. When to stop. Consider holding after loading dose if no further seizures recur and there is no or little evidence of ongoing CNS injury. Decrease to phenobarbital monotherapy as acute CNS injury resolves. Discontinue before discharge if neurologic status otherwise returns to normal. If discharged on medication, reevaluate 1 to 3 months after discharge, and consider discontinuation if no seizures occur while patient is on treatment, EEG is favorable, and if probability of chronic epilepsy is relatively low.

V. HYPOTONIA

N.B.: Acute spinal cord injury presents as hypotonia, and infants with neuromuscular disease are at risk for hypoxic-ischemic brain injury.

A. Hypotonia with predominantly CNS involvement.

1. Clinical features include diffusely low tone and diminished movement, with one or more signs of CNS involvement, including disturbed consciousness, cranial nerve deficits, normoreflexia, or hyperreflexia.
2. Causes include any acute encephalopathy, congenital CNS malformation, Prader-Willi syndrome, hypothyroidism, or other inborn errors or genetic syndromes.
3. Evaluation should be appropriate for acute or congenital encephalopathies, including complete examination, laboratory and metabolic screens, neuroimaging, and genetic evaluation.

B. Hypotonia with predominantly neuromuscular involvement.

1. Clinical features include true weakness, muscle atrophy, diminished or absent reflexes, and normal level of consciousness. Signs include ptosis, external ophthalmoplegia, bifacial weakness, dysphagia, respiratory insufficiency, limb and trunk weakness, or stridor.
2. Causes include myotonic dystrophy, congenital myopathies, myasthenia gravis, spinal muscular atrophy, infantile botulism, mitochondrial encephalomyopathy, or metabolic muscle disease.
3. Evaluation.
   a. Serum creatine kinase levels are moderately elevated in congenital dystrophy.
   b. A family history and examination of family members (especially the mother) can positively diagnose myotonic dystrophy.
   c. Electromyography and nerve conduction studies are useful to define neuropathic and myopathic patterns and distribution. Interpretation is difficult in neonates.
   d. Muscle ultrasonography is useful in some centers to guide further invasive testing.
   e. Muscle biopsy, in experienced hands, is useful for certain congenital myopathies, but technically limited in neonates.
   f. Look for coexisting CNS injury.
4. Management includes cardiorespiratory support pending definitive evaluation, optimization of nutrition, and minimization of orthopedic deformities. The family should be prepared for chronic care needs.

C. Acute spinal cord injury.

1. Clinical features include flaccid paralysis and hypesthesia (sensory level), usually at the cervical level, with variable respiratory insufficiency; neurogenic bladder; and Horner syndrome. Initially, infants are areflexic, then later hyperreflexic.
2. Obstetric history is compatible with cervical trauma.
3. Evaluation includes plain-film radiographs of the neck, which are usually nondiagnostic; MRI of the spine is abnormal (e.g., reveals edema,

hemorrhage); a paraspinal electromyogram (EMG) may confirm and localize diagnosis.
4. **Management.** Stabilize the neck and avoid further acute neck mobilization; maintain airway and ventilation; support blood pressure; allow conservative fluid administration. Early high-dose steroid administration has been suggested but not studied in the neonate.

BIBLIOGRAPHY

Abdel-Rahman AM, Rosenberg AA: Prevention of intraventricular hemorrhage in the premature infant, *Clin Perinatol* 21:505-521, 1994.

American Academy of Pediatrics Committee on Genetics: Folic acid for the prevention of neural tube defects [see comments], *Pediatrics* 92:493-494, 1993.

Casey AT, Kimmings EJ, Kleinlugtebeld AD, et al: The long-term outlook for hydrocephalus in childhood: a ten-year cohort study of 155 patients, *Pediatr Neurosurg* 27:63-70, 1997.

Chervenak FA, Berkowitz RL, Tortora M, et al: The management of fetal hydrocephalus, *Am J Obstet Gynecol* 151:933-942, 1985.

Cochrane DD, Wilson RD, Steinbok P, et al: Prenatal spinal evaluation and functional outcome of patients born with myelomeningocele: information for improved prenatal counselling and outcome prediction, *Fetal Diagn Ther* 11:159-168, 1996.

David DJ: Cephaloceles: classification, pathology, and management–a review, *J Craniofac Surg* 4:192-202, 1993.

Gamache FWJ: Treatment of hydrocephalus in patients with meningomyelocele or encephalocele: a recent series, *Childs Nerv Syst* 11:487-488, 1995.

Haverkamp F, Wolfle J, Aretz M, et al: Congenital hydrocephalus internus and aqueduct stenosis: etiology and implications for genetic counselling, *Eur J Pediatr* 158:474-478, 1999.

Kellaway P, Mizrahi EM: Clinical, electroencephalographic, therapeutic, and pathophysiologic studies of neonatal seizures. In Wasterlain CG, Vert P (editors): *Neonatal seizures*, New York, 1990, Raven Press.

McLone DG: Care of the neonate with a myelomeningocele, *Neurosurg Clin North Am* 9:111-120, 1998.

Oi S, Matsumoto S, Katayama K, et al: Pathophysiology and postnatal outcome of fetal hydrocephalus, *Childs Nerv Syst* 6:338-345, 1990.

Painter MJ, Scher MS, Stein AD, et al: Phenobarbital compared with phenytoin for the treatment of neonatal seizures, *N Engl J Med* 341:485-489, 1999.

Perlman JM, Lynch B, Volpe JJ: Late hydrocephalus after arrest and resolution of neonatal post-hemorrhagic hydrocephalus, *Dev Med Child Neurol* 32:725-729, 1990.

du Plessis AJ: Posthemorrhagic hydrocephalus and brain injury in the preterm infant: dilemmas in diagnosis and management, *Semin Pediatr Neurol* 5:161-179, 1998.

Pollack IF, Kinnunen D, Albright AL: The effect of early craniocervical decompression on functional outcome in neonates and young infants with myelodysplasia and symptomatic Chiari II malformations: results from a prospective series, *Neurosurgery* 38:703-710, 1996.

Volpe JJ: Brain injury in the premature infant: overview of clinical aspects, neuropathology, and pathogenesis, *Semin Pediatr Neurol* 5:135-151, 1998.

15

Orthopedics

PAUL D. SPONSELLER

I. BASIC PRINCIPLES

A. **Growth occurs in response to forces applied to bone.** Many angular and rotational abnormalities and dislocations occur in response to in utero constraints, and these deformities remodel if constraints are relieved.

B. **Epiphyses and growth plates are located at ends of long-bone metaphyses.** Large, unossified, cartilaginous ends of bone appear empty (radiolucent) on the radiograph of the neonate (Fig. 15-1). The distal femoral ossific nucleus appears at 39 weeks of gestation, and that of the proximal tibia at 40 weeks.

C. **Acute joint dislocations never occur in the neonate in response to trauma.** More common are Salter-1 fractures. The hip and knee dislocations, which are occasionally observed at birth, are the product of prolonged, extreme malposition in utero.

D. **Remodeling potential is great in the neonate,** so exact reduction of fractures is unnecessary. Healing is fast (usually 1 to 3 weeks until bone is clinically solid).

E. **Perinatal ligamentous laxity is greatest within the first 2 to 3 days.** Treatment should be started early in certain deformities (e.g., clubfoot).

II. REGIONAL ABNORMALITIES

A. Upper extremities.
  1. Fractures.
    a. Clavicle. Fracture occurs in 2.5% of live births; mostly with cephalic presentation (particularly with large baby or shoulder dystocia). May be either greenstick (incomplete) or complete.
      (1) Findings include localized tenderness, crepitus, hematoma; later, a firm mass of callus is noted. Pseudoparalysis is present if fracture is complete, but some hand and elbow motion is usually present.
      (2) Diagnosis. Radiographs are indicated only if unsure of diagnosis on physical examination; further radiographs are not necessary as healing is uneventful.

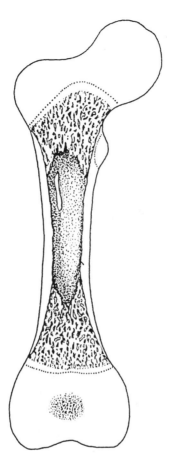

FIG. 15-1. Structure of typical long bone (femur) in the neonate: diaphysis (shaft) is the primary ossification center, but the cortex has not developed full strength; epiphysis (secondary center) is largely cartilaginous at this stage, with small center ossification only in distal femur.

    (3) Treatment. If discomfort is minimal, no treatment is necessary; if fracture is painful, immobilize arm to trunk with elastic bandage or sling support. Clinical healing usually takes about 10 days.

    (4) Differential diagnosis includes brachial plexus palsy, congenital pseudoarthrosis of clavicle (nontender, no healing, right

more often than left), infection, or humeral physeal or shaft fracture.

b. Humerus (proximal).

(1) The etiology of proximal humerus fractures is usually hyperextension or abduction. It is usually a Salter-1 or Salter-2 fracture of the proximal humeral growth plate.

(2) Physical findings show tenderness over the humeral neck; swelling is greater than with a clavicle fracture; it may coexist with brachial plexus palsy.

(3) Radiographic findings show the metaphysis laterally or longitudinally displaced with respect to the glenoid; it often resembles shoulder dislocation because the epiphysis of the humerus is unossified.

(4) Treatment. Using elastic bandage, wrap arm to trunk for 1 to 2 weeks.

c. Humerus (midshaft).

(1) The etiology of midshaft fractures of the humerus is forcible traction or rotation of the arm during delivery.

(2) Findings include decreased mobility, audible snap, and swelling; may have radial nerve palsy (usually resolves in 1 to 3 months).

(3) Treatment. Using elastic bandage, wrap arm to trunk for 2 to 3 weeks and/or apply splints made from tongue depressors.

d. Humerus (distal).

(1) The etiology of distal humerus fractures is elbow hyperextension, usually during a breech delivery.

(2) Findings include decreased mobility, swelling, and crepitus.

(3) Radiographic examination often requires a comparison view because elbow ossification centers have not appeared.

(4) Treatment. Use of a long arm splint in flexion for 2 weeks.

2. Brachial plexus injury.

a. Etiology is a stretch injury to the brachial plexus (Fig. 15-2), usually seen in large infants (e.g., infants of diabetic mothers) or difficult deliveries; occurs in approximately 1:1000 deliveries.

b. Types.

(1) Erb (C5-C6) palsy. Caused by downward force on the shoulder and lateral flexion of the neck; usually a cephalic delivery. Leads to loss of shoulder motion and elbow flexion (arm in "waiter's tip" position).

(2) Klumpke (C8-T1) palsy. Caused by overhead traction on the arm; often in breech position. There is loss of finger and wrist flexion (absent grasp) and Horner syndrome may be present.

(3) Combined. Entire plexus is involved.

c. Differential diagnosis.

(1) Fracture of clavicle/humerus. Generally there is greater swelling, pain, and crepitus, but palsy may *coexist* with the fracture, especially after a difficult delivery.

(2) Central nervous system (CNS) or spinal cord injury; weakness in other extremities.

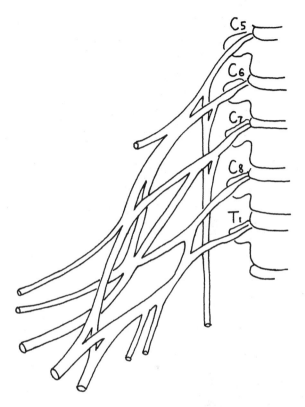

FIG. 15-2. The brachial plexus. Note that the fifth and sixth nerve roots are more vulnerable to stretch. Therefore Erb (upper trunk) palsy is more common.

      (3) Infection. Moro reflex usually not affected by infectious process.

  d. Evaluation.
     (1) Radiographs should be obtained of the upper limb, shoulder girdle, and cervical spine to rule out fracture.
     (2) Muscle examination.
     (3) Electromyography, magnetic resonance imaging (MRI), and myelogram are *not* useful in the neonate.

  e. Natural history.
     (1) Most palsies (90%) resolve spontaneously within the first 4 to 5 months of life. Biceps function is among the earliest to return because the muscle belly is proximal, therefore the dis-

tance for the nerve to regenerate is short. It is the easiest to monitor and is evidenced by return of elbow flexion.

(2) Of those patients whose palsy does not recover if untreated, the most common disability is inability to rotate the arm outwardly or raise it from the shoulder. The scapula may appear to protrude ("winged"). If the palsy is very severe, some weakness of finger and wrist strength may persist.

f. Treatment.

(1) Passive joint exercises through range of motion should be performed by the infant's caretaker with each diaper change to compensate for specific muscle weakness. Exercises should concentrate especially on maintaining elbow extension and shoulder external rotation and abduction.

(2) Surgical plexus repair is an option if return of biceps function is not evident by about 5 months.

(3) Osteotomy or shoulder muscle transfer may be used to help correct residual deformity in those who have not recovered full strength during the first few years of life.

3. Congenital malformations.

a. Polydactyly.

(1) Findings. Polydactyly may be preaxial (thumb side) or postaxial (little finger side) and may or may not be associated with a syndrome. The extra digit may or may not contain bone and tendons.

(2) Treatment.

(a) For a floppy, unstable digit, remove before discharge from the nursery. This may be performed surgically with a local anesthetic if the tissue bridge is substantial, or by tying off if it has just a small skin bridge.

(b) For a duplicated thumb or stable digit, defer resection until the infant is older and function may be better assessed.

b. Syndactyly.

(1) Findings. Fingers are joined by skin and at times bone; Syndactyly may be associated with syndromes, such as acrocephalosyndactyly (Apert syndrome) or congenital constriction band syndrome.

(2) Treatment. No treatment should be done in the neonatal period. Separation can be done early (about 6 months) if deformity develops as a result of asymmetric growth; otherwise separate at 2 to 3 years.

B. Spine.

1. Spinal cord injury.

a. Etiology. Caused by traction at birth; cord is less elastic than vertebral column, so cord damage (tear) often occurs without vertebral fracture or separation. Location is usually at the occiput, C2 (cephalic delivery), or C6-T1 (breech delivery).

b. Findings depend on location and extent of injury and may include diaphragmatic paralysis, initial hypotonia of extremities (spinal shock), absent deep tendon reflexes, and neurogenic bladder. Later, spasticity, contractures, and scoliosis may occur.

c. Evaluation/treatment. MRI and radiographs should be obtained of the entire spine; MRI is most helpful (fracture and dislocation are rare). Immobilize infant if fracture/dislocation is confirmed. There is no role for surgery, and the role of steroids is unclear.

2. Congenital scoliosis.

   a. Intrinsic vertebral malformation includes a wedge-shaped vertebra (failure of formation) or unilateral fusion of several vertebrae (failure of segmentation) (Fig. 15-3); may be associated with other malformations.

      (1) VACTERL association, usually partial. Components of this syndrome include the following: *v*ertebral anomalies, *a*norectal malformations, *c*ardiac defects, *TE* (tracheoesophageal) fistula, *r*enal or *r*adial aplasia, and *l*imb anomalies.

      (2) Klippel-Feil (fusion of cervical vertebrae, Fig. 15-4), Sprengel (undescended scapula).

      (3) Hemiatrophy of extremity.

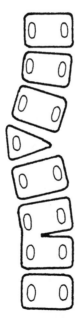

FIG. 15-3. Congenital scoliosis; should be searched for in any newborn having chest radiograph or kidney, ureter, and bladder evaluation because it is often associated with anomalies in cardiac, respiratory, or genitourinary systems. This spine shows examples of both hemivertebra *(upper)* and hemifusion *(lower)*.

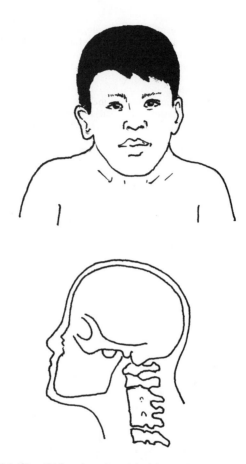

FIG. 15-4. Klippel-Feil syndrome is a triad of short neck, low hairline, and congenital cervical fusion.

    b. Findings. There is often no clinical finding in the newborn period. The back may appear straight; however, congenital scoliosis must be ruled out when patient has one of the associated malformations. Other clues include the following:

       (1) Abnormal hair distribution, vascular marking, or dimple over spine are occasionally seen.

       (2) Radiographic findings include asymmetry of the pedicle number or spacing often noted on a chest radiograph taken for TE fistula or congenital cardiac or renal anomaly.

c. Treatment.
   (1) Observation. Get a good radiograph of the whole spine as a baseline for future comparison.
   (2) Serial follow-up films every 6 months.
   (3) Approximately 50% have significant worsening of curvature. A brace does not help because this is an intrinsic problem of bone growth.
   (4) Ultimately, in situ fusion of the localized area of the abnormality is performed if the curve worsens more than 10 degrees from initial measurement.

3. Myelodysplasia (spina bifida or lipomeningocele).
   a. Obtain baseline anteroposterior and lateral radiographs of the thoracolumbar spine to rule out congenital deformity and kyphosis.
   b. Vertebral resection is sometimes helpful in closing a defect with severe kyphosis.
   c. Perform baseline motor examination and document well for further reference.
   d. Serial casts/splints can be used if a clubfoot deformity is present.
   e. An abduction brace can be used for subluxable hips with *low* lumbar myelodysplasia.

4. Muscular torticollis.
   a. Definition. Sternocleidomastoid muscle contracture causing tilt of ear toward affected side and chin rotation to contralateral side.
   b. Etiology is controversial; may involve a stretch injury to the muscle, usually during difficult birth, or ischemia secondary to in utero compartment syndrome.
   c. Findings. Swelling of sternocleidomastoid muscle in first 3 months, then contracture, torticollis, and eventual plagiocephaly.
   d. Differential diagnosis. In the newborn period, the main differential is congenital cervical vertebral anomaly.
   e. Management. Take extra care to screen for associated congenital hip dislocation. Radiographs of the neck should be obtained to rule out vertebral anomaly. Physical therapy and positioning of the infant to move the head to the opposite side are recommended. Surgical lengthening of muscle is indicated if not resolved by 1 year.

C. Lower extremity.

1. Developmental dysplasia of the hip (DDH) (Fig. 15-5).
   a. Etiology. Gradual, acquired dislocation. There are different levels of severity as a result of malposition and ligamentous laxity. It is more frequent on the left side, in girls, with breech position, and in those with a positive family history.
   b. Physical findings. Not all physical findings are seen in any single instance. All newborns should be evaluated before discharge from the hospital. The baby should be warm and as relaxed as possible. Indications of DDH include the following:
      (1) Adducted position of thigh at rest.
      (2) Deep proximal thigh crease (Fig. 15-6, *A*).

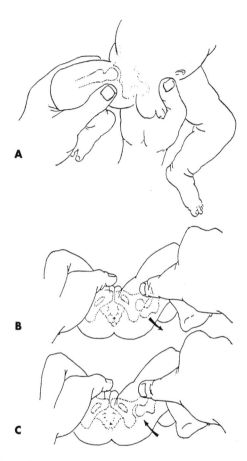

FIG. 15-5. Barlow and Ortolani tests: the definitive tests for unstable hip. **A,** Position: examine only one hip at a time; one hand around flexed thigh; feel greater trochanter with fingertips. **B,** Barlow test: causes *dislocation* by adduction, axial pressure; note sudden "clunk." **C,** Ortolani test: causes reduction by abduction, traction; note clunk with reduction.

(3) Apparent thigh shortening in extension (Fig. 15-6, *B*) or flexion (Allis sign).
(4) Positive Barlow (dislocation) and Ortolani (relocation) tests; should feel a slide or a deep "clunk," not a "click" (Fig. 15-5).
(5) Limited passive abduction (spread of legs apart); clunk with abduction or difficulty diapering in older child.

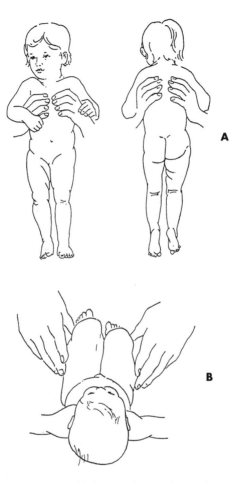

FIG. 15-6. Other signs of unstable hip in newborn. **A,** Asymmetric crease (extra crease in *proximal* thigh). **B,** Allis sign (apparent shortening of one thigh when pelvis is held level and both hips are flexed 90 degrees).

    (6) Document results of examination in chart.
  c. Management.
    (1) Ultrasound if diagnosis is in question (e.g., equivocal Barlow, Ortolani, or Allis sign; asymmetric abduction; consider if breech or if family history positive); *must* be done by sonographer experienced in infant evaluation (Fig. 15-7).

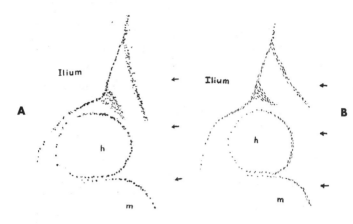

FIG. 15-7. Ultrasound of the neonatal hip in the coronal plane shows cartilaginous structures similar to the way they would appear on a radiograph later, when ossified. Arrows indicate ultrasound source. **A,** Normal hip, with the femoral head well covered by the acetabulum and downward-sloping labrum. The upper oblique line is the plane between the glutei. **B,** Subluxated hip. The femoral head is less than half covered by the acetabulum, and the labrum is elevated.

       (2) Use Pavlik harness if hip is dislocated and child is <6 months old; reduction must be documented with ultrasound or radiograph.

       (3) Traction can be used with closed or open reduction if dislocation is diagnosed after 6 months of age or is not reduced with the Pavlik harness.

  2. Proximal femoral focal deficiency.

    a. Definition/etiology. Focal deficiency or absence of part or all of upper femur. Distal anomalies may coexist; 50% are bilateral. Etiology is unknown.

    b. Diagnosis can be made by plain-film radiograph.

    c. Physical findings include shortening, anterior bowing, and external rotation of the thigh.

    d. Treatment. Obtain orthopedic consultation. Eventual bracing or reconstruction may be necessary.

  3. Congenital subluxation/dislocation of the knee.

    a. Etiology. Caused by in utero hyperextension; may be an isolated finding, or may be associated with myelodysplasia, arthrogryposis, or Larsen's syndrome (multiple joint dislocations).

    b. Findings.

       (1) Hyperextension of knee.

       (2) Limited flexion.

       (3) Posterior prominence of femoral condyles.

       (4) Radiograph distinguishes subluxation from dislocation.

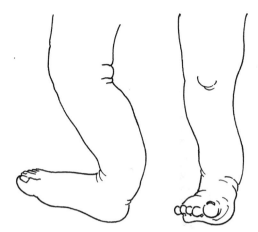

FIG. 15-8. Posteromedial bow. There is a sharp angulation in the distal tibia, with the foot in a position resembling a calcaneovalgus foot.

    c. Treatment. Serial stretching or casting. Hyperextension and subluxation usually respond to these measures; dislocation usually requires open reduction.

4. Leg/foot deformities.
    a. Posteromedial bow of tibia (Fig 15-8).
        (1) Definition. Angulation of distal tibia with a posterior and medial apex; foot appears in valgus, leg shortened.
        (2) Etiology. Unknown.
        (3) Diagnosis can be made by plain-film radiograph.
        (4) Treatment. Observation. There is no risk of fracture; correction usually occurs within 5 years, but slight shortening may persist.
    b. Metatarsus adductus.
        (1) Definition/etiology. Isolated medial deviation of forefoot with normal heel and ankle (Fig. 15-9, *A*) secondary to in utero molding.
        (2) Treatment. In the newborn period, stretching exercises can be done by the infant's parents; serial casts are used if there is no improvement by 8 months.
    c. Clubfoot.
        (1) Definition. Contracture of posteromedial leg muscles and malrotation of foot bones, causing ankle equinus, hindfoot varus and internal rotation, and forefoot adduction (Fig. 15-9, *B*).
        (2) Etiology. Unknown; most cases are isolated, but the condition may be familial or associated with spinal cord anomaly, diastrophic dysplasia, or arthrogryposis.

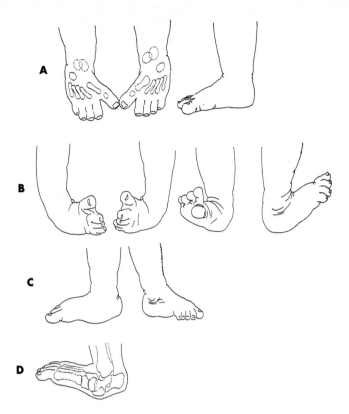

FIG. 15-9. Common foot deformities. **A,** Metatarsus adductus (forefoot medially deviated; normal hindfoot and ankle). **B,** Clubfoot (ankle equinus, hindfoot varus, and internal rotation in addition to forefoot adduction). **C,** Calcaneovalgus foot (excessive dorsiflexion valgus, but can be corrected easily past neutral). **D,** Vertical talus (rigid reversal of arch), with hindfoot plantar flexion, forefoot dorsiflexion, and dislocation of talonavicular joint.

       (3) Treatment. Radiographs are not needed at birth. Serial manipulations can be done from birth. Long leg casts, changed 1 or 2 times per week, can be used if there are no contraindications; taping can be done if casts are not possible (this is a less-desirable option). Surgery can be performed at 6 to 12 months of age if condition is resistant (approximately 50% of cases).

    d. Calcaneovalgus foot.

(1) Definition. Congenital malposition (by stretch) of foot and ankle into valgus and dorsiflexion so that the dorsum of the foot abuts the leg (Fig. 15-9, *C*).

(2) Etiology. In utero malposition.

(3) Findings. Foot rests in extreme calcaneus or dorsiflexion; looks serious but it is not; can be passively plantar flexed to resemble a normal foot having an arch.

(4) Differential diagnosis. Vertical talus (calcaneus remains pulled proximally and curve is in midfoot; reverse of arch), posteromedial bow of tibia.

(5) Treatment. Observation or serial stretching; always resolves by the time the child walks.

e. Vertical talus.

(1) Definition. Plantar flexion of hindfoot and dorsiflexion of forefoot producing subluxation in the middle, with reversal of the normal arch (Fig. 15-9, *D*).

(2) Etiology. May be isolated; approximately 50% of cases are associated with a neuromuscular or chromosomal disorder.

(3) Findings. "Rocker-bottom" sole (reversal of normal arch); head of talus is palpable where arch should be; deep crease in dorsolateral ankle and above heel; not completely correctable by passive manipulation.

(4) Diagnosis. Lateral radiograph of foot in neutral and maximum plantar flexion.

(5) Treatment. Serial stretching/casting to relax dorsal soft tissue; surgery virtually always needed at 6 to 12 months of age.

f. Fibular hemimelia.

(1) Definition. Partial or total absence of fibula, with or without other defects in the limb, primarily on the lateral side.

(2) Findings. Valgus foot. Radiographs demonstrate extent of absence. Shortening of leg.

(3) Treatment. Eventual reconstruction/lengthening if mild; otherwise, ankle disarticulation at age 6 to 12 months.

g. Tibial hemimelia.

(1) Definition. Tibia partially or completely missing; may resemble clubfoot.

(2) Treatment. Depends on how much of proximal tibia is available for the surgical creation of a knee and on the degree of deformity in the foot.

5. Fractures of the lower extremity.

a. Fracture-separation of upper femoral epiphysis.

(1) Etiology. Occurs during difficult delivery, with hyperextension and rotation; analogous to slipped capital femoral epiphysis.

(2) Findings. Swelling, pain, minimal crepitus; leg lies in external rotation; radiograph shows displacement of entire ossified portion of the femur; resembles developmental dysplasia of hip, but acetabulum is normal.

(3) Differential diagnosis. Infection, DDH.

(4) Diagnosis is made by arthrogram.

(5) Treatment. Hip spica cast for 3 to 4 weeks.

b. Fracture of femoral shaft.

(1) Etiology. Difficult delivery, child abuse (rare in newborn period). Also more common in children with a neuromuscular disorder, especially arthrogryposis or myelomeningocele.

(2) Findings. Pain, swelling, crepitus, shortening of leg.

(3) Treatment. Hip spica cast; overhead traction is associated with ischemia and is not recommended.

III. SYSTEMIC/NONREGIONAL CONDITIONS
A. Infection.

1. Osteomyelitis.

   a. Etiology. Hematogenous spread, neonatal sepsis; often no cause is found.

   b. Organisms.

      (1) *Staphylococcus aureus.*

      (2) Group B streptococcus.

      (3) Gram-negative organisms.

   c. Findings.

      (1) Pseudoparalysis. Decreased movement of affected part.

      (2) Multiple sites may be affected, most commonly the proximal humerus, or proximal or distal femur.

      (3) Swelling, pain (appear to be less than in an older child).

      (4) Laboratory findings. Erythrocyte sedimentation rate elevated; white blood cell count variable, may be decreased; blood should be drawn for culture at same time.

      (5) Radiographic findings. May be normal or show soft-tissue swelling only during early phase; osteopenia (later); periosteal reaction (latest).

   d. Diagnosis can be made by bone scan, needle aspiration of bone, MRI.

   e. Treatment.

      (1) If pus is obtained on aspiration, devascularization exists and area should be drained.

      (2) If no pus is present, antibiotics alone are adequate treatment.

      (3) Route. Intravenous antibiotics are given until clinical response is obtained, at which time antibiotics may be given orally if a suitable drug is available. Duration of treatment is 3 to 6 weeks, depending on the stage. Parents should be warned about risk of growth disturbance, which is greater in newborn than in older children.

2. Septic arthritis.

   a. Etiology. Primary hematogenous joint seeding or spread across growth plate from adjacent osteomyelitis.

   b. Organism. Same as for newborn osteomyelitis.

   c. Findings. Pseudoparalysis; swelling is less diffuse than in osteomyelitis; joint effusion; laboratory findings similar to osteomyelitis.

    d. Diagnosis. Ultrasound examination can be obtained if an effusion is suspected; bone scan is not a primary procedure (this is not a *bone* problem); aspiration is key. If one infected joint is found, carefully examine all major joints (physical examination, ultrasound, or both).

    e. Treatment. Surgical drainage can be performed if a major joint is involved; antibiotics should be given for 3 to 6 weeks. The parents should be counseled about possible growth disturbance, stiff joint, and arthritis.

B. Congenital constriction bands.

1. Amniotic bands cause creases, or partial or complete amputation. Distal (fenestrated) syndactyly is common; clubfoot and nerve compression may occur.

2. If lymphedema occurs distal to the constricting band, early Z-plasty is necessary.

3. Otherwise, band revision or syndactyly separation can be performed later in childhood.

C. Arthrogryposis.

1. Definition. Generalized hypoplasia or aplasia of muscle, leading to stiffness of joints, including fingers.

2. Etiology. Presumed to be anterior horn cell disturbance in utero.

3. Risk of fracture is increased because limbs are so stiff.

4. Treatment. Gentle physical therapy to increase joint range of motion to the best extent possible; treatment of clubfoot or other fixed deformity.

BIBLIOGRAPHY

Carson WF, Lovell WW, Whitesides TE Jr: Congenital elevation of the scapula, *J Bone Joint Surg* 63A:1199, 1981.

Dobyns JH, Wood V, Bayne LG: Congenital hand deformities. In Green D (editor): *Textbook of hand surgery,* ed 3, New York, 1994, Churchill-Livingstone.

Farsetti P, Weinstein SL, Ponseti IV: Long-term follow-up of nonoperative and operative treatment of metatarsus adductus, *J Bone Joint Surg* 76:257-264, 1994.

Kling TF, Hensinger RN: Angular and torsional deformities of the lower limbs in children, *Clin Orthop* 176:136, 1976.

Pappas AM: Congenital posteromedial bowing of the tibia and fibula, *J Pediatr Orthop* 4:525, 1984.

Ponseti IV: Current concepts review: treatment of congenital clubfoot, *J Bone Joint Surg* 74:448-454, 1992.

Rushfetti GF: The natural history of hooked forefoot, *J Bone Joint Surg* 60B:8, 1987.

Sponseller PD: Bone joint and muscle problems. In Oski FA (editor): *Principles and practice of pediatrics,* Philadelphia, 1999, Lippincott, Williams and Wilkins.

Staheli LT: *Fundamentals of pediatric orthopedics,* New York, 1992, Raven Press.

Widhe T: Foot deformities at birth: a longitudinal prospective study over a 16-year period, *J Pediatr Orthop* 17:20-24, 1997.

Waters PM: Obstetrical palsy: a comparison of natural history, microsurgical repair, *J Bone Joint Surg* 81A:649, 1999.

Watson BT, Hennrikus WL: Postaxial type-B polydactyly: prevalence and treatment, *J Bone Joint Surg* 79A:65-69, 1997.

Weinstein SL: *The pediatric spine,* New York, 1994, Raven.

16

Skin Care

HENRY M. SEIDEL AND BERNARD A. COHEN

I. GENERAL CONSIDERATIONS

The skin of the healthy, full-term newborn is quite mature. There is relatively more of it as compared with body weight than in the older child or adult (relatively high surface to volume ratio), making it more vulnerable to the toxic effect of topical drugs. Absorption of drugs is greater, and processing and excretion is less efficient. The premature infant, with a greater ratio of surface area to body weight, is at even greater risk. In the full-term infant the outer barrier layer of the epidermis—the stratum corneum—is fully formed. During the last few weeks of pregnancy the skin acquires the additional protection of the vernix caseosa, which is greasy, white, and often copious. These barriers vary in efficiency and amount so that the premature infant is less well protected and, with shedding, the postmature infant is also more vulnerable. Lanugo, the delicate hair found mostly on the shoulders and back, is more prominent in the relatively premature infant (gestational age 31 to 35 weeks) and is quickly shed after birth. Given this variability, full-term infants usually develop parchment-like skin, with cracking and peeling after the first day of life. Postmature babies who develop deep cracking and peeling during the first hours after birth and premature infants with thin transparent skin have decreased skin barrier function and experience increased insensible water loss and heat loss. These babies are also susceptible to cutaneous infections and sepsis.

II. OTHER OBSERVATIONS OF CONSEQUENCE

A. **The healthy baby may be cyanotic at birth** but turns to pink quickly as respirations are established.

B. **Acrocyanosis (cyanosis of the hands and feet, peripheral cyanosis) and mottling of the extremities may appear early** and recur without significance for weeks.

C. **Temporary vascular instability and a cool environment may cause a generalized transient cyanosis or a "harlequin" change** (cyanosis/mottling of half of the baby). Persistent mottling for the first month may be a sign of central nervous system (CNS) dysfunction.

D. The more fat, the less redness of the skin; the greater the transparency (with prematurity), the greater the redness.

E. Yellowed vernix and yellow-to-green meconium staining of fingernails suggest fetal distress.

F. The more premature or postmature the infant, the more likely are fissuring and cracking.

G. The more traumatic the delivery, the more likely are petechiae, ecchymoses, lacerations in a variety of sites, and edema and bleeding in the scalp.

H. The more limited the availability of direct daylight, the more likely jaundice will be overstated.

 I. Melanin is variable and often scant at first in both black and white babies.

J. Postmature babies with longer nails may have superficial scratches on the cheek. No harm; these disappear quickly if ignored. Nails do not need clipping in the newborn period (or for a long time thereafter) and should not be clipped into the corners; at the most, they should be clipped straight across.

III. CARE OF NEONATAL SKIN

The goal of neonatal skin care is to achieve that smooth, soft feel so typical of a baby's derriere. Hydration and lubrication are key and depend on ambient temperature and the dryness of the baby's skin.

A. First bath. After delivery and when vital signs have stabilized, usually at about 2 hours of age, take the baby from the warmer for a bath with comfortably warm water; return to warmer after bath.

B. Subsequent baths require water and gentle sponging; soap is not a necessity, and drying soaps (e.g., Ivory) should not be used.

C. Premature babies may require the humidity and warmth of the isolette (for much more than keeping their skin warm and smooth); the skin of a healthy premature infant matures in 1½ to 2 weeks, regardless of gestational age.

D. Moisturizers will help in a dry environment, but are not usually necessary with humidity. Petrolatum-based ointments without preservatives are best and may be safely used under a warmer (beware of absorption of emulsifiers and preservatives, particularly in premature infants). These products may also be used to decrease insensible water loss.

E. Avoid friction (e.g., with tape, too much Phisoderm or similar preparations, or too-frequent monitor changes, particularly in premature infants).

F. Use semipermeable dressings when wound or other protection is needed. These dressings may also be used in some premature infants to decrease insensible water loss.

G. Hair needs gentle washing only at the time of a bath; no special shampoos are necessary.

H. Powders and corn starch are not necessary or appropriate.
If some mothers insist on their use, suggest good dusting after application, leaving only a trace of powder; otherwise, clumping in the skin folds will facilitate irritation. Watch out for accidental talc aspiration.

IV. COMMON SKIN VARIATIONS IN THE NEWBORN
(Fig. 16-1)

A. Harlequin color change. Signs include erythema and pallor separated at midline when a particularly premature baby is placed on a side. The dependent side reddens, and the color change subsides readily when the baby is moved to the supine position, probably a result of immature autonomic vasomotor control. Do not confuse with harlequin fetus, a life-threatening autosomal recessive condition characterized by scaling, ectropion, and fissures.

B. Mottling (cutis marmorata). Splotchiness with pale red patches forming a sometimes continuous, sometimes discontinuous fishnetlike pattern; macular; more common with cooling, tends to disappear with warming. Persistence for more than a few months suggests hypothyroidism or CNS dysfunction. Lability of appearance and disappearance with warmth are characteristic; poorly developed autonomic vasomotor control is the probable cause.

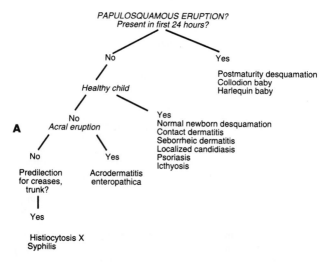

FIG. 16-1. Algorithm for evaluation of neonatal rashes. **A,** Papulosquamous eruption.

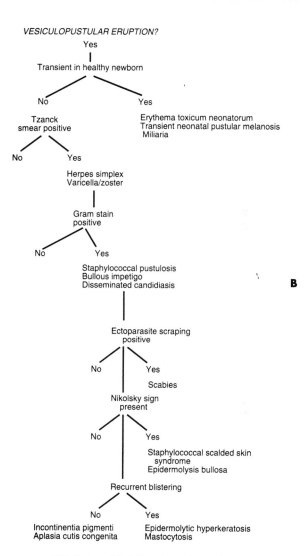

VESICULOPUSTULAR ERUPTION?

Yes

Transient in healthy newborn

No — Yes

Erythema toxicum neonatorum
Transient neonatal pustular melanosis
Miliaria

Tzanck
smear positive

No — Yes

Herpes simplex
Varicella/zoster

Gram stain
positive

No — Yes

Staphylococcal pustulosis
Bullous impetigo
Disseminated candidiasis

B

Ectoparasite scraping
positive

No — Yes

Scabies

Nikolsky sign
present

No — Yes

Staphylococcal scalded skin
syndrome
Epidermolysis bullosa

Recurrent blistering

No — Yes

Incontinentia pigmenti   Epidermolytic hyperkeratosis
Aplasia cutis congenita   Mastocytosis

FIG. 16-1, cont'd. B, Vesiculopustular eruption.

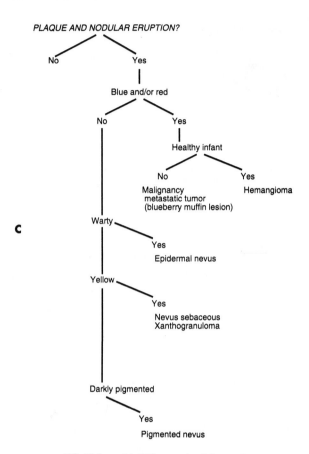

FIG. 16-1, cont'd. C, Plaque and nodular eruption.

FLAT LESIONS WITH COLOR CHANGE ONLY?

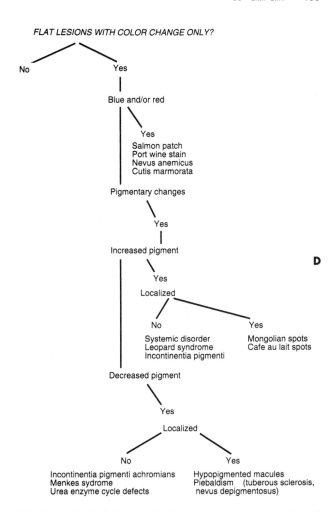

D

FIG. 16-1, cont'd. D, Flat lesions with color change only. (Courtesy Dr. Bernard Cohen.)

C. Milia (color plate 1). Multiple, scattered, white, keratin-filled cysts (miniature epidermal inclusion cysts), about 1 mm in diameter, raised, most often on the face; no "therapy" other than routine cleanliness. They rupture and disappear within days to a few weeks without visible trace. May be confused with sebaceous gland hyperplasia.

D. Sebaceous gland hyperplasia (color plate 2). Multiple scattered, yellowish macules or papules, occurring principally on the nose and cheeks at the site of pilosebaceous follicles. No "therapy" other than routine cleanliness. They tend to disappear within a few days to as many as several months without visible trace. May be confused with milia.

E. Erythema toxicum (color plate 3).

1. Splotchy, reddish macules, scattered on the face, upper body, and upper extremities; may be as much as 3 cm in diameter, many with a tiny central papule or pustule, giving a "flea-bitten" appearance. Wright's stain of contents reveals eosinophils.

2. Lesions appear within about 48 hours of birth and begin to disappear within 4 to 5 days. New ones may appear for up to 10 days. Common, particularly in the full-term infant.

3. Peripheral blood examination, not a routine need, often reveals eosinophilia. No therapy needed. Pathophysiologic significance is unclear.

F. Transient neonatal pustular melanosis (color plate 4).

1. Multiple vesicles and pustules, frequently ruptured, are characterized by a collarette of scale and are scattered over the body, particularly the scalp, face, sacrum, and even the palms and soles. They are more frequent in black boys.

2. Lesions may be present at birth and may last about 5 days. Subsequent pigmented macules may last many more weeks before disappearing. Sometimes macules are the only lesions present at birth.

3. Wright's stain of a pustule reveals neutrophils; pathophysiologic significance is unknown.

4. No treatment necessary.

5. May occasionally be confused with herpes or bacterial infection.

G. Subcutaneous fat necrosis.

1. Relatively hard and well-demarcated subcutaneous plaques and nodules of necrotic fat, appearing within the first few days of life and up to about 2 weeks; trauma and cold are likely contributing factors (e.g., forceps delivery).

2. Cheeks, arms, legs, and buttocks are common sites.

3. No treatment necessary. Resolution is usually within a few weeks, and the babies are usually otherwise healthy and seemingly unconcerned.

4. Might be confused with cellulitis, which is usually accompanied by the appearance of illness.

5. Hypercalcemia is an occasional finding and may be more common than thought. It may not develop until several months of age and may be associated with poor weight gain.

H. Sucking blisters are blisters on fingers, wrists, and forearms that are sometimes seen in the first hours of life and are presumably the result of vigorous in utero or neonatal sucking. No treatment is necessary, but these blisters should not be confused with herpes or impetigo. In bullous disorders, blistering tends to be more widespread.

V. COMMON, USUALLY TRANSIENT SKIN DISEASE OF THE NEWBORN

A. Acne neonatorum (color plate 5).

1. Rarely seen in the newborn, occurs usually at about 2 to 4 weeks of age. Multiple discrete papules and occasionally blackheads are scattered on the face, chest, back, and groin; may evolve into pustules.
2. Will most often subside without treatment. Topical 2.5% benzoyl peroxide gel may help in the severe circumstance.

B. Cutaneous candidiasis.

1. Congenital disease, contracted from an ascending intrauterine infection; evident at birth or within a few hours.
2. Generalized distribution (including palms and soles) of red macules, papules, vesicles, and pustules; may be confused with staphylococcal scalded skin syndrome. Generally self-limited in full-term infants and involves subsequent peeling of skin. May become disseminated in premature infants.
3. Pseudohyphae and budding yeast can be seen on direct microscopy of scales or smear of pustule.

N.B.: Systemic candidiasis, which is much more dangerous, does not usually cause skin rash. A neonatal disease contracted at birth in the vagina, systemic candidiasis does not become manifest for many days to a week. In premature infants, disseminated disease is a much greater risk.

C. Herpes simplex virus (cutaneous) (color plate 6). Grouped vesicles with a red base, anywhere on the body (particularly presenting body parts), often found on the scalp or buttocks; sometimes seen at birth, but onset after several days is more common. Type 2 predominates by far over type 1; more than half of those infected have skin lesions. Maternal birth canal infection is the usual source.

N.B.: Early diagnosis and expeditious therapy are essential. With cutaneous herpes alone, a complete workup is essential: lumbar puncture (LP), chest radiograph, complete blood cell count (CBC), and liver chemistries.

1. Varicella or impetigo, particularly with bullae, may confuse, but they lack the uniform clustered vesicles of herpes.
2. Systemic herpetic infection, particularly involving the CNS, may dominate the clinical picture.
3. On a Tzanck test, or stain cells smeared from the base of a vesicle with Wright's or Giemsa stains, multinucleated giant cells and balloon cells are characteristic; however, only 60% to 70% are sensitive even under the best circumstances.
4. Confirmation is with fluorescein-tagged anti-herpes simplex virus–specific antibody on vesicle smears or snap-frozen biopsy sections of skin. Polymerase chain reaction is even more sensitive.
5. Culture is usually positive at 12 to 24 after birth hours but may take as long as 5 days and should not delay treatment.

6. Treatment of choice is acyclovir, 10 mg/kg intravenously every 8 hours for 10 to 14 days; alternative is adenosine arabinoside, 15 to 30 mg/kg intravenously over 12 hours for 10 to 14 days.

D. Impetigo. Bullae, flaccid, often ruptured, involving any part of the body, particularly the head, periumbilical, and diaper areas. Shallow, erythematous base involving only the outer epidermis; when *Staphylococcus aureus* is present, the erythema may be fringed with remnants of ruptured bullae.

1. Commonly caused by *S. aureus;* at times, group A streptococci or enterococci may be the culprit.
2. Culture of bullous contents can confirm etiology; Gram's stain may give an early lead.
3. Therapy should be immediate with systemic antibiotics appropriate to the organism to forestall spread, sepsis, and staphylococcal scalded skin syndrome.

E. Petechiae and purpura.

1. Petechiae and purpura are frequent harbingers of congenital infection with thrombocytopenia, particularly the TORCH group ("blueberry muffin" rash) (color plate 7).
2. Occasionally there may be a few scattered petechiae on the upper body (after vertex delivery) or lower body (after breech delivery) that are transient and unaccompanied by other evidence of illness.
3. Larger, isolated ecchymotic areas unaccompanied by other evidence of illness suggest trauma (e.g., with forceps). The shape of the bruise may give a clue to the cause.

F. Pustules.

1. Discrete yellow papules or vesicles usually ringed with erythema, up to 1 cm in diameter, that appear in a scattered distribution after delivery, often within a few hours. In erythema toxicum, the pustule is small and the surrounding erythema is large. With bacterial pustules, the pustule is relatively large and the ring of erythema is small.
2. Infection and sepsis (e.g., with prolonged rupture of the membranes) must be a first consideration.
3. Culture of pustule contents is indicated, in addition to other investigations for sepsis guided by history and a full physical examination. Wright's stain of the contents usually reveals neutrophils and, occasionally, bacteria. Although eosinophils are found in the pustules of erythema toxicum, do not be fooled by the presence of eosinophils in bacterial infections.
4. Other common conditions in the differential diagnosis include the following:
    a. Benign pustular eruptions.
        (1) Erythema toxicum (color plate 3).
        (2) Pustular melanosis (color plate 4).
    b. Herpes simplex (usually clustered vesicles, not pustules) (color plate 6).
    c. Candidiasis (usually, but not always limited to diaper and intertriginous areas; sometimes pustular).

    d. Listeriosis, early and late forms; the former is associated with "blueberry muffin" lesions and the latter with disseminated papulopustules, particularly on the back and lumbar area.

G. Sclerema.

1. Diffuse, nonpitting hardening of the skin, more common in the premature infant, characterized by tight immobility and a glistening quality.
2. A very ill infant with severe underlying disease is more susceptible; mortality is apt to be high.
3. Diagnosis tends to be easy.
4. Treatment, guided by the underlying disorder, and maintenance of temperature and nutrition are apt to be difficult.
5. Cold and immature autonomic vasomotor control resulting in cutaneous ischemia and increased fibroblast activity appear to contribute to causation.

H. Staphylococcal scalded skin syndrome (Ritter disease).

1. Generalized erythema appearing as early as 24 to 48 hours of age, followed by scattered superficial bullae, rupture, and widespread exfoliation, particularly involving head, neck, diaper area, skin folds, and periumbilical area.
2. Caused by exotoxins from phage group II staphylococci.
3. Not to be confused with toxic epidermal necrolysis, an immunologic, drug-related form of erythema multiforme, which occurs only rarely in a newborn.
4. Culture of the primary skin lesion (e.g., from the umbilicus or circumcision site) is most often apt to give a positive culture. Most areas of skin do not harbor the organism.
5. Therapy includes immediate administration of systemic antibiotic appropriate to the organism; infant should be isolated. Widespread "scalding" requires meticulous attention to fluid and electrolyte balance. However, the blistering is superficial and reepithelialization occurs quickly in most cases.

I. Varicella (congenital).

1. Rare; may be confused with herpes simplex.
2. There should be a maternal history of infection 14 to 21 days before delivery. Appears in infants as it does in older children and adults, with red macules appearing first and progressing to red papules, delicate vesiculation, rupture, umbilication, and crusting. Lesions may occur anywhere on skin and mucous membranes, beginning usually by 10 days of age.
3. The course may be severe and is occasionally fatal.
4. Herpes simplex or impetigo, particularly with bullae, may confuse. In herpes, vesicles are usually clustered and uniform. Except in areas of trauma, varicella vesicles are in various stages of development and scattered over the entire skin surface.
5. Stain cells smeared from a vesicle that show multinucleated giant and balloon cells are suggestive but not pathognomonic; the Tzanck test will not distinguish between herpes and varicella.

6. Confirmation is with fluorescein-tagged anti-herpes zoster virus-specific antibody on vesicle smears or snap-frozen biopsy sections of skin. Polymerase chain reaction is sensitive and specific.
7. Culture takes 7 to 14 days and should not delay treatment.
8. Therapy. Acyclovir, 10 mg/kg intravenously every 8 hours for 10 to 14 days if the infant is severely ill; varicella-zoster immune globulin may limit the number of vesicles, particularly if maternal infection is within 14 to 21 days of delivery.

N.B.: Varicella-zoster immune globulin should be given to the newborn of any mother who develops varicella within 3 weeks of delivery. It will also have to be given to any accidentally exposed roommates in the nursery.

VI. BIRTHMARKS

Birthmarks are benign hamartomas that may be formed from any component of the skin. They may offer clues to a variety of more generalized diseases (e.g., the café au lait spots of neurofibromatosis or the connective tissue nevi [shagreen patches] of tuberous sclerosis).

A. Vascular birthmarks.

1. Cutis marmorata telangiectatica congenita (congenital phlebectasia). Rare; a reddish-purple vascular malformation, reticulated, spotted with blanching, usually affecting one extremity but occasionally more widespread. Lesions are persistent but may become more subtle in later childhood; may be associated with other congenital defects but is usually isolated. Pathogenesis is not understood; careful attention should be paid to social and emotional impact.
2. Blue rubber bleb nevus syndrome.
   a. Rare; multiple diffuse cutaneous and visceral vascular malformations that are blue, several millimeters to centimeters in diameter, appear in skin and in virtually any other organ.
   b. Gastrointestinal hemorrhage may occur. Accessible lesions can be pressed free of blood, refilling slowly.
   c. Number and location of lesions may influence management and prognosis (e.g., significant intestinal bleeds, compromised cardiovascular efficiency).
   d. Management includes periodic stool guaiac examinations; prednisone, 2 to 5 mg/kg per day for several weeks may be helpful for life-threatening complications. Surgical excision of isolated, delicately situated lesions may be indicated; laser therapy should be considered.
3. Hemangiomas (color plate 8) are not usually apparent in the neonate; a few telangiectases amid blanched skin may be a herald. There is a superficial and/or deep component. Superficial types are bright red, and both are composed of proliferated endothelial cells, mostly unchanneled. Deep lesions are darker, tend to be deep purple or blue, and feel spongy. All become raised, but not necessarily in the neonate. These lesions tend to grow faster than the baby for 2 to 3 months, although growth up to about 1 year is possible; most begin to involute by 12 to 15 months of age; many disappear in a few years, more than 75% by first grade and 90% by 10 years of age.

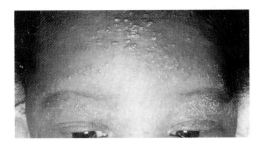

PLATE 1. Milia. (From Cohen BA: *Atlas of pediatric dermatology,* London, 1993, Wolfe Publishing, Mosby.)

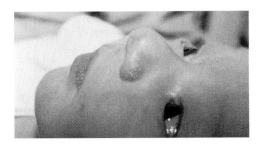

PLATE 2. Sebaceous gland hyperplasia. (From Zitelli BJ, Davis HW: *Atlas of pediatric physical diagnosis,* ed 2, St. Louis, 1991, Mosby.)

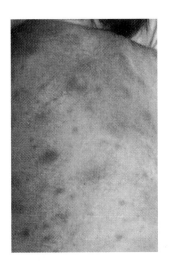

PLATE 3. Erythema toxicum. Blotchy, erythematous macules and plaques with multiple papules and pustules. (From Weston WW, Lane AT: *Color textbook of pediatric dermatology,* St. Louis, 1996, Mosby, p 225.)

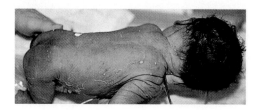

PLATE 4. Transient neonatal pustular melanosis.

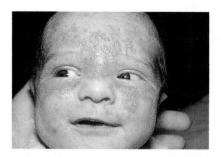

PLATE 5. Neonatal acne. Red papules, closed comedones, and pustules on face of a 1-month-old. (Courtesy Bernard A. Cohen, MD.)

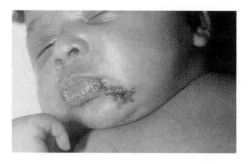

PLATE 6. Neonatal herpes. (From Cohen BA: *Atlas of pediatric dermatology,* London, 1993, Wolfe Publishing, Mosby.)

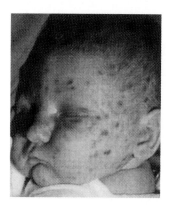

PLATE 7. "Blueberry muffin" rash.

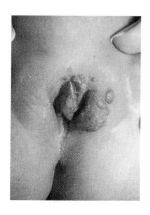

PLATE 8. Hemangioma.

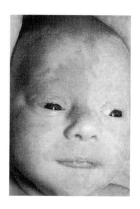

PLATE 9. Nevus flammeus.

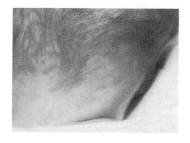

PLATE 10. Salmon patch.

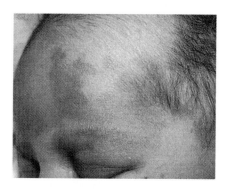

PLATE 11. Café-au-lait spots.

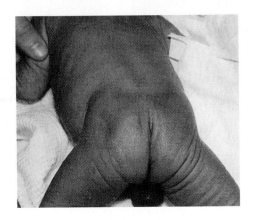

PLATE 12. Mongolian spots.

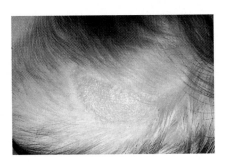

PLATE 13. Nevus sebaceous. Yellow cobblestone-like, hairless plaque on scalp. (Courtesy Bernard A. Cohen, MD.)

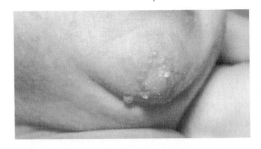

PLATE 14. Juvenile xanthogranuloma. (From Cohen BA: *Atlas of pediatric dermatology,* London, 1993, Wolfe Publishing, Mosby.)

a. Few hemangiomas require treatment in the newborn; bleeding is rarely a problem. A subglottic or intraoral cavernous hemangioma may obstruct the airway, and a large hemangioma external to the trachea may compress it; these require immediate attention. Similarly, hemangiomas in or near vital structures (e.g., eye, ear canal, alae nasi, urethra, or anus) that might obstruct the associated passage require intervention. Rarely, hemangiomas may be associated with Kasabach-Merritt syndrome (disseminated intravascular coagulation [DIC]). Surgery or laser excision may then be first-line treatment; given less urgency, prednisone, 2 to 5 mg/kg daily or every other day, is effective. Tracheostomy may on occasion be necessary. Interferon is an effective alternative but may be associated with neurologic complications.

b. Females are usually more compromised by problem hemangiomas than males. Hemangiomas occur more often in girls than in boys, generally 3 or 4:1.

c. More often, anticipatory guidance is indicated; schooling the parents in the natural history, informing them of available therapy, warning against deleterious radiation or cryotherapy treatments, and planning follow-up examinations in which measurements and photographs will be taken beginning at age 2 weeks is recommended. On consultation with parents, a small hemangioma in a potentially disfiguring location and with uncertainty about its course may be treated.

4. Salmon patch (nevus simplex) (color plates 9 and 10). Often called *stork bites.* Light red, blanching patch, most commonly on glabella, upper eyelids, sacrum, or nape of neck; common in whites; perhaps as many as half gradually disappear, often in a year, sometimes longer. Some adult remnants, particularly at the nape of the neck, are not ordinarily cosmetic problems. No treatment is indicated unless the patch is prominent and persistent in a psychosocially important area.

5. Port-wine stain (nevus flammeus).

a. Port-wine stains are flat, intensely red or purple stains that are usually large. They are often seen on the face, and sometimes on the arms and legs. They are usually unilateral and do not cross the midline. They are cosmetically difficult.

b. A stain on the face, particularly involving the eyelids (distribution of ophthalmic branch of trigeminal nerve), suggests Sturge-Weber syndrome, which includes seizures, cognitive impairment, and glaucoma. A hemangiomatous brain may calcify; computed tomography (CT) or magnetic resonance imaging (MRI) studies are indicated, although most stains are not associated with Sturge-Weber.

c. A stain on an extremity, with associated soft tissue or bony hypertrophy, suggests Klippel-Trénaunay-Weber syndrome; 25% have malformations of the deep venous system.

d. Cosmetic repair can be successfully achieved with pulsed-dye laser. This will also minimize the risk of late complications such as soft tissue hypertrophy and superficial papules, which tend to develop in adolescence or later. Excellent results are probable and therapy is indicated, the earlier the better. Parents need support and counseling; social and emotional impact may be heavy.

B. Lymphatic birthmarks (lymphangiomas).

1. There are a variety of forms of lymphangiomas, from well-demarcated, superficial papular investments of the skin, often in a cluster of thick-walled, skin-colored lesions, ("frog-spawn" appearance; lymphangioma circumscriptum) to deeper, more cavernous, irregular hamartomatous growths of great size (cystic hygromas).

2. Size and location (e.g., the neck) may require immediate surgical intervention (decompression of trachea) or more deliberately considered intervention for cosmetic reasons.

3. There may be hemangiomatous involvement, usually of a cavernous type, which adds a degree of bluish-red color. Recurrent lymphangitis and lymphedema may complicate large lesions.

4. Superficial lesions may be confused with herpes, but they have a more gelatinous substance and do not show multinucleated giant cells on Wright's stain; deep lesions may be confused with nodes, lipomas, or neurofibromas. Sonography is helpful in differentiation.

5. Treatment is generally unsatisfactory; surgery may be complicated depending on the extent of neural and vascular proximities; avoid radiation or steroid therapy. There may be a role for embolization in selected lesions.

C. Pigmented birthmarks.

1. Blue nevus. Rare; bluish or blue-black, well demarcated. Papular, occurring on face, buttocks, dorsum of hands and feet; usually no more than 1 cm in diameter. Although the risk of melanoma is low, unusual changing lesions may require excision.

2. Café au lait spots (color plate 11). Well-demarcated, irregularly shaped, light-brown macules, occurring anywhere on the body, usually solitary; much more common in blacks than whites; six or more with diameters of 0.5 cm or more suggest type I neurofibromatosis. This may be confusing in that numbers can increase with age and the correlation with neurofibromatosis is not absolute. Usually not cosmetically difficult. No treatment. Spots do not generally disappear during childhood.

3. Congenital melanocytic nevi.

   a. Small lesions occur in 1% of newborns; rarely there is large, often grotesque involvement of the skin in a "garment" or "bathing trunk" distribution; may be macular or raised, involving the dermal-epidermal junction (junctional nevocellular nevi) and dermis (compound nevi), or deeper dermis alone (intradermal nevi). Lesions vary in color from light tan to intense black.

   b. Midline lesions on the back may be associated with spina bifida or meningomyelocele; lesions on the head and large lesions on the trunk may be associated with meningeal melanocytosis and seizures or other CNS findings.

c. Malignant melanoma may occur in 5% to 6% of giant nevi, often in the first 5 years; there is uncertain frequency but low risk in smaller nevi, and then usually after puberty.

d. Management is dictated by prevention of malignancy and by the cosmetic requirements. Intervention is not usually indicated in the newborn. Small and medium nevi can be observed and removed with local anesthetic during adolescence if necessary.

4. Mongolian spots (color plate 12).

a. Mongolian spots are almost as common as salmon patches, and are much more so in blacks (90%), Asians (75%), and Native Americans (10%).

b. Large, irregular, blue-green macules can be found almost anywhere on the body, most often on the back and buttocks.

c. Spots will disappear or fade significantly by 2 years of age, particularly as an infant's skin darkens, although there may occasionally be a trace in the adult. Provide parental counseling only; no treatment is required. *Special variants:* Nevus of Ota on the face and nevus of Ito on the shoulder are persistent and respond well to lasers designed for pigmented lesions.

5. Urticaria pigmentosa (mastocytosis).

a. Solitary lesions that occur in about half of affected infants are usually present at birth.

b. Multiple lesions of urticaria pigmentosa tend to develop from a few weeks to about 2 years of age.

c. Mastocytomas are brown or red-brown papules, usually under 2 cm in diameter; the trunk and extremities are most commonly involved, but lesions on the face and scalp are not infrequent.

d. Should be considered in the differential diagnosis of pigmented neonatal lesions.

e. Darier sign (rubbing produces an urticarial wheal as histamine is released) is a helpful, usually diagnostic test; biopsy is definitive.

f. No treatment is indicated unless there is significant histamine release; cutaneous lesions most often resolve by adolescence, sometimes leaving brown spots. Ordinarily, activity decreases with increasing age.

g. Rarely, with diffuse lesions at birth, there may be blistering, flushing, and dermographism with Darier sign.

h. Parents should be counseled to avoid giving the child aspirin, polymyxin, codeine, or other medication with opiates (anything stimulating histamine release).

D. Hypopigmentation. All hypopigmented lesions occur infrequently; none lend themselves to therapeutic intervention.

1. Oculocutaneous albinism. Hair is white and fine, eyes are gray, skin is uniformly white or pink. Nystagmus may be readily detected, along with a suggestion of photophobia. Of several pathogenetic mechanisms, absence or decreased activity of tyrosinase, essential to production of melanin, is most common. There is autosomal recessive inheritance, and the phenotype may be only partially ex-

pressed. Discovery of the related genes has allowed for specific diagnosis of variants.

2. Ash-leaf spots. Hypopigmented macules; classic lesions are leaf-shaped, but may be any shape, and range in size from pinpoint to 4 to 5 cm. Ash-leaf spots are the only neonatal manifestation of tuberous sclerosis. If there is a family history, a Wood's lamp may highlight otherwise hard-to-see macules in light-pigmented infants. In a child with a solitary spot and no other signs of tuberous sclerosis, the term *nevus depigmentosus* should probably be used. Nevus depigmentosus may follow a dermatome distribution and may be present in up to 0.5% of newborns.

3. Chediak-Higashi syndrome. Involves general pigment dilution, with blond hair, blue eyes, and lighter skin than other relatives. Abnormal melanosomes and lysosomes result in defective pigmentation, neurologic deterioration, and increased skin infections.

4. Hypomelanosis of Ito (incontinentia pigmenti achromians). Lesions most often present at birth and may intensify with age. Causes irregular, whorled, widespread areas of hypopigmented skin, often unilateral, involving the whole of one side, or it may be generalized; it is frequently associated with abnormalities of teeth, hair, nails, bone, and CNS. This is a marker of genetic mosaicism that may be demonstrated by chromosomal studies of peripheral lymphocytes and/or involved and normal skin. Stable hyperpigmented lesions (hypermelanosis of Ito) in the same pattern have similar implications.

5. Nevus anemicus. Congenital, pale macule, appearing anywhere on the body; pseudodepigmented. Pallor is result of vasoconstriction of blood vessels, not hypopigmentation. It is a permanent defect that may be transiently highlighted by rubbing; the surrounding area reddens, the macule does not. It does not enhance with a Wood's light.

6. Phenylketonuria. Hair blond, eyes blue, skin pallid. Mandatory screening for phenylalanine should easily differentiate from albinism or Chediak-Higashi syndrome.

7. Piebaldism, a variant of partial albinism. An autosomal-dominant condition characterized at birth by scattered depigmented patches of skin interspersed with bits of normal pigmentation or hyperpigmentation. Severe CNS disorder may become evident with age. Waardenburg syndrome, also autosomal dominant, is a variant characterized by a flip of white frontal hair (white forelock), congenital deafness, hypertelorism, and heterochromia irides, among other features.

E. Organoid nevi. Hamartomatous proliferations of any of the constituents of the epidermis and/or dermis. Usually present at birth but may not become apparent for several months.

1. Epidermal nevi.
   a. Usually linear, oval, streaky; benign papular lesions, sometimes in dermatomal distribution, anywhere on the body.
   b. May be hard to see or feel in the neonate, but will progress from smooth to rough and warty, and from waxy to red or much more intensely pigmented as hyperplasia of skin occurs.

    c. There is no indicated treatment in the neonate. Surgical excision, laser ablation, or keratolytic agents may ultimately be necessary (e.g., 0.05% retinoic acid cream, alpha-glycolic acid cream), depending on cosmetic compromise.

    d. All patients with epidermal lesions, regardless of size, and particularly with head and neck involvement, need careful neurodevelopmental follow-up.

2. Nevus comedonicus.

    a. Present at birth; a proliferation of gaping pilosebaceous follicles stuffed with keratin, generally on the face and scalp but can involve any site; may become pustular.

    b. May require retinoic acid cream, 0.05% twice daily, or possibly meticulous surgical excision.

3. Sebaceous nevi (color plates 13 and 14).

    a. Present at birth; characteristic yellow-orange color; usually linear, sometimes oval; well defined, raised, hairless; commonly found on scalp.

    b. Immediate treatment unnecessary; parental counseling should anticipate growth and intensity with puberty.

    c. Hyperplasia of nevus usually occurs at puberty. Primarily benign neoplasms and occasional malignant changes in adults justify removal when preadolescent or teen will cooperate with local anesthesia.

4. Connective tissue nevi. Rare proliferations of collagen, elastin, or both; scattered skin-colored papules and plaques with thickened skin; those primarily of collagen (collagenomas) may be multiple and follow a dermatomal distribution; those primarily of elastin (elastinomas) are, when multiple, sometimes part of Buschke-Ollendorf syndrome, appearing particularly on the lower trunk and extremities; may be a marker for tuberous sclerosis. No treatment indicated.

VII. APLASIA CUTIS CONGENITA

Rare cutaneous defect of variable depth, not truly a birthmark; hairless, 1 to 2 cm in diameter; primarily in midline of posterior scalp, sometimes on face or trunk; sometimes associated with other readily discernible congenital defects. May appear as healing crust, atrophic scar, or large full-thickness ulcer, and, rarely, extend through skull. Do not confuse with possible trauma during delivery.

VIII. NEURAL TUBE DEFECTS

Tufts of hair, hemangiomas, nevi, or café au lait spots (almost anything) in the midline of the head and down the back suggest defects; hair is usually associated with dimples, and is usually long and black; defects may not be immediately obvious.

IX. ICHTHYOSES

A. Severe variants include lamellar ichthyosis and ichthyosiform erythroderma (diffuse erythema and scale). (Ichthyosis vulgaris, described later in this chapter, is an exception.) Genetically determined, ichthyosis may be heralded in the neonate by a "collodion membrane," an encasement of the baby with a tight, reddish, shiny membrane that restricts movement and may cause ectropion and eclabium. The membrane is shed; normal skin is rarely the result and lamellar ichthyosis generally ensues.

B. X-linked ichthyosis begins with upper-body scaling that is yellowish-brownish and increases in intensity and distribution with age, giving a dirty-scale appearance; palms and soles are not involved. There is a defect in aryl sulfatase A. Mother may have corneal opacities.

C. Lamellar ichthyosis. Autosomal recessive; frequently heralded by a collodion membrane; scales are present of varying degrees of coarseness (do not try to differentiate types by how fine the scales are); palms and soles are thickened. Ectropion and eclabium (eversion of lips) are common.

D. Epidermolytic hyperkeratosis (bullous ichthyosis). Autosomal dominant; significant scaliness at birth, reddened skin, progressing to widespread bullous formations; susceptible to secondary infection in the neonate. Do not confuse with epidermolysis bullosa.

E. Nonbullous ichthyosiform erythroderma. Rare; autosomal recessive; 100% of body surface red and scaly starting at birth, may evolve to more specific clinical variants.

F. Harlequin fetus. Autosomal recessive; most severe of all the ichthyoses; at birth, extensive thick scales invest the entire body; yellow skin with red fissures; there is significant malformation of soft tissues and skeleton; survival is unlikely; condition is probably a result of defects in fat and protein metabolism.

G. Ichthyosis vulgaris. Autosomal dominant; affects 3% to 5% of population; does not appear in the neonate, but may appear by 3 to 5 months of age, generally as dry, scaly skin; not life threatening.

H. The ichthyoses are not readily treated. Occlusive emollients should be used with care. There may be a role for topical organic, acid-containing products (e.g., lactic acid, glycolic acid). Severe variants may respond to oral retinoids. The relatively large surface area of a neonate mandates care before widespread application of anything to the skin. Consultation with a pediatric dermatologist is essential. Parents should be counseled about the long-term follow-up that will be required. These conditions do not modify with age in any meaningful way.

X. NEONATAL SKIN MANIFESTATIONS OF CHRONIC DISEASE

A. Acrodermatitis enteropathica. Autosomal recessive defect of zinc metabolism; indistinguishable from rash of zinc, biotin, or essential fatty acids deficiency; the skin is moist and red, and peeling involves hands and feet, perioral and perianal areas, and creases of the diaper area, arms, and legs. Associated signs are diarrhea, listlessness, hair loss, and failure to thrive. Rare in the newborn; usually becomes manifest at 2 to 3 weeks of age or at a point when a breast-fed baby is weaned. Breast milk contains a protein that helps with zinc absorption even in babies with acrodermatitis enteropathica. May be an early manifestation of cystic fibrosis in which zinc deficiency occurs with calorie and protein malnutrition.

B. Congenital syphilis. Usually manifests as plaquelike scales on the trunk and extremities; occasionally papular or vesicular, particularly on palms and soles; occurs at birth or shortly after (see Chapter 20).

C. Epidermolysis bullosa. Inherited mechanobullous disorders defined by split in skin, inheritance pattern, biochemical markers, and specific gene defect where known; may be manifest at birth. Any easily traumatized area is vulnerable to the development of bullae. Specific diagnosis is based on electron microscopic studies, immunomapping, and identification of the gene in child and parents. Prenatal diagnosis is available for severe variants.

D. Histiocytosis X. Generalized scaly, crusted rash associated with petechiae and purpura, particularly of the head and neck and body creases; frequently seen as a persistent diaper rash. Skin biopsy, even in the newborn, will reveal typical histiocytic cells; hepatosplenomegaly and lymphadenopathy may be present.

E. Incontinentia pigmenti. X-linked dominant, usually lethal in utero to males. At birth, clusters of vesicles are present in a linear, bandlike arrangement, particularly on the extremities and trunk, progressing in 2 to 3 weeks to hyperkeratotic, wartlike lesions, which after several months become hyperpigmented. May be confused with herpes or impetigo in the newborn, but Tzank smear for herpes and cultures can differentiate. Skin biopsy may be helpful. There is no available treatment, but most affected children do well. Associated with eye, dental, and bony anomalies, and rarely with seizure disorder. Genetic counseling is indicated.

ACKNOWLEDGMENT

The outline for this section was originally guided by Neonatal Dermatology. In Weston WW, Lane AT: *Color textbook of pediatric dermatology,* St. Louis, 1991, Mosby.

BIBLIOGRAPHY

Cohen BA: *Atlas of pediatric dermatology,* London, 1993, Wolfe Publishing, Mosby.

Vasiloudes P, Morell JG, Weston WL: A guide to rashes in newborns, *Contemp Pediatr* 14:156, 1997.

Weinberg S, Prose NS: *Color atlas of pediatric dermatology,* ed 2, New York, 1990, McGraw-Hill.

Weston WL, Lane AT: *Color textbook of pediatric dermatology,* St. Louis, 1991, Mosby.

Zitelli BJ, Davis HW: *Atlas of pediatric physical diagnosis,* ed 3, St. Louis, 1997, Mosby.

17

Hematology*†

GREGORY J. KATO, JAMES F. CASELLA,
AND HENRY M. SEIDEL

I. MATERNAL-FETAL RELATIONSHIP: HEMATOLOGIC CONCERNS

A. Iron enters the placenta bound to maternal transferrin and, in the placenta, to transferrin receptors.

1. In full-term neonates, serum iron is initially higher than in the mother, then drops rapidly, and rises in 2 weeks.
2. The fetus leaches iron from the mother; if she is severely iron deficient, the infant may suffer.
3. Prematurity intensifies the problem; there is not enough time to leach iron.
4. On average, a newborn has a total of 0.3 to 0.5 g of iron, an adult about 5 g.
5. Iron gain and stability derive from infant's diet.

B. Transplacental transmission of maternal disease with neonatal hematologic manifestations (Tables 17-1 and 17-2). is possible with the following diseases:

1. Congenital syphilis (see pp. 315-319).
2. Toxoplasmosis (generalized) (see pp. 312-315).
3. Cytomegalovirus (CMV) infection (see pp. 306-307).
4. Rubella (see pp. 307-308).
5. Malaria. In endemic areas, as many as 9% of neonates may have a form of malaria. Congenital malaria causes fever, failure to thrive, a sometimes profound anemia, relentless jaundice, and reticulocytosis; occasionally may cause stillbirth.
6. Coxsackie B virus. 10% to 15% of cases may develop disseminated intravascular coagulation (DIC).
7. Echovirus II. Potentially severe, leading to DIC.
8. Epstein-Barr virus. Probably more common than suspected; transient jaundice and mild to moderate anemia are most likely; severe in utero

---

*Portions of this chapter are from Oski FA, Naiman JL: *Hematologic problems in the newborn,* ed 3, Philadelphia, 1982, WB Saunders.
†Dr. James Casella provided many helpful suggestions in a review of this chapter.

TABLE 17-1
Hematologic Features of Congenital Infection

Infection	Common abnormality	Associated disorders
Rubella	Thrombocytopenia	Hemolytic anemia
Cytomegalovirus	Thrombocytopenia	Hemolytic anemia
Toxoplasmosis	Hemolytic anemia	Thrombocytopenia Eosinophilia
Syphilis	Hemolytic anemia	Thrombocytopenia Leukemoid reaction
Malaria	Hemolytic anemia	
Herpes	Disseminated intravascular coagulation	Hemolytic anemia

From Lukens JN: *Clin Haematol* 7:155, 1978.

infection may cause multiple congenital and hematologic anomalies (e.g., thrombocytopenia, persistent atypical lymphocytosis).

9. Systemic lupus erythematosus (SLE). Intrauterine transfer of autoantibodies can result in thrombocytopenia, sometimes severe anemia, and leukopenia; a rough, red scale involving the face primarily and other parts of the body may leave scars; congenital heart block and hepatosplenomegaly are typical of severe neonatal disease. Transplacentally acquired Ro/SS-A antibody disappears within the first year and the disease subsides. Confirmation is by detection of antinuclear antibodies (ANA) and Ro/SS-A. Protect infant from sunlight. Prednisone administration may be necessary.

10. Malignancy. Maternal disease does not usually spread to the infant; exceptions include malignant melanoma and hematologic malignancy.

11. Maternal hyperthyroidism. Placentally passed thyroid antibodies may result in neonatal thyrotoxicosis with thrombocytopenia, jaundice, hepatosplenomegaly, plethora (sometimes with hyperviscosity), and possibly congestive heart failure.

12. Alloimmune hematologic disease. Red cell hemolysis (e.g., ABO incompatibility [see pp. 212-215], Rh incompatibility [see pp. 209-212], thrombocytopenia [see pp. 232-245]).

13. Diabetes mellitus. Hyperviscosity, hyperbilirubinemia, hyperaggregation of platelets, and increased incidence of thrombosis are all possible. Almost half of infants of diabetic mothers will have hematocrit levels ≥65. These findings are usually transient and seldom require treatment.

14. Maternal drug use.

15. Human immunodeficiency virus (HIV) (see pp. 309-312).

16. Herpes virus (see pp. 301-304).

II. APPROACH TO ANEMIA IN THE NEWBORN

Possible causes of anemia in the newborn include blood loss, hemolysis, or impaired production of red blood cells (RBCs). If, in

TABLE 17-2
Maternal Events Associated With Hematologic Abnormalities in the Newborn Infant

Maternal event		Hematologic abnormalities in the infant
Infection	Cytomegalic inclusion disease	Jaundice, hemolytic anemia, and thrombo-cytopenia
	Toxoplasmosis	
	Syphilis	
	Rubella	
	Coxsackievirus B	
	Herpes simplex	
	Malaria	
Illness	Lupus erythematosus	Thrombocytopenia, leukopenia, and anemia
	Malignant melanoma	Melanoma, hemolytic anemia, and thrombocytopenia
	Hodgkin's disease	Hodgkin's disease in infancy (rare)
	Leukemia	Leukemia in late infancy (rare)
	Diabetes	Polycythemia, jaundice, increase in hemoglobin A_{1c} + F, thrombosis
	Hypertension	Neutropenia
	Hyperthyroidism	Thrombocytopenia, plethora
	Idiopathic thrombocytopenic purpura	Thrombocytopenia
	Autoimmune hemolytic anemia	Hemolytic anemia, thrombocytopenia
	Eclampsia	Thrombocytopenia, disseminated intravascular coagulation

Category	Agent	Effect
Sensitization	Erythrocytes	Hemolytic anemia
	Leukocytes	Leukopenia
	Platelets	Thrombocytopenia
Drug ingestion	Thiazides	Thrombocytopenia (?), leukopenia, hemolytic anemia (?)
	Hydralazine	Thrombocytopenia, leukopenia
	Quinine	Thrombocytopenia
	Mothballs, antimalarials, sulfonamides, fava beans, nitrofurantoins	Hemolytic anemia if infant has G6PD deficiency
	Methylene blue (intra-amniotic insertion)	Hemolytic anemia
	Dicumarol	Hemorrhage
	Hydantoins/barbiturates	Hemorrhage
	Acetylsalicylic acid	Hemorrhage, prolonged bleeding time
	Penicillin	Coombs'-positive hemolytic anemia
	Epidural analgesics	
	prilocaine	Methemoglobinemia
	bupivicaine	Jaundice, decreased red cell deformability
	Oxytocins in excess	Jaundice, increased red cell osmotic fragility
	Methadone	Thrombocytosis

From Oski FA, Naiman JL: *Hematologic problems in the newborn*, ed 3, Philadelphia, 1982, WB Saunders.

the first 24 hours, hypovolemia is present, a severe degree (Hgb ≤5 gm/dl) of anemia may be life threatening; hemorrhage or hemolysis related to alloimmunization is then more likely, and immediate transfusion may be necessary. However, diagnosis unobscured by transfusion is preferable. Once past the first day, other causes become more likely.

A. Hemorrhage.

1. Clinical findings. If bleeding is significant, pallor is often obvious at birth, particularly in the mucous membranes; respiration may be irregular and gasping, but without retractions; pulses are weak and rapid; blood pressure is often unobtainable; notably, there is no edema or organomegaly. This contrasts with asphyxia, in which case the associated pallor improves with oxygen, the pulse is slow, and respiration may be labored or absent. Severe alloimmunization or other causes of severe, chronic anemia may result in pallor associated with hepatosplenomegaly and edema (Box 17-1).

2. Diagnosis.

   a. Obstetric history may include vaginal spotting during the last trimester, placenta previa, abruptio placentae, nonelective cesarean section, and compromise of the umbilical vessels.

   b. Additional considerations.

      (1) Degree of prematurity. Small infants do more poorly with blood loss and the associated hypovolemia and anemia.

      (2) Hemoglobin level. Best determined using venous blood, not a heel stick. An initially high hemoglobin level may be illusory; it may drop quickly as the body compensates for hypovolemia.

      (3) Occult blood loss: fetal hemorrhage into maternal circulation.

         (a) Blood loss may be acute or chronic; for differentiation, see Table 17-3.

         (b) Direct Coombs' test result is negative, and jaundice is generally absent.

         (c) Diagnosis can be confirmed only by demonstrating fetal red cells in maternal circulation (Kleihauer-Betke elution test) and after ruling out alloimmunization (Coombs' test) and evidence of other hemorrhage.

      (4) Occult blood loss: twin-to-twin.

         (a) Most common with monochorionic placenta.

         (b) Donor twin is pale at birth, perhaps in shock, and when the process is chronic, smaller than the usually plethoric recipient.

         (c) Suggested when the hemoglobin difference is >5 g/dl and the donor shows evidence of reticulocytosis, increased numbers of nucleated RBCs, and at times thrombocytopenia.

         (d) Prenatal sonogram might reveal oligohydramnios in the donor amniotic sac, or polyhydramnios in the recipient.

      (5) Occult blood loss: internal hemorrhage.

         (a) Anemia occurring at 24 to 72 hours without jaundice may be the result of internal hemorrhage after traumatic delivery.

BOX 17-1
Types of Hemorrhage in the Newborn

OBSTETRIC ACCIDENTS, MALFORMATIONS OF THE PLACENTA AND CORD

Rupture of a normal umbilical cord
   Precipitous delivery
   Entanglement
Hematoma of the cord or placenta
Rupture of an abnormal umbilical cord
   Varices
   Aneurysm
Rupture of anomalous vessels
   Aberrant vessel
   Velamentous insertion
   Communicating vessels in multilobed placenta
Incision of placenta during cesarean section
Placenta previa
Abruptio placentae

OCCULT HEMORRHAGE BEFORE BIRTH

Fetoplacental
   Tight nuchal cord
   Cesarean section
   Placental hematoma
Fetomaternal
   Traumatic amniocentesis
After external cephalic version, manual removal of placenta, use of oxytocin
   Spontaneous
   Chorioangioma of the placenta
   Choriocarcinoma
Twin-to-twin
   Chronic
   Acute

INTERNAL HEMORRHAGE

Intracranial
Giant cephalhematoma, subgaleal, caput succedaneum
Adrenal
Retroperitoneal
Ruptured liver, ruptured spleen
Pulmonary

IATROGENIC BLOOD LOSS

From Oski FA, Naiman JL: *Hematologic problems in the newborn,* ed 3, Philadelphia, 1982, WB Saunders.

TABLE 17-3
Characteristics of Acute and Chronic Blood Loss in the Newborn

Characteristic	Acute blood loss	Chronic blood loss
Clinical	Acute distress; pallor; shallow, rapid, and often irregular respiration; tachycardia; weak or absent peripheral pulses; low or absent blood pressure; no hepatosplenomegaly	Marked pallor disproportionate to evidence of distress; on occasion signs of congestive heart failure may be present, including hepatomegaly
Venous pressure	Low	Normal or elevated
Laboratory		
Hemoglobin concentration	May be normal initially; then drops quickly during first 24 hours of life	Low at birth
Red cell morphology	Normochromic and macrocytic	Hypochromic and microcytic; anisocytosis and poikilocytosis
Serum iron	Normal at birth	Low at birth
Course	Prompt treatment of anemia and shock necessary to prevent death	Generally uneventful
Treatment	Intravenous fluids and whole blood; iron therapy later	Iron therapy; packed red cells may be necessary on occasion

From Oski FA, Naiman JL: *Hematologic problems in the newborn,* ed 3, Philadelphia, 1982, WB Saunders.

> (i) Cephalohematoma may be large and subaponeurotic blood loss may be great, covering at times the whole of the calvaria, particularly after vacuum extraction or neglect in giving vitamin K. As red cells disintegrate, jaundice results. Estimated blood loss equals 38 ml times the number of centimeter increase over expected head circumference.
>
> (ii) Intracranial hemorrhage (as much as 10% to 15% of blood volume) is more common in the infant who weighs <1500 g.
>
> (iii) Breech delivery may traumatize the perineum and abdominal contents, most commonly the adrenals, kidneys, and spleen.
>
> (b) Hemorrhage into the adrenals may result in precipitous collapse; sonography is helpful.
>
> (c) Rupture of the liver may remain subcapsular or cause free blood in the peritoneal cavity; undetected, shock is common after 24 to 48 hours; a mass contiguous with the

liver may be palpated. Flat radiographs of the abdomen, taken in both erect and supine positions, or paracentesis can confirm blood in the abdomen. Prognosis is guarded.
- (d) Rupture of the spleen is more likely when it is enlarged for any reason (e.g., erythroblastosis fetalis). Pallor, abdominal distention, scrotal swelling, and, noted on radiographs, peritoneal effusion without free air suggest this diagnosis. Rupture may occur during exchange transfusion, leading to a drop in venous pressure rather than the expected rise.

N.B.: Internal hemorrhage should prompt at minimum a detailed family bleeding history and assessment of platelet count, PT, and aPTT; occasionally, neonatal hemorrhage is a presenting sign of a hemorrhagic diathesis, such as hemophilia A or B.
- (6) Placental/cord blood loss.
  - (a) Placental hematoma. Inspection of the placenta may reveal a hematoma large enough to cause significant anemia.
  - (b) Umbilical cord hematoma. Significant hemorrhage into the cord should be readily apparent at birth.
3. Treatment depends on the degree of anemia, hypovolemia, and chronicity of blood loss. Shock may result if there is an acute loss of 20% to 25% of blood volume. Otherwise, hypotension is a relatively late manifestation of blood loss.
   a. If an infant is severely anemic (<8 g/dl) and in distress at birth, get help from a second physician.
      (1) Clear airway, give oxygen, perform artificial ventilation if necessary.
      (2) Obtain blood from umbilical vein for crossmatch and hemoglobin level. Insert catheter into vein and leave in place to measure venous pressure and to provide access for fluids.
      (3) Transfuse with first-available isotonic fluid (e.g., O-negative blood, plasma, Ringer's lactate, D_5 normal saline, or Dextran) after asphyxia has been eliminated as a diagnosis. Give a 20-ml/kg bolus of available fluid. Repeat with 10 to 20 ml/kg of whole blood within 1 hour, particularly if whole blood was not used at first. If whole blood is unavailable, use packed RBCs plus plasma.
      (4) Recheck placenta and umbilical cord for abnormalities; if a bleeding site is not discovered, draw maternal blood to test for fetal hemoglobin.
      (5) Follow transfusion with iron therapy to ensure adequate replacement of iron stores.
   b. If the infant is in congestive heart failure, give furosemide, 1 mg/kg intravenously before transfusion. Alternatively, partial exchange transfusion can be effective.
   c. If the infant is mildly anemic (not unusual in the event of chronic blood loss), transfusion is usually not necessary. Treat with ferrous sulfate, 2 mg/kg elemental iron, three times daily for about 3 months. Check progress with periodic determinations of hemoglobin level.

d. If the problem is twin-to-twin transfusion:
   (1) Do not forget the plethoric twin and the possible need for partial exchange transfusion if the infant is symptomatic and polycythemic (p. 227).
   (2) Check hematocrits on all isosexual twins shortly after birth for clinically inapparent anemia or polycythemia.

B. Hemolytic anemia is a common problem in the first week of life and has multiple etiologies (Box 17-2). The life span of the RBC is shortened, and hyperbilirubinemia is almost always present. It does not take much breakdown of hemoglobin to raise the bilirubin significantly; anemia may not be noted at first. The three etiologic categories are as follows:

1. Alloimmunization. Maternal-fetal incompatibility in Rh, ABO, or other blood-group systems.
2. Congenital defect of the erythrocyte.
   a. Enzymopathy (e.g., glucose-6-phosphate dehydrogenase [G6PD] or pyruvate kinase deficiency).
   b. Membranopathy (or membrane abnormalities) (e.g., hereditary spherocytosis).
   c. Abnormal hemoglobins (or hemoglobinopathy) (e.g., hemoglobin H disease [beta chain defects such as sickle cell disease rarely include anemia before several months of age]).
3. Acquired defect of the erythrocyte (most frequent cause).
   a. Drugs (e.g., penicillin).
   b. Toxins.
   c. Congenital infections, particularly viral.
   d. Profound acidosis, shock, asphyxia; secondary at times to DIC.

C. Impaired RBC production. Rare in the newborn; *always* requires consultation with a pediatric hematologist. Disorders include Diamond-Blackfan syndrome (congenital hypoplastic anemia, congenital pure red-cell aplasia, erythrogenesis imperfecta), Parvovirus B19–induced anemia and hydrops fetalis, transcobalamin II deficiency, and congenital sideroblastic anemia.

D. Differential diagnosis of anemia in the neonate.

N.B.: Profound anemia in the neonate requires rapid action (Fig. 17-1, Box 17-3).

1. Family history should be checked for anemia, jaundice, cholelithiasis, or splenectomy. Hereditary factors to consider include spherocytosis or other cytoskeletal defect, enzymatic red-cell defect, or hemoglobinopathy.
2. Maternal history.
   a. Drug ingestion near term.
      (1) G6PD deficiency (e.g., sulfonamides).
      (2) Recent exposure to naphthalene mothballs.
   b. Obstetric history.
      (1) Vaginal bleeding during pregnancy.
      (2) Placenta previa, abruptio placentae, vasa previa, cesarean section.

BOX 17-2
Causes of a Hemolytic Process in the Neonatal Period

Immune
  Rh incompatibility
  ABO incompatibility
  Minor blood group incompatibility
  Maternal autoimmune hemolytic anemia
  Drug-induced hemolytic anemia
Infection
  Bacterial sepsis
  Congenital infections
  Syphilis
  Malaria
  Cytomegalovirus
  Rubella
  Toxoplasmosis
  Disseminated herpes
Disseminated intravascular coagulation
Macroangiopathic and microangiopathic hemolytic anemias
  Cavernous hemangioma
  Large-vessel thrombi
  Renal artery stenosis
  Severe coarctation of the aorta
Galactosemia
Prolonged or recurrent acidosis of a metabolic or respiratory nature
Hereditary disorders of the red cell membrane
  Hereditary spherocytosis
  Hereditary elliptocytosis
  Hereditary stomatocytosis
  Other rare membrane disorders
Pyknocytosis
Red cell enzyme deficiencies
  Most common are glucose-6-phosphate dehydrogenase deficiency, pyruvate kinase deficiency, 5'-nucleotidase deficiency, and glucose phosphate isomerase deficiency
α-Thalassemia syndrome
Alpha chain structural abnormalities
Gamma thalassemia syndromes
Gamma chain structural abnormalities

From Oski FA, Naiman JL: *Hematologic problems in the newborn,* ed 3, Philadelphia, 1982, WB Saunders.

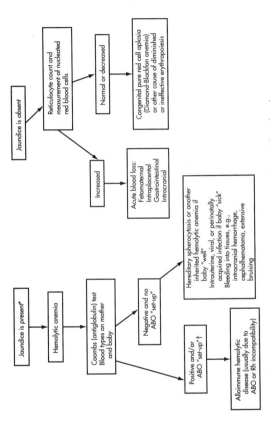

FIG. 17-1. Diagnostic approach to anemia in the newborn infant (hemoglobin ≤14 g/dl, with or without symptoms). The most likely diagnoses are provided in the boxes. (Modified from Oski FA, Naiman JL: *Hematologic problems in the newborn,* ed 3, Philadelphia, 1982, WB Saunders.)

*In addition, reticulocyte count and number of circulating nucleated red blood cells are nearly always elevated.
†Mother group O and baby group A, B, or AB.

BOX 17-3
Differential Diagnosis of Pallor in the Newborn

ASPHYXIA

1. Respiratory findings: retractions, response to oxygen, cyanosis
2. Moribund appearance
3. Bradycardia
4. Stable hemoglobin

ACUTE SEVERE BLOOD LOSS

1. Decrease in venous and arterial pressure
2. Rapid, shallow respirations
3. Acyanosis
4. Tachycardia
5. Drop in hemoglobin

HEMOLYTIC DISEASE

1. Hepatosplenomegaly, jaundice
2. Positive Coombs' test
3. Anemia

Modified from Kirkman HN, Riley HD Jr: *Pediatrics* 24:97, 1959.

      (3) Traumatic delivery.
      (4) Cord rupture.
      (5) Multiple birth.
   c. Age of onset.
      (1) At birth: generally hemorrhage or alloimmunization.
      (2) First 2 days: hemorrhage, external or internal.
      (3) After first 2 days: hemolytic, usually associated with jaundice.
3. Laboratory studies.
   a. Hemoglobin level, white blood cell (WBC) and platelet counts.
   b. RBC indices; if hypochromic or microcytic, consider iron deficiency.
      (1) Fetomaternal or twin-to-twin chronic transfusion.
      (2) α-Thalassemia trait.
   c. Reticulocyte count.
      (1) If elevated, consider hemorrhage or hemolysis.
      (2) If depressed, consider Diamond-Blackfan syndrome or Parvovirus infection.
   d. Peripheral blood smear.
   e. Direct Coombs' test on infant's blood; if positive, alloimmunization is likely.
   f. Maternal blood smear for fetal erythrocytes (Kleihauer-Betke test).
   g. Blood typing of infant and mother if result of direct Coombs' test on infant is positive. Search for maternal antibodies.
   h. Blood and urine cultures if infection is suspected.

   i. Bone marrow aspirate, particularly in the presence of reticulo-cytopenia.
4. Relatively uncommon findings include the following:
   a. Spherocytes or elliptocytes, indicating hereditary disorders of RBC cytoskeleton.
   b. Pyknocytes, suggesting pyknocytosis or G6PD deficiency.
   c. Normocytic, normochromic RBCs, suggesting possible acute blood loss or congenital enzymatic defect of RBCs.

N.B.: Jaundice or hepatosplenomegaly does not usually accompany acute blood loss; pallor or shock may. Fetal cells in maternal circulation can confirm a traumatic delivery with internal hemorrhage.

   d. In the presence of hemolytic anemia and jaundice without evidence of alloimmunization, enzymatic defect of RBCs is likely.
      (1) G6PD deficiency, particularly in Mediterranean and Asian male infants.
      (2) Pyruvate kinase deficiency.
      (3) Hexokinase deficiency.

N.B.: Infection (e.g., from STORCH complex) can disrupt RBC morphology and cause anemia and jaundice. Cultures and serologic studies are necessary. Neutropenia and thrombocytopenia should be a red flag. DIC is a strong possibility with sepsis, acidosis, or hypoxia.

   E. Physiologic anemia of infancy. The hemoglobin concentration of full-term infants decreases over the first 8 to 12 weeks of life—the so-called *physiologic anemia of infancy*—then rises slowly to expected levels after that age. It is not associated with discoverable abnormalities; there is a greater decrease in premature infants, corresponding to the degree of prematurity; hemoglobin generally returns to expected levels by 5 months of age.
1. Iron. Supplementation for prevention of iron deficiency anemia is indicated, certainly by 2 months of age; dosage of elemental iron is 2 to 3 mg/kg per day.
2. Vitamin E (α-tocopherol). The newborn is in a state of relative vitamin E deficiency; the smaller the infant, the greater the deficiency. Hemolytic anemia is a possibility, particularly in infants <1500 g. Correction of anemia is possible with 50 to 200 units of vitamin E per day for 14 days. Prevention is possible with 10 to 15 mg per day for 6 to 8 weeks. Currently available commercial formulas are generally adequate in this regard.
3. Folic acid (pteroylglutamic acid). Deficiency results in megaloblastic anemia. Diarrhea and prematurity contribute. Prevention is possible with 20 to 50 μg per day, which is available in commercial formulas. Parenteral supplementation may be necessary in infants with diarrhea or infection.

III. HEMOLYTIC DISEASE OF THE NEWBORN: ERYTHROBLASTOSIS FETALIS

Blood-group incompatibilities are the most common and, if undetected and untreated, potentially the most severe of the hemolytic anemias. Most common is ABO incompatibility; however, the potential for harm from Rh incompatibility (usually D epitope) is by far the greatest if not prevented. Minor blood-group incompatibilities (e.g., C, Kell, Duffy, Kidd, E) are infrequent, but can be severe.

A. General considerations.

1. Boys are more likely to be severely affected than girls.
2. Racial differences are clear: 15% of whites are Rh negative, compared with 5.5% of blacks in the United States and 0% of Asians.
3. The potential of a clinical problem is increased by an increase in maternal-fetal sharing of blood resulting from obstetric determinants (e.g., toxemia, trauma, amniocentesis, cesarean section, breech delivery).
4. The size and configuration of maternally produced antibody molecules is also a determinant (e.g., anti-A and anti-B in IgG will cross over; naturally occurring anti-A and anti-B in IgM will not).
5. Antibody destruction of red cells results in anemia and hyperbilirubinemia; the degree of anemia depends on the infant's ability to keep pace with the hemolytic process.
6. The principal risk with hyperbilirubinemia is to the central nervous system (CNS); the amount of unconjugated bilirubin deposited in nerve tissue determines the extent of brain damage (kernicterus).
7. The liver of the normal newborn, particularly that of the premature infant, is unable to deal effectively with an increased bilirubin load. Thus even minimal degrees of hemolysis may result in pronounced hyperbilirubinemia. Age, individual variation, prematurity, and concurrent illness can all contribute. Improved bilirubin binding capacity does not begin until the third to fifth day of life and may not be fully achieved until 5 to 6 months of age.

B. Rh incompatibility.

1. Clinical findings.
   a. Jaundice. Generally absent at birth, may be evident at 4 to 5 hours, reaching a peak by 3 to 4 days. Daylight is best for detection, a white fluorescent lamp is second best. Finger pressure to blanch skin is helpful. If jaundice first appears after 24 hours of age, causes other than hemolytic anemia must be considered (see Chapter 19).
   b. Kernicterus. Risk increases as serum indirect bilirubin level approaches or exceeds 20 mg/dl. Lower levels are hazardous in premature infants with acidosis, hypoglycemia, sepsis, or hypothermia. Lethargy, hypotonia, and loss of sucking reflex are early signs. Opisthotonos and generalized spasticity come later. Even mild onset can be followed by severe neurologic problems in time, such as deafness, mental retardation, and choreoathetoid cerebral palsy. Kernicterus as the result of hyperbilirubinemia must be prevented. Once present, it is *not* reversible.

N.B.: Do not be misled by the myth that risk decreases after 4 days of life; fully mature bilirubin binding capacity may take months or longer to achieve.

   c. Anemia. Compensatory erythropoiesis can moderate degree; severe anemia can compromise cardiac function, leading to gener-

BOX 17-4
Nonimmune Hydrops Fetalis: Causes and Associations

FETAL
Hematologic
  Homozygous α-thalassemia (four-gene deletion)
  Chronic fetomaternal transfusion
  Twin-to-twin transfusion (recipient or donor)
  Multiple gestation with "parasitic" fetus
Cardiovascular
  Severe congenital heart disease (atrial septal defect, ventricular septal defect, hypoplastic left heart, pulmonary valve insufficiency, Ebstein, subaortic stenosis)
  Premature closure of foramen ovale
  Myocarditis
  Large arteriovenous malformation
  Tachyarrhythmias: paroxysmal SVT, atrial flutter
  Bradyarrhythmias: heart block
  Fibroelastosis
Pulmonary
  Cystic adenomatoid malformation of lung
  Pulmonary lymphangiectasia
  Pulmonary hypoplasia (diaphragmatic hernia)
Renal
  Congenital nephrosis
  Renal vein thrombosis
Intrauterine infections
  Syphilis
  Toxoplasmosis
  Cytomegalovirus
  Leptospirosis
  Chagas disease
  Congenital hepatitis
  Parvovirus
Congenital anomalies
  Achondroplasia
  E trisomy
  Multiple anomalies
  Turner syndrome
Miscellaneous
  Meconium peritonitis
  Fetal neuroblastomatosis
  Dysmaturity
  Tuberous sclerosis
  Storage disease
  Small bowel volvulus

BOX 17-4
Nonimmune Hydrops Fetalis: Causes and Associations—cont'd

PLACENTAL
Umbilical vein thrombosis
Chorionic vein thrombosis
Chorioangioma

MATERNAL
Diabetes mellitus
Toxemia

IDIOPATHIC

From Etches PC, Lemons JA: *Pediatrics* 64:326, 1979.

alized edema, failure, weak heart sounds—the picture of hydrops fetalis.

N.B.: Hydrops may occur from nonimmune causes (Box 17-4).

   d. Hepatosplenomegaly. Varies with severity of disease, from none to the huge enlargement noted with hydrops.
   e. Hemorrhage. Petechiae and purpura are bad prognostic signs, suggesting onset of a condition simulating DIC.
   f. Maternal polyhydramnios and preeclamptic toxemia are frequent precursors.
   g. Degree of severity increases with subsequent sensitized pregnancies.
2. Laboratory findings.
   a. Hemoglobin concentration. Values <14 g/dl are worrisome. Determinations are best done using venous blood (e.g., from the cord). Capillary blood may give inappropriately high result.
   b. Reticulocyte count. May be as high as 30%.
   c. Nucleated RBCs. Concentrations of >10:100 WBCs are common.
   d. Spherocytes. Usually seen only with ABO incompatibility.
   e. Platelets. Number may be decreased if anemia is severe.
   f. Hypoglycemia. Hyperinsulinism is common in severely affected babies; mechanism remains unclear. Blood glucose level should be closely followed.
   g. Coombs' test. Direct test with infant's washed RBCs is usually clearly positive with Rh incompatibility, but not at all or only weakly so with ABO incompatibility. An indirect test searches for free anti-A or anti-B antibodies in infant serum and is usually positive with clinically significant ABO incompatibility.
   h. Serum bilirubin levels. Cord blood value at birth >4 mg/dl suggests severe disease. The concern is with indirect bilirubin. It is helpful to know the level of direct bilirubin before initiating any type of therapy. The figure of 20 mg/dl as the "risk point" for

kernicterus refers to indirect bilirubin in Rh hemolytic disease. That risk point drops with increasing prematurity.

i. Bilirubin binding capacity of serum albumin. Indirect (unconjugated) bilirubin bound to albumin in the serum is harmless; only the amount unbound or "free" is toxic to the CNS. There is no clinically useful test for this binding capacity.

N.B.: Diagnosis can be facilitated with an approach suggested in Fig. 17-1.

3. Treatment. Prevention of RH incompatibility is the first goal.

a. Injection of the mother with RhoGAM (Rh immunoglobulin), 300 μg, within 72 hours of delivery after the first Rh-incompatible pregnancy; highly effective, with a protection rate of at least 90%; although some babies have been reported to be sensitized during a first pregnancy, this is not common. A larger RhoGAM dose is required for fetomaternal hemorrhage.

b. Exchange transfusion. Not an innocuous procedure, with an estimated mortality rate of 1%; hyperkalemia, hypocalcemia, hypomagnesemia, introduction of citrated blood, acidosis, and hypoglycemia are potential complications; hemodynamic changes may result in myocardial dysfunction; serum IgG levels in the first year of life tend to be lower. Still, a bilirubin level >4 mg/dl at birth and a hemoglobin concentration <14 g/dl suggest the need for urgent exchange transfusion. Portal vein thrombosis and necrotizing enterocolitis (NEC) are possible complications; moderate anemia is not uncommon after exchange.

N.B.: Effective use of RhoGAM prophylaxis has rendered Rh hemolytic disease so rare today that many primary care pediatricians have never performed exchange transfusion in the neonate, or have not done so for many years. Because of the significant mortality rate of the procedure, its use should be determined and undertaken only by highly trained and experienced personnel.

c. Intrauterine intraperitoneal transfusion. Should be used only in fetuses with early evidence of severe incompatibility and who are seriously ill; an experienced operator is essential.

d. Intrauterine plasmapheresis. Should be used only with fetuses otherwise certain to die and in the hands of an experienced operator. A good indication is a previous pregnancy ending in stillbirth before 24 to 26 weeks of gestation.

e. Phototherapy (see p. 214).

f. Persistent reticulocytopenia after birth can result in late anemia for months after birth. Erythropoietin therapy may shorten the period of postnatal transfusion requirement.

C. ABO incompatibility. Currently, ABO incompatibility is the most common cause of alloimmune hemolytic disease of the newborn. It is the result of interaction between maternal anti-A and anti-B antibodies and the corresponding A and B erythrocytes in the baby. A potential for it exists in about 15% of white and black births in the United States; Asian babies are at less risk. The clinical manifestations are generally relatively mild. Only one infant in five develops clinically significant jaundice, which is generally more severe in blacks.

1. Clinical findings. (For comparison with Rh incompatibility, see Table 17-4.)

   a. Jaundice. Usually appears within the first 24 hours; usually mild, rarely sufficiently intense to cause kernicterus.

   b. Pallor. Uncommon.

   c. Anemia. Mild or absent.

   d. Hydrops fetalis/stillbirth. Extremely rare.

   e. Hepatosplenomegaly. Minimal, if at all.

TABLE 17-4
Comparison of Rh and ABO Incompatibility

	Rh	ABO
Blood group setup		
Mother	Negative	O
Infant	Positive	A or B
Type of antibody	Incomplete (IgG)	Immune (IgG)
Clinical aspects		
Occurrence in firstborn	5%	40%-50%
Predictable severity in subsequent pregnancies	Usually	No
Stillbirth or hydrops	Frequent	Rare
Severe anemia	Frequent	Rare
Degree of jaundice	+++	+
Hepatosplenomegaly	+++	+
Laboratory findings		
Direct Coombs' test (infant)	+	+ or −
Maternal antibodies	Always present	Not clear-cut
Spherocytes	0	+
Treatment		
Need for antenatal measures	Yes	No
Value of phototherapy	Limited	Great
Exchange transfusion		
Frequency	Approximately two thirds	Approximately 1%
Donor blood type	Rh-negative; group specific when possible	Rh same as infant group O only
Incidence of late anemia	Common	Rare

From Oski FA, Naiman JL: *Hematologic problems in the newborn,* ed 3, Philadelphia, 1982, WB Saunders.

    f. Half of affected infants are firstborn; there is no predictor for subsequent infants.

    g. Degree of severity is not directly related to the number of pregnancies; there is no predictable progression of severity with succeeding pregnancies.

  2. Laboratory findings.

    a. Hemoglobin concentration. Usually normal, rarely as low as 8 g/dl; may be accompanied by an increase in nucleated RBCs.

    b. Microspherocytosis. Common, accompanied by increased osmotic fragility; can help to distinguish from Rh alloimmunization, in which spherocytes are uncommon.

    c. Bilirubin levels. The earlier the rise, the more likely there is to be a high ultimate bilirubinemia.

    d. Serologic findings. Incompatibility is almost always O with A or B, rarely A with B or B with A. Direct Coombs' test result is usually weakly positive, and may even be negative. Indirect Coombs' test may be helpful in such cases.

N.B.: A positive direct Coombs' test suggests greater need for therapeutic intervention. The indirect Coombs' test is more frequently positive, but the positive direct Coombs' test suggests greater severity.

  3. Treatment. Directed toward control of hyperbilirubinemia. Routine blood typing and direct Coombs' test should be performed on all infants born of type-O mothers; follow-up with serial bilirubin levels can readily identify the baby at risk. The first appropriate intervention is phototherapy. Exposure to blue light (overhead lamp or fiber optic vest) will reduce serum bilirubin concentration promptly and safely in many infants. Phototherapy is more effective with the milder hyperbilirubinemia of ABO incompatibility than with that of Rh; it drastically reduces the need for exchange in the former condition and limits the number of exchanges in the latter.

    a. Cautions.

      (1) Bronze baby syndrome is an infrequent complication in babies with impaired biliary secretion and a greater level of direct bilirubin.

      (2) Side effects (e.g., rash, diarrhea, lethargy, mild hypocalcemia and mild drop in platelets) are transient and usually not significant.

      (3) Eyes must be protected when overhead lamp is in use.

      (4) Phototherapy must *not* be used as a substitute for accurate diagnosis.

    b. Indications.

      (1) Phototherapy for ABO incompatibility in the full-term neonate should usually be instituted when the bilirubin level reaches 10 by 12 hours of age, 12 by 18 hours, 14 by 24 hours, and 15 or more after 24 hours; it should be started earlier in the older premature infant, and earlier still in the younger premature.

      (2) Phenobarbital enhances bilirubin conjugation and excretion; however, the slow rise in blood level over several days limits

its value. Phenobarbital cannot be substituted for phototherapy.

   (3) Exchange transfusion should be considered in ABO hemolytic disease when the rate of bilirubin increase exceeds 1 mg/dl/hr, hemoglobin concentration is 10 g/dl or less, or if bilirubin level exceeds 15 mg/dl in the first 24 hours of life; all are possible but infrequent occurrences.

D. Minor blood-group incompatibilities. Since the introduction of Rh immunoglobulin (RhoGAM), the proportion of cases of hemolytic disease caused by "minor group" antibodies (e.g., Kell, C, E, Duffy [Fya], and Kidd [JK^a]) has increased. Most infants affected by these antibodies show only mild evidence of hemolysis. Diagnosis depends on the clinical picture of jaundice, some evidence of hemolysis, and a positive direct Coombs' test that cannot be explained by an Rh or ABO incompatibility. Consult with a hematologist to pursue exact identification of the antibody.

   1. Prenatal management. Screening of all pregnant women for atypical antibodies early in pregnancy and, if negative, at 28 and 34 weeks of gestation. If serial titers indicate a significant rise, intrauterine transfusion or plasmapheresis may rarely be indicated.

   2. Postnatal management is similar to that of infants with ABO incompatibility.

N.B.: In the unusual event of a need for exchange transfusion, donor blood lacking the antigen to which antibodies have developed must be used.

IV. DISORDERS OF RBC METABOLISM

A. Inherited, transient, or acquired RBC defects may cause hemolytic disease of the newborn. These defects are characterized by shortened RBC life span and variable clinical manifestations depending on the infant's ability to compensate with increased erythropoiesis and bilirubin clearance.

B. Generally, the destruction of 1 g of hemoglobin will result in the production of 35 mg of bilirubin.

C. Because of the neonate's limited ability to compensate, significant hyperbilirubinemia can occur with even minimal hemolysis. Kernicterus is generally a risk only with Rh hemolytic disease; profound anemia is always a possibility; hepatosplenomegaly is a variable finding.

D. Fetal erythrocytes differ from those of older infants and children in their membrane properties, hemoglobins, unique metabolic profile, and much shorter life span. Genetic factors, acquired disease, and maternal and gestationally derived factors may contribute; the clinical picture can vary from that of the older child or adult.

E. The newborn's red cells are osmotically and mechanically more fragile and more prone to hemolysis in the presence of drugs, acidosis, and genetic and congenital metabolic defects (Box 17-5).

BOX 17-5
Causes of Hemolytic Disease in the Newborn

Isoimmunization (erythroblastosis fetalis)
Enzymatic deficiencies of the red cell
  Glycolytic enzymes
    Hexokinase
    Glucose phosphate isomerase
    Phosphofructokinase
    Aldolase
    Triose phosphate isomerase
    2,3-DPG mutase
    Phosphoglycerate kinase
    Pyruvate kinase
    Glucose-6-phosphate dehydrogenase
    Galactose 1-phosphate uridyltransferase deficiency—galactosemia
  Nonglycolytic enzymes
    Glutathione peroxidase (?)
    Glutathione synthetase
γ-Glutamyl-cysteine synthetase
    ATPase
    Adenylate kinase
    Adenosine deaminase
    Pyrimidine-5`-nucleotidase
Drugs and toxins
  Heinz body anemia
Defects characterized by abnormalities of red cell morphology
  Hereditary spherocytosis
  Hereditary elliptocytosis
  Hereditary stomatocytosis
  Infantile pyknocytosis
  Pyropoikilocytosis
Infections
  Bacterial
  Viral (cytomegalic inclusion disease, hepatitis)
  Toxoplasmosis
  Syphilis
Defects in hemoglobin synthesis
  Hemoglobin Barts (α-thalassemia)
  Unstable hemoglobins (congenital Heinz body anemias)
Miscellaneous
  Erythropoietic porphyria
  Disseminated intravascular coagulation

From Oski FA, Naiman JL: *Hematologic problems in the newborn,* ed 3, Philadelphia, 1982, WB Saunders.

F. Enzymatic deficiencies in the neonatal red cell. Enzymatic deficiencies are a heterogeneous group, each of which is capable of causing congenital nonspherocytic hemolytic anemia. They demonstrate normal osmotic fragility, few or no spherocytes, and normal hemoglobin; many do not respond to splenectomy. They can all cause jaundice and anemia, usually mild and possibly escaping detection until later in life. Except for G6PD deficiency, which affects as many as 100 million or more persons in the world, these disorders are rare. Consultation with a pediatric hematologist is needed.

1. Defects of the Embden-Meyerhof pathway. More than 90% of red cell glucose is metabolized by this pathway; hyperbilirubinemia, anemia, and reticulocytosis may occur, possibly with bilirubin levels >20 mg/dl and hemoglobin concentrations <10 g/dl; blood smear reveals a few spherocytes, a random poikilocyte, and a variety of morphologic disorders typical of hemolysis. Pyruvate kinase deficiency is the most common of these defects. Therapy requires control of hyperbilirubinemia and correction of anemia. The use of transfusion, phototherapy, and exchange transfusion is guided by principles similar to those outlined in the treatment of blood-group incompatibilities (see pp. 212-215).

2. Defects of the pentose phosphate pathway and disorders of glutathione metabolism.

   a. Hemolysis is the result of oxidative injury to the red cell, usually mild unless triggered by a drug, infection or acidosis; G6PD deficiency is by far the most common among several otherwise rare conditions and is discovered primarily in the Mediterranean region and among blacks, Sardinians, Greeks, Iranians, and Sephardic Jews.

   b. Fewer than 10% of affected neonates have clinically significant jaundice or anemia. If present, the jaundice usually becomes apparent after the first 24 hours and sometimes not for several days. Bilirubin levels may exceed 20 mg/dl by 3 to 5 days, sometimes into the second week. If there is early-onset jaundice, note the mother's drug history.

N.B.: The risk of kernicterus does not necessarily diminish with time.

   c. Hemoglobin levels may drop.

   d. Reticulocytes will increase.

   e. Blood smear will show nucleated red cells, blister cells, spherocytes, poikilocytosis, and other morphologic disruptions.

   f. Screening tests will reveal sharply diminished G6PD activity. In patients with unstable enzymes, activity levels may be falsely normal if reticulocytosis is present, a result of the higher enzymatic activity of young cells.

   g. Screening is indicated in any baby with clinical evidence of hemolysis who is a member of a high-incidence ethnic group (African or Mediterranean descent).

   h. Treatment may involve phenobarbital, phototherapy, and exchange transfusion. There is some evidence that phototherapy may be less helpful and phenobarbital more so in avoiding or reducing the number of exchange transfusions. In any event, avoidance of "trigger" drugs and careful tracking of hyperbilirubinemia are essential (see Chapter 19).

3. Additional uncommon RBC metabolic abnormalities.
    a. Adenosine triphosphate deficiency.
    b. Adenylate kinase deficiency; probably autosomal recessive.
    c. Adenosine deaminase deficiency.
    d. Pyrimidine-5`-nucleotidase deficiency. Basophilic stippling of red cells is a striking characteristic; autosomal recessive.
    e. Galactose-1-phosphate uridyltransferase deficiency (galactosemia). Not generally considered a primary red-cell disorder but may cause hemolytic anemia; the mechanism is unclear. When hyperbilirubinemia is unexplained, urine should be examined for a non–glucose-reducing substance.

N.B.: The clinical manifestations and treatment approaches for these disorders parallel those for the other hemolytic anemias.

V. DEFECTS ASSOCIATED WITH ABNORMALITIES IN RBC MORPHOLOGY

These disorders may all occur in the neonate, although often they present after the neonatal period.

A. Hereditary spherocytosis. RBCs are spherocytic and abnormally fragile. Inheritance is usually autosomal dominant and is probably more common in northern Europeans. Autosomal recessive mutations with no parental anemia cause a minority of cases.

1. Clinical findings.
    a. Neonatal jaundice is common, usually occurring by 48 hours but as late as 7 days after birth.
    b. Hyperbilirubinemia may exceed 20 mg/dl and be sufficient to cause kernicterus.
    c. Splenomegaly is usually minimal.
    d. Anemia is generally mild; hemoglobin level is rarely <10 g/dl.
    e. Reticulocytes are increased.
    f. Peripheral blood smear reveals characteristic spherocyte, but some neonates may not have many at first. The spherocyte is smaller in diameter and the central pallor is absent, indicating a dense cell.
    g. The red-cell osmotic fragility test is usually strongly positive. Neonatal controls are required.
    h. Haptoglobin levels are not helpful. The haptoglobin level is low in most normal newborns, rendering such test results difficult to interpret in the newborn with anemia, although it is a useful test after 1 year of age.
    i. The most helpful diagnostic findings are spherocytes, reticulocytosis, and low haptoglobin in a parent; this may be confirmed by osmotic fragility test.

2. Treatment parallels that for ABO incompatibility; in this instance, severe and chronic anemia can be avoided with splenectomy; surgery before 4 to 6 years of age should be avoided if possible.

N.B.: ABO incompatibility in the presence of spherocytes does not necessarily establish the incompatibility as the cause of hemolytic anemia. A negative Coombs' test can be helpful. Chronicity may be the ultimate determinant; hereditary spherocytosis is lifelong.

  B. Hereditary elliptocytosis. A group of rare disorders characterized by variable numbers of oval and elliptical red blood cells in the peripheral blood; often autosomal dominant, but genetically heterogeneous.
  1. Neonatal anemia and jaundice are uncommon.
  2. Demonstration of elliptical cells in the infant and at least one of the parents may be diagnostic, although the blood smear may be confusing, requiring hematology consultation. An unusual number of pyknocytes may obscure the diagnosis.
  C. Hereditary pyropoikilocytosis. Rare membranopathy; occurs in early infancy as severe, transfusion-dependent hemolytic anemia with significant disruption of RBC morphology. RBCs are heat labile. Call for consultation.
  D. Hereditary stomatocytosis (hydrocytosis). Rare; an area of pallor in the RBC resembles a mouth and disrupts cell morphology; probably variable inheritance. Call for consultation.
  E. Infantile pyknocytosis. Transient abnormality of the first few months of life. Pyknocytic RBCs are smaller than the normal red cell, misshapen, irregular in outline, densely stained, and contain spiny projections. A few are seen in all infants, more so in premature infants, and disappear after about 3 months. The disorder is caused by an increased number of pyknocytes and is characterized by jaundice, anemia, reticulocytosis, and frequently splenomegaly. It may be clinically evident in the first week, and rarely may require exchange transfusion.
  F. Heinz body anemia. Neonates, particularly premature infants, are susceptible to the development of a hemolytic anemia characterized by Heinz bodies within the RBCs. These inclusions, when stained with a supravital dye, appear as minute, refractile, irregularly shaped bodies, usually near the periphery of the cell. They are not seen in routinely stained smears. They represent hemoglobin precipitation caused by oxidative damage. Heinz bodies can be seen in G6PD deficiency, disorders of the pentose phosphate pathway, and some unstable hemoglobin disorders.
  1. Triggers in the neonate (swallowed by the neonate or mother, or applied to the neonate's skin) include the following:
    a. Naphthalene.
    b. Phenylhydrazine.
    c. Primaquine.
    d. Menadione (vitamin K_3).
    e. Synthetic water-soluble analogs of K_3, Synkayvite, and menadione.
    f. Henna (commonly used in Middle Eastern neonatal skin dyes).
    g. Aniline dyes.
    h. Nitrobenzene derivatives (formerly used for making diapers).
    i. Skin lotions with resorcin.
    j. Sulfonamides.

2. Clinical findings.
   a. Jaundice usually appears after 24 hours and may be prolonged.
   b. Severe anemia takes 2 to 3 weeks to develop.
3. Diagnosis.
   a. Identification of the Heinz bodies with supravital stains.
   b. Usually, red-cell fragmentation, blister cells, and some spherocytosis; G6PD deficiency and the presence of an unstable hemoglobin should be evaluated.
4. Treatment.
   a. Removal of the offending trigger agent.
   b. Exchange transfusion for hyperbilirubinemia.
   c. Simple transfusion for progressive and severe anemia.

VI. DISORDERS OF HEMOGLOBIN SYNTHESIS AND METABOLISM

A. Normal hemoglobin physiology.

1. Hemoglobin enables the RBC to transport oxygen from lungs to tissues. Oxygenation results from the combination of oxygen with the ferrous iron (Fe^{++}) of heme, a totally reversible, non–energy-dependent reaction essential for oxygen transport. Should ferrous iron be oxidized to a ferric (Fe^{+++}) state, methemoglobin incapable of oxygen transport is the result. Normal adult hemoglobins (A, A_2) may vary somewhat in the constitution of their polypeptide chains without loss of oxygenation capacity. Some abnormal hemoglobins can interfere with this function in a manner dependent on their individual characteristics. Hemoglobin F, unlike adult hemoglobins, resists denaturation by strong acid or alkali solutions.
2. The cord blood of the normal neonate contains Hb F, Hb A, and Hb A_2 in varying fractions, with F predominating by far. Hb A is present in small amounts in the first trimester and begins to rise in the third trimester.
3. As the fetus approaches term, Hb A begins to replace Hb F. The process is slower in small-for-gestational-age (SGA) babies. Normally, Hb F declines to levels of 10% to 15% in the first few months, then more slowly after that to levels of <1% at 6 months of age.
4. The γ polypeptide chains of intrauterine life are replaced by the β polypeptide chains of adult life, the γ-β switch. This relatively delicate process can be confounded in a number of ways. Embryonic hemoglobins typical of the first trimester of pregnancy (e.g., Hb Gower 1, Hb Gower 2, Hb Portland) may persist in trisomy 13 or other D-group translocations.

B. Disorders of heme synthesis.
Congenital erythropoietic porphyria is rare and is characterized by skin vesicles, red urine, and hemolytic anemia. Red urine is possible in normal neonates of mothers with porphyria; "passive porphyria" disappears within 48 hours.

C. Disorders of globin synthesis.
Many disorders of globin synthesis may be detected in the neonate.

1. Hemoglobinopathies are qualitative disorders in which an amino

acid substitution in one of the polypeptide chains results in a variant hemoglobin; more than 400 have been described; only a few cause disease and have significant prevalence.

a. Sickle hemoglobin (Hb S) is the most important and prevalent.

b. Hb C is also common. Sickle cell syndromes are inherited, predominantly in blacks but also in Arabs, Asians, Native Americans, and persons of Mediterranean background. The heterozygous form (Hb S with Hb A) occurs in 8% of blacks in the United States; the homozygous form (Hb SS) occurs in 1:500. The homozygous disease tends to be severe; Hb SC is less so but still has the potential for handicap; Hb AC is not clinically significant; Hb CC causes moderate hemolytic anemia that is generally easily managed.

2. Thalassemia syndromes. Characterized by a decreased rate of synthesis of one of the normal polypeptide chains.

a. α-Thalassemia syndromes. Reduced rate of synthesis of α chains; inherited; variable clinical manifestations; common in Southeast Asia and in black populations; most cases require no therapy although occasional transfusion may be necessary.

(1) Homozygous (four alpha gene deletion) infants generally die in utero with profound hydrops, which is sometimes detectable with sonography. Infants with increased, though not predominant levels of Hb Bart's (tetramers of γ chains) at birth may have a lifelong hypochromic, microcytic anemia requiring no diagnostic or therapeutic intervention. Five syndromes have been defined (Table 17-5).

(2) Silent carrier.

(3) α-Thalassemia trait. Newborns may show mild anemia, microcytosis.

(4) Hb H disease. Newborns may show anemia and hemolysis, striking microcytosis, hypochromia, and target cells; there is a significant percentage of unstable Hb Bart's.

(5) Fetal hydrops. Most severe of the α-thalassemias; total absence of α-chain synthesis; fetuses born prematurely, stillborn, or die soon after birth; particularly noted in Southeast Asia; universal edema, profound anemia, massive hepatosplenomegaly, microcytosis, hypochromia, negative Coombs' test. Hb Bart's predominates. Intrauterine transfusion can be lifesaving.

(6) Hb Constant spring. A minor Hb variant associated with α-thalassemia. Newborns, usually Asians, may have mild anemia and microcytosis.

b. β-Thalassemia syndromes. Reduced synthesis of β-hemoglobin chains; autosomal inheritance.

(1) Thalassemia major (Cooley anemia). Homozygous, severe, requiring frequent blood transfusions to sustain life; marked hepatosplenomegaly; failure to thrive; significant compensatory elevations in Hb F in neonate delay clinical manifestation beyond newborn period for as long as 6 months.

TABLE 17-5
Features of α-Thalassemia Syndromes

Syndrome	Clinical Features		Hemoglobin Pattern			Number of genes affected by Thal mutation
	Birth	Late life	Birth	Later life	β/α ratio	
Silent carrier	No anemia or microcytosis	No anemia or microcytosis	1%-2% Hb Bart's	Normal	SI >1	1
Thalassemia trait	Mild anemia and microcytosis	Mild anemia and microcytosis	3%-10% Hb Bart's	Normal	1.2/1	2
Hb H disease	Moderate microcytic hypochromic hemolytic anemia	Same	20%-40% Hb Bart's	5%-30% Hb H	2.5/1	3
Fetal hydrops syndrome	Moderate to severe hypochromic microcytic anemia	Lethal	≈80% Hb Bart's 0%-20% Hb H Small amount of Hb Portland	—	∞	4

From Oski FA, Naiman JL: *Hematologic problems in the newborn*, ed 3, Philadelphia, 1982, WB Saunders.

     (2) Thalassemia minor. Heterozygous, mild microcytic, hypochromic anemia, not usually clinically significant; can be nonanemic with erythrocytosis; notably in individuals of Greek and Italian descent.

     (3) γδβ Thalassemia. Rare; occurs in the neonate with a clinical picture resembling erythroblastosis fetalis; milder presentations are possible.

  3. Diagnosis. These disorders present only rarely in the neonate. Nevertheless, intrauterine diagnosis and early confirmation or detection in the neonate are important to the medical care of the affected individual; some important diagnostic signs (e.g., elevated hemoglobin Bart's in α-thalassemia minor) may be detected only in the neonatal period.

    a. Chorionic villus biopsy at 10 to 12 weeks of gestation is the method of choice for detection, provided the parental mutations are known and detectable by genetic testing.

N.B.: Chorionic villus biopsy is not recommended before 10 weeks of gestation because of potential for congenital abnormalities of digits.

    b. Fetal blood sampling by fetoscopy or placental aspiration offers another method of detection; in the second trimester, β-chain synthesis can be detected by 12 weeks of gestation. Sensitivity and specificity are high.

    c. Amniocentesis for fetal fibroblasts may be used as for chorionic villus sampling above.

    d. Hemoglobin electrophoresis or isoelectric focusing is reliable in the neonate: ordinary screening tests with metabisulfate or dithionate are insensitive to the scant amount of Hb S in neonatal red cells; Hb C and α- and β-thalassemias can be readily detected with cord-blood electrophoresis. Many states have sophisticated newborn hemoglobin screening programs to detect hemoglobinopathies at birth.

N.B.: Fatal intravascular sickling is rare but is more likely in a premature infant transfused with blood from a donor with sickle trait. A prior sickle test on donor blood is preventive.

  D. Methemoglobinemia. Excessive red-cell methemoglobin is unable to transport oxygen, resulting in slate-gray, diffuse cyanosis in the neonate; it should always be included in the differential diagnosis of neonatal cyanosis.

    1. Causes.

      a. Hereditary deficiency of enzymes needed for reduction of methemoglobin.

      b. Presence of abnormal Hb M.

      c. Triggers. Drugs or toxic agents that oxidize hemoglobin directly (e.g., nitrates [contaminated well water; conversion to nitrites required], benzocaine, aniline dyes) (Table 17-6).

    2. Clinical features.

      a. Generalized cyanosis, including mucous membranes, nose, fingers, and toes.

TABLE 17-6
Agents That May Cause Methemoglobinemia in the Newborn

Agent	Source
Nitrates ($\rightarrow$ nitrites)	Well water (contaminated)
	Bismuth subnitrate (antidiarrheal)
Nitrites (ethyl)	Sweet spirit of nitre
Aniline derivatives	Diaper-making dyes
	Disinfectants (e.g., TCC, or trichlorocarbanilide)
	Benzocaine (skin applications)
Resorcin	Skin applications
Acetophenetidin	Analgesic compounds
Prilocaine	Local obstetrical analgesic
Sulfonamides (older)	Sulfanilamide, sulfathiazole, sulfapyridine

From Oski FA, Naiman JL: *Hematologic problems in the newborn,* ed 3, Philadelphia, 1982, WB Saunders.

    b. No respiratory distress unless methemoglobin level is extraordinarily high.
    c. Onset of cyanosis in a previously pink infant (suggests a toxic agent).
  3. Confirmation.
    a. At bedside. Expose a drop of infant's capillary blood on filter paper to air for 30 seconds. Use a drop of normal adult blood as a control. The infant's blood appears chocolate brown as compared with the red color of the control; methemoglobin level may be high enough to warrant treatment.
    b. Normal arterial Po_2 is associated with low oxygen saturation by pulse oximeter or co-oximeter.
    c. Spectroscopic examination of blood, performed on some arterial blood gas machines. Levels of methemoglobin sufficient to cause cyanosis may range from 10% to as high as 60% to 70% in the severely affected infant.
  4. Treatment.
    a. Start with a single intravenous dose of methylene blue, an effective reducing agent, 1 to 2 mg/kg in a 1% solution in normal saline. Cyanosis will generally disappear within 60 minutes, confirmed by a sharp drop in methemoglobin level.
N.B.: Larger or more concentrated doses may damage red cells. Lack of response may be seen with G6PD deficiency.
    b. Search for and remove potential toxic agent; after its elimination, there should be no recurrence and no further need for treatment.
    c. With hereditary methemoglobinemia, continued therapy is indicated with oral methylene blue (anticipate stained diapers) or ascorbic acid, 300 to 400 mg per day orally.

5. Hemoglobin M disease. Rare; autosomal dominant inheritance, may be familial in occurrence. Clinically obvious cyanosis does not respond to treatment with methylene blue; confirm with hemoglobin electrophoresis. This eliminates the need for more extensive pulmonary or cardiac workup.

N.B.: Methylene blue may be used in the differential diagnosis of neonatal cyanosis when an obvious source is unclear.

VII. POLYCYTHEMIA AND HYPERVISCOSITY (NEONATAL THICK BLOOD SYNDROME)

Hyperviscosity and polycythemia are not synonymous. Viscosity relates to hematocrit, deformability of red blood cells, and plasma viscosity; the hematocrit is the most important variable. Viscosity increases exponentially at higher hematocrit levels, leading to poor peripheral flow and perfusion and occasional persistent pulmonary hypertension.

A. Definition. *Venous* hematocrit level ≥65 (hemoglobin ≥22); occasionally, hematocrit level of 60 to 64 may result in hyperviscosity.

N.B.: Measurements of venous hematocrit are more reliable than capillary levels and should always serve as a check on the capillary, particularly at the extremes of the normal range.

B. Incidence. Occurs in 1% to 2% of newborns; half of these may be symptomatic; there is a higher incidence (4% to 5%) at higher elevations.

C. Predispositions to polycythemia (asterisk indicates particular risks).

1. Active (increased intrauterine erythropoiesis).
   a. Intrauterine hypoxia.
      (1) Intrauterine growth retardation (IUGR).*
      (2) SGA (rarely in the very premature).*
      (3) Postmaturity.*
      (4) Placental insufficiency.
      (5) Toxemia of pregnancy.
      (6) Drugs (propranolol).
      (7) Severe maternal heart disease.
      (8) Maternal smoking.
      (9) Cyanotic congenital heart disease.
   b. Maternal diabetes.*
   c. Neonatal thyrotoxicosis.
   d. Congenital adrenal hyperplasia.
   e. Chromosome abnormalities.
      (1) Trisomy 13.
      (2) Trisomy 18.
      (3) Trisomy 21 (Down syndrome).*
      (4) Hyperplastic visceromegaly (Beckwith syndrome).
   f. Decreased fetal erythrocyte deformability.
   g. Pregnancy at high altitude.
2. Passive (secondary to erythrocyte transfusion).
   a. Delayed cord clamping.*

          (1) Intentional.

          (2) Unassisted delivery.

      b. Maternal-fetal transfusion.

      c. Twin-twin transfusion.

N.B.: Infants actively responding to prolonged intrauterine hypoxia are often born with increased numbers of reticulocytes and nucleated red blood cells in peripheral circulation.

N.B.: Idiopathic is probably the most common diagnosis.

    D. Clinical findings. There is considerable variability in the clinical picture; symptoms and signs usually appear in 48 to 72 hours and may include the following:

1. Plethora (most common).
2. Lethargy; hypotonia; weak suck; poor feeding.
3. Difficult to arouse; irritable when aroused.
4. Cyanosis while active.
5. Vomiting.
6. Tremulousness; easily startled; myoclonic jerks.
7. Hepatomegaly.
8. Jaundice (more RBCs to break down).
9. Poor response to light.
10. Increased respiratory rate.
11. Oliguria.

    E. Laboratory findings, which can have considerable variability, include the following:

1. Venous hematocrit ≥65%.
2. Hyperviscosity.
3. Thrombocytopenia.
4. Reticulocytosis.
5. Normoblastemia.
6. Hypoglycemia (one third of affected infants).
7. Hypocalcemia (less common).
8. Hyperbilirubinemia.
9. Abnormal electroencephalogram (EEG) (not generally indicated).
10. Abnormal electrocardiogram (ECG) (only on indication).
11. Urinalysis may reveal hematuria, proteinuria, hemoglobinuria.
12. Evidence of increased vascularity, pleural fluid, hyperaeration, alveolar infiltrates, and cardiomegaly on chest radiograph.

    F. Possible complications, which can have great variability, include the following:

1. Respiratory distress.
2. Congestive heart failure.
3. Convulsions and a variety of neurologic sequelae (e.g., spastic diplegia, hypotonia, tremor).
4. Peripheral gangrene.
5. Priapism.
6. Necrotizing enterocolitis (especially in SGA babies).
7. Ileus.
8. Acute renal failure (hemoglobinuria, hematuria, proteinuria, oliguria, rarely azotemia).
9. Thromboses (CNS, renal).

G. Management.

1. Obtain careful prenatal and perinatal history for risk factors (see list of causative or related factors).
2. Obtain capillary hematocrit on all infants at 4 to 6 hours of life.
3. Measure venous hematocrit level if capillary hematocrit level is ≥65.
4. Perform careful repeat examination of every infant with a venous hematocrit level ≥60.
5. Obtain blood glucose and calcium levels on all infants with a venous hematocrit level ≥65.

H. Treatment.

1. The symptomatic baby should be treated; however, the decision to treat an asymptomatic baby is controversial. Some evidence suggests at least subtle difficulty, particularly neurologic, in later childhood for the presumably asymptomatic newborn. In the face of controversy, the higher the hematocrit level, the more likely treatment becomes.
2. Partial exchange transfusion is the recommended procedure. The goal is to reduce the venous hematocrit level to about 50% to 55%, using 5% albumin, normal saline, or lactated Ringer's solution. Avoid fresh frozen plasma; *never* use simple phlebotomy without volume replacement.
3. Volume of exchange (ml) (approximate) =

$$\text{(Weight in kg} \times 80 \text{ ml/kg)} \times \text{(Current Hct} - \text{Desired Hct)} \div \text{Current Hct}$$

4. Perform exchange in 10- to 20-ml aliquots; do *not* exceed 5% of the blood volume (approximately 4 ml/kg).
5. Repeat measurement of hematocrit level before exchange is ended and catheter is removed.
6. Repeat exchange if there is recurrence or persistence of symptoms.

VIII. DISORDERS OF LEUKOCYTES
A. Neutropenia.

1. Definition. Absolute neutrophil count <1500/mm³; a count <500/mm³ is extraordinarily worrisome.
2. Neutrophil function. At best, the neutrophil in the newborn does not function up to par, thus putting the neonate at considerable risk for infection. Deficiencies may be quantitative, qualitative, or an interplay of both. Qualitative defects may involve the phagocytic process, including the following:
   a. Motility. Random motility may be reduced (delayed detachment of cord suggests this defect) or chemotaxis limited.
   b. Defective opsonization (deficiencies in IgM antibodies and various complement components, including alternative pathway).
   c. Defective phagocytosis and pseudopod formation under stress.
   d. Defective intracellular bactericidal capability, particularly during stress (e.g., sepsis, meconium aspiration, hemolytic jaundice).
3. Reaction to infection. Ordinarily, the total neutrophil count during first day of life peaks at 12 to 14 hours with a range of 7800 to

14,500 cells/mm^3. By 72 hours, the count can be as low as 1750, with a gradual return to as many as 5500 by 5 days of age. Bands may range from 0 to 1400, averaging 500 by 5 days of age. The ratio of immature cells to total neutrophils in the first few hours is 0.16, dropping gradually to 0.13 by 5 days, and after that averaging about 0.12.

  a. Infection alters these numbers; the incidence of infection varies inversely with neutrophil count; neutropenia is more common than leukocytosis; band count increases; an elevated ratio, as much as 0.4 is common, and may even be 0.8 with sepsis.
  b. Infection also (but not always) alters WBC morphology (e.g., increased toxic granulation, vacuolization, Döhle bodies).
4. Conditions with neutropenia. Disorders may involve immune or metabolic disturbance, genetic predetermination, decreased neutrophil survival, myelodysplastic processes; no unifying pathogenic classification.
  a. Infection, viral or bacterial; bacterial sepsis is the most common cause, but consider herpes simplex virus (HSV).
  b. Maternal drug-induced neutropenia (e.g., thiazides, sulfonamides, propylthiouracil, methimazole, gold salts [common]).
  c. Maternal hypertension (common, usually not severe).
  d. Transplacental transfer of maternal IgG against antigens on infant's neutrophils.
    (1) Alloimmune. Maternal sensitization to fetal neutrophil antigen, analogous to Rh or ABO red cell alloimmunization or platelet alloimmunization.
    (2) Maternal autoimmune. Mother with autoimmune neutropenia, often subclinical.
    (3) Infection (e.g., omphalitis) may occur but is not frequent.
  e. Cyclic neutropenia (autosomal dominant when familial; not usually diagnosed in the neonate).
  f. Benign congenital neutropenia (a variety of heritable or random conditions, rarely a clinical problem in the newborn).
  g. Kostmann syndrome (severe congenital neutropenia, ordinarily autosomal recessive; may be clinically obvious on first day of life).
  h. Concurrent immune deficiencies (IgG, IgA); occasionally eczema/polyarthralgia/infection, neutropenia, eosinophilia (similar to Wiskott-Aldrich syndrome).
  i. Exocrine pancreatic insufficiency/dwarfism/malabsorption (Shwachman-Diamond syndrome); probably autosomal recessive; normal sweat test result. (Treatment of malabsorption does not relieve the neutropenia.)
  j. Cartilage hair hypoplasia syndrome.
  k. Reticular dysgenesis (rare, severe, *all* leukocytes deficient).
  l. Severe asphyxia.
  m. Periventricular hemorrhage.
  n. Repeated exchange transfusion (transient; not a worrisome circumstance).
  o. Maternal lupus erythematosus (rare).

5. Conditions that may be associated with increased band/ neutrophil ratio (all of these ratios generally return to normal quickly).
   a. Maternal diabetes.
   b. Hypoglycemia.
   c. Meconium aspiration.
   d. Apgar score <6 at 5 minutes.
6. Diagnosis and management.
   a. Consideration of infection a first priority; sepsis is the most common cause in the neonate, therefore one should presume infection until it is ruled out.
   b. Neutrophil count and band-to-neutrophil ratio should be followed carefully.
   c. Obtain erythrocyte sedimentation rate (ESR), C-reactive protein (optional).
   d. Obtain appropriate cultures, bacterial and viral (e.g., blood, urine, spinal fluid, and others as suggested by history and physical examination).
   e. Initiate antibiotic therapy based on findings, history, clinical judgment.
   f. If infection is not found and neutropenia persists, check for maternal hypertension, familial history of antineutrophil antibody formation, or maternal drug history.
   g. If these factors are absent and neutropenia persists, examine the following:
      (1) Maternal neutrophil counts.
      (2) Does mother have disease or history of drug use?
      (3) Family member neutrophil counts.
      (4) Antineutrophil antibody determinations on infant and mother.
      (5) Consider immune-mediated disease.
      (6) Bone marrow aspirate.
      (7) Consider leukemia, neoplasm, aplastic anemia.
      (8) In vitro granulocyte colony cultures to classify mechanism of neutropenia.
      (9) Follow neutrophil counts twice weekly for 2 months.
      (10) Consider cyclic neutropenia.
7. Specific therapy.
   a. Geared to the particular diagnosis.
   b. Meticulous attention to good hygiene (e.g., hand washing, gloves).
   c. Granulocyte-colony stimulating factor (G-CSF) often can stimulate transient neutrophil production in many neutropenic disorders.
   d. Granulocyte transfusions (only during life-threatening sepsis).
   e. Prophylactic antibiotic schedules when infection is not discovered (to be considered individually, based on severity).

B. Disorders of neutrophil function generally express themselves clinically beyond the newborn period and are generally uncommon (e.g., leukocyte adhesion disorder, lazy leukocyte syndrome, impairment of phagocytosis, degranulation [Chédiak-

Higashi syndrome], neutrophil killing [chronic granulomatous disease]).

C. Lymphocytes in the newborn.

1. Infants generally have more lymphocytes than older children and adults; the range is 3000 to 5000/mm³ at birth, with a transitory decline and a rise to about 6000 around the tenth day. There is a predominance of large and medium cells as compared with those of an adult; the proportion of B cells in cord blood is greater than in adults and relatively mature in function; T cells are relatively inefficient at birth but can release interferon.

2. Lymphopenia.
   a. Definition. Absolute count <1500/mm³.
   b. Causes.
      (1) Infection. There are many viral processes (e.g., CMV, rubella).
      (2) Maternal collagen vascular disease (e.g., the hematologic and serologic findings observed in women with SLE) may be seen in the infant.
      (3) Immunodeficiency syndromes.
      (4) Reticular dysgenesis.
      (5) Agammaglobulinemia of the Swiss type.
      (6) Agammaglobulinemia associated with short-limb dwarfism.
      (7) X-linked recessive agammaglobulinemia (thymic alymphoplasia).
      (8) Lymphopenia with dysgammaglobulinemia (Nezelof syndrome).
      (9) Wiskott-Aldrich syndrome (sometimes lymphopenic).
      (10) Adrenocorticoid excesses.
      (11) Iatrogenic, from steroid treatment (in mother, infant, or both).
      (12) Some instances of congenital adrenal hyperplasia.
      (13) Excessive lymphocyte losses.
         (a) Intestinal lymphangiectasia.
         (b) Thoracic duct drainage (including congenital and acquired chylothorax).
   c. Diagnosis and management.
      (1) Perform immunologic studies for defects of cellular and humoral immune function, including serum immunoglobulin determination and B-cell evaluation.
      (2) Withhold live virus vaccines until clinical picture is clarified.
      (3) Use only irradiated blood products for transfusion (prevent graft-host disease after engraftment with donor lymphocytes).

D. Eosinophilia in the newborn.

1. Definition. Normal infants have <1200 cells/mm³ during first few days of life. At birth, a peak number of 1000/mm³ is common, with 1200/mm³ by 1 week and a drop to 600/mm³ by 4 weeks. Anything in excess should be considered abnormal.

2. Incidence. Common, particularly in premature infants.

3. Significance. Uncertain. The usual causes in older children and infants are not usually detectable or considered in the neonate.

The day of peak eosinophilia is consistently related to the day birth weight is regained. May be related to endotracheal intubation or parenteral nutrition, but there is no consistency in any finding. It may be a response, presumably immature, to foreign antigens.

4. Management. Watchful waiting; keep immune deficiency in mind but do nothing further during newborn period without complementary clinical findings.

E. Leukemia in the very young infant.

1. Definition. Congenital leukemia, indistinguishable from that in older children and adults, may occur in the first few days of life; neonatal leukemia, a semantic hair-splitting, occurs in the first 4 to 6 weeks and is equally undifferentiated.

   a. Acute myeloid leukemia (AML) is far more frequent than other types. The etiology is unknown; a relationship exists with heritable disorders, including Down syndrome, Bloom syndrome, trisomy 13, Turner syndrome, Ellis-van Creveld syndrome.

   b. AML in patients with Down syndrome is often of the megakaryocytic subtype.

2. Clinical findings.

   a. Skin. Large, blue-gray nodules with fibroma-like feel, petechiae, ecchymoses; nodules are an early manifestation.

   b. Hepatosplenomegaly.

   c. Lymphadenopathy (infrequent).

   d. Failure to thrive.

   e. Fever.

   f. Diarrhea; after several days to a few weeks of age.

   g. Pallor; after several days.

   h. Clinical presentation does not distinguish type.

3. Laboratory findings.

   a. Sharply increased WBC count (as high as several hundred thousand/mm^3; may also be in normal range).

   b. Predominance of immature forms.

   c. Distorted RBC morphology.

   d. Thrombocytopenia at times.

   e. Confirmatory bone marrow study is hypercellular, with immature forms, decreased megakaryocytes, and erythrocyte and granulocyte precursors; cytochemical staining or flow cytometry may be necessary to distinguish type.

4. Differential diagnosis.

   a. Frequent confusion with bacterial infection, erythroblastosis fetalis, congenital syphilis, CMV infection, toxoplasmosis, histiocytosis X, metastatic neuroblastoma, and overwhelming viral disease.

   b. Down syndrome patients can have a transient myeloproliferative disease resembling acute myeloid leukemia, but they also are predisposed to bona fide acute myeloid leukemia, often of megakaryocytic lineage.

N.B.: Accurate diagnosis is needed to guide therapy; bone marrow aspiration *must* be undertaken in parallel with steps to exclude other possibilities.

  5. Treatment. The prognosis for neonates with congenital leukemia is generally poor, and optimal outcome is dependent on the most current treatment protocols.

IX. DISORDERS OF PLATELETS

Deficiency of platelet numbers, qualitative impairment of platelet function, or a generalized systemic illness may lead to bleeding. This is often signaled by generalized petechiae and purpuric spots that recur in crops over the first few days of life and is usually much more dramatic than the few, nonrecurring petechiae limited to the head and chest of normal newborns after vertex delivery and to the lower limbs after breech presentation. Newborn platelets are highly susceptible to maternal influences, particularly in premature infants. Associated bleeding is common from mucous membranes and at needle puncture sites.

A. Thrombocytopenia.

  1. Definition.

    a. Platelet counts in healthy, full-term newborns. Most infants have counts >150,000/mm³; a small number are in the 100,000 to 150,000/mm³ range. Recheck of a somewhat lower count is mandatory in a potentially ill infant. Counts <100,000/mm³ are always abnormal; however, severe bleeding is unlikely with counts >30,000/mm³.

    b. Platelet counts in otherwise healthy preterm newborns. Unrelated to the degree of prematurity; there is a somewhat greater tendency to lower counts than in the full-term baby, but at rates insufficient to change approach; recheck counts <150,000/mm³; define significant thrombocytopenia as a count <100,000/mm³.

    c. Severe thrombocytopenia at birth (platelet count <30,000/mm³) is rare and usually the result of alloimmune disease.

  2. Pathogenesis. The numbers of platelets related to rates of production and destruction. Ordinarily, platelets survive about 8 to 10 days; larger platelets may be seen in cases of rapid platelet turnover; defects may be heritable or acquired, and the acquired ones may be subject to a great variety of perinatal influences (Boxes 17-6 and 17-7).

  3. Immune thrombocytopenia. May be autoimmune (passive transfer of maternal antiplatelet autoantibody) or alloimmune (passive transfer of maternal antibody formed against antigen on neonate's platelets).

    a. Autoimmune.

      (1) Maternal idiopathic thrombocytopenia purpura (ITP). There is a risk to the newborn if there is a maternal history of ITP before pregnancy, ITP treated with splenectomy, or circulating antibodies detectable in the mother; it is usually tran-

---

BOX 17-6
Perinatal Influences on Neonatal Thrombocytopenia

Maternal
  Drugs
  Antibodies
  Infections
  Procoagulants (DIC)
  Severe hypertension (HELLP–hypertension, elevated liver chemistries,
    low platelets)
Placenta
  Chorangioma
  Vascular thrombi
  Abruptio placentae
Infant susceptibility
  Illness associated with thrombocytopenia
    Hypoxic (with or without DIC)
    Sepsis (with or without DIC)
    Localized thrombonecrotizing enterocolitis, renal vein thrombosis, etc.
    Giant hemangioma
    Polycythemia
  Therapeutic measures causing thrombocytopenia
Exchange transfusion
Phototherapy
Indwelling vascular catheters (thrombi)

From Oski FA, Naiman JL: *Hematologic problems in the newborn,* ed 3, Philadelphia, 1982, WB Saunders.

sient over a period of weeks to 4 months; may be fatal; the presence of a circulating antibody in a mother with a normal platelet count still places an infant at risk.

(a) The greatest risk is during and immediately after birth; risk of intracranial hemorrhage may be reduced by delivering at-risk babies by cesarean section if the mother's hemorrhagic tendency allows it; objective evidence for this approach is lacking.

(b) Test the mother for platelet count and circulating antiplatelet antibody when there is a history of ITP. Consultation with a pediatric hematologist is advisable.

(c) Platelet count can be obtained on fetal scalp blood, but reliability is limited; umbilical vein sampling to determine infant's platelet counts may be considered in selected cases but involves significant risk to fetus.

N.B.: Scalp blood sampling may result in falsely low counts because of platelet clumping or clotting. It should be relied on only when performed by experienced personnel; a low count may justify cesarean section.

BOX 17-7
Etiologic Classification of Neonatal Thrombocytopenia

Immune disorders
    Passive (acquired from mother)—ITP, drug-induced thrombocytopenia, systemic lupus erythematosus
Active
    Isoimmune—platelet group incompatibility
    Associated with erythroblastosis fetalis—caused by the disease or exchange transfusion
Infections
    Bacterial
    Nonbacterial
        TORCH group
        Congenital syphilis
        Echovirus II
Drugs (administered to mother) (e.g., thiazides [?], tolbutamide, hydralazine)
Congenital megakaryocytic hypoplasia: associations
    Congenital anomalies (chromosomes normal)
        Absent radii (TAR syndrome)
        Microcephaly
        Rubella syndrome
    Pancytopenia
        With congenital anomalies (Fanconi anemia)
        Without congenital anomalies
        Trisomy syndromes—13, 18
Bone marrow disease
    Congenital leukemia
Disseminated intravascular coagulation (DIC)
    Obstetric complication—abruptio placentae, toxemia, amniotic fluid embolism, dead twin fetus
    Hypoxia
    Sepsis
    Giant hemangioma (including placental chorioangioma)
Inherited thrombocytopenias
Miscellaneous
    Extensive localized thrombosis/stasis—intracardiac thrombosis, vascular catheters, renal vein thrombosis, placental vascular thrombi, necrotizing enterocolitis, polycythemia, thrombotic thrombocytopenic purpura
    Inherited metabolic disorders
    The high-risk infant—respiratory distress syndrome, perinatal aspiration, sepsis
Phototherapy
Congenital thyrotoxicosis

From Oski FA, Naiman JL: *Hematologic problems in the newborn,* ed 3, Philadelphia, 1982, WB Saunders.

(d) Consider prenatal intravenous immunoglobulin (IVIgG) to mother, or steroid therapy; the effect is uncertain and insufficient by itself to avoid cesarean section unless the infant's platelet count is determined to be normal.

(e) Platelet counts in infants may be as low as $5000/mm^3$ or, in asymptomatic infants, close to normal; there is poor correlation with maternal platelet counts.

(f) Platelet transfusion, IVIgG, and possibly steroids should form the basis of treatment (in consultation with a hematologist).

(g) Repeat counts should be obtained in an infant with near-normal counts at birth because there may be a significant drop after several hours to days.

(h) Anemia is not ordinarily a factor unless blood loss is great.

(i) Hepatosplenomegaly is not ordinarily seen.

(j) Most infants are mildly affected and recover without specific therapy; risk diminishes after the first few days of life.

(2) Drug-induced thrombocytopenia in the mother is the result of a postulated immune reaction with antibody formation and passive transfer to baby (e.g., quinidine, sulfonamides, thiazide diuretics, phenytoin, methyldopa, ampicillin, cephalexin, meprobamate).

(3) Maternal SLE. Placental transmission of LE factor is well documented; relatively few babies become thrombocytopenic; those that do attain normal counts in 3 to 4 weeks and may not demonstrate clinical signs; those that do not may require therapy, usually with steroids.

b. Alloimmune.

(1) Neonatal alloimmune thrombocytopenic (NAIT) purpura. Not as rare as originally thought, NAIT is the most common cause of severe thrombocytopenia in the first day of life. The mother forms antibodies to infant platelets and then transfers antibodies passively. There is a wide variation in clinical presentation, with greater severity than in autoimmune disease. The firstborn child is often affected. Platelet antigens are genetically determined (e.g., mother is Pl^{A1}-negative, baby and father are positive [not unlike Rh incompatibility]).

(2) Petechiae may appear almost immediately after birth or in a few hours; purpura, ecchymoses, and cephalohematoma are not uncommon. Thrombocytopenia can occur during the second trimester. Intrauterine intracranial hemorrhage is common with Pl^{A1} antibody and can occur with other antigens.

(3) In subsequent pregnancies, the infant of a sensitized mother may be delivered by cesarean section to avoid birth trauma; this is not always successful. Severity of thrombocytopenia tends to increase with subsequent pregnancies.

(4) Hepatosplenomegaly is not ordinarily a factor.

    (5) Platelet count may be as low as 1000/mm³.

    (6) Anemia is ordinarily not a factor unless blood loss is great.

    (7) Jaundice is common and may require therapy.

    (8) Platelet transfusion with P1^A1^ negative platelets (i.e., from the mother) and intravenous immunoglobulin are the therapeutic options (in consultation with a hematologist). Both can be used prenatally as well as postnatally.

c. Thrombocytopenia with erythroblastosis or exchange transfusion may occur as a result of bilirubin toxicity, DIC, or possibly on an alloimmune basis. Occasionally independent of the severity of the hemolytic disease, platelet counts may drop well below 50,000/mm³. Most often, thrombocytopenia with erythroblastosis is corrected by exchange transfusion. The hazard of the transfusion can be minimized by the use of fresh whole blood collected within 12 hours of the transfusion. Freezing blood destroys platelets.

d. With infection (common in newborns).

    (1) Bacterial infection. Platelet counts can fall rapidly with the onset of infection; serial counts can be helpful in diagnosing sepsis; the peak drop usually occurs by 4 days and is the result of increased platelet destruction, possibly with DIC, or bacterial exotoxins. Bleeding tends not to be severe and is generally limited to infants with counts <20,000/mm³. Petechiae are the most common manifestation. Need for treatment is rare; at most, 1 U of platelet concentrate is needed to raise the platelet count above 40,000/mm³.

    (2) Nonbacterial infection. Most commonly occurs with TORCH group of infections, syphilis, and echoviruses. These infants are generally otherwise ill, depending on the specific organism. Hemolytic anemia is common, with reticulocytosis and increased nucleated RBCs on smear. With greater severity, DIC is a risk. Treatment with platelet concentrate is suggested for counts <20,000/mm³, with goal of ≥40,000. One unit usually suffices.

e. Thrombocytopenia with DIC is possible in a variety of circumstances; platelets and other coagulation factors are depleted during the clotting process.

    (1) Obstetric complications, including abruptio placentae, toxemia, amniotic fluid embolism, or dead twin fetus.

    (2) Hypoxia.

    (3) Sepsis.

    (4) Giant hemangioma, obvious at birth, usually huge and solitary, but may be disseminated; thrombocytopenia and associated bleeding correlate with sudden increase in size and firmness of hemangioma. Bleeding is rare. Platelet count is commonly <50,000/mm³; sequestered and destroyed in tumor. Extreme variability in response to therapy. Treatment options to consider include surgical or laser excision, steroids, fibrinolytic inhibitors, anticoagulants, antiplatelet agents, platelet transfusion, perhaps fresh frozen plasma or

cryoprecipitate for coagulation factors, RBC transfusion for anemia, and α-interferon.

N.B.: Consultations with a hematologist and surgeon are necessary. Fatalities can occur secondary to airway compression, hemorrhage, or infection.

- f. Thrombocytopenia with use of antepartum drugs is not common; maternal platelet count is normal and platelet antibodies are absent (nonimmune). Thiazides can be a cause when given over many weeks during preeclampsia, as can tolbutamide and hydralazine. Purpura is seen at or soon after birth; platelet counts are often well under 30,000/mm³; leukopenia is associated. Steroids are not usually helpful.
- g. With megakaryocytic hypoplasia, platelets are not produced; bone marrow is deficient in megakaryocytes or megakaryocyte release is inhibited. Purpura is usually an early manifestation; platelet counts are in the range of 10,000 to 30,000/mm³. There is occasional leukocytosis; anemia is possible if blood loss is severe. Steroids and splenectomy are not helpful. Transfusion with platelet concentrates is recommended for severe bleeding and with RBCs for anemia. It is most commonly associated with obvious anomalies; the causative factor is often obscure.
    - (1) Thrombocytopenia, absent radius (TAR). May be associated with other skeletal, renal, cardiac abnormalities.
    - (2) Microcephaly.
    - (3) Trisomies 13 and 18.
    - (4) Fanconi's anemia (pancytopenia, short stature, microcephaly, thumb, skin, and renal defects).
    - (5) Congenital rubella syndrome.
    - (6) Noonan syndrome, often associated with splenomegaly.
    - (7) Possibly other congenital anomalies.
    - (8) Pancytopenia.
- h. Inherited thrombocytopenia. Bleeding in the newborn is uncommon. Inheritance is usually autosomal dominant or sex-linked recessive. The degree of thrombocytopenia generally is not severe, with counts ranging from 20,000 to 100,000/mm³; diagnosis is difficult in newborns unless there is a positive family history or associated findings to provide the clue; definitive diagnosis is usually made in the older infant who has unexplained thrombocytopenia.
    - (1) Sex-linked recessive.
        - (a) Wiskott-Aldrich syndrome (eczema, immune deficiency). The patient is ill from infancy; melena in the neonatal period often is a first clue. Platelet life is shortened by intrinsic defect; platelets are smaller than in other conditions, and are the most common laboratory abnormality. Splenectomy should be considered but delayed until later in life, if possible, because of concurrent immune deficiency.
        - (b) Without associated findings (milder form of Wiskott-Aldrich).

(2) X-linked or autosomal dominant.
  (a) May-Hegglin anomaly (giant platelets; Döhle bodies in neutrophils).
  (b) Alport syndrome (nephritis and nerve deafness, along with May-Hegglin anomaly); similar to Fechtner and Epstein syndromes.
(3) Autosomal recessive.
  (a) Hermansky-Pudlak syndrome (giant platelets, ceroid accumulation in marrow, albinism).
  (b) Bernard-Soulier syndrome (deficiency of von Willebrand factor receptor on platelets).
  (c) Alport syndrome (same as above, but some cases recessive).
i. Thrombocytopenia with associated findings. Causal relationships are not necessarily clear.
  (1) Localized thrombi with respiratory distress syndrome and severe hypoxia.
  (2) Large thrombosis of umbilical vessels and chorion (usual range is 15,000 to 20,000/mm^3).
  (3) NEC (usual range is 50,000 to 60,000/mm^3).
  (4) Hyperviscosity, polycythemia; platelets return with resolution of hyperviscosity.
  (5) Inborn errors of metabolism, probably related to severe acidosis: methylmalonic acidemia, ketotic glycinemia, isovaleric acidemia, holocarboxylase synthetase deficiency.
  (6) Phototherapy. Thrombocytopenia may occur in infants with meager marrow reserves as platelets are destroyed by phototherapy.
  (7) Hemolytic-uremic syndrome.
  (8) Cyanotic congenital heart disease.
  (9) Hypersplenism.
  (10) Hypertension.
  (11) Down syndrome.
  (12) Intravascular catheter (often associated with thrombi).
  (13) High-risk infant. Increasing survivability of the very premature and very ill infant has enabled more frequent finding of thrombocytopenia than in the past. These infants are more apt to be found to be thrombocytopenic and, if so, are more likely to die. A mother with a high-risk pregnancy (e.g., preeclampsia, eclampsia, placenta previa, abruptio placentae, hypertension) is at greater risk for thrombocytopenia; the infant's platelet counts may correlate with hers.
4. Diagnosis and management of neonatal thrombocytopenia (Tables 17-7 and 17-8, Fig. 17-2).
  a. Maternal history and laboratory evaluation.
    (1) Previous bleeding (idiopathic thrombocytopenia purpura) (e.g., easy bruising, frequent nosebleeds).
    (2) Illness, previous infants with purpura, rubella in first trimester, SLE, drugs (e.g., quinidine, quinine, hydralazine, tolbutamide, thiazides).

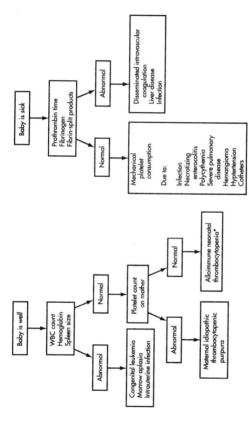

*WBC count may be low in alloimmune thrombocytopenia because of an anti-HLA antibody.

FIG. 17-2. Diagnostic approach to the newborn infant with thrombocytopenia (platelet count <150,000/mm³, with or without symptoms). The most likely diagnoses are provided in the boxes. (Modified from Oski FA, Naiman JL: *Hematologic problems in the newborn*, ed 3, Philadelphia, 1982, WB Saunders.)

TABLE 17-7
Diagnostic Features of Various Types of Neonatal Thrombocytopenic Purpura

	History			Physical Findings		
	Previous infants affected	Maternal illness	Maternal drugs	Jaundice*	Hepatosplenomegaly	Congenital anomalies
Immune disorders						
Maternal ITP	+/0	Purpura	0	0	0	0
Drug purpura	+/0	Purpura	Quinine, quinidine Sedormid	0	0	0
Maternal SLE renal	+/0	Rash, arthritis,	0	0	0	Congenital heart block
Isoimmune	+/0	0	0	+/0	0	0
Infections						
Bacterial	0	+/0	0	+	+	0
Viral						
Protozoal						
Drugs (nonimmune type)	+/0	0	+	0	0	0

						Associated anomalies
Congenital Megakaryocytic Hypoplasia						
Absent radii	0	0	0	0	+/0	Cardiac, skeletal, etc.
Rubella syndrome	0	Rash in T_1	0	+/0	+/0	Eye, cardiac
With pancytopenia (no anomalies)	0	0	0	0	0	0
Bone marrow disease						
Congenital leukemia	0	0	0	+/0	+	0
Giant hemangioma (including chorioangioma)	0	0	0	0	0	Hemangioma
Inherited						
Thrombocytopenia	+/0	Purpura only if carrier	0	0	0	0

From Oski FA, Naiman JL: *Hematologic problems in the newborn*, ed 3, Philadelphia, 1982, WB Saunders.
ITP, Idiopathic thrombocytopenic purpura; *SLE*, systemic lupus erythematosus.
*May occur in any types from enclosed hemorrhage.

TABLE 17-8
Laboratory Study Results Typical of Neonatal Thrombocytopenic Purpura

	LABORATORY STUDIES				
	Associated hematologic abnormalities*	Bone marrow megakaryocytes	Platelet antibodies (mother)	Maternal thrombocytopenia	Duration of thrombocytopenia
Immune disorders					
Maternal ITP	0	↑ (or ↓)	+	+	Up to 3-4 mo
Drug purpura	0	↑ (or ↓)	+	+	Up to 1 wk
Maternal SLE	± Anemia, neutropenia	?	+	+	Up to 1 wk
Isoimmune	0	↑ (or ↓)	+	0	Above 60,000 mm^2 by 2-3 wk
Infections					
Bacterial	± Coagulation defects				Parallels activity of infection; often months
Viral	Anemia (hemolytic)	?	0	0	
Protozoal					

Drugs (nonimmune type)	± Leukopenia	→		0	2-12 wk
Congenital					
Megakaryocytic					
Hypoplasia					
Associated anomalies					
Associated anomalies					
Absent radii	Leukemoid reaction	↓↓ or 0		0	Lifelong
Rubella syndrome	± Leukopenia	→		0 0	Up to 2 mo
With pancytopenia (no anomalies)	Late pancytopenia	↓↓ or 0		0	Lifelong
Bone marrow disease					
Congenital leukemia	Anemia, leukocytosis	(↓ Blasts ++)		0	Fatal
Giant hemangioma	Coagulation	↑		0	Disappears with hemangioma
(including chorioangioma)	defects				
Inherited					
Thrombocytopenia	0	Normal or decreased		+/0	Lifelong, may remit with splenectomy

From Oski FA, Naiman JL: *Hematologic problems in the newborn*, ed 3, Philadelphia, 1982, WB Saunders.

ITP, Idiopathic thrombocytopenic purpura; *SLE,* systemic lupus erythematosus.

*Anemia in any type if bleeding is severe.

(3) Placenta. Possibility of chorioangioma.
(4) Serologic test for syphilis.
(5) Low platelet count.
    (a) Maternal ITP, SLE.
    (b) Drug-induced purpura.
    (c) Inherited thrombocytopenia.

b. Physical examination of the infant; findings may include the following:
    (1) Nothing unusual; does not exclude the following:
        (a) Alloimmune purpura.
        (b) Drugs.
        (c) Inherited thrombocytopenia.
        (d) Early congenital aplastic anemia.
        (e) Metabolic disorders.
        (f) Hepatosplenomegaly (with or without jaundice).
        (g) Bacterial infections.
        (h) Nonbacterial infections.
            (i) TORCH group.
            (ii) Echovirus II.
            (iii) Human immunodeficiency virus (HIV).
        (i) Congenital syphilis.
        (j) Congenital leukemia.
        (k) Congenital anomalies.
        (l) Giant hemangioma.
        (m) Rubella syndrome.
        (n) Absent radii.
        (o) Trisomy syndromes.
        (p) Noonan syndrome.
        (q) Constitutional aplasia (e.g., Fanconi anemia).

c. The general approach should emphasize the following:
    (1) Careful consideration of the mother's history and her platelet status.
    (2) Determination of risk in the pregnancy.
    (3) Those ill with respiratory disorders, NEC, and other serious, even life-threatening conditions.
    (4) Consideration of particular diagnostic features (see Tables 17-7 and 17-8).
    (5) Consultation with pediatric hematologist.

d. Laboratory studies should include some or all of the following:
    (1) Complete blood cell count (CBC).
        (a) Platelet count.
        (b) Hemoglobin level. Associated anemia may be caused by blood loss, concurrent hemolysis, marrow infiltration (e.g., congenital leukemia).
        (c) WBC count. Leukocytosis or neutropenia suggest infection; may be associated with hemolysis or blood loss.
        (d) Smear.
    (2) Bone marrow test. Increased megakaryocyte count suggests consumptive coagulopathy, immune thrombocytopenia

(bone marrow may not be necessary if latter diagnosis seems clear and infant is otherwise well).

   (3) Serologic tests can indicate immune disorders. These are complex and require consultation with a hematologist.

  e. Treatment.

    (1) When intervention is necessary.

      (a) Platelet transfusion (stored at room temperature); should be undertaken with hematology consultation; usually, 1 unit is sufficient to result in a rise to at least 40,000 to 50,000/mm^3, more often as high as 75,000 to 100,000/mm^3; after transfusion, count will drop by about 10% per day; follow-up counts are necessary to judge the need for repeat transfusion; washed maternal platelets may be helpful in the event of alloimmunization from maternal/fetal platelet incompatibility.

      (b) Infusion in any event should be warm and slow.

    (2) Specific therapy is indicated by the underlying disease, as discussed previously.

B. Platelet dysfunction.

1. Drug-induced.

  a. Aspirin and other salicylates may cause platelet dysfunction as a result of irreversible inhibition of platelet cyclooxygenase, which is essential for normal platelet function; they can prolong the bleeding time for days.

  b. Other nonsteroidal antiinflammatory drugs (NSAIDS), including indomethacin, cause reversible inhibition of platelet cyclooxygenase; effects wane 12 to 24 hours after the drug is discontinued.

  c. β-Lactams. Ticarcillin, carbenicillin, and rarely, some cephalosporins have been implicated.

2. Uremia. This has been clearly known for many years, but the precise mechanism is unknown.

3. Liver disease. Unclear defects in platelet function have been reported and these complicate the coagulopathy and thrombocytopenia that often accompany liver failure.

4. Congenital. These are quite rare. Temporary hemostasis may usually be obtained by platelet transfusion, but sometimes this runs the risk of inducing immunization to a congenitally absent platelet protein.

  a. Glanzmann thrombasthenia. A deficiency of the fibrinogen receptor on platelets; there is a relatively high prevalence in Middle Eastern countries.

  b. Bernard-Soulier syndrome. Large platelets; deficiency of the receptor on platelets that binds von Willebrand factor.

  c. Wiskott-Aldrich syndrome. Small platelets, thrombocytopenia, defective adhesion.

  d. Gray platelet syndrome. Absence of alpha granules.

  e. Storage pool syndrome. Deficiency of dense granule contents; includes Hermansky-Pudlak and Chédiak-Higashi syndromes.

  f. Cyclooxygenase deficiency. Clinically resembles drug-induced platelet dysfunction.

  g. Scott syndrome. Unknown defect in platelet procoagulant activity.

C. Thrombocytosis.

1. Definition is difficult because the upper limits of normal are not well defined.
2. Provocative conditions include the following:
   a. Low birth weight. Generally apparent after 2 weeks of age and up to several months of age in a range up to about 700,000/mm³. Etiology is unknown; there is an apparently physiologic change, generally not complicated by thrombosis.
   b. Acute inflammation.
   c. Acute blood loss.
   d. Hemolysis.
   e. Nutritional deficiency (e.g., iron, vitamin E, hyperalimentation with lipid emulsions).
   f. Asplenia.
   g. Leukemia-like syndromes (e.g., as with Down syndrome).
   h. Neuroblastoma.
   i. Maternal abuse of many drugs.
3. Management.
   a. Watchful waiting and therapy directed to the underlying condition are generally appropriate.
   b. No direct intervention is ordinarily necessary.
   c. Thrombosis is an extremely rare event.

TABLE 17-9
Blood Clotting Factors

Procoagulants	Synonyms
Factor I	Fibrinogen
Factor II	Prothrombin (vitamin K–dependent protein)
Factor III	Tissue factor, thromboplastin
Factor IV	Calcium
Factor V	Proaccelerin, labile factor
Factor VI	Number no longer employed, previously recognized as active form of factor V
Factor VII	Proconvertin, stable factor (vitamin K–dependent protein)
Factor VIII	Antihemophilic factor (AHF), antihemophilic globulin (AHG)
Factor IX	Plasma thromboplastin component (PTC), Christmas factor (vitamin K–dependent protein)
Factor X	Stuart-Prower factor (vitamin K–dependent protein)
Factor XI	Plasma thromboplastin antecedent (PTA)
Factor XII	Hageman factor
Factor XIII	Fibrin-stabilizing factor
Prekallikrein	Fletcher factor
High molecular weight kininogen	Fitzgerald, Flaujac, Williams factor

From Oski FA, Naiman JL: *Hematologic problems in the newborn,* ed 3, Philadelphia, 1982, WB Saunders.

    d. Preventive drug therapy (e.g., aspirin, dipyridamole) is not well tested in neonates and not proven efficacious in older children.

X. DISORDERS OF BLOOD COAGULATION

As many as 1 neonate in 100 will have a problem with bleeding or thrombosis; the numbers are probably higher in intensive care nurseries.

A. Bleeding results from the following:

1. Transient "immaturity" of coagulation mechanism in the newborn period (Table 17-9).
2. Transient insult to coagulation mechanism (e.g., DIC).
3. Inherited, permanent coagulation disorders.
4. Abnormal or insufficient platelets.
5. Vascular abnormalities.
6. Trauma with or without associated abnormality.

B. Laboratory testing for coagulation defects.
Because the infant can be bleeding at birth or shortly thereafter, be sure the blood is the infant's and not the mother's.

1. If there is any question, the Apt test (Box 17-8) can be used to settle the issue with any bloody body discharge (e.g., vomitus, stool).
2. Additionally, great care must be taken with collection of blood:
    a. Too much squeezing may contaminate the sample with tissue factor, which activates clotting.
    b. Samples may be contaminated by heparinized catheters.
    c. When anticoagulant is added, the proper amount is determined relative to the hematocrit level (discuss with laboratory).
    d. Collect minimal amounts of blood; microtechniques allow many studies on as little as 1 ml or less.
    e. Collect blood to test for fibrin degradation products in tubes containing a fibrinolytic inhibitor.
    f. Cord-blood collection requires double clamping as soon as possible after delivery (be sure clamps are not too close together), with blood drawn quickly from the intervening segment using a tube with anticoagulant.

BOX 17-8

Apt Test for Differentiation of Fetal and Adult (Maternal) Hemoglobin in Stool or Vomitus

1. Mix 1 part discharge with 5 parts water.
2. Centrifuge 3-4 minutes at 2000 rev/min.
3. Decant pink supernate (contains hemoglobin).
4. Add 1 ml 1% NaOH to 4 ml supernate.
    a. Adult blood: supernate becomes yellow-brown (hemoglobin A).
    b. Infant blood: pink supernate remains (hemoglobin F).
5. Run control tube with infant's peripheral blood.

Modified from Apt KL, Downey WS: *J Pediatr* 47:6, 195 5.

3. Screening tests.
   a. Cover slip smear of peripheral blood. Clumped platelets or many in one oil immersion field suggests *no* significant thrombocytopenia (clumping will not be seen if anticoagulant has been added); examine both cover slip preparations from a single drop of blood because platelets may adhere to only one cover slip.
   b. Whole-blood coagulation time. Generally not a useful test; requires a large volume of blood and the test is not highly specific.
   c. Bleeding time.
      (1) Basically, the time needed for a standardized wound to stop bleeding; prolonged in thrombocytopenia, von Willebrand's disease, functional platelet disorders, and DIC; usually normal in hemophilia and other congenital factor deficiencies.
      (2) Not recommended when thrombocytopenia is already documented or highly probable.
      (3) Not thoroughly standardized for neonates.
   d. Activated partial thromboplastin time (aPTT).
      (1) Sensitive for most plasma procoagulant factors, except VII and XIII.
      (2) Prolonged with factor XII, Fletcher factor, kininogen deficiencies, and other deficiencies not associated with bleeding; also with heparin and other circulating anticoagulants.
   e. Prothrombin time (PT) (Quick's test). Measures activity of factors II, V, VII, X, and fibrinogen; less disturbed by heparin than aPTT.
   f. Thrombin clotting time. Measures plasma clotting time after addition of thrombin; prolonged with fibrinogen deficiency, heparin, or fibrin split products.
   g. Fibrin degradation products (FDP).
      (1) Formed by the lysis of fibrin or fibrinogen by plasmin. FDP accumulate in DIC and thrombotic states. D-dimers are a subset of FDP, seen only in fibrinolysis (not in fibrinogenolysis).
      (2) Can also accumulate without DIC with functional impairment of the liver or kidney, sites where fibrin degradation products are normally cleared.

C. Principles of neonatal blood coagulation.
1. Coagulation status represents a balance between procoagulant and anticoagulant systems. On the whole, neonates appear to be in a relatively prothrombotic state.
2. Almost immediately at birth, there is a decrease in vitamin K–dependent factors, which, if profound after the first few days of life, may result in hemorrhage.
3. The clotting activity of all factors involved in initial activation of intrinsic clotting system is decreased in varying degrees.
4. Illness may further depress naturally low levels of some factors.
5. Fibrinogen levels, on the other hand, approximate those of the adult, except in the rare case of congenital afibrinogenemia.
6. Regardless, thrombin time is generally abnormal, for obscure reasons.

7. Overall, fibrinolytic activity is increased at birth and decreases to adult levels within about 6 hours of age. It is somewhat less in premature babies, particularly those with respiratory distress.

8. Whole-blood clotting time is shortened in healthy newborns.

D. Vitamin K is required for conversion of precursor proteins into proteins with procoagulant and anticoagulant activity; it is additionally involved in protein conversion in bone, kidney, spleen, pancreas, lung, and placenta.

1. Coumarin and coumarin analogs block its action; heparin does not cross the placenta and is preferable if the mother requires anticoagulation therapy; coumarin can be resumed after delivery because it does not appear in breast milk in significant amounts.

2. If precursor protein is diminished, sufficient vitamin K cannot prevent hemorrhage; however, administration of vitamin K to a healthy full-term infant prevents decrease in prothrombin activity and the prolonged PT generally found in the first hours and days of life.

3. The premature infant, especially when very small, responds to vitamin K less predictably and often minimally. An immature liver unable to synthesize precursor proteins is the probable reason.

4. Large doses of synthetic, water-soluble, vitamin K analogs may provoke hyperbilirubinemia, or even kernicterus. Small doses of natural vitamin K do not. In any event, giving large (not recommended) doses does not increase activity or response.

5. Vitamin K administration to the mother during pregnancy may be helpful to the infant, but timing relevant to delivery is hard to judge. It must be given at least 12 hours before delivery to be sure transplacental passage is affected; this is difficult to ensure and is the reason it is given to the baby.

6. The recommended approach to safe and easy prevention of hemorrhage resulting from neonatal vitamin K deficiency is immediate administration of vitamin K (K_1, phytonadione) to the newborn immediately after birth, 0.5 to 1 mg intramuscularly.

7. Repeat doses may be necessary for offspring of mothers treated with anticoagulants or anticonvulsants; these infants are particularly susceptible; clotting studies may be normal in the mother but abnormal in the infant.

N.B.: Oral vitamin K administration, in use in several countries, is not recommended in the United States.

E. Hemorrhagic disease of the newborn is a form of self-limited, generalized hemorrhagic disease usually clinically evident on the second or third day of life, but possible on the first day or many days later; rarely, it can occur weeks or months later. The gastrointestinal tract is the most common site of bleeding; other sites (e.g., adrenal, CNS, nose, skin, umbilical cord; indeed, any body area) may also be involved.

1. Cause. Vitamin K deficiency and a consequent deficiency of factor II, VII, IX, and X activities. The activities of protein C and S are also diminished.

   a. Diet has an impact on the coagulation process; the earlier the feeding the better; cow's milk has four times the vitamin K of breast milk; hemorrhagic disease is more common in breast-fed babies not provided preventive vitamin K (phytonadione, 0.5 to 1 mg intramuscularly).

    b. Vitamin K is not well transported across the placenta.

    c. Response to treatment is rapid, within a few hours.

2. Diagnosis.

    a. Bleeding anywhere in the neonate.

    b. Prolonged PT and aPTT.

    c. CBC otherwise noncontributory.

3. Treatment. Intravenous or intramuscular administration of 1 mg of vitamin K (K_1, Konakion), preferably intravenously; expectation is of rapid response, certainly within 6 to 12 hours. If hemorrhage is serious, fresh frozen plasma should be administered while waiting for vitamin K effect.

F. DIC is an acquired dysfunction distinguished by intravascular consumption of platelets and of plasma clotting factors; fibrinogen; factors II, V, VIII, and XIII; and protein C. Intravascular coagulation leads to widespread deposition of fibrin, thrombi, and hemorrhage as platelets and clotting factors are exhausted. Intravascular fibrinolysis and fibrinogenolysis lead to accumulation of fibrin degradation products. Red cells are fragmented and decreased in number, leading to anemia. DIC is common in sick newborns, much more so than other causes of bleeding; it is characterized particularly by hemorrhage in the lungs and brain.

1. Cause. DIC occurs only in response to an associated disorder. Obstetric, respiratory, and septic processes predominate.

2. Clinical findings are variable and depend on the associated disease process. Oozing may be noted at puncture sites; petechiae and bleeding anywhere and everywhere—umbilicus to CNS—may be present, with symptoms and signs dependent on site and extent of bleeding.

3. Diagnosis.

    a. Prolonged PT and aPTT.

    b. Thrombocytopenia.

    c. Abnormalities of several coagulation factors, particularly reduced factor V and VIII activities, low fibrinogen, and elevated fibrin degradation products, including D-dimer.

    d. Hemolytic anemia. RBC fragmentation on peripheral smear (microangiopathy).

    e. Toxic granulation in leukocytes.

    f. Probable elevated WBC with many immature forms.

    g. Additionally, findings related to associated disease factors (e.g., liver disease) can confuse the picture and make diagnosis more difficult.

4. Treatment consists of attention to the underlying disease process and the repair of coagulation deficiencies. In general, success with the first will correct the second: antibiotics, appropriate fluid and electrolyte maintenance, adequate oxygen, and maintenance of blood pressure may be indicated. Among therapeutic possibilities

for coagulation repair, consider exchange transfusion, fresh frozen plasma/platelets, and cryoprecipitate (limits volume expansion, increases factor VIII and fibrinogen). Fresh frozen plasma helps to maintain appropriate levels of antithrombin needed for heparin effectiveness. None of these has been uniformly successful if the associated disease process does not respond; hemostatic support provides time to give primary therapy a chance. Appropriate schedules include the following:

a. Fresh frozen plasma, 10 to 15 ml/kg every 12 hours.

b. 1 U of platelets every 12 hours when count is ≤50,000/mm³.

c. Exchange transfusion with anticoagulated fresh blood, repeated every 12 hours if coagulation deficiency persists; exchange helps avoid fluid overload in very sick premature infants.

d. Heparin should be used in the event of thrombosis of an artery or deep vein or purpura fulminans, 75 U/kg in initial intravenous bolus and 28 U/kg every hour in a constant intravenous drip; adjust to keep aPTT 1.5 to 2 times normal control; premature babies may need a larger initial bolus and faster drip; maintain platelets at a minimum of 50,000/mm³.

N.B.: Consultation with a hematologist or neonatologist is mandatory. The process may play havoc with a variety of the coagulation factors in unanticipated ways.

  G. Liver disease and neonatal bleeding. The liver is the site of manufacture of most clotting proteins; severe compromise of liver function by any underlying process may lead to bleeding; ascites is a complicating factor because the coagulation proteins may "drain" into the ascitic fluid.

  1. If there is associated bleeding, the following factors must be considered:

a. PT and aPTT are prolonged; sometimes the PT is disproportionately prolonged relative to the aPTT.

b. Factors V, VII, and fibrinogen are reduced.

c. Factor VIII is usually increased or normal, a point that distinguishes this from DIC.

d. Platelets are normal or decreased; associated DIC or splenic sequestration may be seen.

  2. Treatment parallels that of DIC; ensure vitamin K administration. Consultation with hematologist may be important.

  H. Thrombosis. Sick infants are particularly susceptible, often after vascular catheterization. Catheters require careful attention.

  1. Other predisposing pathophysiologic events include the following:

a. Protein C, protein S, AT III (antithrombin) deficiencies, factor V Leiden, plasminogen or plasminogen activator abnormalities, prothrombin 20210 mutation.

b. Maternal diabetes, toxemia, hypertension, antiphospholipid antibody syndrome.

c. Polycythemia.

d. Sepsis.

e. Dehydration.

      f. Congenital nephrosis.

      g. Vascular injury or stasis.

      h. Placental vascular anomalies or thrombosis.

      i. Hyperhomocystinemia or homocystinuria.

2. The clinical picture depends on the extent and site of thrombosis; gangrene is a possibility.

3. Treatment considerations include the following:

    a. Remove catheters or other potential inciting factors; specific attention should be paid to the particular area compromised by the thrombosis.

    b. Provide heparin in a 75-U/kg bolus followed by 28 U/kg/hr in a constant intravenous drip; adjust the infusion to keep the aPTT 1.5 to 2 times control.

N.B.: Preterm infants may require a slightly larger loading dose and infusion rate. Consider urokinase or tissue plasminogen activator (tPA) therapy, depending on the site of thrombosis and risk of intracranial hemorrhage.

    c. Fresh frozen plasma. Some inherited disorders (e.g., severe protein C deficiency) do not respond to heparin; consider replacement therapy if specific deficiency is known.

    d. Ensure that platelet count is maintained at about 50,000/mm^3; platelet transfusion may be necessary.

    e. Consultation with a hematologist. Heparinization can be extraordinarily difficult in the newborn.

I. Congenital deficiencies of procoagulant factors may be manifest in the newborn; often, clinical presentation is delayed several weeks, even into toddler time. Circumcision is a common precipitating event; intracranial and umbilical cord bleeding are relatively uncommon. Massive cephalohematoma, intracranial hemorrhage, or protracted bleeding from scalp puncture, circumcision, or other laceration, no matter the size, should suggest the possibility of a deficiency. The reason for relatively fewer occurrences during the neonatal period is not clear.

1. Hemophilias. Hemophilia A (factor VIII deficiency) and hemophilia B (Christmas disease, factor IX deficiency) are X-linked recessive traits; females are heterozygous carriers and are generally free of symptoms. Prenatal diagnosis is possible in most cases, requiring chorionic villus sampling, amniocentesis, or fetoscopy. Hemophilia C (factor XI deficiency) is autosomal recessive, occurring most often in Ashkenazi Jews; it should be considered if an infant bleeds excessively after ritual circumcision. Hemophilias A and B are most common, but other deficiencies among the factors must be considered, particularly von Willebrand disease, fibrinogen, and factors II, V, VII, X, and XIII deficiency. Factor XIII deficiency may cause delayed bleeding after cord separation or circumcision (with normal PT and aPTT).

2. Diagnosis. A neonate's aPTT is generally somewhat prolonged. Therefore prolongation of aPTT with normal PT cannot be used to confirm hemophilia in the newborn. Confirmation comes from a positive family history and from specific factor assays performed on the infant's and mother's blood, starting with factors VIII and IX.

3. Treatment. Replacement of deficient factors is essential and should be guided by a pediatric hematologist.

a. Hemophilia A. Concentrates that have undergone viral inactivation have replaced cryoprecipitate; recombinant factor VIII is now considered the treatment of choice by most hematologists for newborns diagnosed with hemophilia A. The dose should be 10 to 50 U/kg, depending on the severity of bleeding. One unit of factor VIII activity equals the activity in 1 ml of average normal human plasma. In general, 1 U/kg body weight will yield a 2% rise in circulating factor VIII level; half-life after infusion may be as long as 14 hours, but initial half-life is usually shorter (6 to 8 hours). Administration of 10 to 20 U/kg should achieve the usual goal, a minimum level of 20% to 40%. Concentrates allow this with smaller volumes. In the event of more serious bleeding (e.g., large cephalohematoma or constant umbilical or gastrointestinal loss), continuous infusion may facilitate maintenance of a level of at least 40% for at least 48 hours.

b. Hemophilia B. Recombinant factor IX concentrate should be used at a dose of 20 to 100 U/kg, depending on the severity of bleeding. Factor IX deficiency requires the same approach as factor VIII deficiency; however, 1 U factor IX/kg body weight will generally yield a 1% rise in level; initial half-life may be 6 hours or less, but subsequent half-life is approximately 24 hours.

c. von Willebrand's disease. Viral inactivated concentrates containing von Willebrand factor are preferred to cryoprecipitate for safety reasons.

d. Cryoprecipitate may, with hematologic consultation, be considered for afibrinogenemia.

e. Fresh frozen plasma (FFP) (10 ml/kg) may be necessary with significant hemorrhage in an unidentified coagulopathy.

f. Precautions are necessary to avoid the transmission of hepatitis B and HIV infection.

g. Mandates immediate hepatitis B immunization (administer subcutaneously unless factor replacement has been given).

h. Suspected or known hemophiliacs should receive vitamin K prophylaxis subcutaneously or by mouth instead of intramuscularly because of the risk of muscle hematoma. Avoid or defer circumcision until the infant can receive appropriate factor dosing for the procedure.

XI. DIAGNOSTIC AND THERAPEUTIC APPROACH TO THE BLEEDING INFANT

A. Diagnosis. Bleeding infants may, aside from the hemorrhage, give the impression of either "wellness" or "illness."

1. If a bleeding infant looks "well," the differential diagnosis includes the following:

a. Hemorrhagic disease of the newborn.

b. Inherited coagulation disorders.

c. Immune-induced thrombocytopenia.

    d. Drug-induced thrombocytopenia.

    e. Trauma (e.g., local vascular lesion, superficial or deep [gastrointestinal tract, abdominal cavity, retroperitoneal space]).

    f. Collagen disorders such as Ehlers-Danlos syndrome.

2. If the bleeding infant seems "ill," consider the following:

    a. DIC.

    b. Liver disease.

    c. Platelet consumption (e.g., infection, NEC, renal vein or other thrombosis).

    d. The impact of associated prematurity, acidosis, hypoxia, hyperosmolarity.

    e. Mechanical or immune-complex mediated thrombocytopenia.

    f. Local vascular lesions (e.g., periventricular hemorrhage).

3. The diagnostic workup includes the following (Fig. 17-3):

    a. Family history; often the most helpful factor. More than 50% of patients with factor VIII, IX, and XIII deficiencies have a positive family history.

    b. Maternal history.

        (1) History of hemorrhagic symptoms or disorder, especially autosomal dominant (e.g., von Willebrand disease).

        (2) Drug ingestion (e.g., coumarin, anticonvulsants, barbiturates, or aspirin).

        (3) Recent or past history of thrombocytopenia, rubella, or syphilis.

        (4) Preeclampsia.

        (5) Repeated abortion (factor XIII deficiency).

        (6) Splenectomy for ITP.

    c. Neonate's history.

        (1) Vitamin K_1 administered.

        (2) Trauma.

        (3) Prolonged anoxia.

        (4) Degree of prematurity.

        (5) Sites of bleeding.

    d. Physical examination.

        (1) Type and sites of bleeding.

            (a) In hemophilia, skin lesions seem to be ecchymoses; they are often palpable and not petechiae; muscle and joints may be involved rarely; symptoms are not typical of hemophilia in older individuals.

            (b) Oozing from circumcision, umbilical cord, puncture sites, or lacerations suggests DIC or deficiency of vitamin K or factors VIII, IX, or XIII.

            (c) Hemorrhage in more than one area makes a hemostatic disorder more likely.

            (d) Vomiting of blood with no other site involved may suggest swallowed maternal blood. The Apt test helps differentiate maternal from fetal blood (Box 17-8).

        (2) Indicators of sepsis.

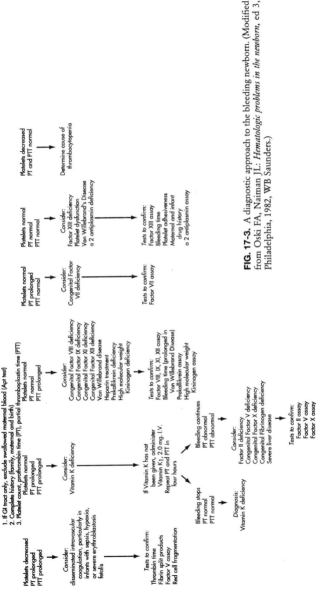

FIG. 17-3. A diagnostic approach to the bleeding newborn. (Modified from Oski FA, Naiman JL: *Hematologic problems in the newborn,* ed 3, Philadelphia, 1982, WB Saunders.)

    (3) Jaundice (may be the result of cephalohematoma or other large, enclosed hematoma).

    (4) Hepatosplenomegaly. Sepsis indicators, jaundice, and hepatosplenomegaly may together or singly suggest hepatosplenomegaly (e.g., toxoplasmosis, herpes simplex, syphilis, or cytomegalic inclusion disease).

    (5) Syndactylism (factor V deficiency).

    (6) Cephalohematoma (e.g., vitamin K deficiency, congenital disturbances of coagulation, trauma).

    (7) Hemangiomas; may trap platelets, leading to consumptive coagulopathy; sonogram may reveal retroperitonea site.

    (8) General clinical status.

  e. Laboratory studies (Table 17-10).

    (1) To determine platelet adequacy, use a well-prepared cover slip smear of peripheral blood, or determine direct platelet count; determine PT and aPTT.

N.B.: Give vitamin K, 1 to 2 mg subcutaneously or orally, while waiting for results.

    (2) If platelet count is abnormal, consider causes of isolated thrombocytopenia.

    (3) If platelet count is decreased and PT and aPTT are prolonged, consider DIC, particularly in a very sick infant with sepsis, hypoxia, or acidosis. Confirmation of this diagnosis requires a decrease in factor V or VIII or fibrinogen, the presence of fibrin degradation products in plasma, and RBC fragmentation.

    (4) If the platelet count is normal and PT and aPTT are prolonged, consider vitamin K deficiency. Prothrombin time should be significantly prolonged, more than 25 seconds. Repeat tests 4 hours after vitamin K is given; cessation of bleed-

TABLE 17-10
Laboratory Evaluation of the Bleeding Infant

	Platelet count	PT	APTT	Fibrinogen	Factor VIII
Well infant					
Thrombocytopenia	↓	N	N	N	N
Vitamin K deficiency	N*	↑	↑	N	N
Classic hemophilia	N	N	↑	N	↓↓
Sick infant					
DIC	↓	↑	↑	↓↓	↓↓
Liver disease	N–↓	↑	↑	Sl↓	N–↑
Infection	N–↓	N	N–↑	↑	↑

From Fanaroff AA, Martin RJ: *Neonatal-perinatal medicine: diseases of the fetus and infant,* ed 4, St. Louis, 1987, Mosby.
N, normal; Sl, slightly.

ing and drop in PT and aPTT times are confirmatory. Liver dysfunction may contribute to a sluggish response to vitamin K therapy.

(5) If the platelet count is normal and PT and aPTT remain prolonged after vitamin K is given, consider congenital deficiencies of factors II, V, or X or fibrinogen. If all vitamin K–dependent factors are normal but one, there is probably a congenital deficiency in that one.

(6) If a prolonged PT is the sole abnormal test result, and it does not normalize after vitamin K treatment, consider congenital deficiency of factors VII or II.

(7) If a prolonged aPTT is the sole abnormal test result, consider von Willebrand disease and, among others, congenital deficiencies of factors VIII, IX, XI, or XII. Also, heparin administration or contamination should be ruled out. Specific factor assays can help determine a particular coagulation defect.

(8) If a congenital defect is a strong possibility or confirmed, study the family. A genetic pattern can provide a clue.

(9) If there are no abnormal platelet, PT, or aPTT results, consider congenital deficiency of factor XIII or antiplasmin, or a defect in platelet function. Disorders of connective tissue (such as Ehlers-Danlos syndrome) and vascular anomalies (such as Osler-Weber-Rendu syndrome) can cause hemorrhage without disorders in the platelets or coagulation factors. Transient platelet dysfunction may be associated with maternal aspirin ingestion.

B. Management. The immediate approach depends on the site and extent of the bleeding.

1. Red cell transfusion if bleeding is extensive.

2. Vitamin K_1 if it has not been administered; give anyway if there is uncertainty.

3. In the event of DIC, consider administration of plasma, platelets, heparin, or exchange transfusion (see pp. 250-251).

4. In the event of congenital disturbance of coagulation, provide fresh frozen plasma (10 to 15 ml/kg every 12 hours) or fresh whole blood in similar amounts until specific abnormality is detected; if anemia is profound, supplement plasma (administered more rapidly) with packed RBCs.

5. At the time of identification of specific coagulation abnormality, substitute specific replacement (when it is available) for fresh frozen plasma. Determine frequency of administration by the severity of the bleeding. In this regard, pediatric hematology consultation is essential.

6. Topical therapy may include thrombin or an absorbable gauze (e.g., Gelfoam or Oxycel).

   a. Do not use nonabsorbable materials. They stick and cause further bleeding on removal.

   b. Do not suture or cauterize, if possible; avoid further trauma.

c. Anticipation and prevention. In the event of a contemplated circumcision, careful maternal and family histories are helpful; bleeding times and other, more sophisticated studies generally are not and should not be done routinely.

BIBLIOGRAPHY

American Academy of Pediatrics: Controversies concerning vitamin K and the newborn, *Pediatrics* 91:1001, 1993.

Committee on Nutrition, American Academy of Pediatrics: Vitamin K compounds and the water-soluble analogs: use in therapy and prophylaxis in pediatrics, *Pediatrics* 28:501, 1961.

Casella JF, Bowers, DC, Pelidis MA: *Disorders of coagulation.* In McMillan JA, DeAngelis JA, Feigin RD, Warshaw JB (editors): *Oski's pediatrics,* ed 3, Philadelphia, 1999, Lippincott, Williams & Wilkins.

Fanaroff AA, Martin RJ: *Neonatal-perinatal medicine: diseases of the fetus and infant,* ed 5, St. Louis, 1992, Mosby.

Nathan DG, Oski FA: *Hematology of infancy and childhood,* ed 4, Philadelphia, 1993, WB Saunders.

Osborne LM, Lenarsky C, Oakes RC, et al: Phototherapy in full term infants with hemolytic disease secondary to ABO incompatibility, *Pediatrics* 74:371, 1984.

Oski FA, Naiman JL: *Hematologic problems in the newborn,* ed 3, Philadelphia, 1982, WB Saunders.

Samuels P, Bussell JB, Braitman LE, et al: Estimation of the risk of thrombocytopenia in the offspring of pregnant women with presumed immune thrombocytopenia purpura, *N Engl J Med* 323:229, 1990.

18

Birth Injuries

BERYL J. ROSENSTEIN

I. RISK FACTORS FOR NEONATAL BIRTH INJURIES
A. Maternal factors.
1. Diabetes.
2. Obesity.
3. Undersized pelvis.
4. Postmaturity.
5. Primiparity.
B. Fetal factors.
1. Macrosomia.
2. Increased ratio of chest circumference to head circumference.
3. Breech position.
C. Obstetric factors.
1. Shoulder dystocia (major factor in pathogenesis of birth injuries).
2. Forceps (especially midforceps) delivery.
3. Vacuum extraction.
4. Prolonged second stage of labor.
5. Precipitous delivery.

N.B.: Infants who are large for gestational age (>4500 gm) and who are delivered vaginally (especially with forceps or vacuum extraction) are at increased risk for fractured clavicle, fractured humerus, brachial plexus injury, asphyxia, and cephalhematoma.

D. Vacuum extraction.
1. May be safer than forceps, but reported complications include the following:
   a. Cephalhematoma (10%).
   b. Scalp abrasions and lacerations (1% to 2%).
   c. Necrosis and avulsion of the scalp.
   d. Subaponeurotic hemorrhage (1% to 2%).
   e. Skull fractures.
   f. Intracranial bleeding (0.5%).
   g. Supratentorial hemorrhage; subdural hematoma.
2. There is no evidence of increased incidence of neurologic sequelae after use of vacuum extraction; however, whenever there are clinical

signs of neurologic compromise after vacuum extraction, evaluation by computed tomography (CT), magnetic resonance imaging (MRI), or ultrasonography is indicated.

II. HEAD TRAUMA
A. Caput succedaneum.
1. Caput succedaneum is a collection of edema fluid in the subcutaneous tissues of the scalp involving the portion of the head that presents in a vertex delivery.
2. Swelling is not limited by suture lines; discoloration of the scalp may occur secondary to ecchymosis.
3. There is spontaneous resolution, without sequelae, over a period of several days.
4. Rarely, there may be massive hemorrhage in the scalp secondary to bleeding within the subaponeurotic layer (sometimes classified as a *hemorrhagic caput succedaneum*).

B. Cephalhematoma.
Traumatic subperiosteal hemorrhage usually involving a parietal bone; seen in 0.5% to 1.5% of births; rare in <36-week gestation.
1. Predisposing factors: large size, primiparity, prolonged labor, male gender, vacuum extraction, forceps delivery (most important).
2. Clinical features.
   a. More than 95% involve parietal bone; 90% to 95% are unilateral, right more than left (2:1).
   b. There is firm swelling fixed at the suture lines; the overlying skin is not discolored.
   c. May not become apparent until several hours to several days after birth.
   d. Any neurologic signs and symptoms are probably related to underlying central nervous system (CNS) trauma.
   e. An underlying skull fracture occurs in 1% to 5% of cases, almost always in association with use of forceps; the fracture is usually linear, nondepressed, and clinically insignificant; routine skull radiographs are not indicated.
3. Course and prognosis.
   a. Spontaneous resolution occurs over a period of several weeks; 1% to 2% will calcify.
   b. Complications include hyperbilirubinemia and anemia (rare), exostoses, and infection.
4. Treatment.
   a. None required, except for associated complications.
   b. If neurologic signs and symptoms are present, workup for underlying CNS trauma is indicated.
   c. Primary infection is rare; infection is usually seen in association with sepsis or meningitis. The most frequently isolated pathogen is *Escherichia coli*. Aspiration of the cephalhematoma is indicated if there is evidence of local infection (e.g., increasing size, local erythema, fluctuance, or osteomyelitis of the underlying calvarium), relapse of systemic infection, or a delay in the resolution of clinical symptoms of systemic infection.

C. Skull fractures.

1. Linear.
   a. Linear fractures are seen in 1% to 5% of patients with cephalhematoma; they are secondary to forceps pressure or pressure against the maternal symphysis or ischial spines and usually involve the parietal bone.
   b. These fractures are rarely clinically significant, but a follow-up radiograph is recommended at several months of age to ensure that healing has occurred and that the fracture has not increased in width.
2. Depressed.
   a. Depressed fractures are the result of excessive molding and compression of the fetal skull by the maternal symphysis or ischial spines or occur secondary to forceps pressure; they are usually "Ping-Pong ball" type fractures and are secondary to inward buckling of the resilient bone.
   b. The need for treatment remains controversial.
      (1) Fractures almost always spontaneously elevate over a period of months.
      (2) If patient is neurologically and behaviorally asymptomatic, treatment probably is not needed.
      (3) Surgical elevation may be indicated if the depression is >5 mm.

D. Intracranial hemorrhage. Rare in the full-term newborn. May be secondary to birth trauma, severe asphyxia, or a coagulation defect.

1. Subarachnoid hemorrhage is the most frequent form of traumatic intracranial bleeding in the term neonate. It is usually of limited degree and rarely of clinical significance. It is probably secondary to birth trauma.
   a. Clinical features.
      (1) May be asymptomatic.
      (2) Intermittent seizures beginning on second or third day.
      (3) Lethargy, irritability, retinal hemorrhages.
   b. Diagnosis.
      (1) Red blood cells (RBCs) in cerebrospinal fluid (CSF) may be hard to interpret because of the frequency of traumatic taps; look for xanthochromia in centrifuged supernatant and count the RBCs in the first and third tubes of CSF.
      (2) CT is the neuroradiologic study of choice; ultrasound is not useful.
   c. Prognosis.
      (1) There are usually no long-term sequelae, but hydrocephalus is a late complication.
      (2) With evidence of other bleeding or cerebral contusion, prognosis is poor.
2. Subdural hemorrhage, now a rare occurrence, is caused by severe molding of the cranium with dural venous lacerations or rupture of the bridging veins over the convexities.
   a. Predisposing factors.
      (1) Large infant delivered to a primipara mother.

(2) Infant born in breech position or with difficult forceps delivery.

(3) Precipitous delivery in a multipara mother.

(4) Macrosomia.

b. Clinical features

(1) Posterior fossa.

(a) Lethargy, irritability, vomiting, irregular respirations, tense anterior fontanel, split sutures, increasing head circumference, anemia, blood in CSF, hypertonia or hypotonia, nystagmus, cranial nerve palsies, seizures.

(b) With a slowly expanding hematoma, symptoms may be delayed up to 96 hours.

(2) Over cerebral hemispheres.

(a) May be clinically silent.

(b) Signs of increased intracranial pressure with anemia and jaundice.

(c) Increased head circumference, poor feeding, vomiting, altered mental status, seizures.

c. Diagnosis.

(1) Ultrasound may be diagnostic; can be done as initial screen.

(2) CT is the definitive diagnostic study.

(3) Lumbar puncture (LP) should be avoided because of risk of herniation.

d. Treatment depends on symptoms, from supportive treatment to craniotomy with removal of subdural collections of blood; one third of cases require a subsequent shunt procedure because of hydrocephalus.

3. Intraventricular hemorrhage.

a. Rare in full-term neonates—*not* related to trauma. May be associated with intrapartum asphyxia or bleeding diatheses.

b. Usual site of bleeding is the choroid plexus, but it may arise from subependymal germinal matrix.

c. Hemorrhage is often clinically silent but may cause hypotonia, hyperreflexia, decreased activity, irritability, poor feeding, seizures, and hyperpyrexia.

d. May be associated with pulmonary hemorrhage and cardiac defects.

e. CT is the best diagnostic procedure.

f. Treatment is supportive, including seizure control.

4. Epidural hemorrhage. Rare in the full-term neonate, epidural hemorrhage is secondary to bleeding from a laceration of the middle meningeal artery after fracture of the temporal bone.

a. Predisposing factor: difficult forceps delivery.

b. Clinical features.

(1) Signs of increased intracranial pressure.

(2) Anemia.

(3) Asymmetric or focal neurologic signs.

c. Diagnosis is by CT.

d. Treatment includes evacuation of blood and ligation of the bleeding vessel.

5. Intracerebral hemorrhage.
   a. Intracerebral hemorrhage is a rare type of bleeding in the full-term neonate.
   b. Clinical features include convulsions, hemiparesis, signs of increased intracranial pressure, lethargy, and irritability.
   c. Diagnosis is by CT.

III. EYE INJURIES

Birth injuries to the eye and its adnexa are common. These include the following:

A. Retinal hemorrhage is seen in up to 50% of vaginal deliveries. It resolves over several days to 2 weeks and requires no specific intervention.

B. Subconjunctival hemorrhage.

C. Corneal edema.

D. Eyelid ecchymosis.

E. Rupture of Descemet's membrane.

F. Orbital hemorrhage with proptosis.

G. Fracture of the orbit.

H. Injuries to the extraocular muscles.

I. Dislocation of the globe outside the eyelids.

J. Eversion of the eyelids.

K. Blepharoptosis.

L. Marginal eyelid lacerations.

M. Laceration of the lacrimal canaliculus.

N. Hyphema.

N.B.: In cases of suspected eye injury, other than retinal hemorrhage, lid ecchymosis, and subconjunctival hemorrhage, *immediate ophthalmologic consultation is mandatory.*

IV. NERVE INJURIES

A. Brachial plexus injury is a mechanical disruption of the brachial plexus nerve roots secondary to traction and lateral flexion during a difficult vaginal delivery; avulsion of the roots is rare.

1. Incidence. 0.5 to 2 per 1000 live births; may occur in up to 10% of cases of shoulder dystocia.
2. Predisposing factors. The major risk factor is shoulder dystocia. Associated factors include fetal macrosomia, breech delivery, multiparity, prolonged second-stage labor, and midforceps delivery.

N.B.: Neonatal injuries are most frequent when shoulder dystocia is unanticipated or unrecognized.

3. Clinical features.
   a. Erb palsy. Secondary to injury of C5-C6 nerve roots; accounts for 90% to 95% of brachial plexus injuries.
      (1) Absence or decreased spontaneous movement of involved extremity; asymmetric Moro reflex.
      (2) Shoulder is internally rotated, forearm prone, elbow extended, and wrist and fingers flexed (waiter's tip position); winging of the scapula; diminished to absent deep tendon reflexes (DTR); hypesthesia.

(3) Right side predominates 2:1; usually unilateral, but in breech delivery may be bilateral.

(4) Associated findings include fetal asphyxia, facial palsy, fractured clavicle, fractured humerus, cephalhematoma, cervical cord injury, and diaphragmatic paralysis (5% of cases).

b. Klumpke paralysis. Secondary to injury to C7, C8-T1 nerve roots.

(1) Hand is flaccid; loss of wrist movement and grasp.

(2) Associated findings are those outlined for Erb, plus ipsilateral Horner syndrome (ptosis, miosis, anhidrosis).

c. Combination paresis.

4. Diagnosis.

a. Physical examination.

b. Electromyography (EMG) and nerve conduction studies can be helpful in delineating the location and extent of the injury and in assessing the degree of recovery.

c. Radiographs of the clavicle, shoulder, and humerus may help in the diagnosis of associated injuries.

5. Treatment.

a. For the first 7 to 10 days the arm should be wrapped against the body to prevent further injury.

b. After 10 days, passive range-of-motion exercises should be carried out.

c. Hand/wrist splints may help prevent contractures in Klumpke paralysis.

d. The role of early microsurgical nerve repair is controversial and is not indicated in the first 3 months.

6. Prognosis.

a. Generally good; 75% to 90% of injuries resolve spontaneously without sequelae; recovery is better for Erb than for Klumpke or mixed pareses (the presence of Horner syndrome is a bad prognostic sign).

b. In most cases, recovery takes place within weeks to 3 months, but there may be gradual improvement up to 1 to 2 years of age. All cases that show complete recovery show some improvement by 2 weeks.

N.B.: There is evidence that if perceptible muscle contractions have not returned to the deltoid and the biceps by the end of the third month, the ultimate functional recovery of the shoulder and arm will be unsatisfactory.

B. Facial nerve palsy may be developmental or acquired; it is seen in approximately 1 to 2:1000 births.

1. Clinical features.

a. Developmental (rare); seen in association with the following:

(1) Möbius syndrome, includes bilateral facial palsy, failure to abduct eyes, multiple cranial nerve abnormalities (3, 4, 6, 7, 10, 12), micrognathia, club feet, and absence of pectoralis muscles.

(2) Hemifacial microsomia.

(3) Agenesis of the depressor anguli oris muscle. Unilateral facial palsy; prominent asymmetry when baby cries (asymmetric crying facies syndrome); thinning of lateral portion of lower lip;

forehead wrinkling, eye closure, and nasolabial folds are symmetric; may be associated with cardiovascular, skeletal, or genitourinary anomalies.
  b. Acquired (common).
    (1) Unilateral; all divisions of the facial nerve are involved.
    (2) Secondary to birth trauma; compression of the facial nerve within the mastoid segment or just outside the sternomastoid foramen.
    (3) Predisposing factors, including large size, primiparity, prolonged second stage labor, and use of forceps (most important).
    (4) Clinical features include decreased forehead wrinkling, increased eye opening, decreased nasolabial fold, and flattening of the corner of the mouth.
    (5) Often associated with facial bruises or lacerations, hematotympanum, temporal bone fracture, or other birth injuries.
    (6) 90% show full recovery, most often within days to weeks, but some may take up to 2 years; 10% show only partial or no return of function.
2. Diagnosis.
  a. Based on birth history, physical examination, radiographic studies, and associated findings.
  b. Facial nerve conduction studies can be helpful and are indicated starting on day 1 or 2 in any newborn in whom the etiology of the palsy is uncertain.
3. Management.
  a. Developmental. Patient should have complete neurodiagnostic evaluation to guide treatment decisions.
  b. Acquired. 90% show complete resolution within 1 month without treatment, but surgical intervention may be helpful in highly selected cases. Criteria for surgical exploration of the facial canal and nerve decompression include the following:
    (1) Unilateral complete paralysis.
    (2) Hematotympanum and depressed fracture of the petrous bone.
    (3) Absence of voluntary and evoked motor unit responses in all muscles innervated by the facial nerve by 3 to 5 days of life.
    (4) No return of facial nerve function clinically or electrophysiologically at 5 weeks of age.

N.B.: It is prudent to observe every patient for at least 5 weeks for evidence of spontaneous recovery before considering surgical exploration (some experts would wait even longer).

C. Miscellaneous nerve injuries.

1. The hypoglossal nerve may be injured during a difficult delivery. Clinical features include weak or hoarse cry (vocal cord paralysis), difficulty feeding, difficulty with secretions, and fasciculations and deviations of the tongue. The injury is usually self-limited.
2. Phrenic nerve.
  a. There may be stretch injury of anterior cervical nerve roots 3, 4, and 5 after a traumatic delivery (breech delivery or shoulder dys-

tocia) leading to paralysis of the diaphragm. Symptoms may begin on the first day of life or may be delayed for as long as a month.

b. Most cases occur in association with an ipsilateral Erb palsy, but isolated phrenic nerve injury has been reported.

c. Clinical features include respiratory distress, cyanosis, and flaring of the chest on the involved side during inspiration. Most cases involve the right side.

d. Fluoroscopy (elevated diaphragm with paradoxic movement) is diagnostic.

e. On EMG there is failure of diaphragmatic response to phrenic nerve stimulation.

f. Initially, the patient may require oxygen, chest physical therapy (PT), continuous positive airway pressure (CPAP), or ventilatory support, but in most cases there is complete recovery over a period of several months. If early recovery of diaphragmatic function is going to occur, it will usually be evident within 2 weeks. In the rare case in which recovery does not occur, surgical plication or partial excision of the involved diaphragm may be helpful.

3. Peripheral nerve injuries. The radial, median, sciatic, and peroneal nerves may rarely be injured, either prenatally (constriction by umbilical cord or amniotic bands) or perinatally (pressure on the nerve during the delivery by bony compression, forceps trauma, or fracture).

D. Spinal cord injury. Spinal cord injury in newborns results from the general laxity of the infantile spine in relation to the more inelastic and fragile cord. Excessive longitudinal stretch and torsional and flexion-extension forces can result in disruption of the dura, vascular supply, and neuronal structures. The lower cervical and upper thoracic areas are usually involved. As many as 10% of all neonatal deaths may have an associated spinal cord injury.

1. Predisposing factors.
   a. Difficult vaginal delivery of a breech presentation.
   b. Mid-to-high forceps delivery.
   c. Prematurity, shoulder dystocia, precipitous delivery.

2. Clinical features.
   a. A "snap" or "pop" may be heard at the time of delivery.
   b. Profound hypotonia, absent deep-tendon reflexes, obvious sensory level, flaccid extremities, Horner syndrome.
   c. Temperature instability.
   d. Absent respiratory effort, paradoxic breathing, bell-shaped thorax.
   e. Neurogenic bladder (urinary retention).
   f. May be associated with hypoxic-ischemic encephalopathy (i.e., neonatal seizures, cranial CT abnormalities, and subsequent developmental delay).

N.B.: Fracture or dislocation of the spinal column is seen in <1% of cases of spinal cord injury.

3. Differential diagnosis.
   a. Hypotonia secondary to birth asphyxia.

    b. Neuromuscular disease.

    c. Congenital spinal cord tumor; syringomyelia.

4. Diagnosis.

    a. Plain-film radiograph of the spine is rarely helpful.

    b. Myelography with CT, ultrasound, nerve conduction studies, EMG, and somatosensory evoked potentials may be helpful but often fail to localize or define the lesion.

    c. MRI is the best diagnostic test available. It is the only modality that produces a direct image of the spinal cord. Advantages of MRI include the following:

      (1) MRI provides excellent soft-tissue definition.

      (2) It can differentiate an extramedullary from intramedullary lesion.

      (3) It can be performed even in ventilator-dependent patients.

5. Treatment.

    a. If there is a possibility of spinal instability, immobilization of the head and neck is mandatory.

    b. Management is best carried out in a tertiary-care facility.

    c. Treatment is usually conservative (reduction obtained with light traction); laminectomy and surgical exploration are rarely of any benefit.

    d. Patient may eventually require a posterior stabilization procedure.

6. Prognosis depends on the extent of neurologic injury.

V. FRACTURES AND DISLOCATIONS

A. Fractured clavicle. This is the most frequently fractured bone in the neonate and is present in 1.5% to 3.0% of vaginal deliveries.

1. Clinical features.

    a. Predisposing factors include large size and shoulder dystocia; most fractures occur after traumatic vaginal deliveries.

    b. Usually involves the lateral segment of the clavicle.

    c. There is a higher frequency on the right (2:1).

    d. The most common finding is minimal swelling or fullness over the fracture site; there may also be crepitus, decreased arm movement, irritability during movement of the arm, and asymmetric Moro reflex. However, 80% have no symptoms and only minimal physical findings; displacement is rare.

    e. The diagnosis is often missed on the initial newborn examination and becomes obvious only when a calcified swelling (callus) is noted at the 2- to 4-week examination.

    f. An associated Erb palsy is present in 2% to 5% of cases.

2. Diagnosis.

    a. Based on careful physical examination.

    b. Radiographs or ultrasound studies are not usually indicated, but ultrasound may be helpful to rule out brachial plexus injury.

3. Differential diagnosis.

    a. Brachial plexus injury.

    b. Traumatic separation of the proximal humeral epiphysis.

    c. Humeral shaft fracture.

    d. Shoulder dislocation.

4. Treatment.
    a. Specific intervention not indicated (if both ends of the bone are in the same room, good healing will occur!).
    b. Advise parents to avoid tension on the affected arm.
    c. Prognosis is excellent; sequelae are rare.
B. Long bone fractures may involve diaphyseal or metaphyseal fractures of the humerus and femur, although other bones may be affected.
1. Predisposing factors.
    a. Usually seen after difficult extraction of infant in breech position.
    b. Most occur during vaginal deliveries but can occur secondary to difficult extraction at cesarean section.
2. Clinical features.
    a. Swelling and tenderness of the extremity.
    b. Decreased mobility.
    c. Audible or palpable click; crepitus.
3. Diagnosis.
    a. Physical examination.
    b. Radiographs.
4. Treatment.
    a. Splinting, soft cast, or hard cast, depending on location and severity of fracture.
    b. Prognosis is excellent.
C. Nasal septal deformities are seen in 0.1% to 1% of births; they are secondary to slipping of the triangular cartilage of the nasal septum from its proper position in the vomerine groove.
1. Etiology. The nasal septum is mainly cartilaginous in the newborn. The tip of the nose is particularly vulnerable to trauma during rotation of the head during delivery. Deformities may also occur secondary to intrauterine forces.
2. Clinical features.
    a. Outward deformity of the nose to one side accompanied by leaning of the columella to the side opposite the dislocation.
    b. Loss of nasal tip stability.
    c. Flattening of the nasal aperture on the side of dislocation.
    d. Diminished movement of ala during inspiration.
3. Diagnosis.
    a. Physical examination. Pass a probe or cotton-tipped applicator along the floor of the nose and feel the subluxated septum.
    b. Compression on the tip of the nose will accentuate asymmetry of the nares.
N.B.: Septal deviation must be differentiated from the more common transient flattening or twisting of the nose that resolves spontaneously over several days.
4. Treatment. The septal cartilage should be replaced in the vomerine groove by the third day of life. This manual reduction can be done in the nursery by an otolaryngologist using a special elevator instrument.
5. Prognosis. If untreated, there is no spontaneous resolution. Although the nose may appear to straighten, there is an increased incidence of septal and cosmetic deformities.

D. Mandibular fracture.
1. Usually secondary to traumatic forceps delivery.
2. Clinical features include facial asymmetry, swelling and ecchymosis over the fracture site, poor feeding, and palpable bony deformity.
3. Diagnosis is by physical examination and radiographs.
4. Treatment consists of immediate reduction followed by maxillo-mandibular fixation.

VI. MISCELLANEOUS INJURIES
A. Myoglobinuric renal failure.
Rarely, rhabdomyolysis and subsequent myoglobinuric renal failure have been reported in newborns secondary to asphyxia and birth trauma.
B. Hemoperitoneum.
1. Intraabdominal bleeding is rare. Risk factors include large size, hepatomegaly, breech extraction, and forceful manipulation during delivery.
2. Bleeding can occur from the liver, adrenals, spleen, mesentery, umbilical vein, or kidney, but the liver is the most common site. There is usually a slowly expanding subcapsular hematoma that ruptures into the free peritoneal cavity.
3. Hemoperitoneum should be suspected in the newborn with pallor, abdominal distention, anemia, and shock without an obvious source of bleeding. A bluish discoloration of the overlying abdominal skin and scrotal ecchymosis and enlargement may be present. Diagnosis is confirmed by paracentesis and laparotomy.
4. Subcapsular hematoma is the most common form of liver injury; rupture may occur up to 1 week of age.
   a. If the hematoma is large there may be nonspecific prerupture symptoms of poor feeding, lethargy, jaundice, and slowly progressive anemia; a right-upper-quadrant mass may be palpable.
   b. Differentiation from a solid tumor can be made by ultrasonography or CT.
   c. Treatment includes prompt resuscitation, correction of any coagulation defect, evacuation of the hematoma, and repair and drainage of the lacerated liver.
   d. In cases in which the laceration or hematoma is small, careful observation with serial ultrasonography may be appropriate.
5. Adrenal injuries may occur in large babies and those born by breech or otherwise difficult delivery; 90% are unilateral, with 75% occurring on the right side.
   a. Symptoms, which usually appear in the first week, relate to the degree of hemorrhage; when small in amount there may be poor feeding, lethargy, and irritability; when large there may be signs of shock.
   b. When both glands are involved there may be signs and symptoms of adrenal insufficiency.
   c. Abdominal ultrasonography may show a suprarenal mass with downward displacement of the kidney and compression of its upper pole. Calcification may occur as early as 12 days and is usually rimlike in distribution.

   d. Treatment depends on the degree of bleeding; it may vary from expectant (blood loss is mild and within the capsule) to evacuation of the hematoma or adrenalectomy.

C. Pneumoperitoneum.

1. Pneumoperitoneum occurs rarely as a direct result of birth injury, but it may also be the indirect result of birth asphyxia and mucosal ischemia.
2. Symptoms include abdominal distention and vomiting.
3. Diagnosis is by abdominal radiograph, especially the left lateral decubitus view.
4. Treatment includes resuscitation and immediate surgical exploration and repair.

D. Pharyngeal injury.

1. Pharyngeal perforation may be restricted to the mucosa and submucosa or may extend into the mediastinum or pleural cavity; it occurs secondary to postpartum suctioning, digital injury during a breech delivery, or attempts to pass a nasogastric or endotracheal tube.
2. Symptoms include excessive oropharyngeal secretions and regurgitation of feedings.
3. Diagnosis is established by water-contrast radiography.
4. Treatment of superficial injuries consists of antibiotics and placement of a soft nasogastric tube. More extensive injuries may require drainage, tube thoracostomy, closure of the perforation, and parenteral nutrition.

E. Limb ischemia and gangrene.

1. Limb ischemia and gangrene may be due to a variety of prenatal or perinatal events that result in occlusive vascular disruption. The etiology is usually not evident but may be secondary to compression by an encircling umbilical cord, compound presentation of the arm and head, acute asphyxia, or thromboembolic events (possibly related to poorly controlled maternal diabetes).
2. When gangrene is established at birth, surgical amputation, autoamputation, or some loss of function is the usual outcome.
3. In cases in which ischemia develops within hours of birth secondary to a thromboembolic event, surgical thrombectomy may be successful.

F. Testicular injury. Among newborns who are delivered vaginally in the breech position, approximately 10% show injury to the genital area, half of whom have testicular damage. In many of these cases the injured testis will remain abnormal. There is no specific treatment.

BIBLIOGRAPHY

Falco NA, Eriksson E: Facial nerve palsy in the newborn: incidence and outcome, *Plast Reconstr Surg* 85:1, 1990.

Gonik B, Hollyer VL, Allen R: Shoulder dystocia recognition: differences in neonatal risks for injury, *Am J Perinatol* 8:31, 1991.

Hazbi B: Subluxation of the nasal septum in the newborn: etiology, diagnosis, and treatment, *Otolaryngol Clin North Am* 10:125, 1977.

Hernandez C, Wendel GD: Shoulder dystocia, *Clin Obstet Gynecol* 33:526, 1990.

Joseph PR, Rosenfeld W: Clavicular fractures in neonates, *Am J Dis Child* 144:165, 1990.

Lanska MJ, Roessmann U, Wiznitzer M: Magnetic resonance imaging in cervical cord birth injury, *Pediatrics* 85:760, 1990.

LeBranc CMA, Allen UD, Ventureyra E: Cephalhematomas revisited: when should a diagnostic tap be performed? *Clin Pediatr* 34:86, 1995.

Ngan HY, Tang GWK, Ma HK: Vacuum extractor: a safe instrument? *Aust NZ J Obstet Gynaecol* 26:177, 1986.

Painter MJ, Bergman I: Obstetrical trauma to the neonatal central and peripheral nervous system, *Semin Perinatol* 6:89, 1982.

Schullinger JN: Birth trauma, *Pediatr Clin North Am* 40:1351, 1993.

Serfontein GL, Rom S, Stein S: Posterior fossa subdural hemorrhage in the newborn, *Pediatrics* 65:40, 1980.

Siegel MJ, Gado MH, Shackelford G, et al: Cranial computed tomography and real-time sonography in full-term neonates and infants, *Pediatr Radiol* 149:111, 1983.

Tiwary CM: Testicular injury in breech delivery: possible implications, *Pediatr Urol* 34:210, 1989.

Turpenny PD, Stahl S, Bowers D, Bingham P: Peripheral ischemia and gangrene presenting at birth, *Eur J Pediatr* 151:550, 1992.

Yasunaga S, Rivera R: Cephalhematoma in the newborn, *Clin Pediatr* 13:256, 1974.

19

Jaundice

AMBADAS PATHAK

I. INDIRECT HYPERBILIRUBINEMIA
A. General considerations.
1. Jaundice is a common occurrence in the newborn period. Two of three full-term newborns develop clinical jaundice; most of them have unconjugated hyperbilirubinemia. Male infants tend to have higher levels of bilirubin than female infants; Asians, whites, and blacks develop hyperbilirubinemia with decreasing frequency.
2. The newborn's susceptibility to jaundice is the result of shortened red cell life span and immaturity of liver function. If one newborn has significant jaundice, subsequent siblings are at significantly increased risk.
3. Breakdown of 1 gm of hemoglobin results in production of 35 mg of bilirubin.
4. A normal full-term infant produces 8 to 10 mg/kg per day of bilirubin.
5. There is a considerable variation in serum bilirubin levels in normal full-term and near-term infants as shown in Fig. 19-1. Factors contributing to this are ethnic background and feeding practices.
6. There is considerable variation in measured bilirubin from laboratory to laboratory. Accuracy of this measurement is ±5%.
7. Serial measurements to determine rate of rise are sometimes necessary.
8. The degree of jaundice may be assessed initially by the number of dermal zones involved (Table 19-1). As jaundice begins, it advances from head to toe; it fades uniformly throughout without significant progression.
B. Causes of indirect hyperbilirubinemia are summarized in Box 19-1.
1. Hemolytic disease of the newborn. Erythroblastosis fetalis is discussed fully in Chapter 17 (see pp. 208-215).
2. Extravascular blood. Cephalhematomas, cerebral and pulmonary hemorrhage, and severe bruising secondary to breech presentation contribute to prolonged hyperbilirubinemia.
3. Polycythemia. Result of twin-twin transfusion, maternal-fetal transfusion, or delayed clamping of cord; the additional bilirubin load for the liver causes hyperbilirubinemia.

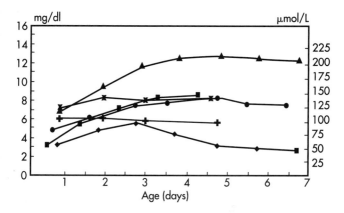

FIG. 19-1. Mean total bilirubin concentrations in normal full-term and near-term infants. ▲, Fifty healthy Japanese newborn infants, 37 to 42 weeks of gestation, all breast-fed. Excludes Rh and ABO incompatibility. (Data from Yamauchi Y, Yamanouchi I: *Acta Paediatr Jpn* 31:65, 1989.) ×, One hundred seventy-six term breast-fed Canadian infants. Excludes Rh hemolytic disease, but includes nine ABO incompatible infants with positive Coombs' tests. Seventeen infants received phototherapy. +, One hundred sixty-four Canadian term formula-fed infants, seven ABO incompatible with positive Coombs' tests, and three received phototherapy. (Data from Maisels MJ, 1999.) ■, One thousand eighty-seven term Israeli infants, 78% fully or partially breast-fed. (Data from D. Seidman, *personal communication*, 1988.) ●, Fifty-six Nigerian term appropriate for gestational age (AGA) infants. Excludes ABO or Rh incompatibility and G6PD deficiency. Infants were "largely breast-fed." (Data from Maisels MJ, 1999.) ◆, Twenty-nine full-term American infants, all formula-fed, about 50% African-American and 50% Caucasian. (Data from Maisels MJ: Neonatal jaundice. In Avery BG, Fletcher MA, MacDonald MG (editors): *Neonatology, pathophysiology, and management of the newborn,* ed 5, Philadelphia, 1999, Lippincott Williams & Wilkins.)

TABLE 19-1
Dermal Zones and Serum Bilirubin Levels

Dermal zone	Mean serum bilirubin (mg/dl)
1. Head and neck	6
2. Trunk to umbilicus	9
3. Groin including upper thighs	12
4. Knees and elbows to ankles and wrists	15
5. Feet and hands including palms and soles	>15

Modified from Kramer LI: *Am J Dis Child* 118:454, 1969.

BOX 19-1
Causes of a Pathologic Indirect Hyperbilirubinemia in Newborn Infants

INCREASED PRODUCTION OR BILIRUBIN LOAD ON THE LIVER
Hemolytic Disease
Immune
   Rh, ABO, and other blood group incompatibilities
Heritable
   Red cell membrane defects (hereditary spherocytosis, elliptocytosis, stomatocytosis, and pyknocytosis)
   Red cell deficiencies (glucose-6-phosphate dehydrogenase [G-6PD] deficiency,* pyruvate kinase deficiency, and other erythrocyte enzyme deficiencies)
   Hemoglobinopathies (α-Thalassemia, β-γ-thalassemia)

Other Causes of Increased Production
Sepsis*†
Extravasation of blood; hematoma; pulmonary, cerebral, or occult hemorrhage
Polycythemia
Macrosomic infants of diabetic mothers

Increased Enteropathic Circulation of Bilirubin
Breast-milk jaundice
Pyloric stenosis*
Small or large bowel obstruction or ileus

Decreased Clearance
Prematurity
G6PD deficiency

Inborn Errors of Metabolism
Crigler-Najjar syndrome, types I and II, and Gilbert syndrome
Galactosemia†
Tyrosinemia†
Hypermethioninemia†

Metabolic
Hypothyroidism
Hypopituitarism†

Modified from Maisels MJ: Neonatal jaundice. In Avery BG, Fletcher MA, MacDonald MG (editors): *Neonatology, pathophysiology, and management of the newborn,* ed 5, Philadelphia, 1999, Lippincott Williams & Wilkins.
* Decreased clearance also part of pathogenesis.
†Elevation of direct-reading bilirubin also occurs.

4. Pyloric stenosis. The absolute decrease in glucuronyl transferase activity and increased enterohepatic circulation in this condition leads to prolonged jaundice.
5. Congenital nonhemolytic unconjugated hyperbilirubinemia. Crigler-Najjar syndrome and Gilbert syndrome are examples; bilirubin uridine diphosphate glucuronosyltransferase (UDPGT) activity is undetectable (in vitro) in the former and is 20% to 30% of normal in the latter.
6. Congenital hypothyroidism. Characteristic prolonged unconjugated hyperbilirubinemia without hemolysis; now easily detectable with neonatal thyroid screening.
7. Sepsis. May occur, though rarely, with jaundice alone; after the first week, elevation of direct fraction is common, but before that nearly all bilirubin is indirect reacting; congenital syphilis, TORCH infections, and coxsackievirus B infection deserve consideration.
8. Galactosemia. Jaundice has a hemolytic and hepatic component secondary to ingestion of galactose.
9. Breast milk jaundice. There is an association between breast-feeding and neonatal hyperbilirubinemia. Studies have shown that breast-fed infants were three times more likely to develop total serum bilirubin levels of 12 mg/dl or higher and six times more likely to develop levels of 15 mg/dl or higher when compared with formula-fed infants. There is a considerable overlap between "breast-feeding jaundice syndrome" and "breast-milk jaundice syndrome." The former appears in the first 2 to 4 days and the latter at 4 to 7 days. In 20% to 30% of all breast-fed infants, indirect hyperbilirubinemia persists beyond 2 to 3 weeks and in some up to 3 months. A decreased caloric intake and an increase in enterohepatic circulation of bilirubin are main contributors. Box 19-2 lists measures to prevent and treat breast-milk jaundice.

BOX 19-2

Approaches to the Prevention and Treatment of Jaundice Associated With Breast-feeding

PREVENTION
1. Encourage frequent nursing (i.e., at least eight times per day)
2. Do not supplement with water or dextrose water

TREATMENT OPTIONS
1. Observe.
2. Discontinue nursing, substitute formula.
3. Alternate feedings of breast milk and formula.
4. Discontinue nursing, administer phototherapy.
5. Continue nursing, administer phototherapy.

From Maisels MJ: Neonatal jaundice. In Avery BG, Fletcher MA, MacDonald MG (editors): *Neonatology, pathophysiology, and management of the newborn,* ed 5, Philadelphia, 1999, Lippincott Williams & Wilkins.

10. Glucose–6 phosphate dehydrogenase/deficiency (G6PD). Seen in infants of African-American, East Asian, or Mediterranean descent, G6PD is accompanied by moderate indirect hyperbilirubinemia and, rarely, kernicterus. These infants have increased bilirubin production caused by hemolysis and abnormal bilirubin elimination.

C. Evaluation of a jaundiced full-term neonate (Table 19-2).

1. History should include details of the pregnancy, including the mother's general health, blood type, diabetes, hemolytic anemia, gallstones, splenectomy, medications, familial disorders, or jaundice in previous children.

TABLE 19-2
Data Collection in the Diagnosis of Neonatal Jaundice

Information	Significance
FAMILY HISTORY	
Parent or sibling with history of jaundice or anemia	Suggests hereditary hemolytic anemia such as hereditary spherocytosis
Previous sibling with neonatal jaundice	Suggests hemolytic disease caused by ABO or Rh isoimmunization
History of liver disease in siblings, or disorders such as cystic fibrosis, galactosemia, tyrosinemia, hypermethioninemia, Crigler-Najjar syndrome, or α_1-antitrypsin deficiency	All associated with neonatal hyperbilirubinemia
MATERNAL HISTORY	
Unexplained illness during pregnancy	Consider congenital infections such as rubella, cytomegalovirus, toxoplasmosis, herpes, syphilis, hepatitis A or B, Epstein-Barr virus
Diabetes mellitus	Increased incidence of jaundice among infants of diabetic mothers
Drug ingestion during pregnancy	Ingestion of sulfonamides, nitrofurantoins, antimalarials may initiate hemolysis in G6PD-deficient infant
HISTORY OF LABOR AND DELIVERY	
Vacuum extraction	Increased incidence of cephalhematoma and jaundice
Oxytocin-induced labor	Increased incidence of hyperbilirubinemia
Delayed cord clamping	Increased incidence of hyperbilirubinemia among polycythemic infants
Apgar score	Increased incidence of jaundice in asphyxiated infants

TABLE 19-2
Data Collection in the Diagnosis of Neonatal Jaundice—cont'd

Information	Significance
INFANT'S HISTORY	
Delayed passage of meconium or infrequent stools	Increased enterohepatic circulation of bilirubin; consider intestinal atresia, annular pancreas, Hirschsprung's disease, meconium plug, drug-induced ileus (hexamethonium)
Caloric intake	Inadequate caloric intake results in delay in bilirubin conjugation
Vomiting	Suspect sepsis, galactosemia, or pyloric stenosis; all associated with hyperbilirubinemia
INFANT'S PHYSICAL EXAMINATION	
Small for gestational age	Infants frequently polycythemic and jaundiced
Head size	Microcephaly seen with intrauterine infections associated with jaundice
Cephalhematoma	Entrapped hemorrhage associated with hyperbilirubinemia
Plethora	Polycythemia
Pallor	Suspect hemolytic anemia
Petechiae	Suspect congenital infection, overwhelming sepsis, or severe hemolytic disease as cause of jaundice
Appearance of umbilical stump	Omphalitis and sepsis may produce jaundice
Hepatosplenomegaly	Suspect hemolytic anemia or congenital infection
Optic fundi	Chorioretinitis suggests congenital infection as cause of jaundice
Umbilical hernia	Consider hypothyroidism
Congenital anomalies	Jaundice occurs with increased frequency among infants with trisomic conditions

LABORATORY DATA

MATERNAL	
Blood group and indirect Coombs' test	Necessary for evaluation of possible ABO or Rh incompatibility
Serology	Rule out congenital syphilis

Continued

TABLE 19-2
Data Collection in the Diagnosis of Neonatal Jaundice—cont'd

Information	Significance
INFANT	
Hemoglobin	Anemia suggests hemolytic disease or large entrapped hemorrhage; hemoglobin above 22 gm/dl associated with increased incidence of jaundice
Reticulocyte count	Elevation suggests hemolytic disease
Red cell morphology	Spherocytes suggest ABO incompatibility or hereditary spherocytosis; red cell fragmentation is seen in disseminated intravascular coagulation
Platelet count	Thrombocytopenia suggests infection
White cell count	Total white cell count less than 5000/mm^3 or band/neutrophil ratio >0.2 suggests infection
Sedimentation rate	Values in excess of 5 during the first 48 hours indicate infection or ABO incompatibility
Direct bilirubin	Elevation suggests infection or severe Rh incompatibility
Immunoglobulin M	Elevation indicates infection
Blood group and direct and indirect Coombs' test	Required to rule out hemolytic disease as a result of isoimmunization
Carboxyhemoglobin level	Elevated in infants with hemolytic disease or entrapped hemorrhage
Urinalysis	Presence of reducing substance suggests diagnosis of galactosemia

From MacMahon JR, Stevenson DK, Oski FA: Management of neonatal hyperbilirubinemia. In Taeusch H, Ballard RA (editors): *Avery's diseases of the newborn,* ed 7, Philadelphia, 1998, WB Saunders.

2. Physical examination should include assessment of cry, color, and activity; check for the presence of petechiae, ecchymoses, or hepatosplenomegaly, and review neurologic status as indicated by tone and reflexes.
3. Critical evaluation of serum bilirubin level. Studies from the National Collaborative Perinatal Project and other recent studies report that about 95% of all infants studied had total serum bilirubin levels under 12.9 mg/dl, leading to the acceptance of this number as the upper limit of "physiologic jaundice." However, more recent studies indicate that the 95th percentile was a level of 17 to18 mg/dl. Thus in a mixed-race population in which 60% to 70% of infants are breast fed, the 95th percentiles are approximately 8 mg/dl, 10 mg/dl, 12 mg/dl,

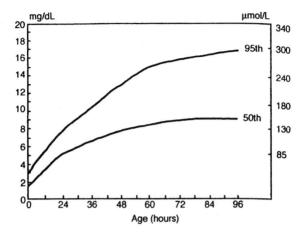

FIG. 19-2. Smoothed curves from studies in diverse populations illustrating the expected velocity of total serum bilirubin (TSB) levels and approximate values for the 50th and 95th percentiles. (From Maisels MJ: Neonatal jaundice. In Avery BG, Fletcher MA, MacDonald MG (editors): *Neonatology, pathophysiology, and management of the newborn,* ed 5, Philadelphia, 1999, Lippincott Williams & Wilkins.)

16 mg/dl, and 17 to 18 mg/dl at 24, 36, 48, 72, and 120 hours of age, respectively. It is therefore imperative that serum bilirubin levels should be considered in conjunction with the infant's age in hours and *not in days.* Fig. 19-2 provides the hourly rate of rise in total serum bilirubin levels. When these exceed the 95th percentile, or the rate of rise crosses percentiles, detailed evaluation, intervention as indicated, and follow-up are necessary.

4. Laboratory studies should include a complete blood count (CBC), including reticulocyte count, peripheral smear, blood group of mother and infant, Coombs' test, and urinalysis.

N.B.: A diagnostic approach proposed by Maisels is recommended (Fig. 19-3). Evaluation and treatment of hyperbilirubinemia in the healthy term infant is presented in a clinical algorithm (Fig. 19-4).

D. Management depends on the cause.

1. Hemolytic jaundice.
   a. Hemolytic jaundice is indicated by anemia, reticulocytosis, and a positive direct Coombs' test.
   b. Hemolytic jaundice resulting from Rh or ABO incompatibility warrants serial measurement of bilirubin level.
   c. Phototherapy is indicated for infants showing a rapid rise in bilirubin (>0.5 to 1 mg/dl per hour) to avoid need for exchange transfusion. In general, the bilirubin level at which exchange transfusion is

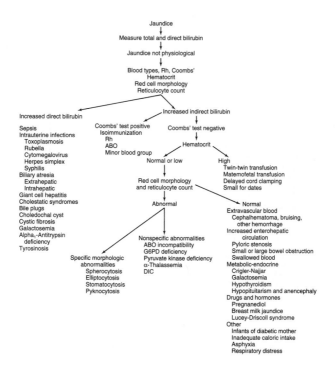

FIG. 19-3. Diagnostic approach to neonatal jaundice. (From Maisels MJ: Neonatal jaundice. In Avery GB (editor): *Neonatology: pathophysiology and management of the newborn,* ed 4, Philadelphia, 1987, JB Lippincott.)

planned is ascertained, and phototherapy commences when the level is 5 mg/dl below that. High-intensity, double-surface phototherapy is more effective than conventional phototherapy. Exchange transfusion is indicated when serum bilirubin rises rapidly (despite phototherapy) to 20 mg/dl (see the section on erythroblastosis fetalis, pp. 208-215).

2. Nonhemolytic jaundice.
   a. The view of management of nonhemolytic jaundice in a full-term infant is undergoing rapid change.
   b. Phototherapy for such infants is indicated for a total serum bilirubin level of 18 to 20 mg/dl at 49 to 72 hours of age. A level of ≥15 mg/dl is used between 25 and 48 hours.
   c. Similarly, exchange transfusion is indicated for a total serum bilirubin level of ≥25 mg/dl at 49 to 72 hours of age if intensive pho-

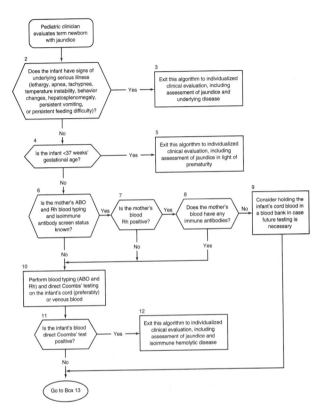

FIG. 19-4. Algorithm for the management of hyperbilirubinemia in the healthy term infant. (Modified from American Academy of Pediatrics Provisional Committee for Quality Improvement and Subcommittee on Hyperbilirubinemia: *Pediatrics* 95:458, 1995.)   *Continued*

    totherapy has failed. A level of ≥20 mg/dl is used between 25 and 48 hours.

N.B.: Attention to fluid and caloric intake, frequency of stools, and general health of the infant is important. Breast-feeding at frequent intervals should be encouraged.

  3. Phototherapy.
    a. Phototherapy converts bilirubin to its photo products, which are less lipophilic and can bypass hepatic conjugation and be excreted without further metabolism.

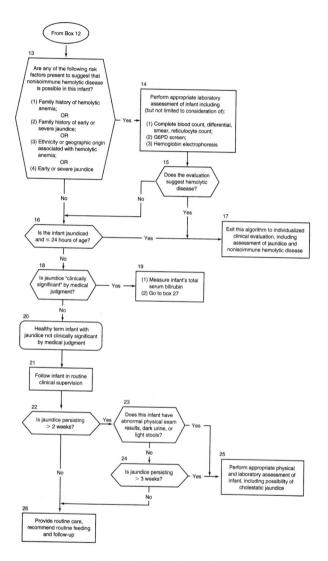

FIG. 19-4. For legend see p. 281.

From Box 19

Management of Hyperbilirubinemia in the Healthy Term Newborn*

Age, hours	TSB Level, mg/dl (µmol/L)			
	Consider Phototherapy†	Phototherapy	Exchange Transfusion if Intensive Phototherapy Fails‡	Exchange Transfusion and Intensive Phototherapy
≤24§	—	—	—	—
25–48	≥12 (170)	≥15 (260)	≥20 (340)	≥25 (430)
49–72	≥15 (260)	≥18 (310)	≥25 (430)	≥30 (510)
>72	≥17 (290)	≥20 (340)	≥25 (430)	≥30 (510)

*TSB indicates total serum bilirubin.
†Phototherapy at these TSB levels is a clinical option, meaning that the intervention is available and may be used on the basis of individual clinical judgment.
‡Intensive phototherapy should produce a decline of TSB of 1-2 mg/dL within 4-6 hours and the TSB level should continue to fall and remain below the threshold level for exchange transfusion. If this does not occur, it is considered a failure of phototherapy.
§Term infants who are clinically jaundiced at ≤24 hours old are not considered healthy and require further evaluation (see text).

FIG. 19-4. For legend see p. 281.

b. A standard phototherapy unit has a bank of eight fluorescent lights: four special blue and four daylight bulbs.

c. For effective phototherapy a minimum irradiance of 4 µW/cm²/nm in the blue spectrum is necessary. Response is dose related; a saturation point is reached at 23 µW/cm²/nm. Irradiance should be monitored by using a photometer.

d. With the infant in a bassinet, lights may be kept at a distance of 10 cm. When halogen phototherapy lamps are used, manufacturer's recommendations should be followed.

e. A wraparound fiberoptic unit is available that has been shown to be effective; it has the advantage of promoting mother-infant bonding and avoiding the complications associated with fluorescent light phototherapy. However, they have a very low spectral power.

f. Bilirubin measurements every 12 hours are necessary; evaluation of skin color is unreliable.

g. Usually 2 to 3 days of continuous therapy is needed; serum bilirubin decreases by 2.5 to 3 mg per day in the absence of excessive production.

h. On discontinuation of phototherapy, primarily in babies with hemolytic jaundice, the serum bilirubin level should be measured after 12 hours to detect rebound phenomenon; rarely this requires restarting of phototherapy.

i. Complications of phototherapy include increased water loss, elevation of temperature, skin rash, hypocalcemia, abdominal distention, displaced eye patches causing respiratory distress, and bronze baby syndrome.

E. Physiologic jaundice.

1. Physiologic jaundice is by far the most common type of jaundice and it accounts for 50% of cases.

2. Proposed criteria.
  a. Jaundice appearing after day 1.
  b. Rate of increase in serum bilirubin <5 mg/dl per day.
  c. Serum bilirubin level does not exceed 13 mg/dl in full-term and 15 mg/dl in preterm infant.
  d. Direct bilirubin fraction is <2 mg/dl.
  e. Jaundice does not last beyond 1 week in full-term and beyond 2 weeks in preterm infant.
3. Infant does not manifest any signs of illness (e.g., lethargy, poor feeding, temperature instability).
4. Elaborate laboratory evaluation and aggressive therapeutic intervention are *not* indicated.
F. Kernicterus. There is an apparent resurgence of kernicterus in the last decade. The reported cases were in infants with G6PD deficiency, very sick newborns with low bilirubin levels, and in apparently healthy term and near-term newborns with very high (usually above 30 mg/dl) bilirubin levels.

II. CHOLESTASIS (REDUCTION IN BILE FLOW)
A. General considerations.
1. Cholestasis results from extrahepatic obstruction or hepatocellular injury, either primary or secondary to many infectious, or metabolic and toxic causes.
2. The newborn is particularly susceptible because of immature hepatobiliary function, with decrease in bile acid pool size, rate of synthesis, intraluminal concentration, and ileal uptake. Consequently, intraluminal fat digestion is impaired, and cholestatic effects of various endogenous and exogenous substances are enhanced.
3. Conjugated hyperbilirubinemia is always a problem and is accompanied by elevation of bile salts and phospholipids, indicating cholestasis. Early recognition allows prompt diagnosis and effective therapy.
B. Clinical syndromes (Box 19-3). Neonatal cholestasis occurs in 1:2500 births, with extrahepatic obstruction accounting for half of the cases. Neonatal hepatitis, biliary atresia and α_1-antitrypsin deficiency are the three most common causes, with an approximate incidence of 1:5000, 1:10,000, and 1:20,000, respectively.
1. Extrahepatic biliary disease.
  a. Extrahepatic biliary atresia. At first, infants with extrahepatic biliary atresia pass "normal-colored" stools. By 3 to 5 weeks, conjugated hyperbilirubinemia develops. In addition to clinical icterus, these infants may have an enlarged liver and, occasionally, an enlarged spleen. Associated anomalies include polysplenia, preduodenal portal vein, malrotation, and congenital heart disease. In established cases, stools are acholic or faintly pigmented. Obstruction to bile flow is at the porta hepatis in the majority of infants. It is important to establish the patency of the extrahepatic biliary tree early to allow prompt surgical intervention. Magnetic resonance cholangiography has been useful in excluding biliary atresia. Postoperative restora-

---

BOX 19-3
Differential Diagnosis of Neonatal Cholestasis

EXTRAHEPATIC BILIARY DISEASE

Extrahepatic biliary atresia
Choledochal cyst
Bile-duct stenosis
Spontaneous perforation of the bile duct
Neoplasm
Cholelithiasis

INTRAHEPATIC BILIARY DISEASE

Intrahepatic bile-duct paucity
   Syndromic form (Alagille syndrome)
   Nonsyndromic forms
Inspissated bile
Caroli disease (cystic dilation of the intrahepatic bile ducts)
Congenital hepatic fibrosis and infantile polycystic disease

HEPATOCELLULAR DISEASE

Metabolic and genetic diseases
   Disorders of amino acid metabolism (tyrosinemia)
   Disorders of lipid metabolism
      Wolman disease
      Niemann-Pick disease
      Gaucher disease
   Disorders of carbohydrate metabolism
      Galactosemia
      Hereditary fructose intolerance
      Glycogenosis type IV
   Peroxisomal disorders
      Zellweger syndrome (cerebrohepatorenal syndrome)
      Adrenoleukodystrophy
      Glutaric aciduria type II
      Olivocerebellar atrophy
   Endocrine disorders
      Idiopathic hypopituitarism
      Hypothyroidism

Continued

    tion of bile flow occurs in up to 80% of infants who undergo surgery before 8 weeks of age as compared with 20% of infants operated on after 12 weeks. Hepatic portoenterostomy (Kasai procedure) is used based on results of the operative cholangiogram and histopathology of the liver.

  b. **Choledochal cyst.** A choledochal cyst is a dilation of the extrahepatic biliary tree that produces signs and symptoms of obstruction

---

BOX 19-3
Differential Diagnosis of Neonatal Cholestasis—cont'd

HEPATOCELLULAR DISEASE—cont'd

Familial with uncharacterized excretory defect
 Dubin-Johnson syndrome
 Rotor syndrome
 Byler syndrome
 Aagenaes syndrome (hereditary cholestasis with lymphedema)
 Familial benign recurrent intrahepatic cholestasis
Defective bile acid synthesis (trihydroxycoprostanic acidemia)
Defective protein synthesis
 α_1-Antitrypsin deficiency
 Cystic fibrosis
Chromosomal disorders
 Trisomy 21
 Trisomy 17-18
 Donahue leprechaunism
Infectious
 Viral
  Cytomegalovirus
  Rubella
  Herpes
  Toxoplasmosis
  Syphilis
  Hepatitis B
  Hepatitis C
  Varicella
  Coxsackievirus
  Enteric cytopathogenic human orphan (ECHO) virus
 Bacterial-sepsis, urinary tract infection, gastroenteritis, listeriosis
Iatrogenic
 Total parenteral nutrition
 Drug or toxin
Idiopathic (neonatal hepatitis)
Miscellaneous (shock or hypoperfusion)

From Haber BA, Lake AM: *Clin Perinatol* 17:483, 1990.

that mimic extrahepatic biliary atresia. It is five times more common in girls than in boys. Complete surgical excision is the treatment of choice and prevents cirrhosis, portal hypertension, and cholangiocarcinoma.

2. Intrahepatic biliary disease.
 a. Paucity of interlobular bile ducts.
  (1) Syndromic. Alagille syndrome (arteriohepatic dysplasia) consists of hypoplastic intrahepatic bile ducts, chronic cholestasis,

and extrahepatic anomalies, including characteristic facies (small, pointed chin; broad forehead; hypertelorism), vertebral defects (butterfly and hemivertebrae), cardiovascular abnormalities (peripheral pulmonary stenosis, coarctation of the aorta), growth retardation, and anomalies of the anterior chamber angle of the eye. Autosomal dominant inheritance with low penetrance is probable. Prognosis is variable but more favorable than the nonsyndromic form.

(2) Nonsyndromic. A progressive cholangiolitic insult leads to paucity of intrahepatic bile ducts; it is also seen as a late complication in infants with biliary atresia and as a feature of liver involvement in graft-versus-host disease. Congenital rubella, cytomegalovirus (CMV), hepatitis B, trisomies 18 and 21, and α_1-antitrypsin deficiency have been associated.

b. Inspissated bile. Results from bilirubin overload in 10% of newborns with hemolytic anemia resulting from Rh or ABO incompatibility, spherocytosis, and G6PD deficiency. Conjugated bilirubin is elevated in cord blood because of intrauterine hemolysis. Hepatosplenomegaly is marked; transaminase levels are normal or mildly elevated, and cholestasis lasts for 4 weeks or longer.

3. Hepatocellular disease.

a. Metabolic and genetic defects.

(1) α_1-Antitrypsin deficiency accounts for 1% to 10% of infants with cholestasis; jaundice appears at about 8 weeks of age and in 15% of cases is resolved by 7 months. Infants may have conjugated hyperbilirubinemia, jaundice, acholic stools, dark urine, and liver enlargement. After a prolonged period of apparent normal health, cirrhosis and its complications may lead to death in late childhood or early adulthood. Diagnosis is confirmed by serum α_1-antitrypsin determination and by protease inhibitor phenotyping. Liver transplantation is the only treatment.

(2) Dubin-Johnson syndrome and Rotor's syndrome are autosomal recessive conditions that cause nonhemolytic conjugated hyperbilirubinemia. Transaminase and bile acid levels are normal; prognosis is excellent.

(3) With benign recurrent intrahepatic cholestasis, infants develop intermittent jaundice, pruritus, dark urine, pale stools, and elevated alkaline phosphatase without progressive liver disease.

(4) Peroxisomal disorders. Zellweger's cerebrohepatorenal syndrome is an autosomal recessive disorder. Clinical features include cholestatic jaundice, hepatomegaly, mental retardation, hypotonia, renal cortical cysts, and abnormal facies with epicanthal folds, hypertelorism, and prominent forehead. The defect consists of absence of peroxisomes and derangement of mitochondria. Other cholestatic disorders in this category include adrenoleukodystrophy, glutaric aciduria type II, and olivocerebellar atrophy.

(5) Cystic fibrosis rarely causes conjugated hyperbilirubinemia. Meconium ileus may be seen in half of the cases. Jaundice resolves gradually, with increased risk of liver disease later in life.

(6) Galactosemia is an autosomal recessive disorder of carbohydrate metabolism resulting from deficiency of galactose-1-phosphate uridyltransferase, with an incidence of 1:100,000. Clinical features include lethargy, emesis, anorexia, growth failure, cholestasis, and lenticular cataract formation. Elimination of lactose- and galactose-containing products from the diet is prudent while erythrocyte enzyme determination is in progress. Galactosemia should be excluded in any infant with septic cholestasis.

(7) Hypopituitarism may cause cholestasis. Hypoglycemia, septo-optic dysplasia, and hypothyroidism may be associated findings.

b. Perinatal infections. Cholestasis in many intrauterine viral infections is a result of hepatic necrosis; CMV, rubella, herpes, hepatitis B, enteroviruses, coxsackievirus B, and echoviruses may produce conjugated hyperbilirubinemia. Toxoplasmosis, syphilis, and bacterial infections that cause neonatal sepsis, pyelonephritis, severe enteritis, and enterocolitis may lead to cholestasis.

c. Iatrogenic disease.

(1) Total parenteral nutrition cholestasis is seen in >50% of infants with birth weights of <1000 gm and in <10% of full-term infants. Prematurity, prolonged fasting, and metabolic alterations (e.g., hyperglycemia and abnormal amino acids) may be contributory.

(2) Cholestasis caused by a drug or hepatotoxin is a possibility. The clinical picture will resemble viral hepatitis.

d. Idiopathic neonatal hepatitis is responsible for 40% of cases of neonatal cholestasis. Prominent physical findings include icterus and hepatomegaly.

C. Clinical presentation. Jaundice, acholic stools, and dark urine are characteristic. Pruritus, lethargy, growth failure, hepatosplenomegaly, and ascites are late signs. Diagnosis includes historical and physical findings (Table 19-3).

D. Laboratory studies (Box 19-4). Evaluation of body fluids, imaging studies, and liver biopsy may be necessary.

E. Management (Box 19-5). It is difficult to provide optimal nutrition to a cholestatic infant. Provision of medium-chain triglycerides results in better caloric intake and growth. Fat-soluble vitamins A, D, E, and K should be supplemented. Ascites and liver failure are managed by low-sodium diet and diuretics (spironolactone, 0.5 to 1.0 mg/kg every 8 hours by mouth; furosemide 1.0 to 2.0 mg/kg per dose by mouth or intravenously every 8 to 12 hours). Phenobarbital (3 to 10 mg/kg per day by mouth) and cholestyramine (0.25 to 0.50 mg/kg per day by mouth) are employed to promote bile flow and excretion of bile acids and cholesterol. Liver transplant is indicated with failure to grow, evidence of liver failure, and poor quality of life.

TABLE 19-3
**Four Most Important Clinical Criteria for Differentiating
Extrahepatic From Intrahepatic Cholestasis**

Clinical data	Extrahepatic cholestasis	Intrahepatic cholestasis	Significance *(P)*
Stool color 10 days after admission			
White	79%	26%	≤0.001
Yellow	21%	74%	
Birth weight (gm)	3226 ± 45*	2678 ± 55*	≤0.001
Age at onset of acholic stools (days)	16 ± 1.5*	30 ± 2*	≤0.001
Clinical features of liver involvement			
Normal liver	1	12	
Hepatomegaly†			
With normal consistency	12	35	≤0.001
With firm consistency	63	47	
With hard consistency	24	6	

Data from Spivak W, Grand RJ: *J Pediatr Gastroenterol Nutr* 2:381, 1983, and
Haber BA, Lake AM: *Clin Perinatol* 17:483, 1990.
*Mean ± SE.
†Number of patients.

BOX 19-4
Diagnostic Evaluation

History and physical examination
Screening assessment of patient's general status and liver sufficiency
    Complete blood count, smear, reticulocyte count
    Liver enzymes (aspartate and alanine aminotransferases, alkaline phos-
        phatase, and γ-glutamyltransferase)
    Total protein and albumin
    Prothrombin and partial thromboplastin times
    Serum bile acids
    Stool pigment
Body fluid examination for etiologic identification
    Blood
        Serology (Cytomegalovirus, herpes, rubella, toxoplasmosis, rapid
           plasma reagin test)
        Hepatitis B markers (infant and mother)
        α_1-Antitrypsin level with protease inhibitor typing
        Thyroxine and thyroid-stimulating hormone
        Plasma amino acids
        Blood culture

From Haber BA, Lake AM: *Clin Perinatol* 17:483, 1990.   *Continued*

BOX 19-4
Diagnostic Evaluation—cont'd

Body fluid examination for etiologic identification–cont'd
  Urine
    Urine culture
    Urine-reducing substance
    Urine metabolic screen (amino acids)
  Sweat chloride test
  Intestine
    Stool culture
    24-hour duodenal intubation
Radiologic examination
  Ultrasound
  Radionuclide examination
  Operative cholangiogram (if operated on for extrahepatic obstruction)
Liver biopsy
  Percutaneous or operative

From Haber BA, Lake AM: *Clin Perinatol* 17:483, 1990.

BOX 19-5
Medical Management

Treat specific etiology
Nutrition
  Provide adequate calories
  Supplement diet with medium-chain triglycerides
  Supplement diet with fat-soluble vitamins A, D, E, and K
Pruritis and xanthoma
  Phenobarbital
  Cholestyramine
Ascites
  Low-sodium diet, 1-2 mEq/kg per day
  Diuretics (spironolactone preferred over furosemide unless acute diuresis is required)
Liver failure, life-threatening portal hypertension, inability to provide adequate growth and development (consider liver transplant)

From Haber BA, Lake AM: *Clin Perinatol* 17:483, 1990.

BIBLIOGRAPHY

American Academy of Pediatrics Provisional Committee for Quality Improvement and Subcommittee on Hyperbilirubinemia: Practice parameter: management of hyperbilirubinemia in the healthy term newborn, *Pediatrics* 94:561, 1994.

American Academy of Pediatrics Provisional Committee for Quality Improvement and Subcommittee on Hyperbilirubinemia: Practice parameter: management of hyperbilirubinemia in the healthy term newborn, *Pediatrics* 95:458, 1995 (erratum).

Haber BA, Lake AM: Cholestatic jaundice in the newborn, *Clin Perinatol* 17:483, 1990.

Kramer LI: Advancement of dermal icterus in the jaundiced newborn, *Am J Dis Child,* 118:454, 1969.

MacMahon JR, Stevenson DK, Oski FA: Management of neonatal hyperbilirubinemia. In Taeusch HW, Ballard RA (editors): *Avery's Diseases of the newborn,* ed 7, Philadelphia, 1998, WB Saunders.

Maisels MJ: Neonatal jaundice. In Avery GB, Fletcher MA, MacDonald MG (editors): *Neonatology: pathophysiology and management of the newborn,* ed 5, Philadelphia, 1999, Lippincott Williams & Wilkins.

Sinatra FR, Rosenthal P: Cholestasis in the neonate. In Avery GB (editor): *Neonatology: pathophysiology and management of the newborn,* ed 3, Philadelphia, 1987, JB Lippincott.

Spivak W, Grand RJ: General configuration of cholestasis in the newborn, *J Pediatr Gastroenterol Nutr* 2:381, 1983.

20

Infection

TIMOTHY TOWNSEND, JANET S. KINNEY
AND MARK C. STEINHOFF

I. INTRODUCTION TO NEONATAL INFECTIONS
A. Bacterial and viral infections are important causes of neonatal morbidity and mortality.
1. Infections with varying outcomes may be caused by pathogenic bacteria or viruses acquired at different times during intrauterine and neonatal life. No agent, no matter how obscure, should be ignored as a possibility when initial probabilities do not seem to be likely.
2. Infection can occur in utero (congenital infection), at the time of delivery (natal infection), and after birth but within the neonatal period (postnatal infection).

B. The choice of antibiotics.
1. Universal coverage is a myth that needs to be dispelled. It is a false concept providing a false comfort, and it must not be substituted for careful observation and careful interpretation of data.
2. Initial coverage, however, is often a must. Start with the following:
   a. Coverage for those organisms that are most likely in the circumstance.
   b. Coverage for those organisms that are likely to pose the greatest threat if not treated.
3. Follow-up coverage is altered as more is learned clinically and in the laboratory.

II. BACTERIAL INFECTION AND SEPSIS
A. General.
1. Invasive bacterial infections primarily involve the bloodstream during the first month of life; meningitis is present in approximately 25% of bacteremic newborns.
2. The occurrence rate is 2 to 3:1000 live births, with a range of 1 to 10:1000 live births.
3. Sepsis is a low-incidence but high-risk problem. Accurate diagnosis is difficult because there is no definitive early diagnostic test. There-

fore a large number of newborns who do not have the disease will of necessity be evaluated and treated for sepsis.

B. Etiology.

1. Group B β-hemolytic streptococcus (especially, for late-onset disease, type III) and *Escherichia coli* (K1 strains) currently account for 60% to 70% of all postnatal infections in most locations in the United States.
2. Other common pathogens include *Staphylococcus aureus, Klebsiella, Enterobacter, Serratia, Citrobacter, Pseudomonas* species, *Staphylococcus epidermidis,* α-hemolytic streptococcus, group D streptococcus (non-*Enterococcus*), *Listeria monocytogenes,* and *Enterococcus.*
3. *Streptococcus pneumoniae, Neisseria meningitidis, Haemophilus influenzae,* and groups A, C, and G streptococci are found, but much less frequently than after the postnatal period.

C. Pathogenesis.

1. Maternal risk factors.
   a. Prolonged rupture of membranes (PROM) (>24 hours) is associated with a 1% incidence of sepsis.
   b. Chorioamnionitis.
      (1) Suggested by the presence of maternal temperature >100.4° F, uterine tenderness, purulent or foul-smelling amniotic fluid, or fetal tachycardia.

N.B.: Epidural analgesia for labor has been associated with a fifteen-fold increase in the incidence of intrapartum maternal fever.

       (2) With chorioamnionitis and PROM, the risk of sepsis increases to 3% to 5%.
   c. Colonization with group B streptococcus.
      (1) Group B streptococcus is isolated from the genitourinary or gastrointestinal tract of 10% to 30% of pregnant women; colonization is persistent throughout pregnancy in 60% to 70% of these women; 40% to 70% of infants of colonized mothers become colonized, and invasive disease develops in 1 of every 50 to 75 of these infants.
      (2) Infant colonization is the result of the following:
         (a) Transplacental transmission in the presence of maternal bacteremia.
         (b) Ascending transmission through leaks in the amniotic membranes or frankly ruptured membranes.
         (c) Surface contamination during passage through the birth canal.
         (d) Intrapartum distress (meconium staining, 5-minute Apgar score <6) with aspiration of infected amniotic fluid.
2. Infant risk factors.
   a. Prematurity. With PROM, gestational age <37 weeks increases the risk of sepsis tenfold.
   b. Depressed immune function in the newborn infant.
      (1) Decreased concentration of antibody to specific organisms (e.g., group B streptococcus).
      (2) Impaired neutrophil function.

        (3) Deficiency of complement, especially in low-birth-weight infants.

        (4) Delayed clearance of organisms from the bloodstream.

        (5) Decreased secretory immunity.

        (6) Impaired ability to respond to capsular polysaccharide.

    c. Gender. Males are two to six times more likely than females to develop sepsis.

N.B.: It is important to note that the preceding risk factors are additive; the presence of two or three of these factors can increase the risk of neonatal sepsis up to 25 to 30 times. It is also appropriate to note that requiring personnel in the nursery to wear gowns is generally unnecessary and offers no benefit in preventing neonatal colonization.

D. Clinical features.

1. The signs and symptoms of neonatal sepsis may be subtle and non-specific. They include respiratory distress, high-pitched cry, lethargy, temperature instability (hypothermia or hyperthermia), hypotonia, vomiting, jaundice, diarrhea, abdominal distention, poor feeding, apnea, cyanotic spells, seizures, poor perfusion, petechiae, and purpura. Although any organ may be involved as part of neonatal sepsis, pneumonia and meningitis are most common. Notably, indirect hyperbilirubinemia (jaundice) in an otherwise well infant should *not* be considered an indicator of bacteremia or incipient sepsis if it is the only manifestation of the problem. Exceptions might be made in the event of late-onset jaundice or total bilirubin with >20% conjugated.

2. Fever.

    a. Ten percent of full-term newborns with a temperature >37.8° C not related to environmental causes have bacterial sepsis. Among afebrile newborns, the incidence of bacterial disease is 1:10,000.

    b. Risk of bacterial infection increases with height of fever; temperature >39° C is associated with a high incidence of infection.

    c. Fever in the first hour of life is usually related to maternal fever.

    d. Newborns with fever and bacterial disease usually, *but not always,* have other symptoms suggestive of infection.

    e. Newborns should be evaluated for infection if they have fever that persists or recurs or a single episode of fever plus any other sign or symptom consistent with infection.

3. Group B streptococcal infection (GBS).

    a. Early-onset disease. Onset occurs from birth to 7 days (accounts for 80% of GBS infections of infants). All serotypes (Ia, Ib/c, Ia/c, II, III, IV, and V) are associated with infections in infants.

        (1) Risk factors include maternal colonization with group B streptococcus, bacteriuria, intrapartum fetal distress, low birth weight, prematurity, and PROM. Risk is increased with "heavy" neonatal colonization, multiple-gestation pregnancy, and history of group B streptococcal infection in a previous sibling. Recent recommendations from the Centers for Disease Control and Prevention (CDC) advocate treatment with intrapartum penicillin if the mother is colonized (determined

through rectoanal and vaginal cultures at 35 to 37 weeks gestation using selective broth media) with group B streptococcus. An alternative strategy is to not culture but to give intrapartum penicillin only to those women with the following risk factors:

(a) Onset of labor or rupture of membranes at less than 37 weeks gestation.

(b) Membranes ruptured 18 or more hours.

(c) Fever (temperature >38° C) during labor.

N.B. This strategy will miss the 25% of early-onset cases born to colonized mothers with no risk factors. All women with GBS bacteriuria during pregnancy and any woman who has delivered an infant who developed GBS disease should have intrapartum penicillin.

(2) GBS may cause pneumonia with or without bacteremia or bacteremia with or without meningitis; there is usually a sudden onset with fulminant course.

(3) Clinical features include tachypnea, bradycardia, shock, cyanosis, apnea, pneumonia, and persistent pulmonary hypertension.

(4) Laboratory findings include hypoxemia, metabolic acidosis, leukopenia, thrombocytopenia, and hypoglycemia.

(5) The course is rapidly progressive; the fatality rate is 5% to 15%.

b. Late-onset disease. Onset occurs from 7 days to 8 to 12 weeks (accounts for 20% of GBS infections of infants).

(1) Not usually associated with the risk factors noted with early-onset disease; almost always serotype III.

(2) May cause meningitis or osteomyelitis with or without bacteremia; other sites of infection include omphalitis, septic arthritis, lymphadenitis, soft-tissue infection, breast abscess, otitis media, endocarditis, and pericarditis.

(3) There is usually an insidious onset with nonspecific signs. Clinical features include signs and symptoms of meningitis or osteomyelitis (especially the right humerus). The fatality rate is 5% to 10%.

4. *L. monocytogenes.*

a. *L. monocytogenes* can cause a flulike illness in the mother just before delivery; maternal blood culture may be positive.

b. The lung is the primary focus of early infection, but infection can also result in hepatosplenomegaly, purulent conjunctivitis, skin rash, and small granulomas on the posterior pharynx. Meningitis is present in 96% of late-onset cases.

c. Fatality rate is 40% to 80%.

E. Differential diagnosis of neonatal sepsis.

1. Metabolic disturbances.

a. Inborn errors of metabolism (e.g., urea cycle defect).

b. Hypoglycemia.

c. Electrolyte imbalance.

2. Maternal drug abuse.

3. Hemolytic disease of the newborn.
4. Congenital heart disease (e.g., hypoplastic left heart syndrome).
5. Other infections.
   a. Congenital and natally acquired infection (e.g., syphilis, herpes simplex virus [HSV], cytomegalovirus [CMV], rubella, toxoplasmosis, tuberculosis, and enterovirus).
   b. Disseminated fungal infection.

F. Laboratory findings.
1. Specific diagnostic tests.
   a. Isolation of bacteria from blood or cerebrospinal fluid (CSF) is the standard method to diagnose neonatal sepsis. However, the rate of proven plus highly suspected infection is undoubtedly greater than the culture-proven rate.
   b. Blood culture.
      (1) Blood may be obtained by venipuncture or from a fresh umbilical artery catheter; samples of cord blood or those from an indwelling umbilical venous catheter or any type of intravascular catheter may be unreliable because of high rates of contamination.
      (2) The optimum amount of blood for culture is unclear; 1 ml is recommended, although lesser amounts may be adequate for high-grade bacteremia.
      (3) Among patients with bacteremia and without antibiotic pretreatment, the vast majority of blood cultures are positive by 48 hours. Late-growing bacteria are usually anaerobes or coagulase-negative staphylococcus or occur in newborns with antibiotic pretreatment.
   c. Cerebrospinal fluid culture.
      (1) Lumbar puncture (LP) is not usually indicated in the evaluation of the full-term newborn who is considered at risk of sepsis based on maternal or obstetric factors.
      (2) In infants who *develop* signs and symptoms suggestive of infection, LP is always indicated. Up to 15% of newborns with positive CSF cultures have a negative blood culture.
      (3) In interpreting CSF results, it is important to note that the CSF has a normal upper limit of 25 cells/mm^3 in the full-term newborn; however, meningitis may occur with lower cell counts. CSF glucose and protein concentrations may be difficult to interpret because of the wide range of normal values.
   d. Urine culture.
      (1) May be useful in the infant with evidence of late-onset or nosocomial infection. Usually not helpful in early-onset sepsis.
      (2) Bagged specimens are unreliable; urine should be obtained by suprapubic bladder tap or, in girls, by straight in-and-out catheterization.
   e. Tracheal aspirate.
      (1) Culture obtained at the time of intubation is useful in the newborn with suspected pneumonia.

(2) A positive culture is found in half of infants who have pneumonia and a negative blood culture.

f. Detection of bacterial antigen.

(1) The latex-particle agglutination test may be carried out in the evaluation of group B streptococcal infection.

(2) May be applied to serum, CSF, or *concentrated* urine (obtained by suprapubic tap or in-and-out catheterization).

(3) Sensitivity is >90%.

(4) Urine specificity is 81% to 99%; may be related to skin or urine contamination with group B streptococci or cross reaction with other bacterial species.

N.B.: A negative result *does not* rule out the possibility of systemic group B streptococcal infection.

2. Nonspecific diagnostic tests.

a. White blood cell (WBC) and differential counts.

(1) The establishment of normal reference values (see Appendix C) has increased the utility of these tests. Note that WBC counts can be higher in capillary than in arterial or venous samples.

(2) Of the nonspecific tests, neutropenia is the best predictor of sepsis; neutropenia in a newborn with fever is highly suggestive of bacterial disease. Maternal hypertension, perinatal asphyxia, and intraventricular hemorrhage may also cause significant neutropenia.

(3) Neutrophilia does not correlate well with neonatal sepsis; it may occur secondary to intrapartum maternal fever, stressful labor, or hemolytic disease of the newborn.

(4) A ratio of immature to total neutrophils (I:T ratio) >0.20 is predictive of neonatal bacterial disease but can also be related to maternal fever and stressful labor.

(5) Neutrophil vacuolization and toxic granulations are also suggestive of bacterial infection.

N.B.: If the total neutrophil count, immature neutrophil count, and I:T ratio are normal, there is a 95% to 100% negative predictive value for sepsis.

b. C-reactive protein (CRP).

(1) CRP is an acute-phase globulin synthesized by the liver within 6 to 8 hours of an inflammatory stimulus; normal value is <1.6 mg/dl on days 1 to 2 and <1.0 mg/dl thereafter.

(2) Sensitivity and specificity are not high enough for the CRP to be used alone as a definitive diagnostic test.

(3) Failure to mount a CRP response may be a poor prognostic sign. Normalization of a CRP elevation may be helpful in determining response to antimicrobial therapy and duration of treatment.

c. Erythrocyte sedimentation rate (ESR).

(1) ESR rate has been used as part of neonatal "sepsis screens."

(2) Normal value is equal to the day of life plus 3 mm/hr up to a maximum of 15 mm/hr.

(3) A false-positive result can occur with hemolysis; a false-negative result may be caused by disseminated intravascular coagulation (DIC).

d. Surface cultures (gastric aspirate). Gram's stain/culture of surface sites are *not* useful indicators of neonatal bacterial infections; they do not distinguish the infected from the colonized infant.

e. Miscellaneous tests. A number of indirect tests, including serum IgM, leukocyte alkaline phosphatase, fibronectin, haptoglobin, and elastase α-proteinase inhibitor levels, and the limulus lysate test for endotoxin detection have been used. They are unreliable when used individually but may be helpful when used in various combinations as part of a sepsis screen. In an individual case, examination of the buffy coat smear by direct staining can be a valuable aid in the early diagnosis of sepsis.

N.B.: No single test or combination of tests has proven superior to the WBC count and differential as an indirect indicator of bacterial infection. No laboratory test result should ever negate a clinical impression of sepsis.

G. Management.

1. The spectrum and severity of symptoms required to prompt a sepsis workup is a matter of clinical judgment and cannot be dictated by protocol. The practitioner must rely on careful maternal and newborn history, physical examination, and laboratory findings. The goal is to identify and treat all infected infants but to avoid excessive investigation and treatment of noninfected infants. If the mother received intrapartum antibiotics for group B *Streptococcus* prophylaxis, clinical management of the infant may be complicated. Clinical judgment is crucial. Institution of intrapartum antibiotics as early as possible after membrane rupture may limit the risk of early-onset group B streptococcal sepsis for the infant.

2. Asymptomatic infant. The decision to treat is based on the perceived level of risk and must be considered independently for each case (Fig. 20-1).

3. Symptomatic infant. Clinical judgment is crucial. The burden of proof is on the practitioner to prove that there is no infection, not on the baby to prove that he or she is infected. Absence of risk factors should never dissuade one from treating a symptomatic neonate (Fig. 20-2).

N.B.: In the asymptomatic premature infant, treatment should be initiated with only a single obstetric or clinical risk factor.

4. Antibiotic therapy.

a. The usual approach is to start with parenteral ampicillin (100 mg/kg per day in two divided doses daily) and gentamicin. (See appendix H for dosage.) The dosing interval of gentamicin should be adjusted according to postconceptional age.

b. It is important to monitor the serum gentamicin levels; trough level should be <2 μg/ml, and peak level should be 5 to 10 μg/ml.

c. Subsequent therapy is guided by culture and sensitivity results.

(1) Group B streptococcus: penicillin alone (preferably) and, at times, gentamicin.

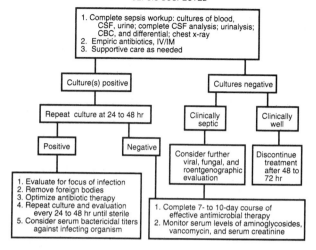

FIG. 20-1. Recommended approach to the diagnostic evaluation and treatment of the neonate with suspected sepsis. (From Siegel JD: Sepsis neonatorum. In Oski FA (editor): *Principles and practice of pediatrics,* Philadelphia, 1994, JB Lippincott.)

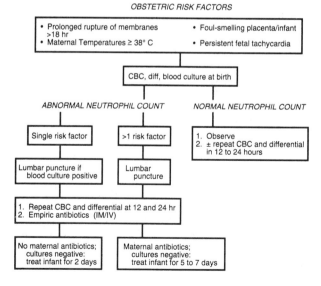

FIG. 20-2. Recommended approach to the diagnostic evaluation and treatment of the asymptomatic term infant with history of obstetric risk factors. (Modified from Siegel JD: Sepsis neonatorum. In Oski FA (editor): *Principles and practice of pediatrics,* Philadelphia, 1994, JB Lippincott.)

(2) *L. monocytogenes:* ampicillin.

(3) *S. aureus:* nafcillin or methicillin (vancomycin if methicillin resistant).

(4) *S. epidermidis:* vancomycin (need to monitor serum levels; trough level should be <10 μg/ml, peak 20 to 30 μg/ml); switch to nafcillin for susceptible organisms.

(5) *Enterobacter, E. coli:* ampicillin plus aminoglycoside (tobramycin, gentamicin); should be guided by susceptibility pattern in individual hospital.

(6) *Pseudomonas* species: aminoglycoside plus ticarcillin or ceftazidime.

(7) *Enterococcus:* ampicillin plus aminoglycoside.

d. Miscellaneous.

(1) Appropriate cultures should be repeated after 24 to 48 hours to document sterile cultures. The usual duration of treatment is 7 to 10 days (with appropriate clinical response), but longer courses are required for meningitis, osteomyelitis, endocarditis, and septic arthritis.

(2) Sulfonamides and ceftriaxone displace bilirubin from albumin and should be avoided.

(3) Chloramphenicol is no longer recommended for treatment of neonatal infection.

(4) Third-generation cephalosporins are inactive against *Enterococcus, L. monocytogenes,* and many staphylococci.

5. Other therapy. Granulocyte transfusions and intravenous immunoglobulin have been used in neonatal sepsis but are not recommended for routine use.

6. Prognosis.

a. Depends on etiologic agent, timing of diagnosis and therapy, complications, and host factors.

b. The fatality rate is 10% to 15%, with substantial morbidity in surviving infants.

III. TORCH

A. Definition. Acronym used to focus on similarities in clinical presentation of intrauterine infections caused by toxoplasmosis (T), other (O), rubella (R), cytomegalovirus (C), and herpes simplex virus (H). Congenital syphilis has been included by some, making the acronym TORCHES.

B. Clinical features associated with TORCH agents (Box 20-1).

1. Infections in newborns share common clinical findings and are clinically indistinguishable from each other.

2. Infected infants may be asymptomatic in the newborn period, yet later develop disabling long-term sequelae.

3. Maternal infections are usually asymptomatic.

4. Diagnosis in the mother and newborn may require special laboratory tests.

C. Diagnostic evaluation. A single TORCH titer is not a complete laboratory evaluation because there are many other agents that cause perinatal infections. The algorithm in Fig. 20-3 gives an ap-

---

BOX 20-1

Common Clinical Features Associated With TORCH Agents in Neonates

---

Growth retardation
Hepatosplenomegaly
Jaundice
Hemolytic anemia
Petechiae, ecchymoses
Microcephaly, hydrocephalus
Intracranial calcification
Nonimmune hydrops
Pneumonitis
Myocarditis
Cardiac abnormalities
Chorioretinitis
Keratoconjunctivitis
Cataracts
Glaucoma

From Steinhoff MC, Kinney JS: Neonatal sepsis and infections. In Reese RE, Betts RF (editors): *A practical approach to infectious diseases,* ed 3, Boston, 1991, Little, Brown.

proach to the laboratory investigation of infants with suspected intrauterine infection.

1. The diagnosis of perinatal infection requires a synthesis of data obtained from the maternal history, the infant's physical examination, laboratory tests, and radiographic findings.
2. Despite detailed evaluation, a definite diagnosis cannot be made immediately because of the problem of passively transferred maternal IgG antibody and the technical difficulties of organism-specific IgM antibody tests.

N.B.: Be reminded that the acronym TORCHES does not go far enough. Among the perinatal infections that must often be considered and that it does not include are coxsackievirus, enterovirus, hepatitis B and C, human immunodeficiency virus (HIV), *Listeria,* parvovirus, and varicella.

IV. VIRAL INFECTION
A. Herpes simplex virus (HSV).

1. The causative agent for HSV is a DNA virus in the herpesvirus family with two antigenically and genomically distinct types.
   a. Type 1 (HSV-1) usually involves the face and skin above the waist.
   b. Type 2 (HSV-2) involves the genitalia and skin below the waist.
   c. However, either type of virus can be found in either site.
2. Epidemiology. The incidence of neonatal HSV infection is low; the estimated rate is approximately 1:3000 to 1:20,000 live births. The seroprevalence of HSV-2 increased 30% from 1976-1980 to 1988-

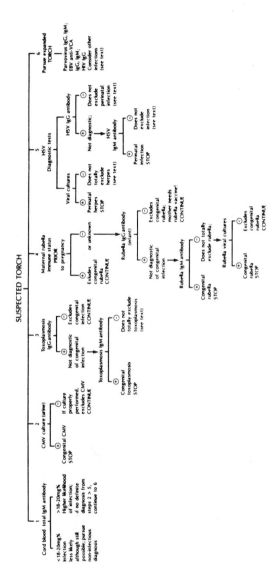

FIG. 20-3. An approach to the laboratory diagnosis of suspected TORCH infection in the neonate. *EBV,* Epstein-Barr virus; *HIV,* human immunodeficiency virus; *HSV,* herpes simplex virus; *VCA,* viral capsid antigen. (From Kinney JS, Kumar ML: *Clin Perinatol* 15:727, 1988.)

1994 and now 1 in 5 persons over the age of 12 has serologic evidence of having been infected with HSV-2.

  a. Risk of neonatal HSV infection is highest (40% to 50%) in infants born vaginally to mothers with primary genital infection as opposed to mothers with recurrent genital infection (at most 3% to 5%).

  b. Most infants with HSV infection have been born to women without history or clinical findings of active herpetic infection during pregnancy.

3. Transmission occurs in utero, intrapartum, or postnatally.

  a. In utero infection is rare.

  b. Intrapartum transmission is the most common (approximately 85% to 90% of cases) and occurs as the infant passes through the infected maternal genital tract or by ascending infection.

   (1) The incubation period is variable. Symptoms usually appear at the end of the first week of life but can appear shortly after birth or as late as 4 to 6 weeks.

   (2) HSV-2 accounts for most neonatal infections; however, 15% to 20% are caused by HSV-1.

  c. Postnatal transmission (less common) occurs from parents, hospital personnel, or an infected infant in the nursery.

4. Clinical findings. Infants with HSV infection acquired intrapartum or postnatally can be divided into three categories.

  a. Disease localized to skin, eye, or mouth, which has the lowest mortality rate.

  b. Encephalitis, with or without skin, eye, or mouth involvement.

  c. Disseminated infection with multiple organ system involvement (e.g., central nervous system (CNS), lung, liver, adrenals, skin, eye, or mouth), which has the highest mortality and morbidity.

N.B.: In utero infection results in the most severely afflicted infants; most common findings at birth: skin vesicles or skin scarring, eye disease (chorioretinitis and keratoconjunctivitis), microcephaly, or hydranencephaly.

5. Outcome.

  a. Long-term prognosis after disseminated infection or encephalitis is poor. Approximately 50% of surviving children have varying degrees of psychomotor retardation, microcephaly, hydranencephaly, porencephalic cysts, spasticity, blindness, chorioretinitis, or learning disabilities.

  b. Disease localized to skin, eye, or mouth is associated with multiple recurrences during the first 6 months of life. Approximately 10% develop evidence of neurologic impairment (spastic quadriplegia, microcephaly, and blindness), which may not be apparent until 6 months to 1 year of life.

6. Diagnostic evaluation (Fig. 20-3).

  a. Virus isolation is the definitive method.

   (1) Obtain cultures from skin vesicles, mouth or nasopharynx, eyes, urine, and blood.

   (2) Polymerase chain reaction (PCR) is the definitive method for CSF and vitreous humor.

b. Serologic methods are not helpful because of the following:
   (1) Commonly available assays cannot distinguish between antibodies to HSV-1 and HSV-2.
   (2) The presence of passively acquired maternal IgG antibody.

7. Treatment. Acyclovir and vidarabine are both effective; however, acyclovir is preferred.
   a. The recommended dose of acyclovir is 30 mg/kg per 24 hours in three divided intravenous doses. Some experts give high doses (45 to 60 mg/kg per day).
   b. Duration of therapy has not been established; recommended minimum is 14 days.
   c. Relapse of disease after therapy can occur.
   d. Treat ocular infection with a topical ophthalmic drug (1% to 2% trifluridine, 1% iododeoxyuridine, or 3% vidarabine) in addition to parenteral antiviral therapy. Ophthalmologic consultation is advised.
   e. The effectiveness of prophylactic antiviral therapy for exposed infants has not been determined.

8. Prevention. Management of a pregnant mother with a history of herpes is in the province of obstetric professionals.
   a. Contact isolation is required for infants while in the nursery.
   b. It is preferable to have the infant room in with its mother until discharge.

B. Hepatitis B virus (HBV).

1. Epidemiology. Mothers who are HBsAg-positive or HBeAg-positive have an 80% likelihood of transmitting the virus to their infants.
   a. Most infants will be asymptomatic, but 90% will become chronic HBV carriers if not given appropriate immunoprophylaxis.
   b. Some groups of women are at particular risk for HBV infection (Box 20-2).

2. Transmission. Transplacental transmission is rare; HBV is usually transmitted during or shortly after delivery. Risk of transmission is greater if maternal infection is symptomatic or occurs late in pregnancy.

3. Clinical findings. The majority of infants are asymptomatic.
   a. A small percentage (1% to 3%) are symptomatic, with jaundice and elevated liver function studies.
   b. HBsAg carriers have an increased risk of developing hepatocellular carcinoma in later years.

4. Diagnosis. All pregnant women should be tested for HBsAg early in pregnancy. A positive HBsAg test result indicates current infection or the presence of a carrier state.
   a. Mothers who have not received prenatal care should be tested at the time of delivery.
   b. If the mother has not been tested and is not available for testing, it is essential that the infant be tested and treated appropriately.

5. Management of the infant born to an HBsAg-positive mother includes immunoprophylaxis with HBV vaccine and HB immune globulin (HBIG).

BOX 20-2

United States Public Health Service's Current Recommendations for Perinatal Screening for Hepatitis B Surface Antigen

---

1. Women of Asian, Pacific Island, or Alaskan Eskimo descent, whether immigrant or U.S.-born
2. Women born in Haiti or sub-Saharan Africa
3. Women with histories of the following:
   a. Acute or chronic liver disease
   b. Work or treatment in a hemodialysis unit
   c. Work or residence in an institution for the mentally retarded
   d. Rejection as a blood donor
   e. Blood transfusion on repeated occasions
   f. Frequent occupational exposure to blood in medical and dental settings
   g. Household contact with a carrier of hepatitis B virus or hemodialysis patient
   h. Multiple episodes of venereal diseases
   i. Percutaneous use of illicit drugs
   j. Prostitution
   k. Sexual partner of the above groups

From Centers for Disease Control and Prevention: *MMWR* 34:313, 1985.

---

   a. HBIG, 0.5 ml intramuscularly, should be given as soon as possible, preferably within 12 hours.
   b. If the infant is born to a high-risk mother whose HBsAg status is unknown, HBIG and vaccine should be given.
   c. Administration of HBIG and HBV vaccine to an at-risk newborn is 90% effective in reducing the probability of chronic infection.
   d. Regardless of maternal status, HBV vaccination should be initiated within 7 days of birth, preferably within 12 hours. Second and third doses are given 1 and 6 months after the first.
      (1) The dose is 0.5 ml intramuscularly for each vaccine product.
      (2) Infants should be tested at 9 months or later for HBsAg and anti-HBsAg. Immunoprophylaxis is not effective in 1% to 2% of cases.
   e. Infants should be bathed immediately to remove maternal blood and secretions from delivery. Universal precautions should be practiced. Mother and infant may room in.
   f. There are no contraindications to breast-feeding for infants who have received immunoprophylaxis of the infant.
6. Preventive measures include prenatal screening of the mother and immunoprophylaxis of the infant.

C. Hepatitis C virus (HCV).

1. HCV is the most common form of non-A, non-B posttransfusion hepatitis; it is also a cause of sporadic non-A, non-B hepatitis.

2. This is an RNA virus in which infection is characterized by persistent viremia.
3. Perinatal and sexual transmission are uncommon; most cases of vertical transmission involve high-risk mothers (intravenous drug abuse, sexually transmitted diseases [STDs], co-infection with HIV, and transfusion recipient). The risk of perinatal transmission is correlated with maternal serum titer of HCV RNA and HIV co-infection.
4. Diagnostic laboratory tests.
   a. Anti-HCV enzyme-linked immunosorbent assay (ELISA) and recombinant immunoblot assay (RIBA). IgG may be positive up to 18 months of age because of passive acquired maternal antibody.
   b. HCV polymerase chain reaction (PCR) is most sensitive but not readily available and is not standardized.
5. Treatment and recommendations.
   a. No immunoprophylaxis is available for the prevention of perinatal disease.
   b. At this time, breast-feeding is not contraindicated.

D. Cytomegalovirus (CMV).
1. Causative agent. Human CMV is a DNA virus that belongs to the herpes virus group.
2. Epidemiology. CMV is ubiquitous and transmitted both horizontally (direct contact with virus-containing secretions, WBCs, or tissues) and vertically. Virus persists in latent form after primary infection, and reactivation can occur.
   a. Three routes of vertical transmission.
      (1) Transplacental passage of maternal blood-borne virus.
      (2) At birth when descending through an infected maternal genital tract.
      (3) Postnatally by ingestion of CMV-positive breast milk.
   b. Latent CMV may be carried in the WBCs and tissues of asymptomatic seropositive persons; thus recipients of seropositive blood, especially the premature infant, are at risk.
3. Epidemiology of congenital CMV. Congenital CMV is the most common intrauterine infection (0.4% to 2.4% of all live births).
   a. In the United States, 10% to 65% of childbearing-age women (depending on race and socioeconomic status) are seronegative and susceptible to primary CMV infection.
      (1) The rate of seroconversion during pregnancy is estimated to be between 1% and 2%.
      (2) Approximately 40% to 50% of pregnant women who develop primary CMV infection transmit the infection to the fetus.
   b. Intrauterine infection can occur regardless of whether the mother had primary infection or reactivation during pregnancy; however, infants infected in utero during maternal reactivation are much less affected than those exposed to maternal primary infection.
4. Clinical findings. About 95% of infected infants are asymptomatic at birth.

    a. Between 10% and 20% develop mental retardation or sensorineural deafness (which is sometimes progressive).

    b. Cytomegalic inclusion disease (CID), the most severe form, occurs in about 5% of infants infected in utero. Frequent findings include hepatosplenomegaly, jaundice, petechial rash/purpura, chorioretinitis, cerebral calcification, microcephaly, and sensorineural hearing loss.

    c. In preterm infants, infection resulting from transfusion with CMV-seropositive blood has been associated with interstitial pneumonia.

    d. Infection from the mother's virus-positive breast milk does not cause clinical disease, most likely because of the presence of passively transmitted maternal antibody; however, symptomatic disease can occur if a seronegative infant is fed CMV-positive milk from milk banks.

5. Diagnostic tests (see Fig. 20-3).

    a. CMV can be isolated from urine, the pharynx, peripheral blood leukocytes, human milk, semen, cervical secretions, and other tissue and body fluids.

    b. Proof of congenital infection requires positive viral cultures or a strongly positive CMV-IgM titer within 3 weeks of birth.

    c. An abnormal CT of the head in the newborn period is highly predictive of an adverse neurodevelopmental outcome in symptomatic CMV-infected neonates.

6. Treatment is supportive.

7. Prevention. No special precautions are recommended. Thorough hand washing after exposure to secretions is important.

    a. Because approximately 1% of infants in newborn nurseries may excrete CMV and be asymptomatic, thorough hand washing should be practiced by all those in contact with infants.

    b. Transmission of CMV to preterm infants via transfusion can be eliminated by the use of CMV-seronegative donors, by removal of the buffy coat, by freezing blood in glycerol before administration, or by filtration to remove the WBCs.

E. Congenital rubella.

1. Causative agent. An RNA virus classified as a rubivirus in the Togaviridae family.

2. Epidemiology. Humans are the source of infection. Postnatal rubella is transmitted via direct or droplet contact of respiratory secretions. The virus can be transmitted from secretions of a child with congenital rubella. Asymptomatic infection can occur. The occurrence of congenital rubella has sharply decreased as a result of routine vaccination in this country.

3. Transmission. Congenital rubella is transmitted in utero during the course of primary maternal infection; fetal infection early in pregnancy may result in teratogenesis or abortion. The risk of fetal infection and congenital anomalies decreases with increasing gestational age.

4. Clinical findings. The majority (approximately 68%) of neonatal infections are subclinical. Clinical findings are similar to those seen with other TORCH infections (see Box 20-1).

a. The most common abnormalities are growth retardation, cataracts, microphthalmia, glaucoma, chorioretinitis, patent ductus arteriosus, peripheral pulmonary artery stenosis, atrial or ventricular septal defects, microcephaly, mental retardation, and sensorineural deafness.

b. Infants classically have a "blueberry muffin" rash with thrombocytopenic purpura, jaundice, and hepatosplenomegaly.

5. Diagnosis (see Fig. 20-3).

a. Knowledge of maternal rubella immune status at onset of pregnancy or previous pregnancies is the most helpful laboratory information. A positive maternal rubella test obtained late in pregnancy does not exclude rubella early in pregnancy.

b. Virus can be isolated from throat, urine, and CSF. Infected infants shed virus in nasopharyngeal secretions and urine for years.

6. Management is supportive. Contact isolation is required for infants with congenital rubella or suspected infection.

7. Prevention. Routine prenatal or antepartum screening for rubella should be done.

a. Vaccine should be administered to susceptible women in the immediate postpartum period.

b. Breast-feeding is not contraindicated.

F. Varicella-zoster (VZ) virus.

1. Causative agent. VZ is caused by the herpesvirus that causes chickenpox during primary infection and herpes zoster when reactivated.

a. VZ spreads by direct contact or by airborne droplet.

b. The incubation period is 14 to 16 days.

2. Clinical syndrome.

a. Maternal infection.

(1) Infection with VZ during early pregnancy is uncommon (<5:10,000 pregnancies) and is associated with a risk of embryopathy of about 2%, including hypoplastic extremities and digits, skin scarring, muscle atrophy, chorioretinitis, and cortical atrophy.

(2) Maternal infection after the first trimester of pregnancy is associated with a lower risk to the fetus.

b. Peripartum infection.

(1) Infants born to mothers with varicella onset within 5 days before or 2 days after delivery are exposed to the virus in the absence of maternal antibody.

(2) Half of these infants develop varicella, with an increased risk of severe disease.

(3) Fatality rate of neonatal varicella may be 5%.

(4) Full-term newborn infants whose mothers develop varicella >5 days before or >2 days after delivery are not at increased risk of severe disease.

3. Diagnosis.
   a. VZ infection must be suspected when there is a generalized vesicular rash, especially if there is a history of exposure to chickenpox or zoster.
   b. A Tzanck smear of the vesicles may show giant cells with intranuclear inclusion bodies.
   c. Viral cultures are usually positive within 3 to 4 days.
4. Treatment.
   a. Varicella-zoster immune globulin (VZIG) (125 units) should be given intramuscularly immediately after birth to newborns of mothers with varicella onset within 5 days before to 2 days after delivery.
   b. Premature infants (<28 weeks) who are exposed to VZ virus should receive VZIG regardless of maternal history because they may not have received maternal antibody transplacentally.
   c. Acyclovir will reduce the severity of varicella and should be administered at 30 mg/kg per 24 hours in three equal doses for 7 days.
5. Prevention.
   a. Infants with varicella-induced fetal malformations do not require isolation.
   b. Infants exposed to maternal varicella should be isolated at birth and, if still hospitalized, until 21 or 28 days of age, depending on whether they received VZIG. Infants with acute varicella should be isolated for the duration of the vesicular rash.
   c. A varicella vaccine has been licensed for routine use.

G. Human immunodeficiency virus (HIV).

1. Causative agent.
   a. HIV infects many cells, including T-helper lymphocytes, and is the cause of acquired immunodeficiency syndrome (AIDS).
   b. HIV is an RNA retrovirus that is transmitted from mother to infant transplacentally and also during birth and through breast milk.
   c. The risk of perinatal infection of a child of an HIV-infected woman, in the absence of antiviral therapy, is estimated at 15% to 40%. With antenatal, perinatal, and postnatal antiviral therapy, the risk of transmission is 8%.
   d. The risk of transmission is increased with advanced maternal AIDS, higher viral loads, low CD4 counts, and maternal vitamin A deficiency.
   e. The incubation period of perinatally acquired AIDS is usually <2 years, but some infected infants do not manifest symptoms until age 5 or older.
2. Clinical syndrome. 10% to 15% of infants born to HIV-positive mothers demonstrate AIDS in early infancy with the following nonspecific signs:
   a. Low birth weight, failure to thrive.
   b. Hepatosplenomegaly, lymphadenopathy.

    c. Candidiasis.

    d. Chronic diarrhea.

    e. Persistent fever.

    f. *Pneumocystis carinii* pneumonia (PCP).

    g. Recurrent bacterial and viral infections.

3. Approximately 15% to 20% of infants born to HIV-positive mothers manifest illness later, typically with the following:

    a. Failure to thrive.

    b. Lymphoid interstitial pneumonia.

    c. Hepatosplenomegaly.

    d. CNS abnormalities.

4. Diagnosis.

    a. Diagnosis, although problematic, is necessary to identify the HIV-infected infant for observation, prophylaxis, and treatment.

    b. All infants born to HIV-infected mothers acquire maternal IgG anti-HIV antibodies. Thus serology is not useful in determination of the infant's status until about 18 months of age.

    c. Advances in laboratory techniques for viral detection have made earlier diagnosis of the HIV-infected infant possible.

        (1) The sensitivity of HIV viral culture or HIV PCR among infants is 60% during the first week of life but increases to >90% by 3 months and to nearly 100% by 6 months.

        (2) The standard p24 antigen-capture assay and the immune-complex dissociated, p24 antigen-capture assay are highly specific, but the sensitivity is low; therefore use of these assays alone is not currently recommended to exclude HIV infection.

        (3) The preferred method of diagnosing HIV infection in infants is the use of HIV culture or PCR.

5. Prenatal management of HIV-infected mothers and their HIV-exposed infants. The AIDS Clinical Trials Group Protocol 076 ZDV regimen (Box 20-3) reduces perinatal HIV transmission. Trials using protease inhibitors and reverse transcriptase inhibitors are underway.

6. Follow-up care of an infant born to an HIV-positive mother.

    a. Infants should be followed closely. Complete blood count (CBC) and differential should be performed at birth as baseline and followed closely. PCR should be obtained within 48 hours of delivery. If positive, it should be repeated; if negative, it should be repeated at 14 days, at 1 to 2 months of age, and at 4 to 6 months.

    b. PCP prophylaxis should not be administered to infants <4 weeks of age. It should be started at 6 weeks of age, when ZDV is discontinued (Table 20-1).

    c. Once HIV infection has been confirmed in the infant, antiretroviral therapy should be started and PCP prophylaxis should be continued.

    d. Infected infants should have serial HIV ELISA, CD4+ lymphocyte counts, and determinations of viral load.

BOX 20-3
Zidovudine Regimen From AIDS Clinical Trials Group Protocol 076

Oral administration of 100 mg of zidovudine (ZDV) five times daily, initiated at 14-34 weeks of gestation and continued throughout the pregnancy.

During labor, intravenous administration of ZDV in a 1-hour loading dose of 2 mg/kg of body weight, followed by a continuous infusion of 1 mg/kg of body weight per hour until delivery.

Oral administration of ZDV to the newborn (ZDV syrup at 2 mg/kg of body weight per dose every 6 hours) for the first 6 weeks of life, beginning 8-12 hours after birth.

TABLE 20-1
Recommendations for PCP Prophylaxis and CD4+ Monitoring for HIV-Exposed Infants by Age and HIV-Infected Status

Age/HIV-infection status	PCP prophylaxix	CD4+ monitoring
Birth to 4-6 wk, HIV exposed	No prophylaxis	1 mo
4-6 wk to 4 mo, HIV exposed	Prophylaxis	3 mo
HIV infected or indeterminate	Prophylaxis	6, 9, and 12 mo
HIV infection reasonably excluded*	No prophylaxis	None

Modified from *MMWR* 44:RR4, 1995.
*HIV infection can be reasonably excluded among children who have had two or more negative HIV diagnostic tests (i.e., HIV culture or PCR), both of which are performed at 1 month of age and one of which is performed at 4 months of age, or two or more negative HIV IgG antibody tests performed at >6 months of age among children who have no clinical evidence of HIV disease.

   e. Studies of prophylactic intravenous immune globulin (IVIG) have shown efficacy in reduction of pyogenic infections.

   f. Infants of HIV-positive mothers who have not been determined to have HIV infection should be investigated and treated aggressively for fever and other signs of infection. Fever, cough, and dyspnea are common presentations of *P. carinii* pneumonia, and this syndrome should be treated presumptively with intravenous trimethoprim-sulfamethoxazole.

   g. Breast-feeding is considered by many to be contraindicated in some areas because there is an as yet unquantified risk of viral transmission through human milk; however, in underdeveloped countries, the benefit of breast-feeding is thought to outweigh any risk.

7. Expert opinion and knowledge about diagnosis and therapy are rapidly changing. It is recommended that consultation with specialists who care for HIV infection and who participate in clinical trials be undertaken.

H. Enteroviruses.

1. Causative agent. An RNA virus.
   a. Viruses include 23 group A and 6 group B coxsackieviruses, 4 types of enteroviruses, and 31 echoviruses.
   b. The viruses are ubiquitous and spread by the fecal-oral route. Infections are more common in summer and fall. Transmission to the newborn may be from the mother, other infants, or hospital staff.
   c. The incubation period is 3 to 6 days.
2. Clinical syndromes.
   a. Inapparent infection and mild febrile illness are the most common syndromes in neonates.
   b. In newborn infants a sepsislike syndrome may occur, with fever, lethargy, rash, and poor feeding. A severe septic shock syndrome with DIC has been reported.
   c. Myocarditis and meningoencephalitis have been described, usually with coxsackieviruses. A severe hepatitis has been seen with echovirus.
3. Diagnosis.
   a. Enteroviruses may be suspected on the basis of season, history of exposure, rash, and the incubation period.
   b. Culture of CSF, pharyngeal secretions, stool, and urine may yield virus.
   c. PCR of CSF, nasopharyngeal secretions, or rectal swab is both sensitive and specific.
   d. Because of the many different serotypes, serology usually is not helpful.
4. Treatment. There is no specific therapy for enteroviruses. There are anecdotal reports of the use of human immunoglobulin to prevent spread in the nursery.

V. CONGENITAL TOXOPLASMOSIS

A. Causative agent. *Toxoplasma gondii.*

B. Epidemiology involves a protozoan parasite that is ubiquitous and infects many warm-blooded animals, especially cats. In the United States, the estimated rate of symptomatic congenital toxoplasmosis is 1 to 4:1000 live births.

C. Transmission. Humans become infected by ingestion of poorly cooked meats or sporulated oocysts in cat feces. Transmission from blood transfusion or organ donor can occur. The incubation period for acquired infection is 4 to 21 days. A fetus is infected by transplacental passage during maternal parasitemia.

1. Approximately 50% of infants born to mothers who seroconvert during pregnancy are infected; however, only 10% are symptomatic.
2. Prenatal diagnosis with PCR testing is rapid, safe, and accurate, but not yet widely available.

D. Clinical findings. Infants are frequently asymptomatic at birth. However, variable findings, including maculopapular rash, generalized lymphadenopathy, hepatosplenomegaly, thrombocytopenia, CSF pleocytosis, microcephaly, chorioretinitis, cerebral calcification, and interstitial pneumonitis, may be present (see Box 20-1).

E. Outcome can be potentially devastating, and may range from severe morbidity and mortality to subtle findings to asymptomatic. Long-term sequelae include hydrocephalus (or microcephaly), mental retardation, chorioretinitis with visual difficulty, convulsions, and varying cognitive development, all as a result of intrauterine meningoencephalitis.

F. Postnatal diagnosis (see Fig. 20-3).

1. If possible, isolation of organism from placenta.

2. Fluorescent antibody tests for IgM often give false-positive results. If available, ELISA techniques to detect specific IgG and IgM are preferred; comparison with mother's serum is always necessary. There may be transplacental transfer of IgG antibodies in an uninfected neonate; in that event, these will disappear, and IgM antibodies, which are not placentally transferable, will not appear as time goes by if they are not present at birth.

3. An infectious disease consultation is recommended. Sensitivities and specificities of this group of tests make this a tricky workup.

G. Treatment.

1. Optimal treatment has not been established. Guidelines are shown in Box 20-4. Neurologic and developmental outcomes are significantly better for treated children compared with those who are not treated.

BOX 20-4
Guidelines for the Treatment of Congenital Toxoplasmosis

DRUGS

1. Pyrimethamine + sulfadiazine:
   - Pyrimethamine: 15 mg/m^2 per day or 1 mg/kg per day (maximum daily dose is 25 mg) orally. Although the half-life of the drug is 4 to 5 days, it should be given on a daily basis unless breaking of the tablets is grossly inaccurate during preparation of the smaller doses. Then, as with small infants (e.g., when a daily dose of 3 mg is indicated), breaking of a tablet may result in a slightly higher dose, which could be administered every 2 days.
   - Sulfadiazine or trisulfapyrimidines: 85 mg/kg per day by the oral route in two divided doses daily.

From Remington JS, Desmonts G: Toxoplasmosis. In Remington JS, Klein JO (editors): *Infectious diseases of the fetus and newborn infant,* ed 4, Philadelphia, 1995, WB Saunders. *Continued*

BOX 20-4
Guidelines for the Treatment of Congenital Toxoplasmosis—cont'd

DRUGS—cont'd

2. Spiramycin: 100 mg/kg per day by the oral route in two divided doses.
3. Corticosteroids (prednisone or methylprednisolone): 1.5 mg/kg per day by the oral route in two divided doses daily. Continue until the inflammatory process (e.g., high level of CSF protein [100 mg/dl before the age of ≥1 month], chorioretinitis) has subsided; dosage should then be tapered progressively and discontinued.
4. Folinic acid: 5 mg every 3 days (intramuscularly in young infants) during treatment with pyrimethamine. If bone-marrow toxicity occurs at this dose, increase to 10 mg every 3 days. If bone-marrow toxicity is severe, discontinue pyrimethamine until the abnormality is corrected, and then begin pyrimethamine again using 10 mg folinic acid every 3 days. In some infants, it may be necessary to administer folinic acid more frequently.

INDICATIONS

1. Overt congenital toxoplasmosis: Treatment is for 1 year in all cases. For infants in whom clinical signs of infection are present, treatment during the first 6 months is with pyrimethamine + sulfadiazine. During the following 6 months, 1 month of pyrimethamine + sulfadiazine is alternated with 1 month of spiramycin. Folinic acid should be started as soon as possible. *No treatment is usually given after 12 months of age except when there is evidence of evolution of the infection, such as a flare-up of chorioretinitis.*
2. Overt congenital toxoplasmosis with evidence of inflammatory process (chorioretinitis, high level of CSF protein, generalized infection, jaundice): Treatment is as in #1 + corticosteroids.
3. Subclinical congenital toxoplasma infection: Pyrimethamine + sulfadiazine for 6 weeks; thereafter, alternate with spiramycin. Spiramycin given for 6 weeks, alternated with 4 weeks of pyrimethamine + sulfadiazine to complete treatment for 1 year.
4. Healthy newborn in whom serologic testing has not provided definitive results but maternal infection was proved to have been acquired during pregnancy: One course of pyrimethamine + sulfadiazine for 1 month. Consultation with appropriate authority to determine necessity for continued therapy and drug and dosage regimen. *Decision to be made on an individual basis depends on multiple factors, including serologic test titers, immune load, and clinical findings.*
5. Healthy newborn born to a mother with high Sabin-Feldman dye test titer–date of maternal infection undetermined: Spiramycin for 1 month. Then regimen as in #4. In certain cases the indication for treatment is difficult to define because of a lack of information about the pregnancy and lack of isolation attempts from the corresponding placenta.

2. Pharmacologic treatment includes a combination of pyrimethamine and sulfadiazine or trisulfapyrimidine with folinic acid to prevent bone marrow suppression. Spiramycin should be given; however, in the United States spiramycin is available only by request to the Food and Drug Administration. CBC and platelet counts should be monitored twice weekly.

3. Corticosteroids (prednisone or methylprednisolone) should be added for patients with chorioretinitis, a high level of CSF protein, generalized infection, or jaundice.

4. Duration of therapy has not been established. An infectious disease consultation should be obtained.

5. Isolation in the nursery is not necessary.

H. Prevention. Pregnant women with negative or unknown serostatus should avoid contact with cat feces, or avoid cats altogether (e.g., working in gardens), and should not eat uncooked meat.

VI. CONGENITAL SYPHILIS

A. Causative agent. *Treponema pallidum* (spirochete).

B. Incidence. Once common, congenital syphilis is much less so since the penicillin era. However, there has been a significant recent increase (100-fold since 1985) as a result of poor or absent prenatal care, poverty, and drug abuse.

C. Pathologic basis. Transplacental invasion of fetus with treponemes occurs in utero and may cause abortion as early as 2 to 3 months of pregnancy; it involves septicemic spread, with potential spirochetal invasion of every body part.

N.B.: Several spirochetes may be transmitted across the placenta (e.g., recent anecdotal evidence for *Borrelia burgdorferi* (Lyme disease) suggests clinically significant neurologic disease not unlike that with congenital syphilis. Other anomalies (cardiovascular, syndactyly) have also been associated.

D. Clinical findings. Half of affected infants are asymptomatic at birth. Depending on the in utero timing of the infection and the extent of spread, the clinical picture may be a combination of some or all of the following:

1. In the child with clinical disease.
   a. Can be severe, even fatal.
   b. Prematurity; small for gestational age (SGA).
   c. Skin rash (may involve palms and soles), maculopapular or vesiculobullous.
   d. Hepatomegaly, splenomegaly.
   e. Jaundice.
   f. Anemia (hemolytic, Coombs' test result negative), thrombocytopenia, leukocytosis.
   g. Persistent snuffles (nasal discharge).
   h. Long-bone invasion (metaphyseal osteochondritis in the first few weeks, diaphyseal periostitis later).
      (1) Periosteal elevation.
      (2) Epiphyseal disruption (e.g., bones of the forearm).
      (3) Radiolucencies (e.g., bones of the hand).
   i. Condylomata lata (particularly in moist creases).

    j. Meningitis (frequent); invasion by treponemes may be unaccompanied by increased CSF cellularity or positive Venereal Disease Research Laboratory (VDRL) test result.

    k. Pneumonia (infrequent).

  2. In the unusual event of an infant *acquiring* syphilis on passage through the birth canal, the familiar stages of adult syphilis are possible in the absence of treatment; no manifestations, however, are noted in the immediate neonatal period.

E. Diagnosis (Fig. 20-4).

  1. Study neonates whose mothers are seropositive and who have the following characteristics:

    a. Have untreated syphilis.

    b. Were treated within 4 weeks of delivery.

    c. Were treated with a drug other than penicillin.

    d. Did not show a serologic response to treatment.

    e. Did not have appropriate follow-up to treatment.

    f. Have a treatment or diagnostic status that is in any way uncertain.

N.B.: Defer discharge of any infant for whom serologic status of the infant or mother is uncertain.

  2. Serologic tests for syphilis.

    a. VDRL.

    b. Rapid plasma reagin (RPR). Nontreponemal screening tests; detect antibody to a cardiolipin; reported at the highest fully reactive dilution; sensitivities and specificities cannot be *fully* trusted; particularly prone to false-positive results (e.g., in the presence of autoimmune disease).

    c. Treponemal tests.

      (1) Fluorescent treponemal antibody absorption test (FTA-ABS), performed on 19S fraction of serum IgM.

      (2) Microhemagglutination test for *T. pallidum* (MHA-TP); reliable but not absolute; once positive, will always be positive.

N.B.: These tests are similar; to use both is redundant.

      (3) *T. pallidum* immobilization test (TPI).

      (4) Treponemal tests are also positive in other spirochetal diseases (e.g., yaws, Lyme disease).

N.B.: IgM does not cross placenta; IgM antibodies are the infant's; beware: often unreliable specificity, sensitivity about 89%.

    d. Dark-field microscopy of available fresh discharges.

      (1) Usually possible with acquired syphilis from chancres or skin lesions; sensitive and specific in *experienced* hands; usually possible with condylomata or vesicular lesions in congenital syphilis.

      (2) Dark-field examination of the placenta is indicated for persons at risk for HIV infection or for those who might not develop an immune response for other reasons.

    e. Direct fluorescent antibody staining of acetone-fixed exudate.

  3. Guiding principles.

    a. Adequate diagnosis relies on full knowledge of the mother's disease status. Transmission of infection occurs almost 100% of the time during primary and secondary stages, usually well within 1 year of appearance of the chancre, but only 10% of the time dur-

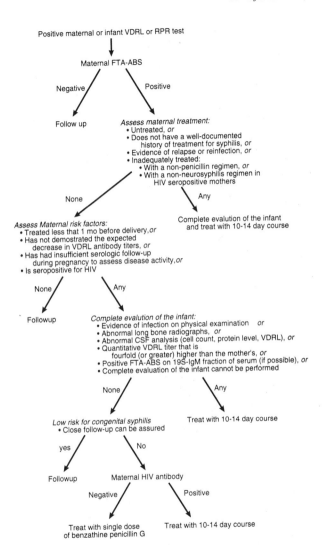

FIG. 20-4. Algorithm for management of a newborn infant born to a mother with positive nontreponemal (VDRL or RPR) test result. (From Ikeda MK, Jenson HB: *J Pediatr* 117:843, 1990.)

ing late syphilis. If the disease has been discovered and treated during or before pregnancy, approach the infant as if therapy has failed.

b. Careful examination should be conducted for clinical findings; unexplained fever alone may be a clue.

c. Use RPR or VDRL on the baby's venous blood (do not use cord blood).

d. Conclude that the infant has congenital syphilis if the titer of the infant's screening test equals or is greater than the mother's or if there is compelling clinical evidence. If there is uncertainty, obtain the following:

    (1) Long-bone radiographs (for periostitis or osteochondritis).

    (2) Chest radiograph (for pneumonitis).

    (3) Lumbar puncture (for CSF cell count, protein level, and VDRL test).

e. If the mother has disease but the baby's workup does not suggest infection, watch without treatment. If the baby's screening titers are initially clearly lower than the mother's, repeat tests at 1- to 2-month intervals until negative, which is most often by 6 months. Consider for treatment, however, if follow-up is uncertain. Do not hesitate to seek consultation in the event of uncertainty.

F. Treatment and subsequent management. Newborns require treatment when there is *any* indication of active disease, uncertainty about the mother's status or treatment history, concern about inadequate or inappropriate maternal treatment (drugs other than penicillin), treatment in the last 4 weeks of pregnancy, the possibility of reinfection, or the anticipation of doubtful compliance.

1. For an asymptomatic neonate who has clear CSF and nontreponemal titers greater than mother's, give intramuscular procaine penicillin 50,000 U/kg as a single daily dose for 10 days.

2. For symptomatic or asymptomatic neonates with abnormal CSF (with or without reactive CSF VDRL, cell count >5/mm^3, or protein >50 mg/dl), give intramuscular procaine penicillin 50,000 U/kg as a single daily dose for 10 to 14 days; repeat spinal tap in 6 months and, if still positive, retreat fully.

N.B.: Anticipate Jarisch-Herxheimer reaction, a temperature elevation, several hours after the first dose of penicillin; this is most often transient and does not require cessation of therapy.

3. Repeat VDRL or RPR at 1, 2, 4, 6, and 12 months until there is a significant drop in titer; decrease should be fourfold in 3 months, eightfold in 6 months; FTA-ABS remains positive and cannot be used in follow-up.

4. Retreat if drop in titer does not occur after third repeat test, titer increases, or clinical findings persist or intensify.

5. Repeat spinal tap in 6 months if it was initially abnormal, or as needed in the event of worsening clinical findings, and every 6 months thereafter until the findings are all clear.

6. All infants with certain or uncertain diagnosis should be reported to the health department (mother and her contacts will need follow-up).

N.B.: An infant successfully treated for congenital syphilis is not immune and may later contract acquired syphilis. Follow-up education and monitoring are important.

VII. TUBERCULOSIS (TB) (CONGENITAL AND ACQUIRED)

A. Definitions.
1. Congenital tuberculosis: infection in utero.
2. Acquired tuberculosis: infection during or after delivery.

B. Causative agents.
1. *Mycobacterium tuberculosis* (most common).
2. Bovine and atypical organisms (rare).

C. Incidence.
TB is rare in the newborn. Detection in early weeks suggests congenital acquisition or infection at delivery via inhalation or aspiration of infected amniotic fluid or bacilli. Women who have pulmonary TB are at risk to infect infant after delivery.

D. Pathology.
1. Infection occurs via respiration; the breathing in of infected amniotic fluid or vaginal secretions leads to a primary complex in lungs.
2. Infection via the umbilical vein leads to a primary complex in the hepatic structures, with likelihood of miliary spread to multiple sites, including the brain and serosal surfaces. Most congenital tuberculosis is the result of hematogenous spread.

E. Diagnostic confirmation.
1. Examine the placenta for tuberculous granulomas (note that their presence does not necessarily indicate disease in the infant).
2. Stain tracheal or gastric aspirates for acid-fast organisms.
3. Culture aspirates and, when indicated, bone marrow, urine, or suggestive nodes.
4. Chest radiograph (a negative film does not rule out disease).
5. A Mantoux skin test (5 TU PPD) is of doubtful value, but is a necessary step; a positive test result may be delayed several weeks or may never occur.
6. LP (examination and culture of CSF is necessary for appropriate assessment of the CNS).
7. Drug susceptibilities of an organism recovered from the mother should be determined. These results will help direct therapy.

F. Management of the infant born to a mother with tuberculosis or into a TB-positive household.
1. Immediate separation at birth is controversial; it is strongly recommended by some, and avoided by others. If it proves necessary, keep this period to a minimum.
2. Confirmation should be made of the presence or absence of infection in other household occupants.
3. A diagnostic workup should be done to seek out infant infection.
4. Specific clinical situations.
   a. Mother (or other household contact) with a positive tuberculin skin test reaction and no evidence of current disease.
      (1) Test infant with Mantoux test (5 TU PPD) at 4 to 6 weeks of age and at 3 to 4 months of age.

(2) If family or mother cannot be tested immediately and situation is high risk for possible TB, consider treating infant with isoniazid (INH) (10 mg/kg per day) pending skin testing of family.

(3) Mother should also be considered for INH preventive therapy. Breast-feeding is not contraindicated.

b. Mother with untreated disease or disease that has been treated for ≥2 weeks and who is considered noncontagious at delivery.

(1) Investigate household members and extended family.

(2) Chest radiograph and Mantoux test should be done at 4 to 6 weeks of age; if negative, repeat at 3 to 4 months of age and at 6 months.

(3) Begin INH (10 mg/kg per day). Once family has been investigated and skin test at 3 to 4 months is negative, INH can be discontinued.

(4) If mother is compliant with therapy, separation of infant and mother is not indicated. Breast-feeding is not contraindicated. However, if mother is noncompliant with therapy, bacille Calmette-Guérin (BCG) vaccine may be considered for infant. Response to vaccine in infants may be inadequate for prevention of TB.

c. Mother with current disease and who is considered contagious at time of delivery.

(1) Infant and mother should be separated until mother begins therapy and is considered noncontagious.

(2) Management is the same as previously outlined.

d. Mother with hematogenous-spread TB.

(1) Congenital TB in the infant is possible. Infant should have Mantoux test and chest radiograph. Begin treatment immediately with INH (10 to 15 mg/kg per day), pyrazinamide (20 to 40 mg/kg per day), rifampin (10 to 20 mg/kg per day), and streptomycin (20 to 40 mg/kg per day) if diagnosis is suspected.

(2) If diagnosis is confirmed, treatment with INH, rifampin, pyrazinamide, and streptomycin daily for 2 months and INH and rifampin daily for 10 months should occur. Infectious diseases consultation is necessary.

(3) If infant's chest radiograph, skin test, or clinical findings do not support diagnosis of congenital TB, infant should be separated from mother (until she is judged noncontagious) and INH (10 mg/kg per day) should be initiated until 6 months of age. If skin test is positive at 6 months of age, INH should be continued for a total of 12 months.

5. When tuberculosis or the possibility of tuberculosis is present, always make an effort to ascertain the HIV status of the mother and infant. In the event of a positive finding, act accordingly.

VIII. NEONATAL MASTITIS

A. **Causative agents** (in usual order of frequency).

1. Staphylococci, particularly *S. aureus*.

2. Group B streptococcus.

3. *E. coli.*
4. *Pseudomonas aeruginosa.*
5. *Proteus species.*
6. Salmonella.
B. Source. Probable invasion of breast ductal system by skin flora.
C. Frequency. Unusual.
D. Time of onset. Age 2 to 4 weeks; rarely within first week.
E. Clinical findings.
1. Erythema.
2. Swelling, more often firm than fluctuant.
3. Tenderness.
4. Unilateral nipple discharge (occasionally bilateral).
5. Abscess formation (uncommon).
F. Differential diagnosis.
1. Milk stasis (witch's milk), hormonally induced (passive transfer from mother).
2. Hormonally induced breast development; usually bilateral, not necessarily symmetric; absence of significant erythema or tenderness.
G. Laboratory studies.
1. If milk can be expressed.
   a. Gram's stain.
   b. Culture and sensitivity.
   c. Leukocyte count ($>10^6$/ml is significant).
2. If there is fluctuation.
   a. Aspirate for smear, culture, sensitivities (incision and drainage to be performed by surgeon).
   b. Blood culture.
   c. CBC count.
3. If there is nipple discharge of any kind, obtain smear, culture, and sensitivities.
H. Treatment.
1. Pending cultures.
   a. Give oxacillin, 50 mg/kg per 24 hours intravenously or intramuscularly (divided into 8-hour doses for infants >2 kg and 12-hour doses for infants <2 kg).
   b. Gentamicin, 2.5 mg/kg intramuscularly every 12 hours in full-term babies.
   c. Further therapy depends on results of culture, sensitivities, and clinical status.
   d. For resistant *S. aureus,* use vancomycin, 15 mg/kg intravenously every 12 hours (potential nephrotoxicity and ototoxicity; as with gentamicin, requires careful monitoring of serum levels).
   e. If streptococcus is cultured, begin administration of potassium penicillin G, 50,000 to 100,000 U/kg per 24 hours, divided into 12-hour doses intravenously or intramuscularly (for infants <2 kg); 50,000 to 150,000 U/kg per 24 hours, divided into 8-hour doses intravenously or intramuscularly (for infants >2 kg).
   f. Hospitalization is appropriate at least until infection is clearly controlled.

IX. MATERNAL MASTITIS
A. Clinical findings.
1. Flulike symptoms.
2. Fever.
3. Erythematous, tender areas in one or both breasts.
B. Management.
1. Rest (if possible).
2. Warm compresses for 10 to 15 minutes, three to four times a day.
3. Frequent nursing, such as every 1½ to 3 hours. This is necessary to prevent stasis and abscess development and to relieve engorgement.

N.B.: Breast abscesses can develop. An obstetrician or surgeon should guide management and judgment regarding drainage and antibiotics. In the event of drainage, nursing may be temporarily interrupted on the affected breast until it is healed. The mother must continue pumping breast milk to maintain an adequate milk supply.

X. OMPHALITIS (PRIMARY INFECTION OF THE UMBILICAL CORD)
A. Causative agents.
1. Group A streptococcus, most commonly.
2. *S. aureus.*
B. The usual expectation. (1) The umbilical stump dries, (2) becomes a hard, dark-brown eschar, (3) separates in about 2 weeks, and (4) epithelializes in about 3 to 4 weeks.

N.B.: Ordinarily, the cord has two arteries and one vein; if there is only one artery, suspect a congenital abnormality, particularly with the kidney, but there is no extra susceptibility to infection.

C. Clinical findings in various combinations.
1. Erythema of varying diameter, ringing cord.
2. Thickened underlying skin.
3. Purulent discharge.
4. Foul-smelling discharge.
5. Moist, fetid cord and bleeding suggest group A *Streptococcus* or *S. aureus* infection.

N.B.: A palpably thickened falciform ligament (a direct route to the liver) is ominous.

D. Major concerns.
1. Extension beyond immediate area of cord.
2. Cellulitis, fasciitis of the abdominal wall.
3. Peritonitis.
4. Bacteremia/sepsis, meningitis.
5. Tetanus neonatorum.
6. Gas gangrene.
7. Ascending infection, umbilical vein to liver and portal system.
   a. Portal vein thrombosis.
   b. Portal hypertension.
   c. Liver abscess.
E. Differential diagnosis.
1. Delayed healing/umbilical granuloma (small, reddened mass; slight purulent discharge; no surrounding erythema).

a. May be the result of infection or irritation from clumps of talcum powder.

b. $AgNO_3$ stick application (one to several times over 2 to 3 weeks) is both diagnostic and therapeutic; failure to subside with this therapy suggests infection or other complication. Some pediatricians prefer cleansing with alcohol and sprinkling with table salt for 2 to 3 days.

2. Embryonic remnants.

a. Allantois (passage of urine through umbilicus). Methylene blue dye placed in umbilicus will be voided in urine.

b. Vitelline duct.

(1) Passage of gas and feces through umbilicus. Carmine red dye given orally and passed through the umbilicus confirms enteric fistula.

(2) Mass, larger and redder than granuloma, unresponsive to $AgNO_3$, may be intestinal mucosa or polyp.

c. Umbilical hernia. Generally, integument is well healed.

3. Meconium-stained umbilical stump is suggestive of fetal distress and not necessarily of umbilical infection.

F. Laboratory studies.

1. Gram's stain should be done of any discharge.

2. Culture and sensitivities should always be obtained when suspicious of infection.

3. CBC with differential and blood culture should be performed if there is more than a simple ring of erythema.

4. A spinal tap may be indicated, depending on the baby's clinical status.

G. Therapy.

1. In the event of a simple ring of erythema in an otherwise clinically well child (often the case), no antibiotics are provided pending culture results (by then, erythema often will have ebbed or subsided).

2. In the event of more serious findings and until laboratory studies are available, treat promptly with the following:

a. Oxacillin, 50 mg/kg per 24 hours intravenously or intramuscularly, administered every 4 to 6 hours for infants >2 kg and every 12 hours for infants <2 kg.

b. Gentamicin, 2.5 mg/kg intramuscularly every 12 hours in term babies.

c. Adjust therapy according to culture results and clinical status; resistant *S. aureus* suggests use of vancomycin, 15 mg/kg intravenously or intramuscularly every 12 hours (potential nephrotoxicity and ototoxicity; as with gentamicin, requires careful monitoring of serum levels); clinical indication of tetanus neonatorum suggests use of potassium penicillin G.

d. Topical antibiotics are not necessary.

3. Hospitalization is indicated until the need for treatment is clarified; rehospitalization after discharge is not usually necessary in the event of a simple ring of erythema.

H. Prevention.

1. Topical antibiotic ointments are inappropriate.

2. Application of triple dye.

3. Alcohol wipe with diaper changes.

4. Sponge bathe with mild, nonperfumed soap; leave area dry and un-
covered. Do not handle cord.

N.B.: It is probably best to leave the cord alone; the more it is bothered,
the longer it will hang on. There is a suggestion that *some* colonization
speeds the process of detachment and subsequent healing. Some cords
may fail to separate when expected; if the time stretches beyond 2 to 3
weeks, suspect some defect in neutrophil mobility. *Do not force separation.*
If problem continues, neutrophil studies are in order.

XI. CANDIDIASIS

A. **Causative agent.** *Candida* species (e.g., *C. albicans, C. pseudotrop-
icalis, C. stellatoides, C. tropicalis, C. parapsilosis*).

B. **Occurrence.** Candidiasis occurs anywhere in the world and anywhere in the body (including the umbilical cord).

N.B.: In a singleton delivery with membranes intact, *Candida* may still be
found in 6% of amniotic fluids.

C. **Sources of neonatal infection.**

1. Mother's vagina during delivery.
2. Intrauterine, ascending from birth canal.
3. Other person-to-person contact (it is ubiquitous).
4. Indwelling intravascular catheters; other instruments.

D. **Clinical findings.** The incubation period is unknown; however,
if lesions are present at birth or within a few hours, infection is intrauterine, ascending from the vagina; if lesions are noted after 3 to
4 days or up to a week after birth, infection occurred during delivery. Lesions localized to the mouth or skin tend to be benign, with
the birth canal as the source; dissemination is more likely to follow
some invasive procedure and to be nosocomial.

1. Diffuse, maculopapular, erythematous, possibly pustular rash or
mucous membrane lesions may be present at birth; they can coa-
lesce into white, cheesy, adherent patches; early lesions may be
vesicular with an areola of erythema; lesions are likely to be found
in warm, moist areas, particularly the diaper area.
2. Poor feeding, regurgitation, vomiting, hematemesis (esophagitis).
3. Notably, significant skin involvement is not usually accompanied
by systemic (e.g., pulmonary) involvement.
4. Infants at increased risk.
   a. Very-low-birth-weight (VLBW).
   b. Other congenital infections.
   c. Abdominal surgery.
   d. Central lines (indwelling intravascular catheters).
   e. Maternal drug abuse.
   f. Prolonged use of broad-spectrum antibiotics.
   g. Immunosuppressive drugs (e.g., corticosteroids).
   h. Immunodeficiency states.
5. VLBW infants may have the following characteristics of sepsis in
whole or in part.
   a. Apnea.
   b. Bradycardia.

    c. Temperature instability.

    d. Shock.

    e. Hypoglycemia; less frequently, hyperglycemia.

    f. Glycosuria.

  6. No part of body is safe (e.g., lungs, kidney, joints, bones [often nosocomial], gastrointestinal [GI] tract [necrotizing enterocolitis], deep or subcutaneous tissues [abscesses]) as a result of penetration of minor vessels, thrombosis, or hematogenous spread. The most common sites include the following:

    a. Oral candidiasis (thrush), most often localized and benign, complicated occasionally by esophagitis and GI colonization.

    b. Skin.

    c. GI tract.

  E. Diagnosis is often difficult. With *extensive* clinical involvement, as many as 35% of cases are discovered only at postmortem, the majority of the remainder are diagnosed too late for effective treatment. Laboratory tests to be considered include the following:

  1. Culture: blood agar, Sabouraud's medium.

N.B.: *Candida* in *any* body fluid or discharge is *not* to be disregarded, and *not* to be considered a contaminant.

  2. Urinalysis: about 6% are positive; half of these culture positive.

  3. KOH preparation of skin scrapings (shows pseudomycelia, spores, pseudohyphae).

  4. Gram's stain of buffy coats (shows budding yeast spores).

  5. Additional tests that are occasionally indicated include the following:

    a. Indirect ophthalmoscopy.

    b. Lung biopsy (pneumonia).

    c. Echocardiography (endocarditis).

    d. Renal ultrasound (positive urine).

    e. Spinal tap (NOTE: CSF may show nothing in the presence of meningitis).

    f. Computed tomography (CT) (brain abscess).

F. Treatment.

  1. Oral. Nystatin suspension, 200,000 U two times a day for 5 to 10 days. Continue until 3 days after thrush is gone.

  2. Cutaneous. Nystatin ointment two times a day for 7 to 10 days; nystatin ointment with a corticosteroid should be used in severe cases. A topical or systemic antibiotic should be used if there is a secondary bacterial infection.

  3. Systemic. Amphotericin B, 0.5 to 1.0 mg/kg; the duration of treatment is determined by the severity of illness and clinical and microbiologic response; usually approximately 4 weeks of treatment is required for disseminated candidiasis.

N.B.: Infectious disease consultation for the development and implementation of an amphotericin-based management plan is strongly recommended.

    a. Caution. Side effects include cardiac arrhythmias, hypokalemia, renal toxicity, and anemia.

    b. Monitor serum electrolytes, blood urea nitrogen (BUN) (discontinue with elevated BUN) and creatinine levels.

4. 5-Fluorocytosine (never give alone in infants; use only as an additional drug in severe cases). 50 to 150 mg/kg per 24 hours orally in divided doses every 6 hours. Monitor CBC count and liver enzymes.
5. Meningitis. Treat as for any other systemic involvement; intrathecal amphotericin B *may* be necessary; use is controversial and should always be preceded by consultation.
6. Bladder infection. Kidney flush with amphotericin B *may* be necessary, again only after consultation.

XII. GUIDELINES FOR INFECTION CONTROL IN NURSERIES

A. Assessment.

1. Obtain mother's obstetric history from obstetrics database and delivery record.
2. Consult with labor and delivery staff about pertinent information related to the infant's need for isolation.
3. Observe infant for signs and symptoms of infectious disease during all contact with the infant.

B. Intervention.

1. Universal precautions should be observed at all times by all staff of the nursery during all routine care (see section on universal precautions later in this chapter). Strict adherence to universal precautions when caring for infants and children cannot be overemphasized. Patients with known risks should be identified in accordance with hospital policy. It should be noted that caregivers who assume no identified risk and who do not comply with universal precautions place themselves, their patients, and their families at increased risk for acquiring disease.
2. For the neonate, most isolettes serve as an isolation facility, and a separate room is not necessary.
3. All specimens sent to the clinical laboratory should be bagged and labeled with the appropriate type of isolation (e.g., by color-coded sticker label); individual nurseries may have different categories of isolation.
4. Contact isolation. Gowns are indicated if soiling is likely; gloves are indicated for touching infective material.
   a. Herpes simplex.
      (1) The infant with active herpes simplex should be isolated in an isolette, with gown and glove technique used.
      (2) The infant born by cesarean section to a mother with herpes without rupture of membranes before delivery requires no isolation.
      (3) The infant of a mother with active herpes lesions at the time of delivery should be identified as requiring thorough hand washing after all contact.
   b. *S. aureus.*
      (1) Place infant in isolette and use gown and glove precautions during all care. Careful hand washing before and after every patient contact is mandatory.
      (2) If organism is methicillin resistant, strict contact isolation is necessary.

    c. Skin infection.

    d. Colonization with gram-negative bacilli.

    e. Impetigo.

    f. Conjunctivitis.

    g. Gonorrhea.

5. Blood and body fluid secretions. Universal precautions are emphasized.

    a. Hepatitis B and C.

      (1) At-risk infants should be bathed immediately to remove maternal blood and secretions.

      (2) Isolation of infants born to HBsAg-positive mothers is not necessary, but their blood should be carefully handled with blood precautions.

      (3) Infant may remain in bassinet.

      (4) Gloves should be used for admission procedures and blood drawing.

      (5) All specimens to lab should be labeled *blood and body secretion precautions.*

    b. AIDS.

      (1) Scrupulously follow universal precautions during all care.

      (2) Eye protection should be worn whenever spattering of blood or body secretions is likely, such as during delivery, arterial puncture, suctioning, rinsing of used surgical instruments, LP, and intubation.

6. Drainage/secretion precautions. Gowns are indicated if soiling is likely. Gloves should be used for touching infective material. Articles contaminated with infective material should be discarded or bagged and labeled before being sent for processing.

    a. Syphilis.

      (1) Precautions are not necessary if no lesions are present.

      (2) If lesions are present, the infant should be isolated in an isolette.

    b. Conjunctivitis, minor or limited abscesses, or wound infections that result in infective purulent material, drainage, or secretion require precautions.

7. Enteric isolation. Gloves are indicated if soiling is likely. Gloves are indicated for touching infective material. Hands must be washed after touching the patient or potentially contaminated articles and before taking care of another patient. Articles contaminated with infective material should be discarded or bagged and labeled before being sent for decontamination.

    a. Hepatitis A. Isolation of the infant born to a mother with hepatitis A is not necessary unless the mother is jaundiced at time of delivery.

    b. Necrotizing enterocolitis.

8. Strict isolation. Masks, gowns, and gloves are indicated for all persons entering the room. Hands must be washed after touching the patient or potentially contaminated articles and before taking care of another patient. Articles contaminated with infective material should be discarded or bagged and labeled before being sent for de-

contamination and reprocessing. Procedures for patients infected with the Varicella (chickenpox) virus include the following:

   a. For a mother who reports exposure to varicella before delivery, the time of exposure and the mother's state of immunity must be established through obstetric records and personal consultation with the mother.

   b. Incubation period can range from 11 to 20 days after contact.

   c. The patient can be contagious for 1 to 2 days before and 5 days after the onset of the rash.

   d. An infant deemed at risk for exposure must be placed in an isolette, transported to and from the mother's room in the isolette, and given VZIG (see p. 309.)

   e. Infants born with varicella embryopathy do not require isolation.

9. Personnel health.

   a. It is generally accepted that a routine culture of personnel for staphylococcal colonization is of little value. Between 20% and 50% of personnel may be carriers at any given time. It is therefore important that the nursery and obstetric personnel assume the responsibility for reporting to their supervisors any communicable disease they might have. If appropriate, they will be excluded from working in the neonatal areas for the duration of that disease. Diseases in this category include any respiratory, skin, conjunctival, gastrointestinal, or hepatic disorders.

   b. Specific disease in personnel.

      (1) Herpes simplex. No essential or nonessential personnel having a herpes simplex lesion anywhere on the face or hands should be permitted to work in the nursery until the lesion is dry.

      (2) Staphylococcal infection. Documented staphylococcal lesions should be handled in an acceptable and individual manner.

10. Procedures to be followed if an epidemic is suspected or proven. An epidemic of staphylococcus may be defined as two documented staphylococcus infections occurring within 2 weeks of each other, including time after discharge from the nursery.

N.B.: Appropriate hospital infection control officers are to be informed of the situation.

   C. Parent teaching. Parents should be taught correct isolation precautions to observe according to the disease identified.

XIII. UNIVERSAL BLOOD AND BODY FLUID PRECAUTIONS

These guidelines apply to health care workers including, but not limited to, nurses, physicians, laboratory and blood bank technologists and technicians, phlebotomists, paramedics, emergency medical technicians, housekeepers, laundry workers, and others whose work involves contact with newborns, their blood, or other body fluids or corpses. These guidelines are derived primarily from the Centers for Disease Control and Prevention (Table 20-2).

TABLE 20-2
Universal Precautions in the Care of All Patients to Prevent Possible Contagion

Because persons of all ages and backgrounds may be sources of infection for the examiner, it is important to take proper precautions when working with blood and body fluids from all patients. **Examples:** Tuberculosis, AIDS, or any potentially infected body fluid or discharge.

- Use gloves when the possibility exists of contact with a patient's blood or potentially infectious body secretions or excretions. **Examples:** Starting intravenous lines, drawing blood, doing cardiopulmonary resuscitation (CPR) or other emergency procedures, handling soiled linen and waste.

- Wash hands after removing gloves (do not wash gloves), and use clean gloves with each patient.

- Do not wear gloves or protective clothing when contact with the patient is unlikely to result in exposure to blood or potentially infectious body secretions or excretions. **Examples:** Shaking hands, delivering supplies and medications, removing trays, holding infants.

- Wear gown, mask, and protective eyewear in addition to gloves during procedures in which spattering of blood or body fluids may occur. **Examples:** Arterial punctures, endoscopies, insertion of arterial lines, hemapheresis, hemodialysis.

- Always be cautious when working with needles, scalpels, or other sharp instruments.

- Always dispose of needles and sharp instruments in the impervious containers readily available in health care facilities. Do not recap, clip, or bend needles or throw them in the trash.

- Use the accompanying chart as a guide in identifying precautions that should be taken in specific situations.

Procedure	Wash hands	Gloves	Gown	Mask	Eyewear
			GUIDELINES		
Talking with patients	—	—	—	—	—
Adjusting IV fluid rate or noninvasive equipment	—	—	—	—	—

Data from Centers for Disease Control and Prevention: MMWR 36(suppl 25):3, 1987.

Continued

TABLE 20-2
Universal Precautions in the Care of All Patients to Prevent Possible Contagion—cont'd

Procedure	Wash hands	Gloves	Gown	Mask	Eyewear
			GUIDELINES		
Examining patient without touching blood, body fluids, mucous membranes	X	—	—	—	—
Examining patient with significant cough	X	—	—	X	—
Examining patient, including contact with blood, body fluids, mucous membranes, drainage	X	X	—	—	—
Drawing blood	X	X			
Inserting venous access	X	X	—	—	—
Suctioning	X	X	Use gown, mask, eyewear if bloody body fluid spattering is likely		
Inserting body or face catheters	X	X	Use gown, mask, eyewear if bloody body fluid spattering is likely		
Handling soiled waste, linen, other materials	X	X	Use gown, mask, eyewear only if waste or linen is extensively contaminated and spattering is likely		
Intubation	X	X	X	X	X
Inserting arterial access	X	X	X	X	X
Endoscopy, bronchoscopy	X	X	X	X	X
Operative and other procedures that produce extensive spattering of blood or body fluids and are likely to soil clothes	X	X	X	X	X

Data from Centers for Disease Control and Prevention: *MMWR* 36(suppl 25):3, 1987.

BIBLIOGRAPHY

A-Kader HH, Balisteri WT: Hepatitis C virus: implications to pediatric practice, *Pediatr Infect Dis J* 12:853, 1993.

American Academy of Pediatrics Committee on Infectious Diseases: Chemotherapy for tuberculosis in infants and children, *Pediatrics* 89:161, 1992.

American Academy of Pediatrics Committee on Infectious Diseases: Hepatitis C virus infection, *Pediatrics* 101:481, 1998.

American Academy of Pediatrics Committee on Infectious Diseases and Committee on the Fetus and Newborn: Guidelines for prevention of group B streptococcal (GBS) infection by chemoprophylaxis, *Pediatrics* 90:775, 1992.

American Academy of Pediatrics and American College of Obstetricians and Gynecologists: *Guidelines for perinatal care,* ed 2, 1988, Elk Grove Village, Ill, AAP and ACOG.

American Academy of Pediatrics: *Report of the committee on infectious diseases,* ed 24, Elk Grove Village, Ill, 1997, American Academy of Pediatrics.

American College of Obstetricians and Gynecologists: Group B streptococcal infections in pregnancy, *ACOG Technical Bulletin* 170:1, 1992.

Boppana SB, Fowler KB, Yaginder V, et al: Neuroradiographic findings in the newborn period and long-term outcome in children with symptomatic congenital cytomegalovirus infection, *Pediatrics* 99:409, 1997.

Caralane DJ, Long AM, McKeever PA, et al: Prevention of spread of echovirus 6 in a special care baby unit, *Arch Dis Child* 60:674, 1985.

Centers for Disease Control and Prevention: Recommendations for protection against viral hepatitis, *MMWR* 34:313, 1985.

Centers for Disease Control and Prevention: Recommendations for prevention of HIV transmission in the health care setting, *MMWR* 36(suppl 25):3, 1987.

Centers for Disease Control and Prevention: Prevention of perinatal transmission of hepatitis B virus: prenatal screening of all pregnant women for hepatitis B surface antigen, *MMWR* 37:341, 1988.

Centers for Disease Control and Prevention: Congenital syphilis in New York city, 1986-1988, *MMWR* 38:825, 1989.

Centers for Disease Control and Prevention: 1989 sexually transmitted diseases treatment guidelines, *MMWR* 38(suppl 8):5, 1989.

Centers for Disease Control and Prevention: 1994 revised classification system for human immunodeficiency virus infection in children less than 13 years of age, *MMWR* 43:1, 1994.

Centers for Disease Control and Prevention: Zidovudine for prevention of HIV transmission from mother to infant, *MMWR* 43:285, 1994.

Centers for Disease Control and Prevention: 1995 revised guidelines for prophylaxis against *Pneumocystis carinii* pneumonia for children infected with or perinatally exposed to human immunodeficiency virus, *MMWR* 44:RR-4, 1995.

Centers for Disease Control and Prevention: Prevention of perinatal group B streptococcal disease: a public health perspective, *MMWR* 45:1, 1996.

Centers for Disease Control and Prevention: Guidelines for the use of antiretroviral agents in pediatrics HIV infection, *MMWR* 7(RR-4), 1998.

Cherry JD: Enteroviruses. In Remington JS, Klein JC (editors): *Infectious diseases of the fetus and newborn infant,* Philadelphia, 1995, WB Saunders.

Ferrieri P: GBS infections in the newborn infant: diagnosis and treatment, *Antibiot Chemother* 35:211, 1985.

Fleming DT, McQuillan GM, Johnson RE, et al: Herpes simplex virus type 2 in the United States, 1976 to 1994, *N Engl J Med* 337:1105, 1997.

Freij BJ, South MA, Sever JL: Maternal rubella and the congenital rubella syndrome, *Clin Perinatol* 15:247, 1988.

Gerber MA, Zalneraitis EL: Childhood neurologic disorders and Lyme disease during pregnancy, *Pediatr Neurol* 11:41, 1994.

Gerdes JS: Clinicopathologic approach to the diagnosis of neonatal sepsis, *Clin Perinatol* 18:361, 1991.

Gershon AA: Chickenpox, measles and mumps. In Remington JS, Klein JC (editors): *Infectious diseases of the fetus and newborn,* Philadelphia, 1995, WB Saunders.

Husson RN, Comeau AM, Hoff R: Diagnosis of human immunodeficiency virus infection in infants and children, *Pediatrics* 86:1, 1990.

Ikeda MK, Jenson HB: Evaluation and treatment of congenital syphilis, *J Pediatr* 117:843, 1990.

Kinney JS, Kumar ML: Should we expand the TORCH complex? A description of clinical and diagnostic aspects of selected old and new agents, *Clin Perinatol* 15:727, 1988.

Krasinski K, Borkowsky W: Laboratory diagnosis of HIV infection, *Pediatr Clin North Am* 38:17, 1991.

Lieberman E, Lang JM, Frigoletto F, et al: Epidural analgesia, intrapartum fever, and neonatal sepsis evaluation, *Pediatrics* 99:415, 1997.

Maisels MJ, Kringe E: Risk of sepsis with severe hyperbilirubinemia, *Pediatrics* 90:741, 1992.

Meyers JD: Congenital varicella in term infants: risk reconsidered, *J Infect Dis* 129:215, 1974.

Miller E, Cradock-Watson JE, Ridehalgh MK: Outcome in newborn babies given antivaricella-zoster immunoglobulin after perinatal maternal infection with varicella-zoster virus, *Lancet* 12:371, 1989.

Modlin JF, Kinney JS: Perinatal enterovirus infections. In Aronoff SC, editor: *Advances in pediatric infectious disease,* vol 2, St. Louis, 1987, Mosby.

O'Connor EM, Sperling RS, Gelber R, et al: Reduction of maternal-infant transmission of human immunodeficiency virus type I with ZDV treatment, *N Engl J Med* 331:1173, 1994.

Pelke S, Ching D, Easa D, Melish ME: Gowning does not affect colonization or infection rates in a neonatal intensive care unit, *Arch Pediatr Adolescent Med* 148:1016, 1994.

Philip AGS, Hewitt JR: Early diagnosis of neonatal sepsis, *Pediatrics* 65:1036, 1980.

Pichichero MD, Todd JK: Detection of neonatal bacteremia, *J Pediatr* 94:958, 1979.

Pitt J: Perinatal human immunodeficiency virus infection, *Clin Perinatol* 18:227, 1991.

Pizzo PA, Wilfert CM: Perinatally acquired human immunodeficiency virus infection, *Pediatr Infect Dis J* 9:609, 1990.

Preblud SR, Alford CA: Rubella. In Remington JS, Klein JC (editors): *Infectious diseases of the fetus and newborn infant,* Philadelphia, 1995, WB Saunders.

Prober CG, Gershon AA: Medical management of newborns and infants to human immunodeficiency virus seropositive mothers, *Pediatr Infect Dis J* 10:684, 1991.

Pylipow M, Gaddis M, Kinney JS: Selective intrapartum prophylaxis for group B *Streptococcus* colonization: management and outcome of newborns, *Pediatrics* 331:631, 1994.

Remington JS, Desmonts G: Toxoplasmosis. In Remington JS, Klein JC (editors): *Infectious diseases of the fetus and newborn infant,* Philadelphia, 1995, WB Saunders.

Roizen N, Swisher CN, Stein MA, et al: Neurologic and developmental outcome in treated congenital toxoplasmosis, *Pediatrics* 95:11, 1995.

Semba RD, Miotti PG, Chiphangwi JD, et al: Maternal vitamin A deficiency and mother-to-child transmission of HIV-1, *Lancet* 343:1593, 1994.

Siegel JD: Sepsis neonatorum. In Oski FA, editor: *Principles and practices of pediatrics,* Philadelphia, 1990, JB Lippincott.

St. Geme JW, Murray DL, Carter J, et al: Perinatal bacterial infection after prolonged rupture of amniotic membranes: an analysis of risk and management, *J Pediatr* 104:608, 1984.

Stagno S: Cytomegalovirus. In Remington JS, Klein JC (editors): *Infectious diseases of the fetus and newborn infant,* Philadelphia, 1995, WB Saunders.

Steinhoff MC, Kinney JS: Neonatal sepsis and infections. In Reese RE, Betts RF (editors): *A practical approach to infectious diseases,* ed 3, Boston, 1991, Little, Brown.

Voora S, Srinivasan G, Lilien LD, et al: Fever in full-term newborns in the first four days of life, *Pediatrics* 69:40, 1982.

Walsh M, McIntosh K: Neonatal mastitis, *Clinical Pediatrics* 25:395, 1986.

Whitley RJ, Nahmias AJ, Visintine AM, et al: The natural history of herpes simplex virus infection of mother and newborn, *Pediatrics* 66:30, 1980.

Whitley RJ, Arvin A, Prober C, et al: Predictors of morbidity and mortality in neonates with herpes simplex virus infections, *N Engl J Med* 324:450, 1991.

Whitley RJ: Herpes simplex virus infections. In Remington JS, Klein JC (editors): *Infectious diseases of the fetus and newborn,* Philadelphia, 1990, WB Saunders.

Yow MD: Congenital cytomegalovirus disease: a new problem, *J Infect Dis* 159:163, 1989.

21

In Utero Drug Exposure

BERYL J. ROSENSTEIN

I. GENERAL CONSIDERATIONS

A. An increasing number of women of childbearing age are using controlled substances; it is estimated that 10% to 15% of newborns are exposed to illicit drugs during pregnancy.

B. Most drugs with high abuse potential cross the placenta and tend to accumulate in the fetus. With drugs with high potential for abuse, dependence develops in the fetus and in the mother.

C. Drug-exposed infants often go unrecognized and may be discharged to homes where they are at increased risk of medical and social problems, including abuse and neglect.

D. Detection of the drug-exposed newborn requires a high index of suspicion.

1. A comprehensive psychosocial history, including specific inquiry concerning maternal drug use, should be part of every obstetric and newborn evaluation.

2. Maternal and newborn urine toxicology testing is a useful adjunct but does not replace a careful maternal history.

3. A positive toxicology result confirms the diagnosis of drug use, but a negative test does not rule out in utero drug exposure.

4. Metabolites of morphine, cocaine, and cannabinoids can be recovered in high concentration in the meconium of drug-exposed infants. This is more sensitive than urine testing, in that meconium accumulates throughout gestation and may be used to establish a profile of drug use by the mother during her pregnancy.

5. Universal maternal toxicology screening is not recommended but may be indicated in areas with high levels of illicit drug use or in conjunction with an early discharge policy.

E. Illicit prenatal drug use should be particularly suspected in the following situations:

1. Maternal history of sexually transmitted diseases, including human immunodeficiency virus (HIV) infection.

2. History of multiple abortions, both spontaneous and elective.

3. Unregistered or late registration for prenatal care or inadequate number of prenatal visits (these are highly predictive of prenatal substance abuse).
4. History of vague or chaotic living arrangements (i.e., homeless, shelter, multiple addresses).
5. Placental abruption (cocaine, amphetamines).
6. Precipitous delivery, especially at home or under unusual circumstances.
7. Unexplained intrauterine growth retardation (IUGR).
8. Neonatal signs and symptoms consistent with in utero drug exposure.
9. History of child neglect or abuse.
10. Hypertensive episode, severe mood swings, myocardial infarction.
11. Previous unexplained fetal demise.

F. It is important to be aware of and screen the mother and newborn for other problems known to be seen in association with illicit drug use, including the following:
1. Acquired immunodeficiency syndrome (AIDS).
2. Tuberculosis.
3. Hepatitis B and C.
4. Syphilis.
5. Other sexually transmitted diseases.

G. Health care workers dealing with drug-exposed newborns must be knowledgeable concerning the following:
1. Details of urine toxicology and meconium-testing procedures performed in their hospital.
2. State and local child protection reporting requirements.
3. Resources available for the treatment and support of the affected mother, newborn, and family.

II. OUTCOMES: GENERAL DRUG USE

A. It is difficult to relate specific neonatal outcomes to specific drug exposures because of multiple associated problems, including the following:
1. Inadequate prenatal care.
2. Multiple drug use, including tobacco and alcohol.
3. Poor nutrition.
4. Chaotic living conditions; physical and sexual abuse.
5. Associated infections, including tuberculosis, AIDS, hepatitis B and C, and other sexually transmitted diseases.

B. Maternal and neonatal outcomes may vary depending on the type, frequency, timing, and intensity of drug use, but there are well-recognized generic effects of prenatal drug use (Table 21-1).
1. Maternal effects.
   a. Increased rates of spontaneous abortion, stillbirth, and shortened gestation.
   b. Placental abruption (cocaine and amphetamines).
2. Fetal/neonatal effects.
   a. Increased neonatal mortality.
   b. IUGR.
   c. Congenital malformations.

TABLE 21-1
Maternal Drug Use—Newborn Outcomes

	Heroin/ methadone	Alcohol	Cocaine	Marijuana	Tobacco
Withdrawal	++	+	+	—	—
Growth retardation	+	++	+	±	++
Birth defects	—	+	+	±	—
Neurobehavioral effects	++	++	++	+	+
Perinatal mortality	↑	↑	—	—	↑
Premature birth	↑	↑	↑	—	↑
Apgar score	↓	↓	↓	±	↓

    d. Microcephaly.
    e. Intrapartum distress (meconium staining, low Apgar scores).
    f. Neurobehavioral abnormalities.
    g. Unexpected infant deaths, especially after in utero exposure to opiates.
    h. Abnormalities of control of respiration.

III. OUTCOMES: SPECIFIC DRUG USE
A. Alcohol.
1. Fetal alcohol levels closely parallel those of the mother; no safe level of alcohol intake during pregnancy has been established. Increased maternal age (>30 years) and binge drinking may significantly increase the risk of adverse neonatal outcomes.
2. Fetal/neonatal effects are probably dose dependent and include the following:
    a. Prenatal and postnatal growth retardation (may be persistent).
    b. Neonatal withdrawal syndrome (tremors, hypertonia or hypotonia, restlessness, inconsolable crying, abnormal reflexes).
    c. Central nervous system (CNS) sequelae, including attention-deficit disorder and mental retardation.
    d. Increased incidence of congenital malformations.
    e. Intrauterine distress (meconium staining, low Apgar scores).
    f. Increased perinatal mortality rate.
3. Maternal effects include increased rates of spontaneous abortion and stillbirth.
4. Features of fetal alcohol syndrome, which affects 1:600 live births and is the third most common cause of mental retardation, consist of the following:
    a. Severe IUGR, including microcephaly.
    b. Neonatal withdrawal syndrome.
    c. Dysmorphic features (microcephaly, short palpebral fissures, ptosis, maxillary hypoplasia; long, smooth philtrum, thin vermilion border of upper lip).

d. Congenital malformations (skeletal, cardiac, genitourinary, cleft lip/palate).

e. Mild to profound mental retardation (average IQ = 65).

5. Treatment.

a. No specific therapy is indicated in the neonatal period.

b. Appropriate long-term follow-up of learning, development, and behavior problems.

B. Marijuana.

1. Tetrahydrocannabinol (THC) crosses the placenta and may lead to fetal hypoxia by increasing the fetal carbon monoxide level and decreasing uterine blood flow.

2. Fetal/neonatal effects.

a. Slight shortening of gestation (average 1 week).

b. Decrease in birth weight by 100 to 150 gm.

c. Transient mild neonatal neurobehavioral abnormalities (increased fine tremors and prolonged startles). At 2- and 3-year follow-up there is no evidence of motor, cognitive, or language abnormalities.

d. There is no evidence of an increased incidence of major or minor physical anomalies.

3. Treatment. No treatment is needed for neonates exposed in utero only to marijuana.

C. Narcotics. Heroin, methadone, codeine, pentazocine (Talwin), and tripelennamine (Pyribenzamine).

1. Maternal effects and common complications.

a. Increased rates of spontaneous abortion, premature labor, premature rupture of membranes.

b. Chorioamnionitis.

c. Preeclampsia.

2. Fetal/neonatal effects.

a. Increased perinatal mortality rate.

b. IUGR, including microcephaly.

c. Intrauterine distress (meconium staining, low Apgar scores).

d. Neonatal withdrawal (abstinence) syndrome.

e. Increased incidence of sudden unexpected death (methadone worse than heroin).

N.B.: During pregnancy, medical withdrawal from opioids should occur in a perinatal unit with fetal monitoring. In general, withdrawal is not advised before 14 weeks gestation because of the potential risk of inducing abortion and should not be performed after the thirty second week because of possible withdrawal-induced stress.

3. Neonatal withdrawal (abstinence) syndrome.

a. Severity depends on type of drug used (methadone is worse than heroin), amount and frequency of use, maternal and infant metabolism and excretion, concomitant drug use, and timing of last use before delivery. (If >1 week has elapsed between the last maternal use and delivery, the incidence of neonatal withdrawal is low).

b. Withdrawal symptoms usually appear soon after birth, reach a peak in 4 to 5 days, and may then occur in a subacute form for weeks to months.

N.B.: The use of naloxone in the delivery room is contraindicated in infants whose mothers are known to be opioid-dependent. However, in the absence of a specific history of opioid abuse, naloxone remains a reasonable option in the delivery room management of a depressed infant whose mother recently received a narcotic.

- c. Manifestations.
  - (1) Irritability, restlessness, tremors, wakefulness, high-pitched cry.
  - (2) Myoclonus, seizures.
  - (3) Poor feeding, frantic sucking, increased weight loss, delay in regaining birth weight.
  - (4) Sneezing, yawning, vomiting, diarrhea, nasal stuffiness, fever, sweating, tachypnea.

N.B.: After in utero methadone exposure, onset of symptoms may be delayed up to 7 to 10 days; withdrawal may be more severe and prolonged than with heroin, and there is a higher incidence of seizures. Infants of women who have been maintained on >25 mg of methadone per day are at particularly high risk.

- d. Treatment.
  - (1) Supportive care; quiet, comforting environment; gentle handling; swaddling (a nonoscillating waterbed has been shown to be effective).
  - (2) Frequent small feedings; in infants with significant weight loss or slow weight gain, high-calorie feedings (24 calories per ounce) are indicated.
  - (3) Pharmacotherapy.

N.B.: Most infants can be managed without drug therapy; all of the drugs used to treat neonatal withdrawal have their own CNS effects.

- e. Indications for drug therapy.
  - (1) Seizures.
  - (2) Vomiting and diarrhea associated with significant weight loss.
  - (3) Marked irritability and tremors that interfere with feedings and sleeping.
  - (4) Fever unrelated to infection.
- f. Abstinence scoring systems (Table 21-2) can be helpful in assessing the need for and response to drug therapy.
- g. Pharmacotherapy. The choice of drugs is somewhat arbitrary. Diazepam, methadone, clonidine, and chlorpromazine have been used, but phenobarbital and tincture of opium are the most frequently used drugs.
  - (1) Phenobarbital. Loading dose is 15 to 20 mg/kg, followed by a maintenance dose of 4 to 5 mg/kg per day, given intramuscularly or orally at 6-hour intervals. Blood levels should be monitored (aim for a peak level of 20 to 30 (μg/ml).
  - (2) Tincture of opium (10 mg/ml) diluted 25-fold to yield a morphine equivalent of 0.4 mg/ml. Starting dose is 0.1 ml/kg or 2 drops/kg with feedings every 4 hours as needed to control withdrawal signs. After stabilization, the dosage can be tapered by gradual decrease in the dose without altering the frequency.

TABLE 21-2
Neonatal Drug Withdrawal Scoring System

Signs	Score* 0	1	2	3
Tremors (muscle activity of limbs)	Normal	Minimally ↑ when hungry or disturbed	Moderate or marked ↑ when undisturbed; subsides when fed or held snugly	Marked ↑ or continuous even when undisturbed, going on to seizurelike movements
Irritability (excessive crying)	None	Slightly ↑	Moderate to severe when disturbed or hungry	Marked even when undisturbed
Reflexes	Normal	Increased	Markedly increased	
Stools	Normal	Explosive, but normal frequency	Explosive, >8/day	
Muscle tone	Normal	Increased	Rigidity	
Skin abrasions	No	Redness of knees and elbows	Breaking of skin	
Respiratory rate/min	<55	55-75	76-95	
Repetitive sneezing	No	Yes		
Repetitive yawning	No	Yes		
Vomiting	No	Yes		
Fever	No	Yes		

From Lipsitz PJ: *Clin Pediatr* 14:592, 1975.
*A score of ≥4 is consistent with neonatal withdrawal syndrome.

(3) The usual duration of therapy is 7 to 14 days. Guides to adequate therapy include a normal temperature curve, ability to sleep between feedings, decrease in activity and crying, decrease in motor instability, and weight gain. Once symptoms have diminished over 2 to 3 days, drug dosage should be tapered over a 7- to 10-day period. Some degree of irritability may persist for weeks to months and is *not* an indication for prolonged drug therapy.

(4) Phenobarbital is effective in treating CNS symptoms but is not effective for the gastrointestinal (GI) manifestations of drug withdrawal.

(5) Paregoric use has declined because of the toxic effects of its many ingredients.

  h. Home cardiorespiratory monitoring is not routinely indicated.

D. Phencyclidine (PCP).

1. Adverse effects.
   a. Increased rate of prematurity.
   b. IUGR, including microcephaly.
   c. There may be jitteriness, tremors, high-pitched cry, irritability, nystagmus, sudden outbursts of agitation, and marked reactivity to auditory stimuli. These neurobehavioral effects represent PCP intoxication rather than drug withdrawal.
2. Treatment is supportive, using swaddling, gentle handling, and a quiet environment. Drug therapy is not usually indicated.
3. By 1 year of age, most exposed infants show normal growth and development.

E. Stimulants. Cocaine, amphetamines.

1. Cocaine is now the illicit drug used most commonly during pregnancy, often in combination with alcohol, tobacco, and other illicit drugs.
2. Pharmacology.
   a. Cocaine inhibits uptake of neurotransmitters at nerve endings, leading to high circulating levels of epinephrine, norepinephrine, and dopamine.
   b. High circulating catecholamine levels lead to vasoconstriction (decreased uterine blood flow, tachycardia, hypertension) and increased uterine contractility.
   c. Decreased uterine blood flow leads to fetal hypoxia, which further stimulates catecholamine release.
   d. Cocaine readily crosses the placenta and fetal blood-brain barrier and enters the fetal CNS.
   e. Evidence indicates that cocaine exerts direct toxic effects on the fetal brain, as evidenced by the following:
      (1) Abnormal neonatal electroencephalogram (EEG).
      (2) Abnormal neonatal computed tomography (CT) scan.
      (3) Presence of neurobehavioral abnormalities in the newborn period even when cocaine use was discontinued after the first trimester.
      (4) Increased incidence of congenital cerebral anomalies.

    f. Results of urine toxicology testing depend on the timing of last cocaine use in relation to testing, drug clearance rates in the mother and fetus or neonate, and the sensitivity of the drug assay. In most cases in which cocaine has been used within several days of delivery, both mother and newborn have positive results; however, in approximately 15% of cases only the mother will be positive, and in 1% to 2% only the neonate will be positive. Meconium is more reliable than maternal or neonatal urine for the detection of cocaine metabolites; however, this type of testing is not yet widely available.

3. Maternal effects.
    a. Increased rates of spontaneous abortion and stillbirth.
    b. Placental abruption.
    c. Shortened gestation.

4. Fetal/neonatal effects depend on the timing, frequency, duration and intensity of drug use, and concomitant drug use. There is evidence that some but not all of the adverse outcomes can be reduced if cocaine use is discontinued during the pregnancy.
    a. IUGR, including microcephaly. Infants usually show "catch-up" growth by 6 to 12 months, but head circumference may remain significantly smaller through 36 months. Postnatal head growth may be an important marker in predicting long-term developmental outcome.
    b. Perinatal cerebral infarction; neonatal myocardial infarction.
    c. Intrauterine distress (meconium staining, low Apgar scores).
    d. Neonatal neurobehavioral abnormalities, including abnormal sleep pattern; startles, tremors, hypertonia; poor feeding; excitability, irritability; high-pitched cry. Most of these symptoms diminish and then disappear within a few months after birth.
    e. Vomiting, loose stools, sneezing.

N.B.: Neurobehavioral abnormalities usually occur soon after birth and last for several days, but there may be a secondary peak of symptoms at 7 to 10 days.

        (1) Effects may be potentiated by concomitant use of other drugs (e.g., heroin).
        (2) On long-term follow-up, cocaine-exposed infants may show evidence of delay in language, visual processing, reasoning, and fine-motor skills; hyperactivity; and behavior problems; however, there is evidence that most early abnormalities improve over time. Studies on the incidence and severity of long-term neurobehavioral sequelae of in utero cocaine exposure are inconclusive.

    f. Increased incidence of sudden unexpected death during infancy.
    g. Increased incidence of necrotizing enterocolitis (in the absence of usual risk factors).
    h. Abnormalities of control of respiration.
    i. Fetal/neonatal arrhythmias (may be symptomatic and resistant to conventional therapy).
    j. Increased incidence of congenital malformations (presumably secondary to fetal vascular disruption).

      (1) Intestinal atresia.
      (2) Genitourinary abnormalities. Hydronephrosis, hypospadias, Eagle-Barrett (prune-belly) syndrome.
      (3) Skeletal. Limb reduction, cranial defects.
      (4) Cardiac.
      (5) Ocular abnormalities. Strabismus, nystagmus, hypoplastic optic disks.

5. Treatment.
    a. Treatment is supportive; pharmacotherapy is rarely indicated. High-calorie (24 calories per oz) formula should be used in infants with large weight loss. Home cardiorespiratory monitoring has not been shown to be effective and is not recommended.
    b. It is important to carry out an in-depth psychosocial evaluation of cocaine users to assess the need for drug treatment, counseling, intensive family services, protective service referral, and specialized pediatric follow-up services.

F. Tobacco.

1. Effects.
    a. Worldwide, maternal smoking is the leading cause of IUGR; there is a close relationship between maternal serum cotinine levels and birth weight. Passive exposure to paternal smoking also decreases birth weight.
    b. Other effects of maternal smoking.
      (1) Increased rates of spontaneous abortion, prematurity, and perinatal mortality.
      (2) Intrauterine distress (meconium staining, low Apgar scores).
      (3) Neonatal neurobehavioral abnormalities (impaired habituation, orientation, consolability, orientation to sound).
      (4) Signs of nicotine toxicity (tachycardia, irritability, poor feeding).
      (5) Possible increased risk of cancer in childhood.

2. Fetal tobacco syndrome.
    a. Mother smoked ≥ 5 cigarettes per day throughout pregnancy.
    b. No evidence of maternal hypertension.
    c. Evidence of symmetric growth retardation at term without any other obvious cause of IUGR.

IV. BREAST-FEEDING

A. Alcohol, marijuana, nicotine, and cocaine cross freely into breast milk. Significant morbidity and even mortality have been described in infants exposed to cocaine via breast-feeding. Moderate use of alcohol or cigarettes is compatible with breast-feeding.

B. Ongoing cocaine use is an absolute contraindication to breast-feeding.

C. Women with a history of substance abuse may breast-feed if they remain drug free as demonstrated by regular urine toxicology testing.

D. Women on low-dose (<20 mg) methadone maintenance may breast-feed as long as no illicit drug use occurs. Methadone should be taken just after breast-feeding.

BIBLIOGRAPHY

American Academy of Pediatrics Committee on Drugs: Neonatal drug withdrawal, *Pediatrics* 101:1079, 1998.

American Academy of Pediatrics Committee on Substance Abuse: Drug-exposed infants, *Pediatrics* 86:639, 1990.

Bauchner H, Zuckerman B: Cocaine, sudden infant death syndrome, and home monitoring, *J Pediatr* 117:904, 1990.

Chasnoff IJ, Griffith DR, Freier C, Murray J: Cocaine/polydrug use in pregnancy: two-year follow-up, *Pediatrics* 89:284, 1992.

Chasnoff IJ, Hunt CE, Kleter R, et al: Prenatal cocaine exposure is associated with respiratory pattern abnormalities, *Am J Dis Child* 143:583, 1989.

Chasnoff IJ, Lewis DE, Squires L: Cocaine intoxication in a breast-fed infant, *Pediatrics* 80:836, 1987.

Chiriboga CA, Brust JCM, Bateman D, Hauser WA: Dose-response effect of fetal cocaine exposure on newborn neurologic function, *Pediatrics* 103:79, 1999.

Coles CD, Smith IE, Fernhoff PM, et al: Neonatal ethanol withdrawal: characteristics in clinically normal, nondysmorphic neonates, *J Pediatr* 105:445, 1984.

Dominguez R, Vila-Coro AA, Slopis JM, Bohan TP: Brain and ocular abnormalities in infants with in utero exposure to cocaine and other street drugs, *Am J Dis Child* 145:688, 1991.

Frassica JJ, Orva EJ, Walsh EP, Lipschultz SE: Arrhythmias in children prenatally exposed to cocaine, *Arch Pediatr Adolesc Med* 148:1163, 1994.

Fried PA: Marijuana use during pregnancy: consequences for the offspring, *Semin Perinatol* 15:280, 1991.

Herzlinger RA, Kandall SR, Vaughan HG: Neonatal seizures associated with narcotic withdrawal, *J Pediatr* 91:638, 1977.

Johnston C: Cigarette smoking and the outcome of human pregnancies: a status report on the consequences, *Clin Toxicol* 18:189, 1981.

Jones KL: Fetal alcohol syndrome, *Pediatr Rev* 8:122, 1986.

Kandall SR, Gaines J, Habel L, et al: Relationship of maternal substance abuse to subsequent sudden infant death syndrome in offspring, *J Pediatr* 123:120, 1993.

Lipsitz PJ: A proposed narcotic withdrawal score for use with newborn infants: a pragmatic evaluation of its efficacy, *Clin Pediatr* 14:592, 1975.

Nieburg P, Marks JS, McLaren NM, et al: The fetal tobacco syndrome, *JAMA* 253:2998, 1985.

Oro AS, Dixon SD: Perinatal cocaine and methamphetamine exposure: maternal and neonatal correlates, *J Pediatr* 111:571, 1987.

Osterloh JD, Lee BL: Urine drug screening in mothers and newborns, *Am J Dis Child* 143: 791, 1989.

Ostrea EM Jr: Testing for exposure to illicit drugs and other agents in the neonate: a review of laboratory methods and the role of meconium analysis, *Curr Probl Pediatr* 29:41, 1999.

Ostrea EM, Chavez CJ: Perinatal problems (excluding neonatal withdrawal) in maternal drug addiction: a study of 830 cases, *J Pediatr* 94:292, 1979.

Rahbar F, Fomufod A, White D, Westney LS: Impact of intrauterine exposure to phencyclidine (PCP) and cocaine on neonates, *J Natl Med Assoc* 85:349, 1993.

Rajegowda BK, Glass L, Evans HE, et al: Methadone withdrawal in newborn infants, *J Pediatr* 81:532, 1972.

Wachsman L, Schuetz S, Chan LS, et al: What happens to babies exposed to phencyclidine (PCP) in utero? *Am J Drug Alcohol Abuse* 15:31, 1989.

Wagner CL, Katikaneni LD, Cox TH, Ryan RM: The impact of prenatal drug exposure on the neonate, *Obstet Gyn Clin North Am* 25:169, 1998.

Wojnar-Horton RE, Kristensen JH, Yapp P, et al: Methadone distribution and excretion into breast milk of clients in a methadone maintenance programme, *Br J Clin Pharmacol* 44:543, 1997.

22

Inherited Metabolic Diseases

ADA HAMOSH

I. GENERAL PRINCIPLES

A limited number of metabolic diseases cause signs and symptoms in the neonatal period. Although individually rare, collectively they represent a significant cause of neonatal morbidity and mortality. Diagnostic delay leads to irreversible central nervous system (CNS) damage or death. The classic presentation of an inborn error of metabolism is that of a normal full-term newborn who becomes acutely ill after the first 24 to 48 hours of life. The signs exhibited by a newborn with metabolic disease are indistinguishable from those seen in sepsis and in disorders of the cardiovascular system and CNS. They include poor feeding, vomiting, lethargy, hypotonia, seizures, and coma. For this reason, any neonate with no risk factors for infection (e.g., prolonged rupture of membranes, maternal fever) who is deemed sick enough to warrant a blood culture warrants an evaluation for metabolic disease.

II. INITIAL EVALUATION
A. Family history.
1. Neonatal deaths in this sibship (most inborn errors of metabolism are autosomal recessive).
2. Male infant deaths on the maternal side (ornithine transcarbamylase deficiency, the most common urea cycle defect, is X-linked).
3. Consanguinity (increases the risk of autosomal recessive disorders).
B. Blood tests.
1. Venous or arterial blood gas for pH, PCO_2.
2. Serum electrolytes; calculate anion gap.
3. Serum glucose.
4. Plasma ammonium.
5. Complete blood cell (CBC) count with differential.
6. Liver function tests. Serum aspartate aminotransferase (AST) and alanine aminotransferase (ALT), total and direct bilirubin.

7. Plasma lactate.

C. Urine tests.

1. Odor (patients with certain inborn errors excrete large amounts of organic acids with distinctive odors).
2. Ketones.
3. Reducing substances.
4. Ferric chloride.
5. Dinitrophenylhydrazine.

III. DIAGNOSIS

Proper diagnosis of metabolic disease is essential.

A. Therapy is specific for each disorder.

B. If therapy is instituted early, a good outcome is more likely.

C. Provide informed genetic counseling; often there is high recurrence risk within a family; prenatal diagnosis is possible for most inborn errors.

D. Plasma ammonium is elevated in several inborn errors that occur in the newborn period (e.g., primary defects of the urea cycle and several organic acidemias). An algorithm for the diagnosis of hyperammonemia of the newborn is shown in Fig. 22-1. Specific diagnosis of the majority of inborn errors of metabolism requires plasma amino acid analysis by quantitative column chromatography and urine organic acid analysis by gas chromatography mass spectroscopy. These studies require proper sample pro-

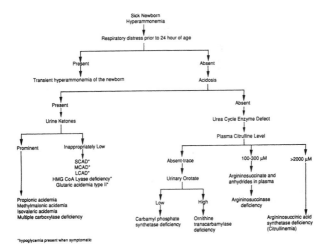

FIG. 22-1. Algorithm for the diagnosis of hyperammonemia in the newborn.

TABLE 22-1
Sample Processing

Specimen	Proper processing
Plasma: Ammonium levels rise rapidly on standing	1-3 ml in a sodium heparin (green top) tube; collect on ice and deliver immediately for analysis
Plasma: Amino acid levels change rapidly on standing and are uninterpretable after feeding	1-3 ml in a sodium heparin (green top) tube, *collected after a 4-hr fast;* deliver on ice, or separate and freeze plasma for later analysis
Plasma: Carnitine	1-3 ml in a sodium heparin (green top) tube; deliver on ice, or separate and freeze plasma for later analysis
Urine: Organic acids	5-10 ml; deliver on ice, or freeze for later analysis
Skin biopsy: Clean a well perfused area* with alcohol, *not* Betadine; use sterile technique	Immerse specimen in tissue culture medium or, if unavailable, patient's own serum; refrigerate; *do not freeze*
Liver biopsy (postmortem):† Obtain specimen as soon as possible for accurate enzyme analysis	"Flash freeze" in liquid nitrogen or on dry ice; store at $-80°$ C for later analysis

*In a viable patient, obtain specimen from the ventral forearm.
† If at all possible, obtain specimen before death.

cessing (Table 22-1) and should be performed only by laboratories proficient in these techniques and able to provide a rapid (1-day) result. Occasionally, skin or liver biopsy (Table 22-1) may be required for diagnosis; however, presumptive therapy should begin as soon as a metabolic disorder is suspected.

IV. MANAGEMENT
A. Immediate interventions.
1. Discontinue protein intake.
2. Provide sufficient calories from glucose (60 kcal/kg per day) to prevent proteolysis and supplemental calories from lipid (60 kcal/kg per day).
B. Any infant in stage II coma (poor muscle tone, few spontaneous movements, but responsive to painful stimuli) or worse is a candidate for immediate hemodialysis, followed by appropriate medical therapy.

N.B.: Hemodialysis is 10 times more effective in removing small molecules than is peritoneal dialysis or arteriovenous hemofiltration. Exchange transfusion does not clear toxins that distribute in total body water and should not be considered therapy for inborn errors of metabolism.

C. Specific therapy for hyperammonemia.

1. Arrange for immediate hemodialysis for any patient with plasma ammonium level more than five times the upper limit of normal or with progressive encephalopathy and elevated ammonia.
2. Simultaneously perform steps listed under immediate interventions.
3. Administer a priming intravenous infusion of sodium benzoate, 250 mg/kg, sodium phenylacetate, 250 mg/kg, and arginine HCl 10% solution, 6 ml/kg, diluted in 35 ml/kg of 10% dextrose solution over 90 minutes; the same solution should then be infused over the next 24 hours (sustaining infusion).
4. Check plasma ammonium level 2 hours after completion of the priming infusion; if normal, continue maintenance infusion (cancel hemodialysis). If elevated, start hemodialysis. If hemodialysis is still not available, start peritoneal dialysis.

N.B.: These disorders are best treated by physicians experienced in the diagnosis and treatment of neonatal metabolic disease. It is usually advisable to transport sick patients to centers with specialized diagnostic facilities. Prompt transfer to a tertiary-care center equipped to perform neonatal hemodialysis may prevent CNS damage and be lifesaving.

V. DISORDERS OF THE UREA CYCLE
A. Carbamoyl phosphate synthetase deficiency (CPSD).

1. Signs and symptoms. Vomiting, irritability, lethargy, seizures, coma.
2. Laboratory findings. Respiratory alkalosis, hyperammonemia (severe), undetectable plasma citrulline, low plasma arginine, low urinary orotic acid.
3. Therapy. Initial therapy as outlined in section IV, except that the arginine HCl should be reduced to 2 ml/kg in sustaining infusion. *Longterm:* Severe protein restriction (0.5 to 0.7 gm/kg per day from natural protein, 0.5 to 0.7 gm/kg per day from essential amino acids; sodium phenylbutyrate, 600 mg/kg per day; citrulline, 175 mg/kg per day).

B. Ornithine transcarbamylase deficiency (OTCD).

1. Signs and symptoms. Vomiting, irritability, lethargy, seizures, coma.
2. Laboratory findings. Respiratory alkalosis, hyperammonemia (severe), undetectable plasma citrulline, low plasma arginine, high urinary orotic acid.
3. Therapy. Initial and long-term therapies are the same as for CPSD.

C. Argininosuccinic acid synthetase deficiency (ASAD).

1. Signs and symptoms. Vomiting, irritability, lethargy, seizures, coma.
2. Laboratory findings. Respiratory alkalosis, hyperammonemia (moderate to severe), high plasma citrulline (>2000 μM), increased urinary orotate.
3. Therapy. Initial, as outlined in section IV; long-term therapy includes protein restriction of 1.5 to 2.0 gm/kg per day, sodium phenylbutyrate 600 mg/kg per day, arginine (freebase) 350 to 750 mg/kg per day.

D. Argininosuccinase deficiency.

1. Signs and symptoms. Vomiting, irritability, lethargy, seizures, coma, hepatomegaly.

2. Laboratory findings. Respiratory alkalosis, hyperammonemia (moderate to severe), high plasma citrulline (>100, <1000 μM), argininosuccinate and anhydrides in plasma.

3. Therapy. Initial as outlined in section IV, except only intravenous arginine HCl 10% solution, 6 ml/kg or 12 gm/m^2 over 90 minutes in 25 to 35 ml/kg 10% Dextrose, and then repeat this infusion over the next 24 hours (i.e., no phenylacetate or benzoate required). Long-term therapy includes protein restriction to 1.5 to 2.0 gm/kg per day, arginine (freebase) 400-700 mg/kg per day or 8.8 to 15.4 gm/m^2 per day.

VI. DISORDERS OF AMINO ACID METABOLISM

A. Maple syrup urine disease (MSUD).

1. Etiology. Branched-chain ketoacid decarboxylase deficiency.

2. Signs and symptoms. Vomiting, lethargy, hypotonia alternating with spasticity, seizures, coma, maple syrup odor of sweat and urine.

3. Laboratory findings. Metabolic acidosis, ketosis, usually increased anion gap, gray-green color of urine with the ferric chloride test, positive 2,4-dinitrophenylhydrazine test on urine, positive blood test for leucine by bacterial inhibition assay (included in some state newborn metabolic screens), and elevated leucine, isoleucine, and valine on plasma amino acid determination: urine organic acids positive for 2-ketoisocaproic, 2-ketoisovaleric, and 2-keto-3-methylvaleric acid.

4. Therapy. For initial therapy, eliminate natural protein from the diet, provide sufficient calories from glucose and lipid to prevent catabolism, and hemodialysis to prevent CNS damage from leucine accumulation. Long-term therapy requires a special diet with restricted leucine, isoleucine, and valine; condition may be responsive to thiamine.

B. Isovaleric acidemia.

1. Etiology. Isovaleryl coenzyme A (CoA) dehydrogenase deficiency.

2. Signs and symptoms. Vomiting, lethargy, hypotonia, seizures, coma, "sweaty feet" odor of urine.

3. Laboratory findings. Metabolic acidosis, ketosis, increased anion gap, occasional mild hyperammonemia, urine organic acids positive for isovalerylglycine and 3-hydroxyisovaleric acid.

4. Therapy. Initial therapy is the same as for MSUD. Long-term therapy involves a special diet restricted in leucine and supplemental glycine to promote excretion of isovaleric acid as isovalerylglycine.

C. Propionic acidemia.

1. Etiology. Propionyl CoA carboxylase deficiency.

2. Signs and symptoms. Vomiting, lethargy, hypotonia, seizures, coma.

3. Laboratory findings. Metabolic acidosis, ketosis, elevated anion gap, neutropenia, occasional thrombocytopenia, occasional hyperammonemia (may be severe), twofold to fourfold elevation in plasma glycine; 3-hydroxypropionate and methylcitrate in urine.

4. Therapy. Initial therapy is to eliminate protein, prevent catabolism,

treat acidosis (usually requires bicarbonate), and treat hyperammonemia as outlined in section IV. Long-term therapy involves a special diet restricted in valine, threonine, methionine, and isoleucine; provide carnitine supplementation; some forms are responsive to biotin.

D. Methylmalonic acidosis.

1. Etiology. Methylmalonyl CoA mutase deficiency, adenosylcobalamin synthetic defect.
2. Signs and symptoms. Poor feeding, vomiting, lethargy, and hypotonia; rarely, seizures and coma.
3. Laboratory findings. Metabolic acidosis, ketosis, elevated anion gap, occasional hyperammonemia (may be severe), twofold to fourfold elevation in plasma glycine, methylmalonic acid in urine. Some forms also have homocystine in urine.
4. Therapy. Initial therapy is the same as for propionic acidemia. Long-term therapy requires a special diet restricted in valine, threonine, methionine, and isoleucine; some forms are responsive to hydroxycobalamin; carnitine supplementation may be helpful.

E. Multiple carboxylase deficiency.

1. Etiology. Holocarboxylase synthetase deficiency.
2. Signs and symptoms. Poor feeding, vomiting, lethargy, hypotonia, seizures, mild to moderate hyperammonemia, coma, urine odor of cat's urine; later, erythematous rash, alopecia, and seizures.
3. Laboratory findings. Metabolic acidosis, ketosis, elevated anion gap, occasional moderate hyperammonemia, lactic acidosis, 3-methylcrotonylglycine, 3-hydroxyisovaleric acid, 3-hydroxypropionic acid, methylcitrate in urine.
4. Therapy. Initial therapy as outlined in section IV, usually responsive to oral biotin (10 mg per day).

F. Nonketotic hyperglycinemia.

1. Etiology. Defect in the glycine cleavage system.
2. Signs and symptoms. Poor feeding, seizures (burst-suppression pattern), hiccups, apnea, coma.
3. Laboratory findings. None on routine tests, threefold to fivefold increase in plasma glycine, more than tenfold increase in cerebrospinal fluid (CSF) glycine.
4. Therapy. Initial therapy is supportive. There is no consistently effective therapy, but sodium benzoate 500 to 750 mg/kg per day (orally) reduces seizures; dextromethorphan 5 to 25 mg/kg per day (orally) may be effective.

G. Glutaric acidemia, type 2.

1. Etiology. Electron transport flavoprotein (ETF) or ETF dehydrogenase deficiency.
2. Signs and symptoms. Poor feeding, vomiting, lethargy, seizures, coma, "sweaty feet" odor to urine, hepatomegaly, may have associated anomalies (usually renal cysts).
3. Laboratory findings. Severe metabolic acidosis, hypoglycemia, *no* ketosis, hyperammonemia.
4. Therapy. Supportive; no effective therapy exists.

H. Tyrosinemia.

1. Transient neonatal.
   a. Etiology. Unknown, probably relative deficiency of *p*-hydroxy-phenylpyruvate oxidase.
   b. Signs and symptoms. Poor feeding, lethargy, prolonged jaundice.
   c. Laboratory findings. Metabolic acidosis, hyperbilirubinemia, hypercholesterolemia, elevated tyrosine, phenylalanine, and histidine levels on plasma amino acid analysis.
   d. Therapy. Protein restriction to 2 gm/kg per day (breast-feeding is effective).

2. Hepatorenal.
   a. Etiology. Fumarylacetoacetate hydrolase deficiency.
   b. Signs and symptoms (not usually present until after the first week of life). Failure to thrive, vomiting, diarrhea, "cabbage" odor, hepatomegaly, fever, edema, melena, epistaxis.
   c. Laboratory findings. Normocytic anemia, leukocytosis, occasionally thrombocytosis, hyperbilirubinemia, abnormal liver function tests, prolonged prothrombin time, hypocholesterolemia, elevated alpha-fetoprotein, elevated plasma tyrosine and methionine, hematuria, glycosuria, and generalized aminoaciduria. The presence of succinylacetone in the urine is diagnostic.
   d. Therapy. A special diet restricted in tyrosine, phenylalanine, and methionine; NTBC (2-(2-nitro-4-trifluorobenzoyl)-1.3-cyclohexanedione) 0.1-0.6 mg/kg per day is effective in 90% of patients; liver transplant is curative for the rest.

I. Pyroglutamic acidemia.

1. Etiology. Glutathione synthetase deficiency.
2. Signs and symptoms. Poor feeding, vomiting, lethargy, jaundice, coma.
3. Laboratory findings. Metabolic acidosis, hyperbilirubinemia; urine organic acids show 5-oxoproline.
4. Therapy. Initial therapy as outlined in section IV; long-term, chronic sodium bicarbonate therapy is usually required.

VII. DISORDERS OF CARBOHYDRATE METABOLISM

A. Galactosemia.

1. Etiology. Galactose 1-phosphate uridyltransferase deficiency.
2. Signs and symptoms. Poor feeding, vomiting, diarrhea, jaundice, hepatomegaly, cataracts.
3. Laboratory findings. Hyperchloremic metabolic acidosis, indirect hyperbilirubinemia (early), direct hyperbilirubinemia (later), abnormal liver function tests; often associated with *Escherichia coli* sepsis; urine positive for reducing substances on Clinitest; galactose on paper chromatography of urine.
4. Therapy. Discontinue galactose-containing formula (any formula with lactose), substitute a nongalactose formula (e.g., soy); supportive as necessary.

B. Glycogen storage disease, types 1A, 1B.

1. Etiology. 1A: glucose-6-phosphatase deficiency; 1B: glucose-6-phosphatase translocase deficiency.
2. Signs and symptoms. Hepatomegaly, seizures.
3. Laboratory findings. Hypoglycemia, metabolic acidosis, ketosis, lactic acidosis, hypercholesterolemia, hypertriglyceridemia, hyperuricemia, abnormal liver function tests.
4. Therapy. Long-term therapy involves frequent feeds (every 3 hours) with cornstarch and continuous enteral nightly feedings; allopurinol to treat hyperuricemia.

C. Hereditary fructose intolerance.

1. Etiology. Fructose 1-phosphatealdolase deficiency.
2. Signs and symptoms (require exposure to fructose, which is present in sucrose, fruit juices, Nursoy, and some oral antibiotics). Vomiting, hepatomegaly, jaundice, sepsis, seizures, coma.
3. Laboratory findings. Metabolic acidosis, ketosis, hypoglycemia, elevated lactate; diagnosis later confirmed by intravenous fructose tolerance test or measurement of hepatic enzyme activity.
4. Therapy. Initial therapy is to discontinue fructose and supportive care; for long-term therapy, eliminate fructose and sucrose from the diet.

VIII. DISORDERS OF FATTY ACID METABOLISM

In addition to the disorders listed below there is also a very long chain acyl-CoA dehydrogenase deficiency and for each of the chain lengths there is a hydroxy-acyl-CoA dehydrogenase deficiency. Each may sometimes present with hepatic encephalopathy, with cardiomyopathy/myopathy or with both. This field is rapidly growing. An acylcarnitine profile of dried blood on filter paper is diagnostic or suggestive and should always be performed when this class of disorders is considered.

A. Medium chain acyl-CoA dehydrogenase deficiency (MCAD).

1. Signs and symptoms. Lethargy, seizures, coma, hepatomegaly, dilated cardiomyopathy, sudden infant death syndrome.
2. Laboratory findings. Hypoglycemia with inappropriately low or absent urine ketones, metabolic acidosis, occasionally hyperammonemia, abnormal liver function tests, low plasma carnitine, urine organic acids show medium chain dicarboxylic acids and acyl carnitines, phenylpropionyl glycine, hexanoyl glycine, and subaryl glycine.
3. Therapy. Initial therapy is as described in section IV. If hyperammonemic, as described above, carnitine supplementation (100 mg/kg per day) is required. For long-term therapy, avoid prolonged fasting, add carnitine supplementation, provide intravenous glucose infusion to prevent hypoglycemia associated with catabolism during intercurrent illness.

B. Short chain acyl-CoA dehydrogenase deficiency (SCAD).

1. Signs and symptoms are the same as for MCAD. Examination may reveal only cardiomyopathy, which can be dilated or hypertrophic.

2. Laboratory findings are the same as for MCAD, except urine organic acids show only ethylmalonic acid.

3. Therapy is the same as for MCAD.

C. Long chain acyl-CoA dehydrogenase deficiency (LCAD).

1. Signs and symptoms are the same as for MCAD; hypertrophic cardiomyopathy has been described in some cases.

2. Laboratory findings are the same as for MCAD, except urine shows only dicarboxylic acids.

3. Therapy is the same as for MCAD, but a low-fat diet is recommended.

D. Hydroxymethylglutaryl-CoA lyase deficiency (HMG).

1. Signs and symptoms are the same as for MCAD; urine has an odor similar to cat's urine.

2. Laboratory findings are the same as for MCAD, except urine shows 3-hydroxy-3-methylglutaric acid and 3-methylglutaconic acid.

3. Therapy is the same as for MCAD.

IX. CONGENITAL LACTIC ACIDOSES

A. Pyruvate dehydrogenase complex deficiency (PDH).

B. Pyruvate carboxylase deficiency (PC).

C. Defects of the electron transport chain (ETC).

1. Signs and symptoms may occur before 24 hours of age. Hypotonia and respiratory distress from severe metabolic acidosis, apnea, coma, dilated cardiomyopathy; may have associated dysmorphic features; may be small for gestational age (SGA); abnormal brain imaging.

2. Laboratory findings. Normoglycemic; severe metabolic acidosis caused by sharply elevated lactate, absence of other organic acids, elevated pyruvate (normal lactate/pyruvate ratio of <25) suggests PDH; decreased or normal pyruvate (increased lactate/pyruvate ratio of >35) suggests PC or ETC defects. PC deficiency type B causes lactic acidemia, citrullinemia, and hyperammonemia; ETC defects require muscle biopsy for diagnosis.

3. Therapy. High-dose vitamin therapy may be helpful for PDH or PC; no therapy exists for ETC defects.

X. OTHER DISORDERS

Peroxisomal disorders may present in the newborn period with dysmorphic features and hepatomegaly (Zellweger syndrome) or with isolated neonatal seizures. Very long chain fatty acid and plasmalogen levels in whole blood (EDTA) are diagnostic or suggestive. Rarely, lysosomal storage diseases may present as neonatal hydrops and should be included in the differential. Smith-Lemli-Opitz syndrome (characterized by multiple congenital anomalies including ptosis, upturned nose, heart defects, cryptorchidism, and syndactyly of the second and third toes) is caused by a defect in cholesterol synthesis and can be diagnosed by measuring 7-dehydrocholesterol, which is markedly elevated in plasma. In severely affected infants, serum cholesterol is very low.

XI. THE DEAD OR DYING INFANT

Any infant dying of unknown cause or of suspected metabolic disease requires a diagnosis for genetic counseling and accurate diagnosis in subsequent pregnancies. A full autopsy, including radiographic skeletal survey, should be performed. Specimens required for diagnosis include the following (see Table 22-1 for proper processing):

A. Blood. For assessment of plasma amino acids, plasma carnitine, and an acylcarnitine profile, obtain extra serum (clotted) and plasma (heparinized); separate and freeze; freeze the red blood cells (RBCs) separately.

B. Urine. For organic acids, reducing substances, and ketones; freeze.

C. Skin. Fibroblast culture for enzymatic analysis and for DNA diagnosis.

D. Liver. Freeze a specimen for enzymatic analysis.

XII. NEONATAL METABOLIC SCREENING

Every state screens for phenylketonuria and hypothyroidism, both insidious conditions that lead to preventable mental retardation. Most states also screen for the hemoglobinopathies and galactosemia. Many states screen for MSUD, tyrosinemia, homocystinuria (an enzyme defect causing mental retardation, hypercoagulability, long-bone overgrowth, and ocular lens dislocation), biotinidase deficiency (similar to multiple carboxylase deficiency, but of later onset), and congenital adrenal hyperplasia. Several states screen for cystic fibrosis.

Routine metabolic screening of the newborn should be performed after sufficient nutrient consumption has resulted in the accumulation of toxic metabolites, but before this accumulation has become symptomatic. The former is rarely accomplished before 24 hours of age. The initial screen should occur between 48 and 72 hours of age, except possibly in formula-fed infants, who can be screened as early as 24 hours. Repeat screening should be performed between 2 and 4 weeks of age; earlier repeat screening (1 to 2 weeks) is suggested for those breast-fed infants initially screened before 48 hours and formula-fed infants screened before 24 hours.

BIBLIOGRAPHY

American Academy of Pediatrics Committee on Genetics: Newborn screening fact sheets, *Pediatrics* 83:449, 1989.

Brusilow SW, Valle DL, Arn P: Symptomatic inborn errors of metabolism. In Nelson NM (editor): *Current therapy in neonatal-perinatal medicine,* ed 2, Philadelphia, 1989, Decker.

Burton B: Inborn errors of metabolism in infancy: a guide to diagnosis, *Pediatrics* 102:E69, 1998.

Fernandez J, Saudubray JM, Tada K (editors): *Inborn metabolic diseases,* Berlin, 1990, Springer-Verlag.

Scriver CR, Beaudet AL, Sly WS, et al (editors): *The metabolic and molecular bases of inherited disease,* ed 7, New York, 1995, McGraw-Hill.

23

Metabolism and Endocrinology

MARVIN CORNBLATH

I. GENERAL

A number of congenital, inherited, and adaptive metabolic and endocrine abnormalities may occur in the full-term neonate. Fortunately, they are uncommon or rare. Furthermore, relatively few call for urgent attention and care. In this chapter, the emphasis will be on problems that require immediate decisions to be made regarding advising parents, establishing a proper diagnosis, and ordering or providing appropriate treatment. These problems include ambiguous genitalia and assignment of gender role; seizures of metabolic/endocrine origin that are amenable to therapy; hypoglycemia, hypocalcemia, and hypomagnesemia before or associated with clinical manifestations; and inborn errors of metabolism that benefit from identification during the neonatal period. Although decisions may have to be made for immediate care, the definitive diagnostic investigation of the problem usually involves consultants, specialized diagnostic studies and procedures, and time for the clinical course of the problem to be manifest. Each problem is discussed in the order of the frequency of its occurrence.

II. HYPOGLYCEMIA

The definition of hypoglycemia in the term or near-term newborn infant remains elusive because of the lack of any significant correlation between plasma glucose concentrations with or without clinical manifestations and long-term outcome. Therefore the definition of "significant hypoglycemia" cannot be based on a single blood glucose value for all infants under all conditions, and the concept of a *threshold value* for plasma glucose at which clinical intervention is indicated is more appropriate and correct than "significant hypoglycemia" as a guide to care. Based on available data, regular monitoring and therapeutic intervention to raise the blood glucose level in infants with clinical manifestations should be considered at plasma glucose concentrations of 45 mg/dl (2.5 mM) or less (the *operational threshold*). In an asymptomatic newborn and in those "at risk" for hypoglycemia (see below), plasma glucose levels less than 35 mg/dl (2.0 mM) should be considered as threshold values. The threshold values for surveillance and intervention must be separated from therapeutic goals, which should be significantly higher at 60 to 90 mg/dl (3.3 to 5.0 mM). A reliable serum or plasma glucose value is necessary for establishing the glucose status of a newborn at any specific age.

A. Clinical management is based on four principles: (1) Screening infants at risk (routine screening of normal term newborns is not indicated), (2) confirming that the plasma glucose is low, (3) demonstrating that the low glucose is responsible for the clinical manifestations when these have cleared after blood glucose has been restored to normoglycemia, and (4) observing and documenting all of these events.

1. Screening. Hypoglycemia can frequently be anticipated by screening infants known to be at risk, including those whose history includes any of the following:
   a. Intrapartum glucose administration to mother.
   b. Maternal drug treatment (e.g., terbutaline, beta blockers, oral hypoglycemics).
   c. Infants of insulin-dependent or gestational diabetic mothers, or of massively obese mothers.
   d. Infants who are large for gestational age (LGA) (>90th percentile).
   e. Infants who are small for gestational age (SGA) (<10th percentile, or the smaller of discordant twins).
   f. Significant hypoxia, perinatal distress, or Apgar scores <5 at 5 minutes, requiring resuscitation.
   g. Severe erythroblastosis (cord blood hemoglobin level <10 g/dl).
   h. Polycythemia.
   i. Isolated hepatomegaly.
   j. Congenital cardiac malformations.
   k. Sepsis.
   l. Any infant with microphallus or anterior midline defect, especially with hyperbilirubinemia.
   m. Infant with exomphalos, macroglossia, and gigantism.
   n. Family history of neonate with hypoglycemia or unexplained death in infancy.
   o. Inborn errors of metabolism.
2. Screening can be done beginning at 2 to 4 hours of age and then before feeding for 12 to 48 hours of age, or whenever a baby becomes symptomatic with any of the following clinical manifestations:
   a. Change in level of consciousness.
   b. Episodes of tremors, cyanosis, seizures, apnea, limpness, irregular respirations, listlessness, difficulty in feeding, exaggerated Moro reflex, irritability, high-pitched cry, or coma.

3. Clinical manifestations should subside within minutes to hours in response to adequate treatment with intravenous glucose if hypoglycemia alone is responsible. The clinical manifestations are not specific and have been associated with a number of neonatal problems. In addition, the hypoglycemia may be associated with or may be secondary to other diseases (e.g., meningitis, intraventricular hemorrhage, intracranial hemorrhage, gram-negative sepsis, congenital heart disease, maternal drugs, or TORCH infections), which by themselves may be responsible for the observed clinical manifestations.

B. Screening procedure.

1. All glucose oxidase strip tests, whether read by meter or by eye, are too variable and unreliable to establish the diagnosis. However, bedside glucose screening is feasible by quantitative techniques such as the glucose oxidase analyzer or the newer optical bedside glucose sensors.

2. When glucose oxidase strip tests are used, any value <40 mg/dl should be confirmed by a reliable laboratory method before making the diagnosis in a symptomatic newborn or initiating therapy in the asymptomatic neonate.

C. Operational thresholds are an indication for action, but are not diagnostic of a disease. These thresholds are based on clinical and experimental data, are conservative approximations, and designate the lower level of normoglycemia. The operational threshold for surveillance and therapeutic intervention vary among the following specific groups of infants:

1. Symptomatic infants. Glucose values of 45 mg/dl (2.4 mM) or less require a response.

2. Asymptomatic infants and those at risk for hypoglycemia. Whether the infant is full term or preterm (34 to 37 weeks gestational age), plasma glucose values less than 30 to 35 mg/dl (1.7 to 2.0 mM) require close monitoring and intervention if these low levels persist. It appears that during the establishment of adequate feedings, breast-fed infants who otherwise have no abnormalities often have lower plasma glucose values associated with elevated ketone bodies. Unless they are symptomatic, these infants usually do not require any intervention.

3. Plasma or serum glucose values less than 20 to 25 mg/dl indicate significant hypoglycemia requiring parenteral glucose therapy and careful monitoring.

D. Diagnosis is based on the following: (1) the presence of clinical manifestations (noted above), (2) a laboratory-confirmed glucose concentration (<35 to 45 mg/dl), and (3) the clearing of all clinical manifestations after raising the level of glucose over 45 mg/dl (Whipple triad). Only by satisfying all of this triad and documenting the results is it reasonable to consider the diagnosis of significant neonatal hypoglycemia.

1. Diagnosis requires a reliable laboratory determination of plasma glucose obtained and kept in a manner to avoid increased glycolysis known to occur in newborn red blood cells.

2. Whether plasma values between 25 and 45 to 50 mg/dl are of any significance or consequence remains unanswered at this time. The evidence suggests they are not, except in medicolegal litigation.

E. Therapy.

1. To maintain glucose levels in the 40 to 50 mg/dl range, oral glucose (10 ml/kg 5% dextrose water) may be given by nipple or gavage in the asymptomatic infant. The plasma glucose should be checked again in 30 to 60 minutes and thereafter as necessary to ensure that the glucose values are normal.

2. In the symptomatic infant unable to take a nipple, or in those with a glucose level of <25 mg/dl, parenteral glucose should be given. Initially a bolus of 0.25 gm/kg or 2.5 ml/kg of 10% glucose, or 1.0 ml/kg of 25% glucose can be given at the rate of 1 to 2 ml per minute. Continue the intravenous glucose at the rate of 6 to 8 mg/kg per minute as 5%, 10%, or 15% glucose in water, depending on the fluid needs and clinical condition of the infant. Plasma glucose levels should be maintained above 50 mg/dl (2.8 mM) in these infants.

3. After 12 hours, add sodium chloride (40 mEq/L, or quarter-strength saline) to provide 1 to 2 mEq/kg per day to prevent iatrogenic hyponatremia. After 48 hours, add potassium (as KCl or buffered potassium phosphate) to provide 1 to 2 mEq/kg per day.

4. Plasma glucose values should be followed at 1- to 3-hour intervals initially to determine the effectiveness of therapy and then at 4- to 8-hour intervals to ensure that normoglycemia has been maintained.

5. If it is too difficult or impossible to give parenteral glucose, glucagon (300 µg/kg, *not to exceed 1.0 mg total*) may be given subcutaneously or intramuscularly while the infant is being transferred to a neonatal intensive care unit (NICU).

6. If the hypoglycemia persists after 10 to 12 mg/kg per minute of glucose, give prednisone 2 mg/kg per day orally or hydrocortisone 5 mg/kg per day either orally or intravenously; obtain a consultation and, if indicated, transfer the infant to a NICU for diagnosis and care.

F. Prognosis.

1. Hypoglycemia of short duration (<12 to 18 hours), even if symptomatic, does not appear to have well-documented long-term sequelae.

2. If hypoglycemia is severe, persistent, or recurrent, there may be long-term consequences. More often than not, the hypoglycemia is associated with or is secondary to a multiplicity of problems, ranging from central nervous system (CNS) congenital anomalies to hypocalcemia or polycythemia, and the outcome may be more directly related to the primary disease than to the secondary hypoglycemia.

N.B.: Be sure to document in the chart all of the glucose values, their source and method of analysis, and all clinical manifestations related to the hypoglycemia. Finally (most important and most often neglected), be sure to note the response of the clinical manifestations and that of the plasma glucose level to the therapy that has been initiated. Clinical manifestations should subside within minutes to hours in response to adequate treatment. This is critical to establish the clinical significance of the hypoglycemia.

III. HYPERGLYCEMIA

A. **Hyperglycemia (plasma glucose >150 to 180 mg/dl),** although relatively frequent in the "micropremie" (<1000 g or <30 weeks of gestation), is rare in the full-term neonate and occurs under three distinct conditions.

1. Iatrogenic transient hyperglycemia. Secondary to glucose administration, especially if associated with stress (intraventricular hemorrhage [IVH], sepsis, meningitis, and hypoxic ischemic encephalopathy).

2. Transient neonatal diabetes mellitus.
   a. Usually in SGA infants.
   b. Can be familial.
   c. May require insulin for varying periods of time.
   d. Normal or transient reduction in C-peptide levels in serum or urine.
   e. Ketonuria absent.
   f. Rarely, follows transient hypoglycemia.
   g. Good prognosis; it is extremely rare for it to occur as true insulin-dependent diabetes at an older age.

3. Insulin-dependent diabetes mellitus (IDDM), or permanent diabetes.
   a. Requires insulin throughout life.
   b. Low to absent C-peptide levels, which do not recover.
   c. Rare.

B. **Clinical presentation.**

1. Significant hyperglycemia is manifest by weight loss, dehydration, polyuria, and glucosuria, usually in the presence of a good food intake and the absence of diarrhea or vomiting. A plasma glucose value >150 to 200 mg/dl establishes the diagnosis. In both transient and permanent diabetes mellitus, the plasma glucose may range between 300 and 2000 mg/dl.

2. Symptoms and signs may occur anytime after starting parenteral glucose at 10% or higher concentrations at rates exceeding 8 to 10 mg/kg/min, but they are usually present during the first 48 to 72 hours of therapy. Transient or permanent diabetes usually manifests itself at a mean of 12 days but can occur anytime between days 1 and 42. Both may be associated with infections or vomiting.

C. **Diagnosis is confirmed by a reliable laboratory determination of a plasma glucose value >150 to 200 mg/dl at the time of symptoms.** A glucose oxidase strip test, although more reliable at hyperglycemic than at hypoglycemic levels, is a screening test only and must be confirmed by a laboratory glucose determination to establish the diagnosis. Von Muhlendahl and Herkenhoff have redefined neonatal diabetes mellitus as hyperglycemia requiring insulin treatment, occurring during the first month of life, and lasting more than 2 weeks. They point out that the diabetes may represent an underlying congenital metabolic defect or Wolcott-Rallison syndrome. These findings remain to be confirmed. Not everyone agrees with the definition.

D. **Treatment.**

1. For transient hyperglycemia secondary to parenteral fluids, reduce the concentration or rate of the infusion slowly. It may be necessary to discontinue the fluids if hyperglycemia persists.

2. In the absence of parenteral glucose therapy, the infant should be referred to a consultant with experience in managing neonates or young infants with diabetes mellitus or should be managed in consultation with such an individual.

E. Prognosis is excellent for the infant with transient hyperglycemia and transient diabetes mellitus. Rarely, the infant with the latter may develop IDDM during adolescence or in early adulthood. Too few neonates have IDDM to permit any definitive statement.

N.B.: Until the complete clinical course of the hyperglycemia has been observed, it is often impossible to differentiate between the three conditions just noted. By and large the outcome is excellent, but it is still necessary to await the recovery of the infant to be relatively sure of the prognosis. However, current studies to identify specific markers and antibody characteristics of type 1 insulin-dependent diabetes should permit a specific diagnosis in these infants early in their clinical course.

IV. TETANY—HYPOCALCEMIA (HYPOMAGNESEMIA)

A. Hypocalcemia (a total serum calcium value of <8.0 mg/dl in full-term and <7.0 mg/dl in preterm infants, or an ionized calcium concentration of <3.0 to 3.5 mg/dl) is unusual in full-term infants.

1. Early neonatal hypocalcemia in the first 24 to 48 hours of life occurs with a frequency of 25% to 30% in preterm infants and in full-term infants of diabetic mothers, infants delivered by cesarean section, infants with birth asphyxia, and infants of mothers taking anticonvulsant medications not supplemented with vitamin D. Rarely, hypocalcemia is secondary to maternal hyperparathyroidism and may be the clue to the diagnosis in the mother.

2. Late neonatal hypocalcemia (presenting after 3 days of age) is now relatively rare and is usually formula related.

3. Because these infants may be asymptomatic, screening high-risk infants is indicated, as well as establishing the diagnosis in symptomatic infants.

B. Clinical presentation. Neonatal hypocalcemia is characterized by increased neuromuscular irritability or activity ("jitteriness"), jerky movements of one or more limbs (twitching), and generalized convulsions. The classic signs of a high-pitched cry, facial muscle twitching when stimulated (Chvostek sign), and carpal spasm after constricting the upper arm (Trousseau sign) are seen more often in older infants but may occur in the neonate.

C. Diagnosis.

1. A laboratory determination of a total serum calcium value of <8.0 mg/dl or an ionized calcium level of <5.0 mg/dl is confirmatory. Abnormalities in the electrocardiogram (ECG) with a prolonged Q-T interval (corrected for heart rate) >0.40 second or a corrected Q_0-T interval of >0.20 second may be present with hypocalcemia.

2. Because the clinical manifestations of hypomagnesemia are similar to those of hypocalcemia, it is prudent to obtain a serum magnesium

value as well. A value of <1.2 to 1.6 mg/dl is considered abnormally low.

3. The differential diagnosis includes hypomagnesemia, hypoglycemia, narcotic withdrawal, CNS abnormalities, and sepsis.

D. Treatment.

1. In the symptomatic infant, parenteral calcium (10% calcium gluconate, 2 ml/kg; 18 mg of elemental calcium per kilogram) is given in a peripheral vein over 10 minutes while monitoring the heart rate to avoid bradycardia or cardiac arrest. Care must also be taken to avoid extravasation of the calcium because a tissue slough can occur.

2. Therapy is then continued with either oral or parenteral calcium gluconate at a dose of 75 mg/kg of elemental calcium per day (8 to 9 ml 10% calcium gluconate per kilogram per day) until normocalcemia is achieved. If given parenterally, reduce the calcium by 37.5 mg/kg per day, giving 18 mg/kg on the last day to avoid rebound hypocalcemia. Oral 10% calcium gluconate should also be discontinued over a period of several days. Diarrhea can occur with oral calcium salts.

3. Failure to respond may indicate concurrent hypomagnesemia, which can be treated by the intramuscular administration of 0.1 to 0.2 ml of 50% magnesium sulfate solution every 12 hours. Magnesium levels should be monitored every 12 hours.

E. Prognosis is excellent for the infant with transient hypocalcemia and hypomagnesemia.

N.B.: Until the complete clinical course of the patient with hypocalcemia has been observed, it is often impossible to differentiate between the transient neonatal type of hypocalcemia and the persistent or recurrent type that might represent underlying disease. It is necessary to await the recovery of the infant to be relatively sure of the prognosis.

V. HYPOTHYROIDISM

Congenital hypothyroidism, defined as a serum T_4 concentration <6 μg/dl and a thyroid-stimulating hormone (TSH) level >20 μU/Uml on day 2 to 5 on a filter paper screen, occurs in approximately 1:3000 to 4000 live births. It may be the result of thyroid dysgenesis or agenesis, inborn defect in hormone synthesis or metabolism, maternal iodine ingestion (often resulting in an infant with goiter), or antithyroid medication or autoimmune disease, or it may occur secondary to TSH or thyrotropin-releasing hormone (TRH) deficiencies. Almost every patient has been detected by the metabolic screening test done routinely on discharge from the nursery. Rarely, an infant may have clinical manifestations of neonatal cretinism before the result of the metabolic screen is reported.

N.B.: In Maryland, parental consent is required for the test to be performed.

A. Clinical manifestations and management.

1. Screening. Essentially all neonates are screened for hypothyroidism in the majority of states in the United States and worldwide in industrialized countries. If a low T_4 or a high TSH value is reported, it is crit-

ical to confirm the result by a laboratory measurement of T_4 and TSH to establish the diagnosis and the baseline for therapy.

2. Because low thyroid hormone concentrations may be caused by multiple defects, both primary and secondary to intrinsic and extrinsic abnormalities, referral to a pediatric endocrinologist for definitive diagnosis and treatment is indicated.

3. Although usually asymptomatic, the rare neonate may show delayed bone maturation (e.g., abnormally large fontanels); poor feeding; vomiting; moderately elevated or prolonged jaundice (often with an elevated direct component); lethargy; poor peripheral circulation; cool, mottled skin; and facial edema. These rarely occur before 4 to 6 weeks of age, long after the screening and confirming results should be known.

B. Diagnosis. After a positive screening test, reliable laboratory determinations of T_4 levels <6.5 μg/dl and of TSH >20 μU/ml are diagnostic of primary congenital hypothyroidism. If TSH is normal (<10 to 15 μU/ml) with an abnormally low T_4, the infant may have transient hypothyroidism secondary to iodides taken by the mother, or hypothalamic-hypopituitary hypothyroidism. Follow-up studies are indicated to determine the exact etiology.

C. Treatment. Once the diagnosis is established and often before clinical manifestations appear, L-thyroxine is given as a starting dose of 5 to 15 μg/kg per day depending on the severity of the hypothyroidism. Frequent monitoring of T_4 levels is necessary to determine the optimal dose. Required dosage may be as high as 25 to 50 μg/kg per day.

D. Prognosis. Thyroid hormone actions in the fetus are to stimulate cellular metabolism and growth and maturation of a variety of organs. Most important, thyroid hormone is critical for the growth and development of the brain from early in fetal life throughout the first 2 to 3 years of life. Therefore early diagnosis and prompt, adequate treatment are essential to obtain the best possible outcome. Because those deficiencies, if any, that occurred in utero are unknown, a definitive prognosis cannot be given in the newborn period, even with the current advantages of early diagnosis and therapy as a result of newborn screening.

N.B.: Expediting confirmatory laboratory diagnosis of an abnormal screening value and prompt consultation with a pediatric endocrinologist to enable initiation of therapy are clearly indicated. Documented communications with the parents and carefully dated and timed laboratory results and therapeutic decisions are important. Recent reports indicate that untreated or even mild maternal hypothyroidism in pregnancy may adversely affect fetal brain development, resulting in reduced IQ scores and other abnormalities of intelligence, aptitude, and visual motor skills.

VI. HYPERTHYROIDISM

Although extremely rare, hyperthyroidism occurs in approximately 2% of pregnancies complicated by maternal Graves' disease. With an estimated prevalence of Graves' disease of 1:500 pregnancies, approximately 1:25,000 live-born infants may have thyrotoxicosis. A history of Graves' disease in the mother, either during or before the current pregnancy, and maternal hypothyroidism secondary to Hashimoto's thyroiditis plus fetal tachycardia (>160 beats per minute) are indications to obtain serum T_4, T_3, TSH, and thyroid-stimulating immunoglobulin-G (TSI) titers either on the cord blood or on day 2 to 3 of life. T_4 values >30 to 50 μg/dl, T_3 >400 ng/dl, TSH <8 μU/ml, and high titers of TSI are present concurrently.

A. Clinical manifestations and management.

1. Evidence of fetal hyperthyroidism includes growth retardation, goiter (highly variable in size), advanced bone age, and craniosynostosis.

2. Neonatal manifestations may occur within 24 to 48 hours of age and are usually transient, but they may be chronic or delayed, or persist as evidence of familial Graves' disease. Symptoms can also occur at 1 week of age when maternal antithyroid medications have been eliminated from the neonatal circulation. These include irritability, flushing, tachycardia, poor feeding, failure to thrive, and prolonged jaundice, as well as a small goiter and exophthalmos.

3. Thrombocytopenia with hepatosplenomegaly and hypoprothrombinemia have been reported. Cardiac arrhythmia and failure are associated with severe disease.

4. In view of the varied manifestations and clinical courses that occur in these infants, referral to a pediatric endocrinologist is indicated.

B. Therapy.

1. For controlling acute manifestations and tachycardia and preventing cardiac failure, give propranolol, 2 mg/kg per day in two or three divided doses.

2. For thyrotoxicosis, propylthiouracil (PTU), 5 to 10 mg/kg per day in divided doses every 8 hours; iodides, sodium ipodate, and dexamethasone may be necessary but should be used only in consultation with a pediatric endocrinologist.

C. Prognosis.

1. Although it usually subsides after 3 to 6 weeks of life (half-life of TSI), thyrotoxicosis may persist for months to over a year. This may represent a high titer of a potent TSI, a delayed onset, subacute or chronic disease, or even early-onset familial Graves' disease.

2. The prognosis, in the absence of cardiac failure, is good with transient disease. In subacute or chronic disease, the prognosis is guarded. Growth retardation and mild to moderate mental retardation may occur.

3. Severe neonatal disease with cardiac failure, delay in diagnosis, and inadequate treatment has been associated with a 15% to 20% mortality rate.

N.B.: History of maternal thyrotoxicosis or Graves' disease before or during the current pregnancy is important if the fetal heart rate exceeds 160 beats per minute. Cord blood measurements of TSI titers, T_4, and TSH are indicated. If clinical manifestations occur during the first days of life, repeat studies plus a T_3 level are indicated. Consult a pediatric endocrinologist for management.

VII. AMBIGUOUS GENITALIA

A. An infant born with ambiguous genitalia is an extremely rare event that represents both a social and medical emergency and requires prompt attention for two main reasons.

1. To obtain the agreement of the health professional delivering the baby *not to assign a gender to the newborn* until a definitive diagnosis has been made.

2. To obtain blood for electrolytes and glucose concentrations in female infants with signs of masculinization or "males" with hypospadias and nonpalpable testes, in anticipation of hypoglycemia or a salt-losing adrenogenital syndrome caused by a severe 21-hydroxylase enzyme deficiency. Although an adrenal crisis with hyponatremia and hyperkalemia rarely occurs before 6 to 14 days of age, it has been reported as early as 3 to 4 days of age.

B. The diagnosis, management, gender assignment, and treatment of the newborn infant with ambiguous genitalia require the collaboration of a pediatric endocrinologist, geneticist, radiologist, urologist, and psychologist before definitive recommendations are made.

N.B.: Recent advances in identifying, diagnosing, and treating newborns with ambiguous genitalia caused by androgen receptor gene mutations and congenital adrenal hyperplasia, as well as outcomes from assigning specific gender roles, makes it more important than ever to obtain appropriate consultations before assigning a gender in such a newborn.

BIBLIOGRAPHY

Al-Alwan I, Navarro O, Daneman D, Daneman A: Clinical utility of adrenal ultrasonography in the diagnosis of congenital adrenal hyperplasia, *J Pediatr* 135:71, 1999.

Coran AG, Polley TZ Jr: Surgical management of ambiguous genitalia in the infant and child, *J Pediatr Surg* 26:812, 1991.

Cornblath M, Ichord R: Hypoglycemia in the neonate, *Semin Perinatol* 24:136, 2000.

Cornblath M, et al: Controversies regarding definition of neonatal hypoglycemia: suggested operational thresholds, *Pediatrics* 105:1141, 2000.

Fisher DA: Maternal-fetal thyroid function in pregnancy, *Clin Perinatol* 10:614, 1983.

Fisher DA: Neonatal thyroid disease in the offspring of women with autoimmune thyroid disease, *Thyroid Today* 9:1, 1986.

Haddow JF, et al: Maternal thyroid deficiency during pregnancy and subsequent neuropsychological development of the child, *N Engl J Med* 341:549, 1999.

Hawa MI, et al: Antibodies to IA-2 and GAD65 in type 1 and type 2 diabetes, *Diabetes Care* 23:228, 2000.

Loughead JL, et al: A role for magnesium in neonatal parathyroid gland function? *J Am Coll Nutr* 10:123, 1991.

Ong YC, Wong HB, Adaikan G, Yong EL: Directed pharmacological therapy of ambiguous genitalia due to an androgen receptor gene mutation, *Lancet* 354:1444, 1999.

Rovet JF, Ehrlich RM: Long-term effects of L-thyroxine therapy for congenital hypothyroidism, *J Pediatr* 126:380, 1995.

Specker BL, Tsang RC, Ho ML: Changes in calcium homeostasis over the first year postpartum: effect of lactation and weaning, *Obstet Gynecol* 78:56, 1991.

Von Muhlendahl KE, Herkenhoff H: Long-term course of neonatal diabetes, *N Engl J Med* 333:704, 1995.

24

Prenatal Diagnosis and Screening

KRISTYNE M. STONE

I. GENERAL PRINCIPLES

All couples, regardless of parental age and family history, have an approximate 2% to 3% risk of having a child with a serious birth defect. Some couples may be at higher risk based on their personal and family histories. For the past 25 to 30 years, prenatal diagnosis and screening have afforded pregnant women the option of detection of some of these conditions before birth. Because prenatal diagnosis is invasive and involves some risk to the fetus and/or mother, it is generally reserved for couples whose risk of having a child with a particular condition is greater than the risk associated with the diagnostic testing. Alternatively, prenatal screening (which does not diagnose or rule out a particular condition but instead identifies patients at increased risk for having a child with the condition) is typically offered to all pregnant women. Although some birth defects and genetic conditions can be diagnosed before birth, the majority are not detected through routine prenatal diagnosis and/or screening.

Fortunately, the majority of babies are healthy, and the information gained from prenatal diagnosis and screening is most often reassuring. When an abnormality is diagnosed, however, couples are faced with the difficult decision of terminating the pregnancy, continuing the pregnancy and caring for the infant, or in some cases placing the infant for adoption. If the parents elect to continue the pregnancy, knowledge of the diagnosis before delivery often helps to prepare both the parents and medical care providers for the birth of a child with special needs. In some cases (e.g., after the birth of one child with an abnormality), prenatal diagnosis provides an option for couples that would otherwise not attempt pregnancy or would terminate *any* pregnancy for fear of having an affected child.

Because prenatal testing may reveal a fetal abnormality and involves potential risks to the fetus and/or mother, decisions regarding prenatal diagnosis are quite personal and can be very difficult for some patients. Genetic counseling is therefore helpful *before* prenatal diagnosis to help patients understand the risks, benefits and limitations of testing, to facilitate autonomous decision making, and to provide psychologic support.

II. COMMON INDICATIONS FOR PRENATAL DIAGNOSIS

A. The American College of Obstetrics and Gynecology recommends that prenatal diagnosis be *offered* to women who will be 35 years or older at the time of delivery (some centers may offer testing at a younger age). The risk for a fetal chromosome abnormality increases with advancing maternal age, and at age 35 the risk of a chromosome abnormality is greater than the risk of miscarriage associated with amniocentesis.

B. Couples who have had a child with a nondisjunctive chromosome abnormality, such as Down syndrome, may be at increased risk for having another child with a chromosome abnormality. This risk is likely to be 1% or less until the maternal age-related risk exceeds 1%. Parents of a child with a de novo unbalanced chromosome rearrangement may also be at some increased risk for having another affected child because one of the parents may have germline mosaicism (i.e., the presence of two or more genetically different types of germline cells in an individual) for the rearrangement.

C. An individual with a balanced chromosome rearrangement should be offered prenatal diagnosis; they are at increased risk for having a live-born child with physical and mental abnormalities. The magnitude of risk varies with the specific chromosome rearrangement.

D. Individuals with a previous child with a genetic condition (e.g., cystic fibrosis, muscular dystrophy) or birth defect (e.g., neural tube defect), have a close family member with such a condition, or are known carriers for an inherited condition should be offered genetic counseling and prenatal diagnosis.

E. Women with an increased risk for having a baby with a fetal chromosome abnormality or neural tube defect based on maternal serum screening results should be offered prenatal diagnosis.

F. Women whose fetuses have a fetal anomaly (e.g., heart defect) or structural variant (e.g., choroid plexus cysts) on obstetric ultrasound may be offered invasive prenatal diagnosis.

G. Women with a teratogenic risk secondary to an exposure or maternal health condition (e.g., diabetes) may be offered prenatal diagnosis.

III. DIAGNOSTIC PROCEDURES

A. Chorionic villus sampling (CVS). CVS involves analysis of villus tissue from the developing placenta. This procedure is advantageous in that it provides a method of prenatal diagnosis during the first trimester of pregnancy, thereby allowing for earlier termination of pregnancy if a fetal abnormality is detected. Termination of pregnancy during the first trimester is medically safer and is psychologically easier for many patients than a second trimester termination. Early diagnosis may also allow for prenatal treatment in some cases (e.g., for 21-hydroxylase deficiency).

1. CVS is best performed between 70 and 91 days after the first day of the last menstrual period.
2. A preprocedure ultrasound is necessary to confirm fetal viability, gestational age, and sampling method.
3. CVS can be performed transcervically (with a catheter) or transabdominally (with a needle) depending on placental location and relative position of the cervix and uterus; active vaginal herpes lesions or other sexually transmitted diseases may be a contraindication to the transcervical procedure.
4. The vaginal or abdominal area is prepped with an iodine solution and the procedure is performed using simultaneous ultrasound guidance.
5. Safety.
   a. Pregnancy loss. Most centers quote a 0.5% to 1% procedure-associated risk for miscarriage that is usually secondary to placental injury, infection, and/or rupture of membranes; the rate of pregnancy loss secondary to CVS is difficult to assess because of the relatively high background rate of loss at this gestational age.
   b. Complications. Vaginal bleeding may occur after CVS, but it is usually mild and without long-term complications; RhoGAM is given to Rh-negative unsensitized women after the procedure.
   c. Fetal malformations. There is not likely to be an increased risk of fetal malformations caused by CVS if the procedure is performed after 10 weeks gestation; earlier sampling may be associated with increased risk for transverse terminal limb defects and oromandibular-limb hypogenesis syndrome.
6. Laboratory issues.
   a. Types of analysis. Cytogenetic studies are most commonly performed; DNA and/or biochemical testing may also be available on villus tissue.
   b. Accuracy of cytogenetic results. Cytogenetic studies are greater than 99% accurate (they cannot be 100% accurate because of the possibility of human error and undetected low-level mosaicism); discrepancies may arise between mesenchymal core cells and cytotrophoblasts, which are used for long-term cultures and "direct" analysis, respectively; long-term cultures are more likely to be representative of the fetus.
   c. Timing of cytogenetic results. "Direct" analysis can yield a karyotype within 24 hours; cultured results are usually available within 10 to 14 days; because of inherent inaccuracies in "direct" analyses, cultured results are usually reported to the patient; culture failure rarely occurs.
   d. Placental mosaicism occurs in approximately 1% of samples; it is often confined to the placenta, with normal outcome; amniocentesis is recommended to rule out fetal trisomy or mosaicism; pla-

cental mosaicism may lead to uniparental disomy (i.e., inheritance of both members of a chromosome pair from the same parent) via "trisomy rescue"; confined placental mosaicism may alter placental function, leading to intrauterine growth restriction or fetal death.

e. Maternal cell contamination is unlikely to be a problem in experienced centers when an adequate sample quantity is available; experienced personnel are able to visually distinguish maternal decidua from villus material; maternal metaphase spreads are generally not present in "direct" preparations.

7. Follow-up.

a. Maternal serum alpha-fetoprotein (AFP) measurement should be offered to screen for neural tube defects that are not detected through CVS.

b. Detailed obstetric ultrasound should be performed at approximately 18 to 20 weeks gestation to screen for structural anomalies that may not be evident at the time of CVS.

B. Amniocentesis. Amniocentesis involves withdrawal of a small amount of amniotic fluid from the gestational sac for diagnosis of a variety of genetic conditions and/or birth defects.

1. Traditional midtrimester amniocentesis is generally performed at or after 16 menstrual weeks.

2. A preprocedure ultrasound is necessary to confirm fetal viability, gestational age, and location of the placenta and amniotic fluid. A sonographic screen for fetal anomalies is often performed in conjunction with the procedure.

3. The abdominal area is prepped with an iodine solution and a 20- to 22-gauge spinal needle is inserted through the maternal abdomen and uterus into the amniotic fluid using simultaneous ultrasound guidance. Twenty to thirty milliliters of fluid are collected; the first few drops are discarded because they may contain blood and/or maternal cells.

4. Safety.

a. Pregnancy loss. Most centers quote ≤0.5% procedure-associated risk for miscarriage.

b. Complications. Vaginal bleeding and/or leakage of amniotic fluid may occur after amniocentesis and may be mild and without long-term complications or may lead to miscarriage; infection after amniocentesis is rare; RhoGAM is given to Rh-negative unsensitized women after the procedure.

c. Fetal malformations. Case reports of fetal malformations caused by amniocentesis exist in world literature; most large studies do not reveal an increased risk for fetal malformations.

5. Laboratory issues.

a. Types of analysis. Cytogenetic studies are most commonly performed; DNA and/or biochemical testing may also be available; AFP measurement detects approximately 98% of open neural tube defects; amniotic fluid can be analyzed for the presence of acetylcholinesterase if there is an elevated AFP level.

  b. Accuracy of cytogenetic results. Amniocentesis has a greater than 99% accuracy rate (it cannot be 100% accurate because of the possibility of human error and undetected low-level mosaicism).
  c. Timing of cytogenetic results. Cultured results are usually available within 10 to 14 days; culture failure rarely occurs.
 6. Early amniocentesis. Early amniocentesis at 10 to 14 weeks gestation is currently being investigated. Recent studies suggest that the procedure-associated risk for miscarriage is higher than that associated with midtrimester amniocentesis and CVS. In addition, early amniocentesis may increase the risk of clubfeet in the fetus.

C. Fetal tissue sampling.

 1. Fetal blood sampling.
  a. The most common indication for fetal blood sampling is rapid cytogenetic analysis when a fetal anomaly is diagnosed late in pregnancy or when a mosaic result is obtained through CVS or amniocentesis.
  b. It was commonly used in the past to diagnose some hemoglobinopathies and coagulopathies; more recent advances in DNA methodology allow for diagnosis of the majority of these conditions via CVS or amniocentesis.
  c. Fetal blood sampling can be used to determine hematocrit levels in fetuses at risk for anemia, to diagnose some immunologic conditions, and to evaluate for some fetal infections.
  d. The blood sample is usually obtained from the umbilical or hepatic vein at ≥18 to 20 weeks gestation.
  e. The procedure-associated risk of miscarriage is estimated to be 1% to 2%.
 2. Other fetal tissue sampling. Although rarely used today, fetal skin, liver, and muscle samples can be obtained for diagnosis of fetal conditions (e.g., epidermolysis bullosa, muscular dystrophy) in cases in which DNA diagnosis is not possible or informative.

D. Ultrasound.

Many structural fetal anomalies can be diagnosed through obstetric ultrasonography. Examples include neural tube defects, congenital heart defects, polycystic kidneys, hydrocephalus, duodenal atresia, limb defects, and diaphragmatic hernias. Prenatal diagnosis of such anomalies allows for optimal prenatal and postnatal management and, in some cases, provides the option for termination of pregnancy. The detection rate of congenital anomalies varies depending on the experience and training of the sonographer, the type of equipment used, and the thoroughness of the examination.

IV. SCREENING TOOLS

There are several screening methodologies that provide an alternative to invasive prenatal diagnosis. These tools are attractive in that they do not involve a risk to the pregnancy. Patients and physicians should approach these screening tools with caution because they may increase a patient's anxiety and lead to invasive prenatal testing.

N.B.: Normal screening results do not rule out fetal abnormalities.

A. Maternal serum screening. The measurement of particular chemicals in blood during pregnancy allows for patient-specific risk assessment for a variety of fetal abnormalities. This technology is commonly used to screen for open neural tube defects, Down syndrome, and trisomy 18. Standard of care in the United States dictates that maternal serum screening be offered to all pregnant women during the second trimester. First-trimester maternal serum screening has more recently become commercially available.

1. Second-trimester screening. All analytes (the samples of blood taken for testing) are reported as multiples of the median (MOM) (median = 1.0). The amount of each analyte varies with the gestational age of the pregnancy; therefore, a common reason for "abnormal" serum screening is inaccurate dating of the pregnancy. Screening for neural tube defects and Down syndrome is most reliable between 16 and 18 weeks gestation.

   a. AFP screening. AFP is synthesized by the fetal yolk sac, gastrointestinal tract, and liver; AFP levels are adjusted for maternal weight, race, and diabetic status; AFP levels are typically elevated in the presence of an open neural tube defect; however, there is significant overlap with levels in unaffected pregnancies (measurement of maternal serum AFP detects 80% to 90% of incidents of open spina bifida and more than 90% of anencephaly, with a 2% to 5% false positive rate; sensitivity and false positive rates vary depending on cutoff used). High levels may be predictive of pregnancy complications (e.g., fetal/neonatal death, preterm birth, low birth weight and preeclampsia); high levels are also associated with abdominal wall defects, kidney abnormalities, and other more rare conditions. There is an association between low maternal serum AFP levels and fetal Down syndrome (average = 0.7 MOM in affected pregnancies); however, there is a great deal of overlap between levels in affected and unaffected pregnancies. AFP levels also tend to be low in trisomy 18.

   b. Human chorionic gonadotropin (hCG). hCG is a glycoprotein made by the placenta; there is an association between high levels and fetal Down syndrome (average = 2.1 MOM in affected pregnancies). However, there is a great deal of overlap between levels in affected and unaffected pregnancies; high levels may be predictive of pregnancy complications (e.g., fetal/neonatal death, preterm birth, low birth weight and preeclampsia). hCG levels tend to be low in trisomy 18.

   c. Unconjugated estriol (uE3). uE3 is a steroid hormone that is a major estrogen of pregnancy. There is an association between low levels and fetal Down syndrome (average = 0.7 MOM in affected pregnancies); however, there is a great deal of overlap between levels in affected and unaffected pregnancies. Very low levels may also be indicative of trisomy 18, Smith-Lemli-Opitz syndrome, and X-linked ichthyosis.

   d. Triple screen. AFP, hCG, and uE3 are independent predictors of Down syndrome. An algorithm combines information from all three analytes with maternal age to estimate a patient-specific risk for Down syndrome. The screen is considered positive (i.e., the patient should be offered amniocentesis) if triple-screen risk for Down syndrome is ≥1 in 270 (the risk of a 35-year-old woman); because maternal age is included in the algorithm, the chance of an "abnormal" triple screen increases with maternal age. The triple screen detects approximately 60% of cases of fetal Down syndrome, with a 5% amniocentesis rate in women under 35 years of age; the use of serum screening in women over 35 is controversial and is not considered a replacement for amniocentesis. Addition of other analytes, such as inhibin, may increase detection rates and/or decrease false positive rates.

2. First-trimester screening. Screening for Down syndrome in the first trimester is a new procedure and is not yet the standard of medical care. Recent studies indicate that approximately 60% to 65% of fetuses with Down syndrome and 90% of fetuses with trisomy 18 can be detected by combining maternal age risks with serum levels of free β-hCB and pregnancy-associated plasma protein A (PAPP-A) between 10 and 14 weeks gestation. The nuchal translucency (fluid accumulation behind the fetal neck) can also be measured by ultrasound during the first trimester and may be predictive of a fetal abnormality. The addition of the nuchal translucency measurement to first-trimester maternal serum screening increases the detection of Down syndrome to about 90%, with a 5% false positive rate. Measurement of the nuchal translucency is technically difficult and should only be performed by specially trained sonographers.

B. Ultrasound. Variants in fetal development may be detected through obstetric sonography and may be suggestive of an underlying fetal abnormality (e.g., aneuploidy). For example, increased nuchal thickening, shortened femurs/humeri, choroid plexus cysts, dilated renal pelves, and/or echogenic bowel may suggest an increased risk for trisomy 21 in the fetus. Echogenic bowel is also suggestive of cystic fibrosis. Invasive prenatal testing may be warranted in the presence of such variants in fetal development.

C. Carrier testing. To assess the risk of having a child with certain genetic conditions, it is essential to inquire about the ethnic backgrounds of both parents. Carrier testing for various autosomal recessive conditions should be offered if one or both members of the couple are from a high-risk ethnic group. For example, standard of care in the United States dictates that individuals of Eastern European (Ashkenazi) Jewish descent be offered carrier testing for Tay-Sachs disease and Canavan's disease. An individual of French-Canadian descent is also at an increased risk of being a carrier of a mutation in the Tay-Sachs disease gene. Screening for hemoglobinopathies is pertinent among individuals of African/African American, Mediterranean (e.g., Greek, Italian), Middle Eastern, Indian, Southeast Asian, Chinese, and Pacific Islander descent. Carrier testing for cystic fibrosis may soon be offered to all couples, either preconceptionally or in the early part of pregnancy.

N.B.: Current concepts in prenatal diagnosis and genetic testing are constantly evolving and changing. If a patient is interested in such testing or if there are additional questions about the above information, local genetic counselors and The National Society of Genetic Counselors (610-872-7608 or *www.nsgc.org*) are helpful resources.

BIBLIOGRAPHY

Ormond KE: Update and review: maternal serum screening, *J Genet Counsel* 6(4):395-417, 1997.

Reece EA: Early and midtrimester amniocentesis, *Fetal Diagn Ther* 24(1):71-81, 1997.

Simpson JL, Golbus MS: *Genetics in obstetrics and gynecology,* ed 2, Philadelphia, 1992, WB Saunders, pp 201-221.

Wapner RJ: Chorionic villus sampling, *Fetal Diagn Ther* 24(1):83-110, 1997.

25

Breast-Feeding

JUDITH W. VOGELHUT

I. ADVANTAGES
A. Lower renal solute load.
B. Antiinfective properties.
1. Protection against diarrhea. Bifidus factor promotes proliferation of *Lactobacillus bifidus* in infant's intestines, which discourages colonization by pathogens; secretory IgA antibodies to *Escherichia coli* continue to be produced into the second year of lactation.
2. Protection against respiratory infections, including respiratory syncytial virus (RSV) and otitis media.
3. Antiviral properties.
4. Protection against necrotizing enterocolitis (NEC).
5. Promotes phagocytosis by macrophages and leukocytes.

C. Antiallergic properties.
1. Decreased incidence and severity of eczema.
2. Species-specific protein; delays introduction of foreign protein.

D. Bonding.
1. Promotes special closeness between mother and baby.
2. Prolactin response increases maternal relaxation.
3. Increases maternal self-confidence.
4. Meets infant's needs for safety, security, and cuddling.

II. CONTRAINDICATIONS
A. Breast cancer. Mother's need for treatment takes precedence over lactation.
B. Hepatitis B. However, an infant given hepatitis B immune globulin (HBIG) and hepatitis B vaccine may breast-feed.
C. Human immunodeficiency virus (HIV) infection. It is recommended that HIV-infected women in the United States not breast-feed based on the risk of transmitting the virus to the uninfected infant.
D. Life-threatening illness in the mother.
E. Galactosemia in infant.

F. Herpes simplex virus (HSV) infection. Breast-feeding is contraindicated in the presence of active breast lesions.

G. Current maternal substance abuse.

H. Active tuberculosis in mother. May breast-feed after at least 2 weeks of treatment.

III. HUMAN MILK CHARACTERISTICS

A. Colostrum is produced from the second trimester through the first few postpartum days; it is yellow in appearance and has a mean energy value of 67 kcal/100ml. It contains a high concentration of immunoglobulins, especially secretory IgA.

B. Transitional milk contains increasing volume, caloric content, and water-soluble vitamins; there is a decreasing concentration of immunoglobulins.

C. Mature milk contains 75 kcal/100ml; it is in large part water; the fat content is most variable.

1. Foremilk is the early portion of a feeding; it is more dilute and lower in fat.
2. Hindmilk is secreted later in the feeding and has three to five times the fat content of foremilk.

IV. MANAGEMENT

A. Put the infant to the mother's breast as soon as is feasible postpartum because early contact with the mother's breast may have an imprinting effect on mother and baby. The infant's quiet, alert state shortly after birth is conducive to nursing if mother and baby are stable.

B. Encourage rooming-in. Avoid supplemental feeding unless medically indicated; frequent nursing helps establish mother's milk supply, prevent excessive engorgement, and minimize neonatal jaundice.

C. Positioning.

1. Cradle position. Infant's head is in the mother's antecubital fossa, with its body rotated so that the face, chest, and abdomen are against her chest, and the infant's lower arm is behind the mother. Pillows may be needed for support; a footstool is helpful if the mother is in a chair.
2. Clutch (football) position. The infant's body is positioned on pillows to the mother's side; the infant's hips are flexed, with the back of the infant's neck supported by the mother's hand.
3. Side-lying position. The mother is positioned on her side in bed and the infant is placed on its side facing the mother. The lower breast is offered first, then mother rolls toward baby to offer upper breast or rolls to her other side to offer second breast.

D. Latch-on.

1. Mother supports and lifts her breast with her thumb on top and her other fingers below, staying behind the areola; mother strokes the infant's lips gently with her nipple, waits for baby to open mouth wide, and then, with nipple centered toward mouth, draws baby in

close. The tip of the baby's nose should touch the breast; the airway can be maintained by lifting up on the breast or drawing the baby's buttocks in close.

2. Appropriate latch-on and nutritive sucking is accomplished when the infant's jaw excursions are wide, swallows are audible, and the infant's tongue is visible coming forward to the lower gum (visualized by holding down lower lip). The baby should not be pulled off the breast easily; the infant's lips are flanged outward and can be gently pulled out if necessary.

3. If baby latches on correctly and mother does not report pain, there is no need or benefit to limiting feeding time; arbitrarily doing so can limit baby's intake and promote engorgement in the mother by inadequate emptying.

4. Both breasts should be offered at each feeding, although the baby may nurse from only one. The mother should alternate the breast offered first because the baby sucks more vigorously on the first breast at each feeding. Once the milk supply is established, the mother should follow the baby's cues as to when one side is finished.

5. The infant can be removed from the breast by the mother inserting a finger into the corner of the baby's mouth between gums to release suction.

6. The mother should burp the baby after each breast.

7. After feeding, the mother should express a few drops of colostrum or milk onto the nipple and areola and follow by air drying for several minutes.

E. Anticipatory guidance.

1. It is important during prenatal and postpartum visits to identify any barriers to successful breast-feeding (Box 25-1).

2. Expect a full-term infant initially to nurse 8 to 12 times in 24 hours, generally 15 minutes per breast.

3. Infants usually wet at least 6 diapers in 24 hours and have at least 2 or 3 soft, yellow, seedy stools per 24-hour period; some breast-fed babies stool with each feeding initially and then less frequently after the first month. A significant variation from this pattern should be brought to the practitioner's attention.

4. In most cases, avoid supplementary bottles for the first month to allow mother and infant time to become skilled at breast-feeding, to allow for optimum milk production, and to allow time for mother's milk ejection reflex (letdown) to become conditioned.

5. Several letdowns may occur during the course of a feeding. The milk ejection reflex is characterized by slow, long sucks with frequent swallows, milk leaking from the contralateral breast, and possibly a pins-and-needles tingling in the breast. In the early postpartum period, there may be uterine cramping.

6. Infants typically experience growth spurts (milk supply lagging behind increasing demand) at 2 to 3 weeks, 6 weeks, 3 months, and 6 months. Generally, 2 to 3 days of unrestricted nursing will increase the supply enough to meet the increased demand.

BOX 25-1
Barriers to Breast-Feeding

It is important to discover barriers to successful breast-feeding. There are questions which, when asked appropriately and open-endedly, may help in revealing, understanding, and dealing with these barriers.

QUESTIONS TO ASK AT THE PRENATAL VISIT

How will a new baby change your life?
How are you planning to feed your baby?
Have you considered breast-feeding?
What do you know about breast-feeding?
Have you breast-fed another child? If so, how did it go?
How do most of your friends feed their babies?
Are you taking any medications?
Do you have any medical problems?
How does the baby's father feel about your breast-feeding?
May I suggest a list of books you might read about breast-feeding?

QUESTIONS TO ASK AT THE "JUST AFTER DELIVERY VISIT"

How are you planning to feed your baby?
Have you started breast-feeding yet?
Were you able to nurse in the delivery room?
Do you understand the instructions for breast-feeding?
Would you like to see a lactation consultant?
How often do you plan to nurse your baby?
Do you understand how to prevent sore nipples and breast infections?
How is the baby reacting to breast-feeding?
Are you having difficulty with latching on or any other problem getting started with breast-feeding?
Do your breasts hurt or are they tender?
Are you on any medications or drugs?
Would you like to see a video about breast-feeding?

QUESTIONS TO ASK WITHIN THE FIRST WEEK AFTER DISCHARGE*

How is breast-feeding going?
Do you have any worries about it?
Are you enjoying breast-feeding?
Are you feeling tired?
Who spends a lot a time with you, and what do they think about breast-feeding?
Has your health been good since your delivery?
How long do you plan to nurse?
What contributes to that decision?
Would you like to consult a lactation specialist?

Modified from Bennjamin JY, Shariat H: *Contemp Pediatr* 16:73-83, 1999.
*Asking questions within the first week after discharge becomes important. It re-inforces the effort at nursing at a time when many mothers may be discouraged and give it up.

7. Vitamin D supplementation is recommended and is generally dispensed as A, D, C drops. Iron intake from breast milk is adequate for full-term infants until 4 to 6 months of age.
8. Conduct telephone follow-up with mother 48 hours after nursery discharge; the initial office or clinic visit should be within the first week. Full-term breast-fed babies most often regain their birth weight by 2 weeks.

V. MATERNAL CONCERNS
A. Flat or inverted nipples.
1. Plastic breast shells can be worn inside the bra during the last trimester beginning 1 hour per day, with gradually increasing wearing time.
   a. Should not be worn when sleeping to avoid undue pressure on breast.
   b. Shells often increase nipple protrusion.
   c. May be worn postpartum for 30 minutes before feeding unless breasts are engorged.
   d. Milk that leaks into shells should be discarded.
2. May use a breast pump briefly before offering infant the breast to increase nipple protrusion.

B. Engorgement.
1. Engorgement is a physiologic reaction caused by milk accumulation and increased vascularity.
2. Small, firm breasts are prone to more significant engorgement.
3. Frequent nursing during the colostral phase minimizes edema.
4. Areolar edema may flatten the nipple, making latch-on difficult and causing nipple soreness.
5. Advise mother on use of warm compresses, soaks, or showers followed by gentle massage and expression of milk to soften the areola.
6. Frequent nursing maintains drainage and prevents decreased milk production from back pressure on ducts.
7. Cold compresses to breast after feeding may reduce swelling.
8. A bra should be worn for support. Avoid underwire bras.

C. Nipple soreness.
1. Nipple soreness is best prevented by proper latch-on and positioning, alternating breast-feeding positions, and careful air drying of the breast after feedings, with some hindmilk massaged into the nipple and areola before drying.
2. Development of soreness is unrelated to prenatal preparation.
3. Nipple shields (an artificial nipple placed over the breast during feeding) may significantly reduce the amount of milk the baby receives.
4. The mother should nurse first on the less-affected breast.
5. Late-onset soreness may be caused by *Monilia* infection. Treatment consists of nystatin oral suspension to infant's mouth, 2 ml four times daily, and nystatin topically four times daily after feeding to mother's nipple and areola.
6. Remove baby gently without precipitously pulling baby off breast.

D. Maternal diet.
1. Mother should eat an extra 500 kcal per day.
2. Drink to quench thirst (there is no benefit to forcing fluids).
3. Limit caffeine.

E. Plugged ducts.
1. Tender lump in the breast.
2. No systemic symptoms.
3. Possible factors include constricting bra, missed feedings, fatigue, or nursing multiples.
4. Treatment.
   a. Moist heat before nursing.
   b. Frequent feedings.
   c. Remove bra if too tight.
   d. Massage breast during feeding.
   e. Position infant with chin toward the lump to improve drainage of affected area.
   f. Watch for symptoms of mastitis.

F. Maternal mastitis.
1. Mastitis may be preceded by maternal fatigue, a plugged duct, unrelieved engorgement, or nipple trauma.
2. It is usually unilateral, and rarely bilateral. The most common organisms are *Staphylococcus aureus* and *E. coli;* rarely, *Streptococcus* can be found in bilateral mastitis.
3. The highest incidence occurs 2 to 6 weeks postpartum.
4. Systemic symptoms may precede localized ones. Symptoms include fever, chills, malaise and body aches, nausea and vomiting, warm area on breast, tender lump or wedge in breast, or an erythematous streak.
5. Treatment.
   a. Bed rest.
   b. Warm compresses.
   c. Frequent nursing to empty ducts.
   d. Begin feedings on unaffected side.
   e. Antibiotic therapy for 10 days (full course recommended to avoid relapse): dicloxacillin, a cephalosporin, or erythromycin.
   f. Increased maternal fluid intake.
   g. Remove bra and other constrictive clothing.

G. Breast-feeding and returning to work.
1. Assess workplace before return.
   a. Privacy for pumping.
   b. Adequate break time.
   c. Refrigerator or cooler to store pumped milk.
   d. Options concerning full-time versus part-time hours.
2. Mother should choose a supportive babysitter and familiarize caregiver with the proper handling of breast milk.
3. Allow at least 1 month of exclusive breast-feeding before introducing artificial nipples.
4. Familiarize infant with artificial nipples 10 to 14 days before return to work.

  a. Expressed breast milk may be preferred initially to ameliorate new experiences.
  b. Initially, an artificial nipple may be better accepted if offered by someone other than mother at a midday feeding rather than early morning or bedtime. Try it when the baby is drowsy rather than ravenously hungry if he or she is reluctant to take the bottle.
5. Mother should practice expressing or pumping milk and begin freezing it for later use.
6. Milk may be expressed by hand, manually-operated pump, battery-operated pump, small electric pump, or heavy-duty electric breast pump.
7. Pump 10 to 15 minutes per breast.
8. Pump parts are first rinsed in cold water, then washed in hot soapy water (use dishwashing liquid), rinsed well, and air dried.
9. Store milk in clean plastic bottles with lids; date the containers.
10. Milk may be kept refrigerated for 48 hours, frozen in a refrigerator freezer for 3 months, and frozen at 0° F for 6 months. Store away from the fan in a self-defrosting freezer; do not store in the freezer door.
11. Store upright, with most recently pumped milk behind the older milk.
12. Thaw in cool, progressing to warm water before feeding; never boil or microwave.
13. See Box 25-2 for information on breast pumps and other paraphernalia.

BOX 25-2
Breast Pumps and Other Paraphernalia

MANUAL

Most require two hands to operate; have the advantages of being inexpensive and widely available; may be tiring.
1. Kaneson
2. Hollister Egnell (one-handed)
3. Medela (spring express)
4. White River
5. Evenflo
6. Gerber
7. Avent

BATTERY

Approximately 4 hours pumping time on each set of batteries; moderate pricing; convenient if not near an electrical outlet.
1. Gentle Expressions
2. Hollister Egnell
3. Medela
4. Evenflo

BOX 25-2
Breast Pumps and Other Paraphernalia—cont'd

PORTABLE ELECTRIC

Generally noisy, as are the battery pumps; one-handed operation.

1. Gerber
2. Mag Mag
3. Evenflo
4. Nurture 3 (allows double pumping)
5. Medela (available for single or double pumping)

ELECTRICAL PUMPS FOR PURCHASE (CLOSE TO HOSPITAL GRADE)

Expensive; probably worth it if pump is to be used over several months.

1. Medela Pump in Style
2. Egnell Purely Yours

HEAVY DUTY ELECTRIC PUMPS FOR RENTAL (HOSPITAL GRADE)

Expense may be disadvantage; preferable for long-term pumping; more adequate hormone stimulation; available with double-pumping kits to pump both breasts simultaneously.

1. Medela Classic and portable Lactina model
2. Hollister Egnell
3. White River

BICYCLE HORN

Use of this pump should be discouraged; it is less expensive but can damage the breast because the amount of suction is difficult to control with the rubber bulb. Milk that goes into the bulb may be contaminated.

HAND EXPRESSION

Mothers can be taught to express milk by hand. In fact, during long-term pumping occasionally expressing by hand allows skin-to-skin contact, which may increase milk supply.

BREAST SHELLS

Hard plastic cups that can be worn inside the bra prenatally and postpartum to help alleviate flat or inverted nipples; any milk collected in the cups is to be discarded.

FEEDING TUBE DEVICE

To supplement the infant at the breast; may be useful for premature babies, postoperatively, and with adoptive nursing.

HAND EXPRESSION FUNNEL

Catches the sprays; universal threads allows expression directly into bottle.

VI. INFANT CONCERNS.
A. Jaundice.
1. Jaundice may be a pathologic condition if it is visible at 24 hours.
2. Early hyperbilirubinemia may be related to infrequent feeds (<8 per 24 hours), infrequent stools, or prematurity.
3. Treatment.
   a. Early, frequent feedings.
   b. Assess infant for normal suck pattern.
   c. Augment feeds with formula if indicated; mother may need to pump her breasts to increase milk supply.
   d. Phototherapy as necessary.
4. Breast-milk (late onset) jaundice.
   a. Delayed and prolonged hyperbilirubinemia (1:200 births); usually occurs after first 3 to 5 days, peaks at approximately 2 weeks, and, if nursing continues, may persist for several months.
   b. Normal stooling.
   c. Cause is as yet unidentified, but may be related to glucuronyl transferase inhibitor in milk.
   d. A bilirubin level decrease of 2 mg/100 ml on discontinuing breast-feeding reassures that it is breast-milk jaundice; there will be a slight rise in the bilirubin level on resuming breast-feeding, followed by a slow, steady drop.
   e. Not a contraindication to continued nursing.
B. Low birth weight and very low birth weight.
1. Support the mother's decision to provide breast milk for infant.
2. Pumping.
   a. The mother should begin pumping as soon after delivery as possible.
   b. Use of a heavy-duty electric breast pump is preferable.
   c. Pump a total of at least 6 times in 24 hours to equal 100 minutes of pumping time.
   d. Mother can use a double-pump kit to express both breasts simultaneously.
   e. Direct nipple stimulation may improve milk ejection reflex.
   f. Allow mother 6 hours of uninterrupted rest at night.
3. Transition to breast.
   a. Infant should be held to the breast as soon as possible after stability is achieved.
   b. Any contact, even if nonnutritive, provides positive experience to help infant learn and to increase maternal milk supply.
   c. Allow sucking on finger or pacifier by the infant during gavage feedings.
   d. Feedings at breast.
      (1) Position infant with entire body supported by mother's arm.
      (2) The cross-cradle or football hold is often recommended.
   e. Lack of suck pads in cheeks and decreased muscle tone may necessitate support of infant's jaw by mother's hand while at the breast.

       f. In some cases, supplementation of breast-feeding with a feeding-tube device is helpful by decreasing the infant's exposure to artificial nipples while learning to breast-feed.

       g. A human milk fortifier may be used to supplement calories, vitamins, and minerals.

   4. Discharge from the hospital.

       a. Infant may not be feeding totally at breast when discharged.

       b. Continue pumping after feeding while infant is being supplemented.

       c. Gradually decrease amount and frequency of supplements as baby's suck improves.

VII. DRUGS IN BREAST MILK

A. Factors to consider.

1. Dosage. Determine whether drug is a single dose versus long-term use; short-acting drugs are preferable over the long-acting form.
2. Age and maturity of infant.
   a. An infant's liver can metabolize most drugs at 42 weeks of gestational age.
   b. Some compounds (e.g., sulfadiazine) compete for bilirubin binding sites, thus increasing the risk of kernicterus.
3. Quantity of milk consumed by the infant.
4. Experience with giving drug directly to infants: watch infant for unusual signs; weigh risk of drug versus benefit of breast-feeding.
5. Minimize effects. For most medications, schedule maternal dose just after feeding.

B. American Academy of Pediatrics list of drugs contraindicated in nursing mothers.

1. Bromocriptine.
2. Cyclosporine.
3. Lithium.
4. Phenindione.
5. Marijuana.
6. Cocaine.
7. Doxorubicin.
8. Methotrexate.
9. Amphetamine.
10. Nicotine (smoking).
11. Cyclophosphamide.
12. Ergotamine.
13. Phencyclidine (PCP).
14. Heroin.

C. Certain radiopharmaceuticals require temporary discontinuation of breast-feeding.

VIII. NURSING TWINS (OR TRIPLETS)

A. Breast-feed as soon after birth as possible if one or both babies are sufficiently stable; if both babies are unable to nurse, the mother should begin pumping within 24 hours of infants' births; if

one baby is able to breast-feed, the mother can pump one breast and store the milk for the other baby.

B. Positioning. Mother can breast-feed twins simultaneously to save time and increase milk production. She should start the baby that has the more efficient suck first to stimulate the milk ejection reflex, then latch on the other infant. Mother will need several pillows or a nursing pillow for support.

C. Fatigue is the biggest problem. Encourage family members to arrange for help during the first 2 weeks at home if at all possible.

D. There is a higher incidence of plugged ducts and mastitis when nursing twins or multiples secondary to increased milk production and fatigue.

E. Triplets can be exclusively breast-fed, or one baby each feeding may receive a supplement.

F. Provide support. Refer mother to community resources such as peer or breast-feeding support groups or local parents of multiples; maintain telephone contact.

IX. WEANING

A. Baby-initiated weaning is ideal. Weaning should be accomplished as slowly as possible.

B. Replace one feeding with a bottle or cup (depending on the age of the baby); begin with midday feeding rather than early morning, naptime, or bedtime, when baby nurses for comfort as well as nutrition.

C. Allow a few days for milk supply to adjust downward before substituting another bottle or cup feeding.

D. Generally, bedtime feeding is the last to go.

E. There is a risk of plugged ducts or mastitis if weaning is too rapid.

BIBLIOGRAPHY

American Academy of Pediatrics Committee on Drugs: The transfer of drugs and other chemicals into human breast milk, *Pediatrics* 93:137-150, 1994.

American Academy of Pediatrics Work Group on Breastfeeding: Breastfeeding and the use of human milk, *Pediatrics* 100:1035-1039, 1997.

Bennjamin JY, Shariat H: Overcoming impediments to breastfeeding: how pediatricians can help, *Contemp Pediatr* 16:73-83, 1999.

Huggins K: *The nursing mother's companion*, ed 4, Boston, 1999, The Harvard Common Press., LaLeche League International: *The womanly art of breastfeeding*, ed 4, Franklin Park, Ill, 1990, LaLeche League International.

Lawrence R, Lawrence R: *Breastfeeding: a guide for the medical profession*, ed 5, St. Louis, 1999, Mosby.

Riordan J, Auerbach K: *Breastfeeding and human lactation*, ed 2, Sudbury, Mass, 1999, Jones and Bartlett.

26

Childbirth Education, Parent-Infant Bonding, and Continuing Education

HENRY M. SEIDEL

I. CHILDBIRTH EDUCATION

A. General information. Prenatal education, formal and informal, about childbirth education, pregnancy, labor, delivery, and the postpartum period is designed to potentiate all of the positive aspects of the passage to parenthood and to put all of the concerning aspects in context. It recognizes birth as the first basic condition of life, seeks to endow it with the feel of an experience unencumbered by perhaps unnecessary artificial interventions, and assumes that greater knowledge and insight in both parents help achieve goals rightly set by the individuals or couples involved. One dramatic change during recent decades involves the mother's attitude regarding analgesia during labor and delivery. The shift from a desire to sleep through it all to the wish to experience as much of it as possible has been paralleled by the development of formal approaches to education that include both mother and father or, in some instances, mother and an invited partner. Sibling involvement, depending on age, should be encouraged as much and as soon as possible.

B. Benefits.
1. A valid result is the documented reduced need for analgesia and anesthesia during labor and delivery; some women achieve "natural childbirth," avoiding drugs completely.
2. The subjective feeling of satisfaction most couples who participate report.
3. The support provided to the mother by the father or other partner throughout the entire experience.

4. The rapport and mutual support of all of the participants in an education group; an extension of the family.

5. The developing sense in both parents of "belonging" to the obstetric "team."

6. The sense of support to the idea of family.

C. Facilitators. Maternal and newborn care are inextricably linked. If the purposes of education are to be best achieved, a combination labor, delivery, and recovery room (birthing suite) is ideal for an uncomplicated vaginal delivery. It should be set up as a comfortable, clean room with all medical and obstetric necessities readily available. The further the delivery area is from the nursery, the greater the need for support equipment at the delivery site; however, separate labor, delivery, and recovery arrangements should be available for those who wish it.

D. Family-centered birthing. The full involvement of everyone in the immediate family regardless of age (and some in the extended family), at home or at a freestanding birthing center, puts a huge responsibility on the professional attendant, often a nurse-midwife. Childbirth education should include responses to emergencies if this birthing option is chosen.

E. The Lamaze method of childbirth education. Lamaze is one of the most commonly used (there are many variations) formal approaches to childbirth education in the United States. Its process and principles include the following:

1. 12 to 16 hours of classroom instruction.

2. Supplementary reading and home practice.

3. Discussions of relevant subjects.
   a. Anatomy.
   b. Physiology.
   c. Fetal growth and development.
   d. Emotional and behavioral issues, as they apply to pregnancy, labor, and delivery.
   e. Alternatives to drug-dependent labor and delivery.
   f. Issues regarding vaginal and cesarean births.
   g. Postpartum adaptations of mother and child.
   h. Advantages of and alternatives to breast-feeding.
   i. Care of the newborn.
   j. Planned parenthood.

4. Restraint on the part of instructors to imposing their personal preferences. The method does not preach; it seeks to facilitate.

5. Recognition of varying preoccupations over time (e.g., early in pregnancy, parents tend to think about the baby; later on, about the process of labor and delivery).

II. PARENT-INFANT BONDING

A. General information. The term *bonding* used in the context of the development of the primary relationship of an infant with the parents is now fixed in the jargon of baby care. Even the adopted child, deprived of some of the opportunity, is not deprived ultimately of the potential. Bonding is vital, but there is no one event that achieves or ensures it. There are *too many variables* to suggest irretrievability if some are lost or to suggest success if all are experienced.

Each parent has a separate and unique role in establishing a relationship with a new baby and, as a duo, they fulfill yet another role (see Chapter 28). The mother has a "sensitive" period, called by some a "primary maternal preoccupation," which develops during pregnancy and may last for a few postnatal weeks. During this time, because feelings of love are *not* necessarily instantaneous, she may be distressed if she does not feel the expected emotion. Reassurance that she will reclaim the sense of it that she may have had during pregnancy is appropriate.

The father or other partner can complement the activity of this time, providing an emotional "space" during which the mother can indulge her feelings and allow them to "flow" without undue stress. She can focus on the baby as others deal with the environment; such support helps to fortify her skills as a mother, and benefits each of them—and the baby.

During the maternal sensitive period, mother and child have a truly two-way reciprocal relationship. In a positive way their senses mesh. They entertain each other, gurgling and cooing, feeling each other's warmth. The baby cries and has needs; the parent assures and reinforces by feeding and caressing.

B. Barriers to bonding.
1. Blindness, deafness, other physical deprivations or incapacities.
2. Anxiety; "stiffness" in child and parent; maternal "projection" of negative feelings, traits, concerns onto child.
3. Drug-influenced infant (or mother).
4. Difficult labor or other maternal illness, which may make nursing more difficult.
5. Neonatal intensive care unit (NICU) placement or maternal-infant separation caused by prolonged hospital stay of one without the other.
6. Family discord.

C. Facilitators.
1. Fathers, too, feel better about themselves after contact with the baby; parents welcome contact *immediately* postpartum. Try to facilitate it whether delivery is vaginal or by cesarean section.
2. Placing the baby on the mother's abdomen immediately after delivery is nice to do, and some say these babies have fewer adaptive problems at home and in school in the long run. I am all for doing it, but I do not accept as gospel the reported long-term benefit. Again, no one has successfully isolated the variables.
3. Examine the baby in the view of or even in the arms of the mother or, if necessary, the father or other partner.
4. Encourage sucking and closeness soon after birth.
5. Try to keep the family together. Rooming in can be very helpful and satisfying. It helps to keep the baby and the family physically and emotionally at appropriate temperatures.
6. To the extent possible, depending on age, involve siblings as soon as it is feasible.

III. CONTINUING EDUCATION

A. General information.
Pregnancy and delivery are the first stages in a continuing education process. The prenatal visit initiates a relationship that can be enhanced at the time of the examination of the infant in the presence of the parents. From then on, every interaction gives the chance to teach.

B. Barriers to the educational relationship.
1. The sense of isolation many young adults feel.
2. Excessive dependency in a poorly prepared or immature parent.
3. The overworked professional.
4. Inadequate or socially disorganized family and other societal resources.

C. Facilitators for the educational relationship.
1. The energy and desire most new parents bring to the initial attachment to their infants.
2. The innate capacity of the newborn to adapt to the "new" environment.
3. The information gleaned from such measures as the Brazelton behavioral scale (see Chapter 5).
4. The telephone or e-mail, the link with the "teacher."
5. Home visits (usually by nurses) soon after hospital discharge are a marvelous opportunity to learn about the family in its many dimensions.

N.B.: These facilitators do not ultimately create overdependency on the educator in most circumstances. Other variables (e.g., barriers) do. In general, increasing experience, knowledge, and insight breed self-sufficiency in parents.

D. Counseling during the newborn period.
The following topics should be addressed in counseling new parents.
1. Feeding.
2. Voiding and stooling.
3. Skin care.
4. Cord care.
5. Safety.
6. Signs of illness.
7. Expected infant behavior (e.g., sleep pattern).
8. Clothing and other supplies.
9. Going out (e.g., excursions, visits to others, to the supermarket).
10. Involvement of others (e.g., siblings, relatives, friends, support help).
11. Develop insight to parental feelings.

N.B.: The birth of twins (or more) compounds the need for attention to all details of the relationships and the needs of newborns and their parents.

BIBLIOGRAPHY

Becker PG: Counseling families with twins: birth to 3 years of age, *Pediatr Rev* 8(3):81, 1986.

Charney E: Counseling of parents around the birth of a baby, *Pediatr Rev* 4(6):167, 1982.

Kennell JH, Klaus MH: The perinatal paradigm: is it time for a change? *Clin Perinatal* 15:80, 1988.

Klaus MH, Kennell JH: *Parent-infant bonding,* ed 2, St Louis, 1982, Mosby.

LaLeche League International: *The womanly art of breastfeeding,* ed 6, 1997.

Yogman MW: Development of the father-infant relationship. In Fitzgerald HE, Lester BM, Yogman MW (editors): *Theory and research in behavioral pediatrics,* vol 1, New York, 1980, Plenum Press.

27

Indications for Transfer to the Intensive Care Nursery

AMBADAS PATHAK

I. GENERAL CONSIDERATIONS

Capabilities, staffing, equipment, and patient care philosophy vary from nursery to nursery. Hence each nursery must develop its own indications for transferring infants to the intensive care nursery. In general, infants requiring frequent and close monitoring involving placement of intravascular catheters and use of sophisticated monitors, intravenous (IV) therapy, or essentially "intensive" nursing care require transfer to the intensive care nursery. These infants are usually born at <34 weeks of gestation. Following are some general recommendations, presented by category, for transfer to the intensive care nursery.

A. Cardiopulmonary.

1. Central cyanosis requiring oxygen, associated with enlarged heart on chest radiograph, pallor, and hypotension (consider transposition of great vessels, hypoplastic left heart syndrome).
2. Respiratory distress indicated by tachypnea, retractions, flaring, grunting, and hypoxemia (consider respiratory distress syndrome, sepsis, meconium aspiration syndrome, persistent pulmonary hypertension, pneumothorax, diaphragmatic hernia, tracheoesophageal fistula).
3. Stridor at birth or soon thereafter (consider choanal atresia, micrognathia and glossoptosis, laryngeal webs, tracheomalacia, laryngoesophageal defects, vascular rings compressing the trachea).

B. Neurolgic.

1. Seizures (consider asphyxia, metabolic abnormalities, infection, intracranial hemorrhage).
2. Coma (consider metabolic abnormality, heavy maternal sedation).
3. Severe hypotonia (consider birth injuries, congenital myopathies).

C. Gastrointestinal (GI).

1. Abdominal distention accompanied by tenderness, absent bowel sounds, erythema, edema of abdominal wall, bilious vomiting, visible peristalsis (consider GI perforation, necrotizing enterocolitis [NEC], malrotation, GI obstruction).
2. Hematemesis and melena (consider swallowed maternal blood, gastric ulcer, volvulus, enterocolitis).
3. Congenital abnormalities (consider gastroschisis, duodenal atresia, omphalocele, imperforate anus).

D. Genitourinary.
Abdominal mass (consider hydronephrosis, multicystic kidneys, dysplastic kidneys, polycystic kidneys, ovarian cysts, hydrometrocolpos). If the infant is otherwise stable, initial evaluation may take place in the full-term nursery.

E. Hematologic.

1. Anemia (consider Rh or ABO isoimmunization, fetomaternal hemorrhage, internal hemorrhage).
2. Polycythemia with symptoms (consider twin-twin transfusion, small for gestational age [SGA] infant, postmaturity).
3. Petechiae and purpura, especially when generalized and recurrent (consider maternal idiopathic thrombocytopenic purpura, platelet group incompatibility, bacterial and viral infections, and disseminated intravascular coagulation [DIC]).
4. Hyperbilirubinemia early (within 18 hours) and rapidly progressive, needing phototherapy or exchange transfusion (consider erythroblastosis fetalis).

F. Neonatal infections
indicated by lethargy, temperature instability, respiratory distress, poor feedings, petechial or vesicular rash, sclerema (consider bacterial and viral infections).

G. Metabolic.

1. Hypoglycemia, persistent (consider hyperinsulinism, Beckwith-Wiedemann syndrome).
2. Hyponatremia, profound (consider congenital adrenal hyperplasia, maternal administration of salt-free intravenous fluids).
3. Hypermagnesemia (consider tocolysis by magnesium sulphate, preeclamptic toxemia).
4. Hyperammonemia (consider inborn errors of metabolism).

H. Multiple congenital malformations.

1. Chromosomal disorders: trisomies 13, 18, and 21.
2. Pierre Robin syndrome.
3. Osteogenesis imperfecta.
4. Asphyxiating thoracic dystrophy.

I. Miscellaneous.

1. Birth injuries (consider diaphragmatic paralysis, cervical cord injury).
2. Severe abstinence syndrome (secondary to in utero drug exposure).
3. Apnea.

28

Discharge Considerations and Process

Jean S. Wheeler

I. DISCHARGE TEACHING

N.B. These guidelines are not expected to be rigid. The individual circumstance of the patient and the preferences of the practitioner mandate flexibility at all times, with the potential of addition and deletion of items.

A. Assessment.

1. Consider past experience.
2. Evaluate knowledge base.
3. Consider common limitations after delivery.
   a. Maternal sleep deprivation.
   b. Physical discomfort.
   c. Short hospital stay.

B. Intervention.

1. Individual teaching.
2. Written instructions; handouts.
3. Videotapes.
4. Classes.

C. Content.

1. Feeding.
   a. Formula.
      (1) Iron fortified. Low-iron formulas should be avoided (term infants require 1 mg/kg per day of iron, assuming an average rate of absorption of 12% of dietary content; infants weighing 1500 to 2500 g require 2 mg/kg/day).
      (2) Preparation instructions (refer to illustration on can).
      (3) Thoroughly cleanse nipples and bottles before use.
      (4) 1.5 oz minimum of formula every 3 to 4 hours, increased gradually.
      (5) Additional water or juice is not recommended.

    b. Breast-feeding (see Chapter 24).
      (1) Infant should be fed on demand every 2 to 3 hours.
      (2) Average 8 to 10 feeds every 24 hours.
      (3) Infant should feed for 10 to 15 minutes on each side per each feeding.
      (4) Adequate rest and fluid intake by the mother are imperative.
      (5) Sore nipples indicate poor positioning.
2. Voiding and stooling.
    a. Bottle-fed infants' stools are yellow-green and firm to pasty; straining is normal and not necessarily indicative of constipation.
    b. Breast-fed infants' stools are bright yellow and loose; frequency varies from stooling with each feed to every other day. In the first weeks, frequent stools are a good indication of successful nursing.
    c. Four to six wet diapers a day are usually indicative of adequate intake.
3. Jaundice.
    a. Occurs in >50% of normal newborns and occurs more often in breast-fed infants than those who are bottle-fed.
    b. Jaundice is a temporary condition and is most often not associated with disease.
    c. It usually peaks at 3 to 4 days of life.
    d. Scleral icterus should be brought to the physician's attention.
4. Skin.
    a. Sponge bathe every day or every other day per parents' preference.
    b. Tub baths must wait until after the umbilical cord remnant falls off.
    c. Mild, unscented soap is preferable.
    d. Shampoo scalp with each bath.
    e. Lotions, oils, or powders are unnecessary.
    f. Reassure parents that dry, peeling skin is expected and resolves spontaneously.
    g. Diaper rash may be treated with petroleum jelly and air exposure; if persistent, parents should call practitioner.
    h. Mention to parents any rash present at discharge (e.g. erythema toxicum, pustular melanosis).
    i. If applicable, point out fetal scalp electrode site and instruct parents regarding signs of infection.
5. Cord care.
    a. Rubbing alcohol should be applied to the cord with an alcohol-soaked cotton ball several times per day.
    b. The diaper, whether cloth or disposable, should be fastened below the cord.
    c. Sponge baths are given to avoid getting the cord wet.
    d. The cord will usually drop off at approximately 2 weeks.
    e. Redness around the base, foul odor, or drainage from the cord should be reported to the practitioner immediately.
    f. If the infant was circumcised, a petroleum jelly–impregnated gauze strip should cover the penis for 24 hours; after removing

the gauze, apply petroleum jelly to the penis after each diaper change until healed, usually a few days. Parents should notify the practitioner if there is bleeding or signs of infection.

  g. If a Plastibell was used after the circumcision, petroleum jelly should not be used because this could loosen the string.

6. Safety.

  a. Car seats are mandatory for all car rides, including the ride home from the hospital.

  b. Bottle propping is dangerous because of the risks of choking.

  c. The infant should sleep on its back, not on its stomach. The side position is an alternative if necessary.

  d. Infants should never be in a bed with a sleeping adult because of the risk of suffocation or falling from the bed. (There are some who may disagree with this.)

  e. Avoid soft bedding, pillows, stuffed toys, plastic bags, and strings in infant's bed.

  f. Pacifiers should never be placed around the infant's neck on a string or cord; strangulation may occur.

  g. A plain nipple should never be used as a pacifier; the infant may aspirate it and occlude the airway.

  h. Hot liquids should be avoided while handling the baby; babies burn easily.

  i. Direct sunlight should be avoided; suntans are not healthy, and sunscreens contain chemicals that may not be safe for use in newborns.

  j. Smoke detectors should be installed and in working order before discharge of the baby from the hospital.

  k. Cigarette smoking around the infant, both in the house and in the car, should be avoided by all members of the infant's household.

  l. Keep the infant away from crowds and sick individuals for the first 4 to 5 weeks to prevent infection (e.g., excursions to the supermarket, crowded parties should not have high priority).

  m. Overdressing is not necessary for a healthy, full-term baby; thermoregulatory mechanisms are usually in order by several days of age; the home does not need to be super hot, and the amount of clothing can be gauged by what is appropriate for an older child or even an adult.

  n. Never leave the infant alone with a pet.

7. Expected infant behavior.

  a. Hiccups are common and require no treatment.

  b. Sneezing is expected and does not necessarily indicate the presence of a cold.

  c. Sucking on a pacifier helps satisfy the infant's nonnutritive sucking needs and rarely leads to long-term dependency or dental problems.

  d. Crying up to 1 to 1½ hours a day is normal in the first month. Assess hunger, diaper change, burping. Parents should hold infant and rock gently. NEVER SHAKE A BABY.

  e. There are great variations in infant sleep patterns; the cycle may be 45 to 60 minutes in the neonatal period; babies are wiser than

we are—they usually get what they need; there should be reasonable quiet time, but babies often adapt to noise.
8. Signs of illness.
   a. Poor feeding, cyanosis, tachypnea, irritability, lethargy, unusual skin rash, problems with the cord, vomiting, diarrhea, decreased urinary output, rectal temperature >100° F, or a change in the infant's usual behavior should immediately be reported to the practitioner.
   b. Emphasize that neonatal infection is not necessarily accompanied by a fever.

D. Review.
1. Questions.
   a. Encourage the parents to ask questions about the baby.
   b. Clarify any specific areas that are not completely understood; written instructions may be helpful.
2. Reassure new parents that many more questions will probably arise and that it is appropriate to call the practitioner.

E. Follow-up care.
1. Physician follow-up should be arranged before the infant's discharge.
2. Parents should be advised at the time of discharge when the baby is to return to the practitioner for the first visit.
   a. Within 48 to 72 hours if there is an early discharge.
   b. Otherwise 1 to 2 weeks.
3. Provide parents with the phone number of the primary care practitioner.
4. Send newborn records to the primary care practitioner.
5. Factors influencing the time of the first pediatric visit.
   a. The medical condition of the baby.
   b. The length of hospital stay.
   c. Experience of the mother and others caring for the baby.
   d. The baby's size and gestational age.
   e. The social situation.
   f. How well the baby is feeding and whether the baby is breast-feeding (a first-time breast-feeding mother should maintain close contact with the baby's practitioner and have the baby in for a weight check within the first week of life to ensure that excessive weight loss has not occurred and to provide support if commitment to nursing is wavering).
6. Home nursing visit.
   a. Within 24 to 48 hours of discharge.
   b. Should occur for all infants discharged at 24 hours or less.
   c. Useful for breast-feeding infants. (If possible, the nurse should observe the infant nursing.)

II. SOCIAL BARRIERS TO DISCHARGE
N.B.: Whenever a problem is identified that may endanger an infant's safety or well-being, a social work evaluation should be requested.
  A. Referral. If necessary, a referral should be made to the child protective agency in the community, and a home assessment should be completed before discharge.

B. Some problems that may prevent or delay discharge.
1. Maternal history of substance abuse.
2. Present or previous history of psychiatric illness in the mother.
3. Severe illness or physical disability of the mother.
4. History of neglect or abuse of a previous child.
5. History of domestic violence.
6. Inappropriate maternal behavior or poor maternal-infant bonding.
7. Maternal homelessness or inadequate living and support arrangements.

III. PHYSICAL BARRIERS TO DISCHARGE
A. Feedings. All infants must demonstrate good breast-feeding ability or adequate formula intake before discharge.
B. Prematurity.
1. An infant <37 weeks of gestation or <2500 gm should be observed if possible for a minimum of 3 days.
2. A premature infant must demonstrate the ability to maintain a normal body temperature in an open bassinet for 24 hours (36.4° to 37° C or 97.5° to 98.6° F)
3. Jaundice in a premature infant (<37 weeks) is more likely to require treatment.
C. Neonatal drug withdrawal.
1. An infant exposed to drugs in utero should be held for observation.
2. A social work evaluation should be done.
3. If symptoms occur or a urine toxicology screen on the infant is positive, a referral to child protective services should be considered. Some jurisdictions mandate referral.
4. If medication is required to treat severe symptoms, the infant must be held until the medication is no longer necessary.
5. The symptomatic infant should be held until symptoms have subsided.
6. The mother should be encouraged to enter drug treatment.
7. Instruct mother or other caretaker regarding symptomatic and supportive care of the withdrawing infant.
8. Advise mother regarding danger of passive cocaine exposure to infant.
D. Congenital abnormalities.
1. Heart murmurs thought to be pathologic should be evaluated before discharge.
2. Dislocated hips should be seen by an orthopedic specialist, an ultrasound should be obtained, and treatment begun.
3. Clubfeet should be seen and treated by an orthopedic specialist.
4. Abnormal prenatal renal ultrasound results should be evaluated before discharge.
5. Other major malformations (e.g., cleft lip/palate) may require additional time for parental education and adjustment and evaluation and coordination of services by medical subspecialists.
E. Infections.
1. Sepsis.
   a. An infant at increased risk for sepsis, whether on treatment or not, should be observed in the hospital for signs of infection a minimum of 48 hours.

    b. An infant born to a group B streptococcus (GBS)–colonized mother, with or without intrapartum treatment, should be observed in the hospital a minimum of 48 hours (per American Academy of Pediatrics [AAP] *Guidelines for Perinatal Care*).

    c. When antibiotics are started, the treatment should continue in the hospital until the blood culture is negative for 48 to 72 hours.

2. Syphilis.

    a. Infants with congenital syphilis or infants of mothers with syphilis who were untreated, inadequately treated, or treated in the last 4 weeks of pregnancy should receive a spinal tap and be treated for 10 days with intramuscular (IM) or intravenous (IV) penicillin administration (see Chapter 20).

    b. The infant should be held in the hospital for completion of the penicillin course unless outpatient treatment can be arranged and compliance can be ensured.

3. Pneumonia. Infants with pneumonia should be held in the hospital for 7 to 14 days of IM or IV antibiotic administration. Home care may be an option when the infant is stable.

4. Tuberculosis; mother with positive tuberculin test (see Chapter 20).

F. Hyperbilirubinemia.

1. Any jaundice visible in the first 24 hours of life should be investigated. Initial evaluation should include a blood type and direct Coombs' test, a hematocrit or hemoglobin level, and a total bilirubin level (see Chapter 19).

2. Indications for phototherapy are discussed in Chapter 19. Home health care agencies may be able to arrange for phototherapy to be performed at home.

3. Infants with an elevated bilirubin level but without hemolysis can usually be discharged if follow-up levels can be obtained by the infant's practitioner.

IV. EARLY DISCHARGE

Is infant a candidate for early discharge (Box 28-1)?

A. General criteria. After low-risk deliveries, infants may be discharged within 24 hours of birth.

1. A tentative decision should be made before delivery.

2. Discharge should be a joint plan by the obstetrician, pediatrician, and family; it should be physician directed, not insurer driven; many states have laws requiring minimum 48-hour stays after vaginal delivery.

3. Pregnancy, antepartum, intrapartum, and early postpartum periods should be uncomplicated. Any change in the status of the mother, fetus, or neonate at any stage may alter the plan.

4. Mother should have attended prenatal education and neonatal care classes that include information on potential problems in the first 3 to 5 days of life.

5. Pediatric care after discharge must be identified.

6. The mother needs adequate support at home. Both mother and neonate should be examined in 2 to 3 days, preferably at home.

BOX 28-1
Postponing Newborn Discharge: Factors to Consider

MATERNAL MEDICAL FACTORS
Cesarean delivery
Abnormal labor or delivery
Medical conditions such as diabetes mellitus
Elevated temperature
Group B streptococcal colonization
Sexually transmitted disease
O or Rh-negative blood group

MATERNAL SOCIAL FACTORS
No or poor prenatal care
Substance abuse
Adolescence
Poor support system
Mental retardation or psychiatric illness
Planning adoption or foster placement

INFANT FACTORS
Preterm (≤37 weeks)
Small for gestational age
Large for gestational age
Abnormal physical examination
Vital signs, color activity, feeding
Significant congenital malformation

ABNORMAL LABORATORY FINDINGS
Hypoglycemia
Hyperbilirubinemia
Polycythemia
Anemia
Rapid plasma reagin positive

From Hurt H: *Contemp Pediatr* 11:76, 1994.

B. Neonatal criteria.
1. Single birth.
2. Uncomplicated vaginal delivery.
3. Full-term infant (38 to 42 weeks), weight appropriate for gestational age, with a normal examination by a pediatrician or nurse practitioner before discharge.
4. Uncomplicated transition.
5. Normal vital signs, stable temperature.
6. Infant demonstrates a healthy suck and swallow and has fed from breast or bottle at least twice, with coordinated suck, swallow, and breathing.
7. Infant has voided. If circumcised, no bleeding occurs for >2 hours.

8. Infant has stooled. (If meconium has not passed by 24 hours of age, mother should be instructed to call her practitioner.)
9. No jaundice is apparent in the first 24 hours of life.
10. Laboratory tests.
    a. Maternal or cord blood test for syphilis is nonreactive.
    b. Maternal hepatitis B surface antigen is negative.
    c. Cord blood of infant should be tested for blood type and Coombs' test if the mother is Rh-negative or type O.
    d. Hematocrit and blood glucose levels are as clinically indicated.
    e. Metabolic screening. (If obtained at <24 hours, repeat testing should be ensured.)
    f. Hepatitis B vaccine (thimerosal-free) given or scheduled with the primary care practitioner.
11. Stable social situation.
12. Follow-up ensured.
C. Maternal criteria.
1. Demonstrates ability with feeding technique, skin care, cord care, and temperature measurement with a thermometer.
2. Demonstrates ability to assess the infant's well-being and signs of illness.
N.B.: The AAP states that it is "unlikely" the above minimum criteria and conditions can be met before 48 hours.
D. Follow-up.
1. A home nursing or office visit should be scheduled within 24 to 48 hours to assess the following:
    a. Weight. Unclothed infant should not be more than 8% to 10% below birth weight.
    b. Feeding. Ensure infant is receiving an adequate amount; observe breast-feeding if possible.
    c. Elimination. Check frequency of urination; number and color of stools. (Is infant still passing meconium?)
    d. Jaundice.
    e. Signs of illness (e.g., tachypnea, cyanosis, poor feeding, vomiting, irritability).
2. Telephone follow-up may be helpful but *should not* take the place of a visit.

V. DISCHARGE EVALUATION
A. Importance of evaluation. Shorter postpartum hospitals stays for mothers and constricted time for observation make a thorough discharge examination imperative because there is little time to observe the infant for potential problems. According to the AAP and ACOG's 1997 *Guidelines for Perinatal Care,* a newborn should be examined within 24 hours after birth and within 24 hours of discharge, therefore many newborns will only have one physical examination.
B. Guidance. When performed in the presence of the parents, the discharge evaluation allows opportunity for providing education, answering questions, and giving anticipatory guidance.
C. Notations. The discharge evaluation should include a complete examination, with emphasis on any points omitted or any abnormalities noted on the admission examination.

D. The following areas should be of particular note:

1. General.
    a. Check frequency and duration of breast-feedings; if bottle-fed, the frequency and amount of formula feedings.
    b. Check number of voids and stools.
    c. Compare present weight with birth weight.
    d. Observe the infant's color, posture, activity, tone, and temperature.
    e. Review vital signs.

2. Head.
    a. Palpate fontanels and sutures.
    b. Look for a cephalhematoma; may not be present at birth but may become apparent over first few days of life (increases risk of jaundice).
    c. Check any caput succedaneum or cranial molding, which should be resolving.
    d. Inspect any abrasions, lacerations, fetal scalp electrode site, or forceps marks, which should be healing.
    e. Measure head circumference.

3. Eyes.
    a. Note subconjunctival hemorrhages.
    b. Look for chemical conjunctivitis, which may have resulted from eye prophylaxis (unusual with erythromycin).
    c. Perform an ophthalmoscopic examination to look for red reflex, congenital cataracts, or glaucoma.

4. Ears.
    a. Assess pinnae for normal configuration and set.
    b. Check traumatic lesions such as bruises or abrasions.
    c. Note preauricular tags or sinuses.
    d. Check for patent canals.

5. Nose.
    a. Check patency of nares.
    b. Look for asymmetry or septal deviation, flaring.

6. Mouth.
    a. Inspect for natal teeth, mucoid cysts, ranula, or bifid uvula.
    b. Observe palate for cleft.
    c. Check sucking reflex.
    d. Check size and position of tongue.

7. Neck.
    a. Examine for congenital malformations such as fistulas, cysts, lymphangiomas, or goiter.
    b. Check for webbing.

8. Chest.
    a. Count respiratory rate.
    b. Observe symmetry of chest movement and ease of respirations.

9. Heart.
    a. Note cardiac rate and rhythm.
    b. Palpate point of maximum impulse.
    c. Note precordium activity.
    d. Auscultate for murmurs; murmurs that signify congenital heart disease are often not heard until after the first few days of life.
    e. Palpate brachial and femoral pulses.

10. Abdomen.
    a. Observe for distention.
    b. Palpate for enlarged organs or masses.
    c. Assess cord for bleeding or signs of infection.
11. Genitalia.
    a. Inspect female infant for patent vagina, vaginal tags, discharge, or pseudomenses. Palpate labia for gonads.
    b. Check male infant for chordee, hypospadias, undescended testes, or hydroceles; if circumcised, inspect for bleeding or infection.
12. Skeletal.
    a. Inspect for supernumerary digits, syndactyly, metatarsus adductus, clubfoot.
    b. Examine clavicles for fracture.
    c. Check hips for subluxation or dislocation.
    d. Inspect spine for scoliosis, sacral dimple, and/or sinus.
13. Nervous system.
    a. Assess infant's tone and symmetry of Moro reflex.
    b. Observe for tremulousness.
    c. Look for palsies of upper extremities or face.
    d. Assess suck.
14. Skin.
    a. Inspect for rashes, hemangiomas, nevi, café au lait or mongolian spots, or supernumerary nipples.
    b. Note presence and degree of any jaundice.
  E. Follow-up considerations. Any abnormality on discharge examination not requiring immediate evaluation or treatment but needing follow-up should be brought to the attention of the practitioner who will be caring for the infant.
  F. Practitioner. All newborns being discharged from the hospital should have an identified primary care practitioner to whom records should be sent.

VI. NEWBORN METABOLIC SCREENING
A. Newborns in the United States have been screened for metabolic disorders for over 30 years using a technique of blood drops impregnated on filter paper.
B. State regulations. Because there are no federal guidelines regarding newborn metabolic screening, practitioners must be aware of regulations in their state.
C. There is wide variation from state to state in not only what disorders are screened but also whether participation is voluntary or mandatory. (In Maryland, parental consent is required to screen the infant.)
D. Presently, all states screen for phenylketonuria (PKU) and hypothyroidism. Some states screen for up to six different disorders. It is necessary to check locally (see Chapter 22).
E. Metabolic diseases that are screened for in one or more states include the following:
1. Biotinidase deficiency, congenital adrenal hyperplasia, congenital hypothyroidism, cystic fibrosis, galactosemia, homocystinuria, branched-

chain ketoaciduria (maple syrup urine disease), PKU, sickle cell disease, and tyrosinemia.
2. As screening and treatment become available, new tests may be added.
3. As states review their programs and populations, other tests may be deleted.

F. When should screen be done?
1. After 24 hours of age, after feeding is well established and toxic metabolites have a chance to accumulate.
2. Screening is usually done at discharge from the hospital, preferably at 48 to 72 hours of age; a repeat test is recommended at a 2- to 4-week visit.
3. If the initial screen is obtained before 24 hours of age, a second specimen should be obtained at 1 to 2 weeks.
4. Many states have changed the cutoff for normal serum phenylalanine from 4 to 2 mg/dl because of early screening prompted by <24-hour discharge.
5. Regardless of age, a newborn screen should be obtained from all infants at discharge; missing a metabolic disorder is more likely to occur because a sample was never obtained rather than because it was obtained too early.

VII. NEWBORN HEARING SCREENING
A. Prevalence of congenital hearing loss is 1.5 to 6/1000 live births.
B. Identification of hearing-impaired neonates.
1. Average age of identification is 24 to 30 months.
2. Moderate hearing losses frequently are not identified until 5 to 6 years of age.
3. Early identification is important so interventions can be initiated that will affect speech and language acquisition.
C. Universal newborn hearing screening versus screening by risk factors.
1. Screening neonates based on risk factors misses 50% of hearing-impaired neonates.
2. Universal hearing screening is recommended and is becoming mandated by law in many states.
D. Type of screening.
1. Otoacoustic emissions (OAE).
2. Auditory brainstem evoked response (ABR).
3. Improvements in these technologies are making screening more efficient, cost effective, and "user friendly."

BIBLIOGRAPHY

Acosta PB, Yannicelli S (editors): *A practitioner's guide to selected inborn errors of metabolism,* Columbus, Ohio, 1992, Ross Laboratories.

American Academy of Pediatrics: Newborn screening for congenital hypothyroidism: recommended guidelines, *Pediatrics* 91:1203, 1993.

American Academy of Pediatrics: Group B Streptococcal Infections. In Peter G (editor): *1997 red book: report of the Committee on Infectious Diseases,* ed 24, Elk Grove Village, Ill, 1997, the Academy.

American Academy of Pediatrics: Syphilis. In Peter G (editor): *1997 red book: report of the Committee on Infectious Diseases,* ed 24, Elk Grove Village, Ill, 1997, the Academy.

American Academy of Pediatrics: Hospital discharge of the high risk neonate: proposed guidelines, *Pediatrics* 102:411, 1998.

American Academy of Pediatrics Joint Committee on Infant Hearing: 1994 position statement, *Pediatrics* 95:152, 1995.

American Academy of Pediatrics and American College of Obstetricians and Gynecologists: *Guidelines for perinatal care,* ed 4, Elk Grove Village, Ill and Washington DC, 1997, AAP and ACOG.

Barsky-Firkser L, Sun S: Universal newborn hearing screenings: a three-year experience, *Pediatrics* 99(6):1997.

Beebe SA, et al: Neonatal mortality and length of newborn hospital stay, *Pediatrics* 98:321, 1996.

Gibson E, Cullen JA, et al: Infant sleep position following new AAP guidelines, *Pediatrics* 96:69, 1995.

Maisels MJ, Kring E: Length of stay, jaundice and hospital readmission, *Pediatrics* 101:995, 1998.

Sinai LN, Kim SC, et al: Phenylketonuria screening: effect of early newborn discharge, *Pediatrics* 96:605, 1995.

Thilo EH, Townsend SF: Early newborn discharge: have we gone too far? *Contemp Pediatr* 13:29, 1996.

Wheeler JS, Donohue PK: Newborn care after early discharge: role of the primary care provider, *Clin Rev* 9:65, 1992.

29

Adoption

PATRICIA H. SMOUSE

In addition to the needs that every neonate possesses, the baby to be placed for adoption requires special considerations.

I. REASONS WHY ADOPTION MAY BE CONSIDERED
A. Young mother.
B. Unwanted pregnancy.
C. Rape.
D. Parental preference.

II. ADOPTION PROCEDURES
A. Verify maternal decision to place the baby for adoption.
B. **Recognize the complex needs of the birthmother and baby.** Involve a hospital social worker to assist with counseling of the mother, to explore options if prior arrangements have not been made or if the mother is ambivalent about placing the baby for adoption, to identify pertinent community resources, and to coordinate discharge according to hospital policy, which should be in accordance with state laws regarding adoption. Respect the birthmother's wishes for her extent of involvement with the baby and desire for anonymity and privacy. Her involvement may vary from refraining from any contact with the baby to an open arrangement in which the birthparents and adoptive parents have met prenatally and all participate in the infant's hospital course of care. Some involvement of the birthmother may assist her in dealing with feelings of doubt and guilt and aid in the long-term grieving process.
C. **Provide emotional support to the birth mother.** Recognize her need to discuss her feelings; despite this being a voluntary decision, she is likely to experience significant feelings of grief.
D. **Birthmother's rights.** The birthmother has the legal right to name the baby and to sign consent for infant screening tests and procedures, including circumcision.
E. **Release of the baby.** The birthmother should sign for release of the baby to the proper agency or individual before she and the baby

are discharged from the hospital. Early discharge mandates may make this difficult to achieve.

F. Birthfather. Ensure knowledge and consent of the adoption plan by the putative father in states that specify this requirement.

G. Right to medical information. Do not ignore the birthmother's right to medical information regarding her baby.

H. Release of medical information to the adoptive parents. The birthmother should sign a release of medical information for herself and her baby to the adoptive parents or agency.

III. TYPES OF ADOPTION

A. Agency adoption. Adoption involving a licensed adoption agency.

1. Baby is usually discharged to an employee of the adoptive agency and may then be placed in temporary foster care, allowing the birthmother some time to reconsider her decision before the baby is placed with the adoptive parents.

2. Counseling is provided to the birthmother through the adoption agency.

B. Private adoption. Adoption without involvement of a licensed adoption agency. Private adoption is usually arranged prenatally by the birthmother, adoptive family, and an attorney hired by the adoptive family.

1. Baby is discharged directly to the adoptive parents.

2. Visitation of the baby at the hospital by the adoptive family is contingent on approval by the birthmother.

3. It is essential to ensure that the birthmother is not pressured into a decision.

IV. DISCHARGE NEEDS

A. Agency. If the baby is being placed with an agency, the agency should provide a copy of its license and whatever other documents the hospital requires. Picture identification of the worker picking up the baby must be verified; copies of the worker's picture identification should be placed in the medical record.

B. Adoptive parents. If the baby is going directly to adoptive parents, they most often must provide a temporary custody order of which a true test copy remains in the medical record. Picture identification of the adoptive parents must be verified and copies placed in the chart. Some hospitals require only the birthmother's release to allow the adoptive parents to take the baby from the hospital.

C. A complete medical record of maternal history, family history, history of present pregnancy, labor and delivery, neonatal course, and any special health needs should be filled out.

D. Document the results of all medical tests.

E. Provide any special medical instructions and routine baby care information to agency worker or adoptive family.

F. Advise agency or adoptive parents regarding infant's first pediatric visit.

BIBLIOGRAPHY

American Academy of Pediatrics and The American College of Obstetricians and Gynecologists: *Guidelines for perinatal care,* ed 4, Elk Grove Village, Ill, 1997, the Academy and the College.

American Academy of Pediatrics Committee on Early Childhood, Adoption and Dependent Care: Initial medical evaluation of an adopted child, *Pediatrics* 88:642, 1991.

Dewarle BK: Open adoption, *Can Nurse* 88:14, 1992.

McNally C: Adoption: the perinatal social worker's role in the process, *Natl Assoc Perinat Social Workers* 14:1, 1994.

Thaler CH: Personal communication, August 5, 1994.

30

The Importance of
Wasting No Time

HENRY M. SEIDEL

The central nervous system (CNS) of the newborn is marvelously sophisticated, a brain ready to perform and a myriad of neuronal connections eager to be put to constructive use. Nature and nurture have been working together since conception to bring the infant to life, and even at the very beginning they have had a vital partner in the social context that will shape the child's experience.

The mother's contribution to that context is as vital to the fetal experience as are traditionally recognized nature and nurture. We no longer need to be persuaded that hearing is well-established early, usually by 24 to 25 weeks of gestation, or that newborns really do feel pain. Indeed, the fetus hears the mother's voice and can distinguish it from others after birth. Impressively, the sounds of classical music heard during fetal and early postnatal life are said to increase the ability to learn mathematics later on. Too much noise during gestation, however, can contribute to later deafness. The neurophysiologic ability to sense pain and to remember it is also firmly in place by the start of the third trimester.[1,3] Handling and immobilization in the early hours of life can influence a baby's response to a later painful stimulus.[4] The first breath after delivery, the "once in a lifetime event," is the logical next step for a habit established in the third month of gestation.

Thus the full-term newborn is an exquisitely sentient person well-constituted for the tasks ahead. As many as 100 billion neurons, each able to produce 15,000 synapses, are ready to be influenced and firmly set by stimuli that might be healthy or noxious—an intensely realized activity from the first hours and through the first years of life. Only half of those synapses will survive. Repeated early experiences activate synapses that, becoming permanent, more sharply define the brain's patterns. Therefore the social context that is the baby's becomes an important player, ranking right up there with the genes. We must pay close attention to that context prenatally and in the precious hours when the new baby is in our charge in our nurseries.[5]

Every baby is the result of a relationship between two people–a dyad. Baby makes three, a relationship that has as its roots three dyads, mother-baby, father-baby, and mother-father. The whole is greater than the sum of the parts, but that "whole" depends very much on the nature of the trio of dyads. This trio is the simplest construction. Each additional baby increases the number of dyads considerably, and one can imagine the complexity when the original dyad may rupture and a possible welter of new relationships develops. Still, the understanding of what may be going on in the whole of a social system requires a grasp of the issues confronting any one member in the dyad with each of the others.

Consider the original trio. Parents love their children–or do they? What was the nature of the original dyad? How does the mother take to the baby? Does nursing really please her? Does the father resent the intrusion of the child? How do the parents now feel about each other? So many questions, and the answers can be found within each dyad.

We who have responsibility for some of the care of a newborn must understand the plasticity of the infant's nervous system and respect that as we consider how we contribute to the baby's experience. We must educate parents about this as much as about the impressive physiologic adjustments of new life. Long ago, Leo Kanner reminded us that everyone *always* needs the 4 "As": attention, affection, acceptance, and approval. The *always* is as fully relevant to the fetus and newborn as it is to any of us, and the need for the four "As" carries the same urgency as the need for food and water. Understanding this and assessing the availability of these four "As" in each consideration of a dyad will go a long way to abet our effort to help each child have the best possible start in life, the "head start" that Eisenberg reminds us is as vital to our goal in care as is the physical well-being of a baby.[2]

BIBLIOGRAPHY

American Academy of Pediatrics Committee on Environmental Health: Noise: a hazard for the fetus and newborn, *Pediatrics* 100:724, 1997.

Eisenberg L: Experience, brain, and behavior: the importance of a head start, *N Engl J Med* 340:1031, 1999.

Porter FL, et al: Pain and pain management in newborn infants: a survey of physicians and nurses, *Pediatrics* 100:626, 1997.

Porter FL, Wolf CM, Miller JP: The effect of handling and immobilization on the response to acute pain in newborn infants, *Pediatrics* 102:1383, 1998.

Shore R: *Rethinking the brain: new insights into early development (executive summary)*, New York City, 1997, Families and Work Institute.

APPENDIX A

Conversion Tables and Formulas

TABLE A-1
Temperature Equivalents

Celsius*	Fahrenheit†	Celsius*	Fahrenheit†
34.0	93.2	38.6	101.4
34.2	93.6	38.8	101.8
34.4	93.9	39.0	102.2
34.6	94.3	39.2	102.5
34.8	94.6	39.4	102.9
35.0	95.0	39.6	103.2
35.2	95.4	39.8	103.6
35.4	95.7	40.0	104.0
35.6	96.1	40.2	104.3
35.8	96.4	40.4	104.7
36.0	96.8	40.6	105.1
36.2	97.1	40.8	105.4
36.4	97.5	41.0	105.8
36.6	97.8	41.2	106.1
36.8	98.2	41.4	106.5
37.0	98.6	41.6	106.8
37.2	98.9	41.8	107.2
37.4	99.3	42.0	107.6
37.6	99.6	42.2	108.0
37.8	100.0	42.4	108.3
38.0	100.4	42.6	108.7
38.2	100.7	42.8	109.0
38.4	101.1	43.0	109.4

From Hoekelman RA, Friedman SB, Nelson NM, et al: *Primary pediatric care,* ed 3, St Louis, 1997, Mosby.
*To convert Celsius to Fahrenheit: (9/5 × Temperature) + 32.
†To convert Fahrenheit to Celsius: 5/9 × (Temperature −32).

TABLE A-2
Conversion Formula

Height (length)
1 millimeter (mm) = 0.04 inch
1 centimeter (cm) = 0.4 inch
2.54 cm = 1 inch
1 meter (m) = 39.37 inches

Weight
60 milligrams (mg) = 1 grain
28.35 grams (gm) = 1 ounce
454 gm = 1 pound
1000 gm (1 kilogram [kg]) = 2.2 pounds

Milligram-milliequivalent conversions

$$mEq/L = mg/L \times \frac{Valence}{Atomic\ weight}$$

$$mg/L = mEq/L \times \frac{Atomic\ weight}{Valence}$$

$$Equivalent\ weight = \frac{Atomic\ weight}{Valence}$$

Milliosmols

The milliequivalent (mEq) is roughly equivalent to the milliosmol (mosm), the unit of measure of osmolarity or tonicity.

Prefixes for decimal factors

Prefix	Symbol	Factor
mega	m	10^6
kilo	k	10^1
hecto	h	10^2
deka	da	10^1
deci	d	10^{-1}
centi	c	10^{-2}
milli	m	10^{-3}
micro	μ	10^{-6}
nano	n	10^{-9}
pico	p	10^{-12}
fento	f	10^{-15}

From Hoekelman RA, Friedman SB, Nelson NM, et al: *Primary pediatric care,* ed 3, St Louis, 1997, Mosby.

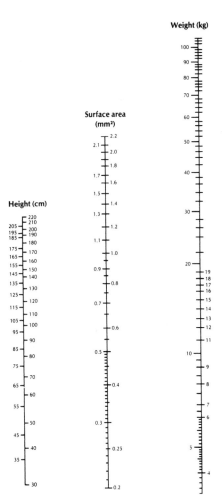

Weight (kg)

Surface area (mm²)

Height (cm)

FIG. A-1 Nomogram to determine body surface area. (Redrawn from Cole CH (editor): *The Harriet Lane handbook,* St Louis, 1989, Mosby. Based on data from Gelian EA, George SL: *Cancer Chemother Rep* 54:225, 1970.)

APPENDIX B

Anthropometric Charts and Tables

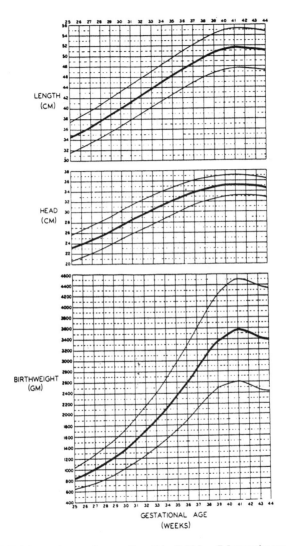

FIG. B-1 Intrauterine growth curves. (From Usher R, McLean F: Intrauterine growth of live-born Caucasian infants at sea level: standards obtained from measurements in seven dimensions of infants born between 25 and 44 weeks of gestation, *J Pediatr* 74:901, 1969.)

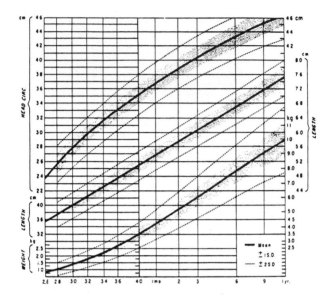

FIG. B-2 Extrauterine growth curves. (From Babson SG, Benda GI: Growth graphics for the clinical assessment of infants of varying gestational age, *J Pediatr* 89:814, 1976.)

TABLE B-1

Distribution of Measurements for White Newborn Male Infants (Controls) by Percentiles According to Gestational Ages

Percentile	37	38	39	40	41	42-43
	GESTATIONAL AGE (WEEKS)					
	CROWN-HEEL LENGTHS (CM)					
95	52.0	53.0	54.0	54.5	55.0	55.3
90	51.5	52.5	53.5	54.0	54.5	54.8
75	50.5	51.5	52.5	53.0	53.5	54.0
50	50.0	50.7	51.5	52.0	52.5	53.0
25	49.0	49.7	50.5	51.0	51.5	52.0
10	48.0	48.7	49.5	50.0	50.5	51.0
5	47.5	48.2	49.0	49.5	50.0	50.5
	OCCIPITOFRONTAL CIRCUMFERENCE (CM)					
95	35.5	36.0	36.4	36.8	37.2	37.4
90	35.2	35.6	35.9	36.3	36.7	37.2
75	34.6	34.9	35.3	35.7	36.0	36.2
50	34.0	34.3	34.6	34.9	35.2	35.5
25	33.4	33.7	34.0	34.3	34.7	35.0
10	32.8	33.2	33.5	33.8	34.2	34.5
5	32.4	32.7	33.1	33.4	33.8	34.2

Percentile	37	38	39	40	41	42-43
	GESTATIONAL AGE (WEEKS)					
	BIRTH WEIGHTS, FIRST-BORN INFANTS (KG)					
95	3.63	3.82	3.97	4.10	4.23	4.34
90	3.50	3.70	3.86	4.00	4.13	4.24
75	3.30	3.48	3.65	3.78	3.92	4.03
50	3.10	3.27	3.43	3.57	3.70	3.82
25	2.85	3.00	3.13	3.26	3.38	3.49
10	2.70	2.84	2.96	3.08	3.18	3.28
5	2.62	2.76	2.88	3.00	3.10	3.20
	BIRTH WEIGHTS, INFANTS OF MULTIPARAS (KG)					
95	3.66	4.00	4.20	4.39	4.50	4.60
90	3.47	3.70	3.90	4.08	4.24	4.37
75	3.30	3.50	3.70	3.87	4.03	4.15
50	3.10	3.27	3.44	3.61	3.75	3.85
25	2.85	3.02	3.18	3.34	3.50	3.62
10	2.71	2.86	3.02	3.19	3.34	3.45
5	2.63	2.78	2.94	3.08	3.31	3.32

From Miller HC: Intrauterine growth retardation: an unmet challenge, *Am J Dis Child* 135:946, 1981.

TABLE B-2
Distribution of Measurements for White Newborn Female Infants (Controls) by Percentiles According to Gestational Ages

	GESTATIONAL AGE (WEEKS)					
Percentile	37	38	39	40	41	42-43
	CROWN-HEEL LENGTHS (CM)					
95	51.5	52.5	53.5	54.0	54.5	54.5
90	51.0	52.0	53.0	53.5	54.0	54.0
75	50.0	51.0	52.0	52.5	52.8	53.1
50	49.0	50.0	50.7	51.3	51.7	52.0
25	48.0	48.9	49.5	50.0	50.5	51.0
10	47.5	48.5	49.0	49.5	50.0	50.5
5	47.0	47.9	48.6	49.1	49.5	50.0
	OCCIPITOFRONTAL CIRCUMFERENCES (CM)					
95	35.0	35.5	35.9	36.2	36.5	36.8
90	34.5	35.0	35.4	35.7	36.1	36.3
75	33.9	34.3	34.7	35.1	35.5	35.8
50	33.2	33.6	34.1	34.5	34.8	35.2
25	32.5	32.9	33.4	33.8	34.2	34.5
10	32.0	32.4	32.8	33.2	33.6	33.9
5	31.8	32.2	32.6	32.9	33.3	33.6

	GESTATIONAL AGE (WEEKS)					
Percentile	37	38	39	40	41	42-43
	BIRTH WEIGHTS, FIRST-BORN INFANTS (KG)					
95	3.44	3.72	3.90	4.03	4.12	4.20
90	3.30	3.60	3.80	3.92	4.02	4.10
75	3.17	3.38	3.57	3.70	3.82	3.94
50	3.00	3.15	3.30	3.43	3.56	3.66
25	2.79	2.93	3.07	3.18	3.29	3.37
10	2.55	2.72	2.85	2.97	3.09	3.17
5	2.46	2.61	2.76	2.89	3.01	3.10
	BIRTH WEIGHTS, INFANTS OF MULTIPARAS (KG)					
95	3.60	3.86	4.02	4.14	4.23	4.31
90	3.50	3.67	3.84	3.95	4.07	4.15
75	3.26	3.48	3.64	3.75	3.85	3.95
50	3.00	3.20	3.34	3.50	3.62	3.72
25	2.80	2.95	3.08	3.23	3.35	3.45
10	2.67	2.80	2.93	3.05	3.16	3.26
5	2.52	2.67	2.80	2.92	3.04	3.15

From Miller HC: Intrauterine growth retardation: an unmet challenge, *Am J Dis Child* 135:946, 1981.

TABLE B-3
Distribution of Measurements for Black Newborn Male Infants (Controls) by Percentiles According to Gestational Ages

Percentile	37	38	39	40	41	42-43
	GESTATIONAL AGE (WEEKS)					
	CROWN-HEEL LENGTHS (CM)					
95	51.5	52.5	53.5	54.5	54.5	54.5
90	51.0	52.0	52.7	53.5	54.0	54.0
75	50.5	51.5	52.0	52.5	53.0	53.0
50	49.5	50.0	50.5	51.0	51.5	52.0
25	48.5	49.0	49.5	50.0	50.5	51.0
10	47.5	48.0	48.5	49.0	49.5	50.0
5	47.0	47.5	48.0	48.5	49.0	49.5
	OCCIPITOFRONTAL CIRCUMFERENCES (CM)					
95	35.3	35.8	36.2	36.7	37.0	37.0
90	35.0	35.5	35.9	36.3	36.7	36.8
75	34.6	34.9	35.3	35.6	36.0	36.3
50	33.6	34.0	34.4	34.7	35.1	35.5
25	33.1	33.4	33.8	34.1	34.5	34.9
10	32.4	32.8	33.1	33.4	33.8	34.1
5	32.1	32.5	32.8	33.1	33.4	33.7
	BIRTH WEIGHTS (KG)					
95	3.44	3.71	3.97	4.13	4.29	4.40
90	3.38	3.62	3.84	3.97	4.10	4.15
75	3.30	3.46	3.62	3.72	3.82	3.92
50	3.08	3.18	3.30	3.40	3.50	3.60
25	2.83	2.93	3.03	3.13	3.22	3.32
10	2.63	2.73	2.82	2.90	2.99	3.08
5	2.54	2.68	2.72	2.82	2.95	3.00

From Miller HC: Intrauterine growth retardation: an unmet challenge, *Am J Dis Child* 135:946, 1981.

TABLE B-4
Distribution of Measurements for Black Newborn Female Infants (Controls) by Percentiles According to Gestational Ages

Percentile	37	38	39	40	41	42-43
	GESTATIONAL AGE (WEEKS)					

| | CROWN-HEEL LENGTHS (CM) | | | | | |
Percentile	37	38	39	40	41	42-43
95	51.0	51.7	52.5	53.3	54.0	54.0
90	50.3	51.0	51.8	52.5	53.5	53.0
75	49.5	50.5	51.0	51.5	52.0	52.5
50	49.0	49.5	50.0	50.5	51.0	51.5
25	48.0	48.5	49.0	49.5	50.0	50.5
10	47.0	47.5	48.0	48.5	49.0	49.5
5	46.5	47.0	47.5	48.0	48.5	49.0
	OCCIPITOFRONTAL CIRCUMFERENCES (CM)					
95	35.0	35.1	35.6	35.9	36.2	36.5
90	34.3	34.8	35.3	35.6	35.8	36.0
75	34.1	34.3	34.6	34.8	35.1	35.3
50	33.4	33.6	33.9	34.1	34.4	34.7
25	32.7	33.0	33.2	33.5	33.7	34.0
10	32.1	32.3	32.6	32.8	33.1	33.3
5	31.7	32.0	32.2	32.5	32.8	33.0
	BIRTH WEIGHTS (KG)					
95	3.44	3.65	3.83	3.97	4.00	4.15
90	3.32	3.53	3.73	3.88	3.98	4.05
75	3.14	3.32	3.48	3.60	3.73	3.85
50	2.93	3.07	3.22	3.34	3.46	3.58
25	2.70	2.83	2.95	3.08	3.03	3.32
10	2.53	2.65	2.77	2.89	3.01	3.10
5	2.43	2.54	2.65	2.77	2.89	3.01

From Miller HC: Intrauterine growth retardation: an unmet challenge, *Am J Dis Child* 135:946, 1981.

APPENDIX C

Laboratory Observations

BLOOD CHEMISTRY VALUES

Acid-Base Response in Respiratory Acidosis and Alkalosis

The nomogram shown in Fig. C-1 provides confidence bands for the normal adjustments in carbon dioxide content and pH made to acute and chronic changes in arterial P_{CO_2}.

1. Determine pH on nomogram from plotted Pa_{CO_2} and carbon dioxide content obtained from blood-gas measurement.
2. If pH value is not within confidence bands, alteration in carbon dioxide content and pH varies from that expected from a pure respiratory condition, and a metabolic abnormality is also present.
3. To estimate the effects of acute and chronic changes in P_{CO_2} on pH, use the following formulas:

Acute change in P_{CO_2}:

$$\Delta P_{CO_2} \times 0.008 = \Delta pH$$

Chronic change in P_{CO_2}:

$$\Delta P_{CO_2} \times 0.003 = \Delta pH$$

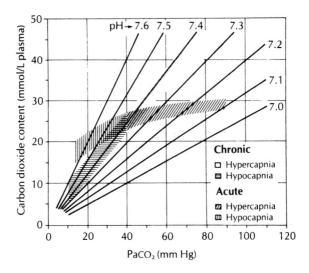

FIG. C-1 Acid-base response in respiratory acidosis and alkalosis. (Modified from Arbus GS: An in vivo acid-base nomogram for clinical use, *Can Med Assoc J* 109:291, 1973.)

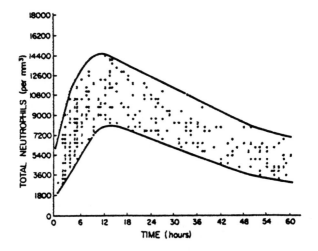

FIG. C-2 The total neutrophil count in normal infants during the first 60 hours of life. Stars represent single values; numbers represent the number of values at the same point. (From Manroe BL, et al: *J Pediatr* 95:89, 1979.)

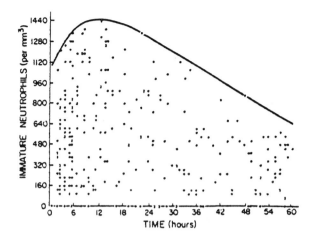

FIG. C-3 The range for immature neutrophils in normal infants during the first 60 hours of life. Stars represent single values; numbers represent the number of values at the same point. (From Manroe BL, et al: *J Pediatr* 95:89, 1979.)

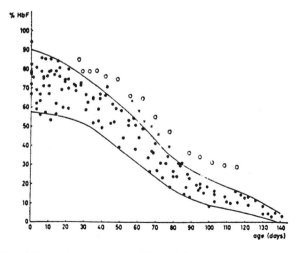

FIG. C-4 The relative concentration of Hb F in infants and its variation with age. The region between the curved lines contains 120 observations in 17 normal children. (From Garby L, Sjolin S: *Acta Paediatr* 51:245, 1962.)

TABLE C-1
Blood Gases: Representative Values in Normal Infants at Term

| | Umbilical vein | ARTERIAL BLOOD | | | | | Reference |
		30 min	1-4 hr	12-24 hr	24-48 hr	96 hr	
pH	7.33	—	7.30	7.30	7.39	7.39	Reardon et al (1960)
P_{CO_2}, mm Hg	43	—	39	33	34	36	Oliver et al (1961)
HCO_3, mEq/L	21.6	—	18.8	19.5	20	21.4	Nelson et al (1962, 1963)
P_{O_2}, mm Hg	28 ± 8	—	62 ± 13.8	68	63-87		
O_2 saturation			95%	94%	94%	96%	

From Taeusch HW and Ballard RA: *Avery's diseases of the newborn*, ed 7, Philadelphia, 1998, WB Saunders, and Bucci G, et al: *Biol Neonate* 8:81, 1965.

TABLE C-2
Acid-Base Status

Determination	Sample source	Birth	1 hr	3 hr	24 hr	2 days	3 days
VIGOROUS TERM INFANTS, VAGINAL DELIVERY							
pH	Umbilical artery	7.26					
	Umbilical vein	7.29					
Pco$_2$ (mm Hg)	Arterial	54.5	38.8	38.3	33.6	34	35
	Venous	42.8					
O$_2$ saturation	Arterial	19.8	93.8	94.7	93.2		
	Venous	47.6					
pH	Left atrial		7.30	7.34	7.41	7.39 (Temporal artery)	7.38 (Temporal artery)
CO$_2$ content (mEq/L)		—	20.6	21.9	21.4		
PREMATURE INFANTS							
	Capillary (skin puncture)						
pH	<1250 g				7.36	7.35	7.35
Pco$_2$ (mm Hg)					38	44	37
pH	>1250 g				7.39	7.39	7.38
Pco$_2$ (mm Hg)					38	39	38

Data from Schaffer AJ: *Diseases of the newborn*, ed 3, Philadelphia, 1971, WB Saunders. Data from Weisbrot IM, et al: *J Pediatr* 52:395, 1958, and Bucci G, et al: *Biol Neonate* 8:81, 1965.

TABLE C-3
Serum Chemistries in Term Infants

Determination	Cord		1-12 hr		12-24 hr		24-48 hr		48-72 hr	
Sodium, mEq/L*	147	(126-166)	143	(124-156)	145	(132-159)	148	(134-160)	149	(139-162)
Potassium, mEq/L	7.8	(5.6-12)	6.4	(5.3-7.3)	6.3	(5.3-8.9)	6.0	(5.2-7.3)	5.9	(5.0-7.7)
Chloride, mEq/L	103	(98-110)	100.7	(90-111)	103	(87-114)	102	(92-114)	103	(93-112)
Calcium, mg/dl	9.3	(8.2-11.1)	8.4	(7.3-9.2)	7.8	(6.9-9.4)	8.0	(6.1-9.9)	7.9	(5.9-9.7)
Phosphorus, mg/dl	5.6	(3.7-8.1)	6.1	(3.5-8.6)	5.7	(2.9-8.1)	5.9	(3.0-8.7)	5.8	(2.8-7.6)
Blood urea, mg/dl	29	(21-40)	27	(8-34)	33	(9-63)	32	(13-77)	31	(13-68)
Total protein, gm/dl	6.1	(4.8-7.3)	6.6	(5.6-8.5)	6.6	(5.8-8.2)	6.9	(5.9-8.2)	7.2	(6.0-8.5)
Blood sugar, mg/dl	73	(45-96)	63	(40-97)	63	(42-104)	56	(30-91)	59	(40-90)
Lactic acid, mg/dl	19.5	(11-30)	14.6	(11-24)	14.0	(10-23)	14.3	(9-22)	13.5	(7-21)
Lactate, mmol/L†	2.0-3.0		2.0							

From Taeusch HW, Ballard RA, Avery ME: *Diseases of the newborn*, ed 6, Philadelphia, 1991, WB Saunders.
*Acharya PT, Payne WW: *Arch Dis Child* 40:430, 1965.
†Daniel SS, Adamsons KJ, James LS: *Pediatrics* 37:942, 1966.

TABLE C-4
Blood Chemistry Values in Premature Infants During the First 7 Weeks of Life (birth weight 1500-1750 g)

Constituent	AGE 1 WEEK			AGE 3 WEEKS			AGE 5 WEEKS			AGE 7 WEEKS		
	Mean	SD	Range	Mean	SD	Range	Mean	SD	Range	Mean	SD	Range
Na (mEq/L)	139.6	±3.2	133-146	136.3	±2.9	129-142	136.8	±2.5	133-148	137.2	±1.8	133-142
K (mEq/L)	5.6	±0.5	4.6-6.7	5.8	±0.6	4.5-7.1	5.5	±0.6	4.5-6.6	5.7	±0.5	4.6-7.1
Cl (mEq/L)	108.2	±3.7	100-117	108.3	±3.9	102-116	107.0	±3.5	100-115	107.0	±3.3	101-115
CO_2 (mM/L)	20.3	±2.8	13.8-27.1	18.4	±3.5	12.4-26.2	20.4	±3.4	12.5-26.1	20.6	±3.1	13.7-26.9
Ca (mg/dl)	9.2	±1.1	6.1-11.6	9.6	±0.5	8.1-11.0	9.4	±0.5	8.6-10.5	9.5	±0.7	8.6-10.8
P (mg/dl)	7.6	±1.1	5.4-10.9	7.5	±0.7	6.2-8.7	7.0	±0.6	5.6-7.9	6.8	±0.8	4.2-8.2
BUN (mg/dl)	9.3	±5.2	3.1-25.5	13.3	±7.8	2.1-31.4	13.3	±7.1	2.0-26.5	13.4	±6.7	2.5-30.5
Total protein (gm/dl)	5.49	±0.42	4.40-6.26	5.38	±0.48	4.28-6.70	4.98	±0.50	4.14-6.90	4.93	±0.61	4.02-5.86
Albumin (gm/dl)	3.85	±0.30	3.28-4.50	3.92	±0.42	3.16-5.26	3.73	±0.34	3.20-4.34	3.89	±0.53	3.40-4.60
Globulin (gm/dl)	1.58	±0.33	0.88-2.20	1.44	±0.63	0.62-2.90	1.17	±0.49	0.48-1.48	1.12	±0.33	0.5-2.60
Hb (gm/dl)	17.8	±2.7	11.4-24.8	14.7	±2.1	9.0-19.4	11.5	±2.0	7.2-18.6	10.0	±1.3	7.5-13.9

Modified from Thomas J, Reichelderfer T: *Clin Chem* 14:272, 1968.

TABLE C-5
Selected Chemistry Values in Full-Term and Preterm Infants

Constituent	Preterm	Term
Ammonia (μg/100 ml)	—	90-150
Base, excess (mmol/L)	—	−10 to −2
Bicarbonate, standard (mmol/L)	18-26	20-26
Bilirubin, total (mg/dl)		
Cord	<2.8	<2.8
24 hr	1-6	2-6
48 hr	6-8	6-7
3-5 days	10-12	4-6
≥1 mo	<1.5	<1.5
Bilirubin, direct (mg/dl)	<0.5	<0.5
Calcium, total (mg/dl), week 1	6.0-10.0	8.4-11.6
Ceruloplasmin (mg/dl)		1-3 mo: 5-18
		6-12 mo: 33-43
		13-36 mo: 26-55
Cholesterol (mg/dl)		
Cord		45-98
3 days -1 yr		65-175
Creatine phosphokinase (U/L)		
Day 1		44-1150
Day 4		14-97
Creatinine (mg/dl)		
Birth	Mother's level	Mother's level
10 days	1.3 ± 0.07 (mean ± SD)	1-4 dy 0.3-1.0
1 mo	0.6 ± 0.05 (mean ± SD)	>4 dy 0.2-0.4
Ferritin (μg/dl)		
Neonate		25-200
1 mo		200-600
2-5 mo		50-200
>6 mo		7-142
Gamma-glutamyl transferase (GGT) (U/L)	—	14-131

From Fanaroff AA, Martin RJ (editors) *Neonatal-perinatal medicine: diseases of the fetus and infant,* ed 5, St Louis, 1992, Mosby.

TABLE C-5
Selected Chemistry Values in Full-Term and Preterm Infants—cont'd

Constituent	Preterm	Term
Glucose (mg/dl)		
<72 hr	20-125	30-125
>72 hr	40-125	40-125
Lactate dehydrogenase (U/L)	—	357-953
Magnesium (mg/dl)	—	1.7-2.4
Osmolality (mOsm/L)	—	275-295 (may be as low as 266)
Phosphate, alkaline (U/L) (mean ± SD)		
26-27 wk	320 ± 142	164 ± 68
28-29	292 ± 87	—
30-31	281 ± 85	—
32-33	254 ± 72	—
34-35	236 ± 62	—
36	207 ± 60	—
Phosphorus (mg/dl)		
Birth		4.5-8.7
Day 5		4.2-7.2
Month 1		4.5-6.5
SGOT/AST (aspartate amino transferase) (U/L)		24-81
SGPT/ALT (alanine amino transferase) (U/L)		10-33
Triglycerides (mg/dl)		10-140
Urea nitrogen (mg/dl)	3-25	4-12
Uric acid (mg/dl)	—	3.0-7.5
Vitamin A (μg/dl)	16.0 ± 1.0	23.9 ± 1.8
(<10 μg/dl indicates very low hepatic vitamin A stores)		
Vitamin D		
25-Hydroxycholecalciferol (ng/ml)*		20-60
1,25-Dihydroxycholecalciferol (pg/ml)*		40-90

*Serum levels affected by race, age, season, and diet.

TABLE C-6
Laboratory Parameters of Acid-Base Disturbances*

	pH	Paco$_2$	HCO$_3$ (mEq/L)	CO$_2$ Content (mEq/L)
Normal values	7.35-7.45	35-45	24-26	25-28
Disturbances				
Metabolic acidosis	↓	↓	↓	↓
Acute respiratory acidosis	↓	↑	↔	Slight ↑
Compensated respiratory acidosis	↔ or slight ↑	↑	↑	↑
Metabolic alkalosis	↑	Slight ↑	↑	↑
Acute respiratory alkalosis	↑	↓	↔	Slight ↓
Compensated respiratory alkalosis	↔ or slight ↑	↓	↓	↓

From Hoeckelman RA, Friedman SB, Nelson NM, et al, editors: *Primary pediatric care,* ed 2, St. Louis, 1992, Mosby.
*Values obtained by arterialized capillary blood or direct arterial puncture.

TABLE C-7
True Blood Sugar Levels in Normal Term and Low Birth Weight Infants

Maternal status	Delivery type	AGE (HOURS)						
		0	0.5	1	2	4	6	24
No fluid administration	Vaginal	66	55	55	48	55	47	—
		44-84	34-90	35-89	22-73	30-71	27-78	—
Saline, IV administration	Cesarean section	64	75	76	70	60	57	54
		38-90	58-107	34-136	45-108	47-101	35-76	43-76
Glucose, IV administration	Cesarean section	109	69	66	56	58	52	68
		61-204	31-125	31-111	35-85	27-86	32-77	35-91
Glucose, IV administration	Vaginal	89	54	47	41	50	51	—
		54-163	27-98	16-82	19-71	34-80	29-80	—

From Cornblath M, et al: *Pediatrics* 27:378, 1961.

TABLE C-8
Age-Specific Indices

Age	Hgb (g %) Mean (−2 SD)	Hct (%) Mean (−2 SD)	MCV (fl) Mean (−2 SD)	MCHC (g/dl RBC) Mean (−2 SD)	Reticulocytes (%)	WBC/mm³ × 1000 Mean (+2 SD)	Platelets/mm³ (× 1000) Mean (Range)
26-30 wk gestation*	13.4 (11)	41.5 (34.9)	118.2 (106.7)	37.9 (30.6)	—	4.4 (2.7)	254 (180-327)
28 wk	14.5	45	120	31.0	(5-10)	—	275
32 wk	15.0	47	118	32.0	(3-10)	—	290
Term† (cord)	16.5 (13.5)	51 (42)	108 (98)	33.0 (30.0)	(3-7)	18.1 (9-30)‡	290
1-3 days	18.5 (14.5)	56 (45)	108 (95)	33.0 (29.0)	(1.8-4.6)	18.9 (9.4-34)	192
2 wk	16.6 (13.4)	53 (41)	105 (88)	31.4 (28.1)		11.4 (5-20)	252

From Johnson KB, editor: *The Harriet Lane handbook*, ed 13, St Louis, 1993, Mosby.

*Values are from fetal samplings.

†Under 1 m/o, capillary Hgb exceeds venous: 1 hr: 3.6 gm difference; 5 days: 2.2 gm difference; 3 weeks: 1.1 gm difference.

‡Mean (95% confidence limits).

TABLE C-9
Leukocyte Values in Term and Premature Infants (10³ Cells/μl)

Age (hours)	Total white cell count	Neutrophils	Bands/Metas	Lymphocytes	Monocytes	Eosinophils
TERM INFANTS						
0	10.0-26.0	5.0-13.0	0.4-1.8	3.5-8.5	0.7-1.5	0.2-2.0
12	13.5-31.0	9.0-18.0	0.4-2.0	3.0-7.0	1.0-2.0	0.2-2.0
72	5.0-14.5	2.0-7.0	0.2-0.4	2.0-5.0	0.5-1.0	0.2-1.0
144	6.0-14.5	2.0-6.0	0.2-0.5	3.0-6.0	0.7-1.2	0.2-0.8
PREMATURE INFANTS						
0	5.0-19.0	2.0-9.0	0.2-2.4	2.5-6.0	0.3-1.0	0.1-0.7
12	5.0-21.0	3.0-11.0	0.2-2.4	1.5-5.0	0.3-1.3	0.1-1.1
72	5.0-14.0	3.0-7.0	0.2-0.6	1.5-4.0	0.3-1.2	0.2-1.1
144	5.5-17.5	2.0-7.0	0.2-0.5	2.5-7.5	0.5-1.5	0.3-1.2

From Oski FA, Naiman JL: *Hematologic problems in the newborn*, ed 3, Philadelphia, 1982, WB Saunders.

TABLE C-10

Changes in Polymorphonuclear Neutrophil Count of Healthy Term Babies With Age (cells/mm^3)

Postnatal age	5th centile	Median	95th centile
Birth	4,120*	7,750	14,600
6 hr	6,640*	12,500	23,500
12 hr	6,640*	12,500	23,500
18 hr	6,370*	11,000	20,700
24 hr	4,830*	9,100	17,100
36 hr	3,820*	7,200	13,400
48 hr	3,080*	5,800	10,900
3 days	2,550	4,800	9,040
4 days	2,260	4,250	8,000
5 days	2,040	3,850	7,250
7 days	1,800	3,400	6,400
10 days	1,730	3,250	6,120
2 wk	1,700	3,200	6,020
3-4 wk	1,650	3,100	5,840

From Gregory J, Hey E: *Arch Dis Child* 47:747, 1972.
*About 5% of healthy preterm babies probably have a neutrophil count of less than 3000 cells/mm^3 at this age.

TABLE C-11
Hemostatic Function

Hemostatic factor or component	Premature infant	Full-term infant	Age adult level is attained
VASCULAR AND PLATELET FUNCTION			
Vasoconstriction	Present	Present	At birth
Capillary fragility	Increased	Normal	At birth
Bleeding time	Normal	Normal	At birth
Platelet count	Normal	Normal	At birth
Platelet function	↓ ↓ Aggregative ability	↓ Aggregative ability ↓ Clot retraction ↓ Platelet factor 3 availability	Not established
COAGULATION			
Whole blood clotting time	Decreased	↓ or normal	At birth
Activated partial thromboplastin time (APTT) (adult normal, 35–45 seconds)	70–145 sec	45–70 sec	2–9 mo
Prothrombin time (PT) (adult normal, 12–14 seconds)	12–21 sec	13–20 sec	3–4 days

Modified from Bleyer WA, Hakami N, Shepard TH: *J Pediatr* 79:838, 1971, and Fanaroff AA, Martin RJ (editors): *Neonatal-perinatal medicine: diseases of fetus and infant*, ed 5, St Louis, 1992, Mosby, p. 969.

Continued

TABLE C-11
Hemostatic Function—cont'd

Hemostatic factor or component	Premature infant	Full-term infant	Age adult level is attained
Thrombin time (TT) (adult normal, 8-10 seconds)	11-17 sec	10-16 sec	Few days
Thrombotest (II, VII, IX, X)	30%-50%	40%-68%	2-12 mo
XII (Hageman factor)	10%-50%	25%-60%	9-14 days
IX (PTA)	5%-20%	15%-70%	1-2 mo
IX (PTC)	10%-25%	20%-60%	3-9 mo
VIII (AHF)	20%-80%	70%-150%	At birth
VII (proconvertin)	20%-45%	20%-70%	2-12 mo
X (Stuart-Prower factor)	10%-45%	20%-55%	2-12 mo
V (proaccelerin)	50%-85%	80%-200%	At birth
II (prothrombin)	20%-80%	26%-65%	2-12 mo
I (fibrinogen) (gm/dl)	150%-300%	150%-300%	2-4 days
XIII (fibrin-stabilizing factor)	100%	100%	At birth
Fibrin split products (µg/ml)	0-10	0-7	
Antithrombin III	48%	55%	

Modified from Bleyer WA, Hakami N, Shepard TH: *J Pediatr* 79:838, 1971, and Fanaroff AA, Martin RJ (editors): *Neonatal-perinatal medicine: diseases of fetus and infant*, ed 5, St Louis, 1992, Mosby, p. 969.

TABLE C-12
Thyroid Function Tests: Routine Studies

Test	Age	Normal	Comments
T_4 RIA (mcg/dl)	Cord	6.6-17.5	Measures total T_4 by radioimmunoassay
	1-3dy	11.0-21.5	
	1-4wk	8.2-16.6	
	1-12mo	7.2-15.6	
	1-5yr	7.3-15.0	
	6-10yr	6.4-13.3	
	11-15yr	5.6-11.7	
	16-20yr	4.2-11.8	
	21-50yr	4.3-12.5	
T_3 RU (%)	—	25-35	Measures thyroid hormone binding, not T_3
T Index	—	1.25-4.20	T_4 RIA $\times$ T_3 RU
Free T_4 (ng/dL)	1-10dy	0.6-2.0	Metabolically active form, the normal range for free T_4 is very assay dependent
	>10dy	0.7-1.7	
T_3 RIA (ng/dL)	Cord	14-86	Measures T_3 by RIA
	1-3dy	100-380	
	1-4wk	99-310	
	1-12mo	102-264	
	1-5yr	105-269	
	6-10yr	94-241	
	11-15yr	83-213	
	16-20yr	80-210	
	21-50yr	70-204	
TSH (mIU/ml)	Cord	<2.5-17.4	TSH surge peaks from 80-90mIU/ml in term newborn by 30 min after birth; values after 1 wk are within adult normal range; elevated values suggest primary hypothyroidism, whereas suppressed values are the best indicator of hyperthyroidism
	1-3dy	<2.5-13.3	
	1-4wk	0.6-10.0	
	1-12mo	0.6-6.3	
	1-15yr	0.6-6.3	
	16-50yr	0.2-7.6	
TBG (mg/dL)	Cord	0.7-4.7	
	1-3dy	—	
	1-4wk	0.5-4.5	
	1-12mo	1.6-3.6	
	1-5yr	1.3-2.8	
	6-20yr	1.4-2.6	
	21-50yr	1.2-2.4	
Reverse T_3 (ng/dL)	Newborns	90-250	Reach adult range by 1 wk
	Children	10-50	
	Adults	10-50	

From Siberry G and Iannone R (editors). *The Harriet Lane handbook,* ed 15, St Louis, 2000, Mosby.
RIA, radioimmunoassay; *RU,* resin uptake; T_3, triiodothyronine; T_4, thyroxine; *TBG,* thyroxine-binding globulin; *TSH,* thyroid-stimulating hormone.

TABLE C-13
Thyroid Antibodies*

Interpretation	Antithyroglobulin	Antimicrosomal
Insignificant	<1:40	<1:400
Borderline	1:80	1:400
Significant	1:160-1:640	1:1600-1:6400
Very significant	<1:640	<1:6400

From Siberry G and Iannone R (editors): *The Harriet Lane handbook,* ed 15, St Louis, 2000, Mosby.
*High titers of thyroid antibodies are consistent with Hashimoto's thyroiditis.

TABLE C-14
Serum T$_4$ (μg/dl) In Preterm and Term Infants

	ESTIMATED GESTATIONAL AGE (WK)				
Age	30-31	32-33	34-35	36-37	Term
Cord	4.5-8.5	3.3-11.7	4.3-9.1	1.9-13.1	4.6-11.8
12-72 hr	7.3-15.7	5.9-18.7	6.2-18.6	10.3-20.7	14.8-23.2
3-10 days	4.1-11.3	4.7-12.3	5.2-14.8	7.7-17.7	9.9-21.9
11-20 days	3.9-11.1	5.1-11.5	6.9-14.1	5.4-17.0	8.2-16.2
21-45 days	4.8-10.8	4.6-11.4	6.7-11.9	3.0-19.8	9.1-15.1
46-90 days	6.2-13.0	6.2-13.0	6.2-13.0	6.2-13.0	6.4-14.0

From Siberry G and Iannone R (editors): *The Harriet Lane handbook,* ed 15, St Louis, 2000, Mosby.

TABLE C-15
Serum Immunoglobulin Levels (mg/dl) in Newborns

Age	Newborn	1-3 mo
IgG	1031 ± 200 (645-1244)	430 ± 119 (272-762)
IgA	2 ± 3 (0-11)	21 ± 13 (6-56)
IgM	11 ± 5 (5-30)	30 ± 1 (16-67)

From Stiehm ER, Fudenberg HH: *Pediatrics* 37:715, 1966.

TABLE C-16
Electrocardiographic Standards in Newborns

Measure	AGE IN DAYS									
	0-1		1-3		3-7		7-30	
Number of patients	189		179		181		119	
Heart rate (beats/min)	122	(99-147)	123	(97-148)	128	(100-160)	148	(114-177)
QRS axis (degrees)	135	(91-185)	134	(93-188)	133	(92-185)	108	(78-152)
P-R duration II (ms)	107	(82-138)	108	(85-132)	103	(78-130)	101	(75-128)
QRS duration V_5 (ms)	50	(26-69)	48	(27-61)	49	(26-63)	53	(27-75)
Q-T duration V_5 (ms)	290	(220-360)	280	(235-330)	272	(272-315)	258	(230-290)
P amplitude II (mV)	0.16	(0.07-0.25)	0.16	(0.05-0.25)	0.17	(0.08-0.27)	0.19	(0.09-0.29)
R amplitude V_{3R} (mV)	1.05	(0.40-1.79)	1.19	(0.52-1.95)	1.02	(0.18-1.80)	0.82	(0.30-1.50)
R amplitude V_1 (mV)	1.35	(0.65-2.37)	1.48	(0.70-2.42)	1.28	(0.50-2.15)	1.05	(0.45-1.81)
R amplitude V_5 (mV)	1.0	(0.25-1.85)	1.1	(0.48-1.95)	1.3	(0.48-1.95)	1.45	(0.60-2.1)
R amplitude V_6 (mV)	0.45	(0.05-0.95)	0.48	(0.05-0.95)	0.51	(0.10-1.05)	0.76	(0.26-1.35)
S amplitude V_{3R} (mV)	0.43	(0.07-1.18)	0.5	(0.05-1.2)	0.36	(0.05-0.8)	0.20	(0.05-0.64)
S amplitude V_1 (mV)	0.85	(0.10-1.85)	0.95	(0.15-1.90)	0.68	(0.10-1.50)	0.4	(0.05-0.97)
S amplitude V_5 (mV)	0.99	(0.38-1.79)	0.98	(0.20-1.59)	0.95	(0.38-1.63)	0.8	(0.24-1.38)
S amplitude V_6 (mV)	0.35	(0.02-0.79)	0.32	(0.02-0.76)	0.37	(0.02-0.80)	0.32	(0.02-0.82)
R/S amplitude V_{3R}	1.5	(0.2-4.8)	1.6	(0.2-4.2)	1.8	(0.2-5.8)	1.9	(0.2-2.5)
R/S amplitude V_1	2.2	(0.4-7.0)	2.0	(0.4-5.4)	2.8	(0.05-7.2)	2.9	(1.1-6.3)
R/S amplitude V_5	0.7	(0-7.0)	1.0	(0-5.0)	1.5	(0-5.0)	2.0	(0-5.1)
R/S amplitude V_6	2	(0-8)	3	(0-9)	2	(0-8)	4	(0-9)
Mean (5% and 95% values)								

From Davignon A, et al: *Pediatr Cardiol* 1:123, 1979-1980.

BOX C-1
Normal Laboratory Values (Cerebrospinal Fluid)

WBC COUNT
Preterm mean (range)
 9 (0-25 WBCs/mm^3)
 57% PMNs
Term mean (range)
 8 (0-22 WBCs/mm^3)
 61% PMNs

GLUCOSE
Preterm mean (range)
 50 (24-63 mg/dL)
Term mean (range)
 52 (34-119 mg/dL)

CSF GLUCOSE/BLOOD GLUCOSE
Preterm mean (range)
 55%-105%
Term mean (range)
 44%-128%

LACTIC ACID DEHYDROGENASE
Mean
 20 (5-30 U/L), or about 10% of serum value

MYELIN BASIC PROTEIN
 <4 ng/mL

OPENING PRESSURE
Newborn
 80-110 (<110 mmH$_2$O)
Infant/child
 <200 mmH$_2$O (lateral recumbent)
Respiratory variations
 5–10 mmH$_2$O

PROTEIN
Preterm mean (range)
 115 (65-150 mg/dL)
Term mean (range)
 90 (20-170 mg/dL)

From Siberry G and Iannone R (editors): *The Harriet Lane handbook,* ed 15, St Louis, 2000, Mosby.

APPENDIX D

Procedures*

I. VENIPUNCTURE
A. Heel or finger stick (Fig. D-1).
1. Warm extremity to provide optimal blood flow and more accurate samples. To prevent burns, do not use a warming towel that is warmer than 40° C.
2. Lance either the lateral or medial side of the heel; avoid the heel pad. For digital artery sampling, use the lateral surface of the distal phalanx of second, third, or fourth finger.
3. Use a 2.5-mm lancet or an Autolet for optimal skin penetration.
4. Wipe away the first drop of blood with dry gauze. Alcohol used in cleansing skin may produce hemolysis.
5. Massage (but do not squeeze) finger or heel.
6. Samples may be inaccurate if patient is poorly perfused or polycythemic.
B. External jugular puncture. Used for blood sampling in patients with inadequate peripheral vascular access or during resuscitation.
1. Restrain infant securely (Fig. D-2).
2. Extend neck and turn head slightly to one side. This accentuates the posterior margin of contralateral sternocleidomastoid muscle. This may be facilitated by positioning the infant so that its head falls over the side of the table or by placing a rolled towel under the infant's shoulders.
3. Prepare the area carefully with povidone-iodine and 70% alcohol.
4. To distend the external jugular vein, occlude its most proximal segment or provoke child to cry. The vein runs from the angle of the mandible to the posterior border of the lower third of the sternocleidomastoid muscle.
5. While continually providing negative suction on the syringe, insert the needle at about a 30-degree angle to the skin. Continue as with any peripheral venipuncture.
N.B.: Hematoma, pneumothorax, and infection can be complications.
C. Femoral puncture. For venous or arterial blood sampling of patients with inadequate vascular access or during resuscitation.

---

*Modified from Siberry G, Iannone R (editors): *The Harriet Lane handbook*, ed 15, St Louis, 2000, Mosby.

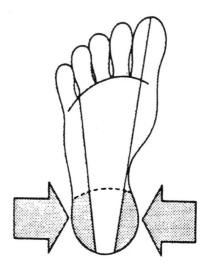

FIG. D-1 Recommended sites *(shaded areas)* for warmed heel puncture. (From Blumenfeld TA, Turi GK, Blanc WA: *Lancet* 1:230, 1979.)

Careful skin preparation is needed to prevent septic arthritis. **Femoral puncture is particularly hazardous in neonates and is not usually recommended or appropriate in this age group. Avoid femoral punctures in children who are thrombocytopenic, have coagulation disorders, or are scheduled for cardiac catheterization.**

1. Have an assistant hold the child securely, with the hips flexed and abducted (in a frog-leg position).
2. Prepare area as for blood culture with povidone-iodine and 70% alcohol.
3. Locate the femoral pulse, then insert the needle 2.0 cm distal to the inguinal ligament and 0.5 cm medial to the femoral pulse.
4. Insert the needle slowly at a 30-degree angle to the skin to a depth of approximately 0.5 to 0.75 cm. Continually aspirate while maneuvering the needle until blood is obtained.
5. Withdraw the needle and apply direct pressure to the puncture site for a minimum of 5 minutes.

D. Internal jugular puncture.

1. Securely restrain the infant.
2. Extend the infant's neck and turn the head slightly to one side. This accentuates the posterior margin of the sternocleidomastoid muscle. This may be facilitated by positioning the infant so that its head falls over the side of the table or by placing a rolled towel under the infant's shoulders.

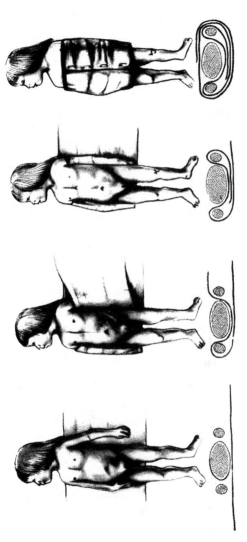

FIG. D-2 Method of mummy-wrapping an infant or child to restrain the upper extremities. The four steps are illustrated with frontal and cross-sectional views. A wider sheet or blanket may be used to restrain the lower extremities. Useful when performing jugular puncture. (From Hoekelman RA, et al: *Primary pediatric care*, ed 2, St Louis, 1992, Mosby.)

3. Prepare the area as for blood culture with povidone-iodine and 70% alcohol.

4. Insert the needle just deep to and behind the posterior margin of the sternocleidomastoid muscle, approximately halfway between its origin and insertion. Advance the needle under the muscle, parallel to the skin surface, and in the direction of the suprasternal notch. Advance for a distance equal to the width of the sternocleidomastoid muscle.

5. While exerting suction, slowly withdraw needle until blood is withdrawn.

6. After obtaining blood, hold child upright and apply pressure to the puncture site.

II. UMBILICAL ARTERY CATHETERIZATION

Umbilical artery catheterization is used to obtain vascular access and monitor blood pressure and blood gas levels in critically ill neonates.

A. Catheter placement.

1. Restrain infant. Prepare and drape umbilical cord and adjacent skin using sterile technique. Place sterile drapes sparingly to expose infant to the radiant warmer.

2. Determine the length of catheter to be inserted for either high (T6 to T9) or low (L3 to L4) position. Place marker (sterile bandage or tape) on catheter at desired length.

3. Flush catheter with sterile saline solution before insertion.

4. Place sterile umbilical tape around base of cord. Cut through cord horizontally approximately 1.5 to 2.0 cm from skin; tighten umbilical tape to prevent bleeding.

5. Identify the large, thin-walled umbilical vein and smaller, thick-walled arteries. Use one tip of open curved iris forceps to gently probe and dilate one artery. Then gently probe with both points of closed forceps and dilate artery by allowing forceps to open gently.

6. Grasp catheter 1 cm from tip with toothless forceps and insert catheter into the lumen of the artery. Gently advance catheter to desired distance. DO NOT FORCE. If resistance is encountered, try loosening umbilical tape, applying steady gentle pressure, or manipulating the angle of the umbilical cord to the skin.

7. Secure the catheter with both a suture through the cord and marker tape and a tape bridge. Confirm the position of the catheter tip radiographically.

8. Look for complications of catheter placement, such as blanching or cyanosis of the lower extremities, ischemia, perforation, thrombosis, embolism, and infection.

B. Catheter position.
Umbilical artery catheters may be placed in either of two positions: low-line position, between lumbar vertebrae 3 and 4, or high-line position, between thoracic vertebrae 6 and 9. The length of catheter required to achieve either position may be

determined using a standardized graph or a regression formula. Catheter length is about one third the crown-heel length.

1. Graphical representation.
   a. Determine the shoulder-umbilical length by measuring the *perpendicular* line dropped from the tip of the shoulder to the level of the umbilicus. Note that a diagonal measurement will be inaccurate.
   b. Use the graph below to determine the catheter length to be inserted for either a high or low line (Fig. D-3). For a low line, the tip of the catheter should lie just above the aortic bifurcation (avoid the renal artery orifice, around L2). With a high line the tip should be above the diaphragm. Add length for the height of the umbilical stump.

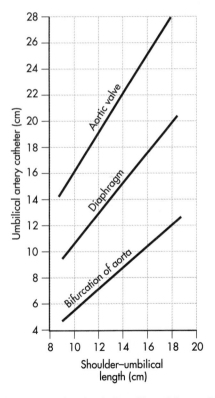

FIG. D-3 Umbilical artery catheter length. (From Siberry G, Iannone R, editors: *The Harriet Lane handbook*, ed 15, St Louis, 2000, Mosby.)

2. Birth weight (BW) regression formula.
   a. High line: Umbilical artery (UA) catheter length (cm) = (3 ×
      BW [kg]) + 9
   b. Low line: UA catheter length (cm) ≈ BW (kg) +7
N.B.: Formula may not be appropriate for infants who are small for gestational age (SGA) or large for gestational age (LGA).

III. UMBILICAL VEIN CATHETERIZATION
Umbilical vein catheterization is used to obtain vascular access in critically ill neonates.
A. Catheter placement.
1. After restraining the infant, clean, drape, and cut the umbilical stump as for umbilical artery catheterization.
2. Determine the length of the catheter needed to place the catheter tip in the inferior vena cava above the level of the ductus venosus or hepatic veins. Place a marker (sterile bandage or tape) on the catheter at desired length.
3. Flush the catheter with sterile saline solution before insertion.
4. Isolate a thin-walled umbilical vein; clear thrombi with forceps, and insert catheter. Gently advance catheter to desired distance. DO NOT FORCE. If resistance is encountered, try loosening umbilical tape, applying steady gentle pressure, or manipulating the angle of the umbilical cord to the skin.

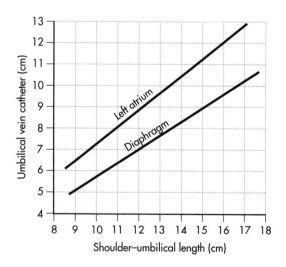

FIG. D-4 Umbilical vein catheter length. (From Siberry G, Iannone R, editors: *The Harriet Lane handbook*, ed 15, St Louis, 2000, Mosby.)

5. Secure the catheter as described for the umbilical artery catheter. Confirm the position of the catheter tip radiographically.

N.B.: Hemorrhage, infection, air embolism, and arrhythmias are possible complications.

   B. Catheter position. The umbilical catheter should be placed in the inferior vena cava above the level of the ductus venosus and the hepatic veins. The length of the catheter necessary to achieve this position can be determined using the graph or regression formula.

   1. Graphical representation.
      a. Determine the shoulder-umbilical length by measuring the *perpendicular* line dropped from the tip of the shoulder to the level of the umbilicus.
      b. Using Fig. D-4, determine the catheter length needed to place the tip between the diaphragm and left atrium. Add length for the height of the umbilical stump.
   2. Birth weight regression formula: UV catheter length (cm) $\times$ (0.5 $\times$ UA catheter length [cm]) + 1. Formula may not be appropriate for SGA or LGA infants.

IV. NEONATAL EXCHANGE TRANSFUSION

   See Chapter 17 for volume calculations.

N.B.: Complete blood count, reticulocyte count, peripheral smear, bilirubin, Ca, glucose, total protein, infant blood type, and Coombs' test should be performed on preexchange samples of blood because they are no longer of diagnostic value on postexchange blood. If indicated, also save preexchange blood for serologic or chromosome studies.

   A. Sensitized cells or hyperbilirubinemia.
   1. Crossmatch donor blood against maternal serum for first exchange and against postexchange blood for subsequent exchanges.
   2. Use type O-negative (low titer) blood; may use infant's type if there is no chance of maternal-infant incompatibility. Blood should be stored at room temperature, either fresh or up to 48 hours old, and anticoagulated with ACD or CPD unless infant is acidotic or hypocalcemic.
   3. Infant should be NPO during and at least 4 hours after exchange. Empty the infant's stomach if it was fed within 4 hours of procedure.
   4. Follow infant's vital signs and temperature closely; have resuscitation equipment ready.
   5. Prepare and drape patient for sterile procedure.
   6. Insert umbilical artery and vein catheters as described. During the exchange, blood is removed through the umbilical artery catheter and infused through the venous catheter. If unable to pass an arterial catheter, use a single venous catheter.
   7. Prewarm blood in quality-controlled blood warmer if available; do not improvise with a water bath.
   8. Exchange 15-ml increments in vigorous full-term infants, smaller volumes for smaller, less stable infants. Do not allow cells in donor unit to sediment.

9. Withdraw and infuse blood at rate of 2 to 3 ml/kg per minute to avoid mechanical trauma to patient and donor cells.
10. Give 1 to 2 ml of intravenous (IV) 10% calcium gluconate solution slowly for ECG evidence of hypocalcemia. Flush tubing with NaCl before and after calcium infusion. Observe for bradycardia during infusion.
11. To complete the double-blood volume exchange, transfuse 160 ml/kg for a full-term infant and 160 to 200 ml/kg for a preterm infant.
12. Send the last aliquot withdrawn for Hct, smear, glucose, bilirubin, potassium, Ca^{++}, and type and crossmatch.

B. Anemic heart failure. Have O-negative concentrated red blood cells (RBCs) in the delivery room. Perform a partial exchange with packed RBCs to correct anemia and failure (30 to 50 ml/kg). Allow infant to stabilize if possible before attempting a full two-volume exchange.

C. Complications.
1. Cardiovascular. Thromboemboli or air emboli, thromboses, dysrhythmias, volume overload, and cardiorespiratory arrest.
2. Metabolic. Hyperkalemia, hypernatremia, hypocalcemia, hypoglycemia, and acidosis.
3. Hematologic. Thrombocytopenia, disseminated intravascular coagulation (DIC), overheparinization (may use 10 μg protamine for each unit of heparin in donor unit), and transfusion reaction.
4. Infectious. Hepatitis, HIV, and bacteremia.
5. Mechanical. Injury to donor cells (especially from overheating), vascular or cardiac perforation, and blood loss.

V. CHEST TUBE PLACEMENT

Chest tube placement is used for evacuation of pneumothorax, hemothorax, chylothorax, large pleural effusion, or empyema for diagnostic and/or therapeutic purposes.

A. Technique.
1. Position the infant with the affected side up. Preferably, chest tubes are placed in the third or fourth intercostal space in the midaxillary line, avoiding breast tissue.
2. If necessary, temporarily decompress the pneumothorax by inserting a "butterfly" or angiocath in the same location in the ipsilateral anterior second intercostal space.
3. After cleaning and anesthetizing the area locally with 0.5% lidocaine, make a 0.5-cm incision directly over the rib below the desired interspace. Insert a small curved hemostat to bluntly dissect a track over the superior margin of the rib through the intercostal muscles and into the pleural cavity.
4. Place a clamp 0.5 to 1.0 cm from the tip of the chest tube and pass through the previously punctured space into the pleural cavity. Angle the tube anteriorly and superiorly and insert it the desired distance.

5. Secure tube to chest wall with suture through skin incision and then around tube. Cover incision with petroleum gauze and a sterile dressing.
6. Connect the chest tube to 15- to 20-cm water suction for decompression via one-way valve. Confirm position and function with chest radiograph.

B. Complications. Lung perforation, hemorrhage, scarring, and tube malposition.

VI. LUMBAR PUNCTURE

Lumbar puncture (LP) facilitates examination of the spinal fluid for suspected infections.

A. Precautions.

1. Increased intracranial pressure. Before LP, perform funduscopic examination. The presence of papilledema, retinal hemorrhage, or clinical suspicion of increased intracranial pressure may be contraindications to the procedure. A sudden drop in intraspinal pressure by rapid release of cerebrospinal fluid (CSF) may cause fatal herniation. If LP is to be performed, proceed with extreme caution.
2. Bleeding diathesis. A platelet count of $\geq 50,000/mm^3$ is desirable before LP. Correct any clotting factor deficiencies.
3. Overlying skin infection. May result in inoculation of CSF with organisms.

B. Technique.

1. Apply a eutectic mixture of local anesthetics (EMLA).
2. Position the child in either the sitting position or lateral recumbent position with hips, knees, and neck flexed. Ensure that a small infant's cardiorespiratory status is not compromised by positioning.
3. Locate the desired interspace (either L3-L4 or L4-L5) by drawing a line between the top of the iliac crests.
4. Clean the skin with povidone-iodine and 70% alcohol. Drape conservatively so as to be able to monitor the infant. Use a spinal needle with a stylet. (Epidermoid tumors from introduced epithelial tissue have been reported.)
5. Anesthetize overlying skin with 0.5% lidocaine.
6. Puncture skin in the midline just below the palpated spinous process, angling slightly cephalad. Advance several millimeters at a time and withdraw stylet frequently to check for CSF flow. In small infants, one may not feel a change in resistance or "pop" as the dura is penetrated.
7. If resistance is met, withdraw needle to the skin surface and redirect angle slightly.
8. Send CSF sample for appropriate studies: cultures, glucose, protein, cell count and differential, antigen detection tests, VDRL.

VII. THORACENTESIS

Thoracentesis is done to obtain diagnosis or relief of an abnormal collection of fluid within the pleural space.

A. Technique.

1. Ideally, perform procedure with the patient sitting and with an assistant standing in front to support the patient.
2. Select the interspace to be tapped on the basis of dullness to percussion and the level of effusion on the erect chest radiograph. Ultrasound examination can help clarify location of the effusion if there is confusion as to its exact location. In the event of a small effusion, the patient may be tilted laterally toward the affected side to maximize the yield.
3. Clean and drape the chest.
4. Use a local anesthetic to infiltrate the skin, the underlying tissue, and the pleura in the interspace above the rib.
5. Attach a large-bore needle or intravenous catheter attached to a three-way stopcock and syringe. With needle bevel down, insert needle directly on the rib below the desired interspace, and "walk" the needle over the superior edge of the rib. Gradually advance the needle; a "pop" is felt on entering the pleural space. Advance the catheter 2 to 3 mm and remove the stylet.
6. Attach a syringe with a stopcock to the hub of the catheter and slowly withdraw the desired volume of fluid.
7. At the end of the procedure, withdraw the needle or catheter and place an occlusive dressing over the thoracentesis site.
8. Obtain a follow-up chest radiograph after thoracentesis to rule out pneumothorax.
9. Send pleural fluid for routine laboratory studies.

VIII. URINARY BLADDER CATHETERIZATION

Bladder catheterization is used to obtain urine for culture when a urinary tract infection or sepsis is suspected.

A. Technique.

1. Prepare the urethral opening using sterile technique.
2. In the male, apply gentle traction to the penis in a caudal direction to straighten the urethra.
3. Gently insert a lubricated catheter into the urethra. Slowly advance the catheter until resistance is met at the external sphincter. Continued pressure will overcome this resistance and the catheter will enter the bladder. In the female, only a few centimeters of advancement is required to reach the bladder.
4. Carefully remove the catheter once the specimen is obtained.

N.B.: Trauma to the urethra or bladder, vaginal catheterization, and infection are possible.

IX. SUPRAPUBIC BLADDER ASPIRATION

Avoid this procedure in children with genitourinary tract anomalies.

A. Technique.

1. The infant's diaper should be dry, and the infant should not have voided in the 30 to 60 minutes before the procedure. Anterior rec-

tal pressure in females or gentle penile pressure in males may be used to prevent urination during the procedure.

2. Restrain the infant in the supine, frog-leg position. Clean the lower abdomen suprapubic area with povidone-iodine and 70% alcohol.

3. The site for puncture is 1 to 2 cm above the symphysis pubis in the midline. Use a syringe with a 22-gauge 1-inch needle and puncture at 10 to 20 degrees to the perpendicular, aiming slightly caudad.

4. Exert suction gently as the needle is advanced until urine enters syringe. The needle should not be advanced more than 2.5 cm. Aspirate the urine with gentle suction.

N.B.: Hematuria (usually microscopic), intestinal perforation, abdominal wall infection, and bleeding are possible.

APPENDIX E

Breast Milk and Chemicals

TRANSFER OF DRUGS AND OTHER CHEMICALS INTO HUMAN MILK*†

In this section, lists of the pharmacologic or chemical agents transferred into human milk and their possible effects on the infant or on lactation, if known, are provided (Tables E-1 to E-7). The fact that a pharmacologic or chemical agent does not appear in the tables is not meant to imply that it is not transferred into human milk or that it does not have an effect on the infant but indicates that there are no reports in the literature. These tables should assist the physician in counseling a nursing mother regarding breast-feeding when the mother has a condition for which a drug is medically indicated.

The following should be considered when prescribing drug therapy for lactating women:

1. Is the drug therapy really necessary? Consultation between the pediatrician and the mother's physician can be most useful.
2. Use the safest drug (e.g., acetaminophen rather than aspirin for oral analgesia).
3. If there is a possibility that a drug may present a risk to the infant (e.g., phenytoin, phenobarbital), consideration should be given to measurement of blood concentrations in the nursing infant.
4. Drug exposure to the nursing infant may be minimized by having the mother take the medication just after completing a breast-feeding or just before the infant has his or her lengthy sleep period.

Data have been obtained from a search of the medical literature. Because methodologies used to quantitate drugs in milk continue to improve, this current information will require continuous updating.

---

*This material is from the American Academy of Pediatrics Committee on Drugs: The transfer of drugs and other chemicals into human breast milk, *Pediatrics* 93:137, 1994. Copyright © 1994 by the American Academy of Pediatrics.
†The recommendations in this statement do not indicate an exclusive course of treatment to be followed. Variations, taking into account individual circumstances, may be appropriate.

Text continued on p. 456

TABLE E-1
Drugs That Are Contraindicated During Breast-Feeding

Drug	Reason for concern, reported sign or symptom in infant, or effect on lactation
Bromocriptine	Suppresses lactation; may be hazardous to the mother
Cocaine	Cocaine intoxication
Cyclophosphamide	Possible immune suppression; unknown effect on growth or association with carcinogenesis; neutropenia
Cyclosporine	Possible immune suppression; unknown effect on growth or association with carcinogenesis
Doxorubicin*	Possible immune suppression; unknown effect on growth or association with carcinogenesis
Ergotamine	Vomiting, diarrhea, convulsions (doses used in migraine medications)
Lithium	One third to one half therapeutic blood concentration in infants
Methotrexate	Possible immune suppression; unknown effect on growth or association with carcinogenesis; neutropenia
Phencyclidine (PCP)	Potent hallucinogen
Phenindione	Anticoagulant; increased prothrombin and partial thromboplastin time in one infant; not used in United States

*Drug is concentrated in human milk.

TABLE E-2
Drugs of Abuse: Contraindicated During Breast-Feeding*

Drug reference	Reported effect or reason for concern
Amphetamine†	Irritability, poor sleeping pattern
Cocaine	Cocaine intoxication
Heroin	Tremors, restlessness, vomiting, poor feeding
Marijuana	Only one report in literature; no effect mentioned
Nicotine (smoking)	Shock, vomiting, diarrhea, rapid heart rate, restlessness; decreased milk production
Phencyclidine	Potent hallucinogen

*The Committee on Drugs strongly believes that nursing mothers should not ingest any compounds listed in Table E-2. Not only are they hazardous to the nursing infant, but they are also detrimental to the physical and emotional health of the mother. This list is obviously not complete; no drug of abuse should be ingested by nursing mothers even though adverse reports are not in the literature.
†Drug is concentrated in human milk.

TABLE E-3
Radioactive Compounds That Require Temporary Cessation of Breast-Feeding*

Drug	Recommended time for cessation of breast-feeding
Copper 64 (^{64}Cu)	Radioactivity in milk present at 50 hr
Gallium 67 (^{67}Ga)	Radioactivity in milk present for 2 wk
Indium 111 (^{111}In)	Very small amount present at 20 hr
Iodine 123 (^{123}I)	Radioactivity in milk present up to 36 hr
Iodine 125 (^{125}I)	Radioactivity in milk present for 12 days
Iodine 131 (^{131}I)	Radioactivity in milk present 2-14 days, depending on study
Radioactive sodium	Radioactivity in milk present 96 hr
Technetium-99 m (^{99m}Tc), ^{99m}Rc macroaggregates, ^{99m}Tc O4	Radioactivity in milk present 15 hr to 3 days

*Consult nuclear medicine physician before performing diagnostic study so that radionuclide that has shortest excretion time in breast milk can be used. Before study, the mother should pump her breast and store enough milk in freezer for feeding the infant; after study, the mother should pump her breast to maintain milk production but discard all milk pumped for the required time that radioactivity is present in milk. Milk samples can be screened by radiology departments for radioactivity before resumption of nursing.

TABLE E-4
Drugs Whose Effect on Nursing Infants Is Unknown but May Be of Concern

Drug	Reported or possible effect
ANTIANXIETY*	
Diazepam	None
Lorazepam	None
Midazolam	—
Perphenazine	None
Prazepam†	None
Quazepam	None
Temazepam	—
ANTIDEPRESSANTS*	
Amitriptyline	None
Amoxapine	None

*Psychotropic drugs, the compounds listed under antianxiety, antidepressant, and antipsychotic categories, are of special concern when given to nursing mothers for long periods. Although there are no case reports of adverse effects in breast-feeding infants, these drugs do appear in human milk and thus could conceivably alter short-term and long-term central nervous system function.

TABLE E-4
Drugs Whose Effect on Nursing Infants Is Unknown but May Be of Concern—cont'd

Drug	Reported or possible effect
ANTIDEPRESSANTS*—cont'd	
Desipramine	None
Dothiepin	None
Doxepin	None
Fluoxetine	—
Fluvoxamine	—
Imipramine	None
Trazodone	None
ANTIPSYCHOTIC*	
Chlorpromazine	Galactorrhea in adult; drowsiness and lethargy in infant
Chlorprothixene	None
Haloperidol	None
Mesoridazine	None
CHLORAMPHENICOL	Possible idiosyncratic bone marrow suppression
METOCLOPRAMIDE†	None described; dopaminergic blocking agent
METRONIDAZOLE	In vitro mutagen; may discontinue breast-feeding 12-24 hr to allow excretion of dose when single-dose therapy given to mother
TINIDAZOLE	See metronidazole

†Drug is concentrated in human milk.

TABLE E-5
Drugs That Have Been Associated With Significant Effects on Some Nursing Infants and Should Be Given to Nursing Mothers With Caution*

Drug	Reported effect
5-Aminosalicylic acid	Diarrhea (1 case)
Aspirin (salicylates)	Metabolic acidosis (1 case)
Clemastine	Drowsiness, irritability, refusal to feed, high-pitched cry, neck stiffness (1 case)
Phenobarbital	Sedation; infantile spasms after weaning from milk containing phenobarbital; methemoglobinemia (1 case)
Primidone	Sedation, feeding problems
Sulfasalazine (salicylazosulfapyridine)	Bloody diarrhea (1 case)

*Measure blood concentration in the infant when possible.

TABLE E-6
**Maternal Medication Usually Compatible
with Breast-Feeding***

Drug	Reported sign or symptom in infant or effect on lactation
Acebutolol	None
Acetaminophen	None
Acetazolamide	None
Acitretin	—
Acyclovir†	None
Alcohol (ethanol)	With large amounts drowsiness, diaphoresis, deep sleep, weakness, decrease in linear growth, abnormal weight gain; maternal ingestion of 1 gm/kg daily decreases milk ejection reflex
Allopurinol	—
Amoxicillin	None
Antimony	—
Atenolol	None
Atropine	None
Azapropazone (apazone)	—
Aztreonam	None
B₁ (thiamin)	None
B₆ (pyridoxine)	None
B₁₂	None
Baclofen	None
Barbiturate	See Table E-5
Bendroflumethiazide	Suppresses lactation
Bishydroxycoumarin (dicumarol)	None
Bromide	Rash, weakness, absence of cry with maternal intake of 5.4 gm/day
Butorphanol	None
Caffeine	Irritability, poor sleeping pattern, excreted slowly; no effect with usual amount of caffeine beverages
Captopril	None
Carbamazepine	None
Carbimazole	Goiter
Cefadroxil	None
Cefazolin	None

*Drugs listed have been reported in the literature as having the effects listed or no effect. The word "none" means that no observable change was seen in the nursing infant while the mother was ingesting the compound. It is emphasized that most of the literature citations concern single case reports or small series of infants.
†Drug is concentrated in human milk.

TABLE E-6
Maternal Medication Usually Compatible
with Breast-Feeding—cont'd

Drug	Reported sign or symptom in infant or effect on lactation
Cefotaxime	None
Cefoxitin	None
Cefprozil	—
Ceftazidime	None
Ceftriaxone	None
Chloral hydrate	Sleepiness
Chloroform	None
Chloroquine	None
Chlorothiazide	None
Chlorthalidone	Excreted slowly
Cimetidine†	None
Cisapride	None
Cisplatin	Not found in milk
Clindamycin	None
Clogestone	None
Clomipramine	—
Codeine	None
Colchicine	—
Contraceptive pill with estrogen/progesterone	Rare breast enlargement; decrease in milk production and protein content (not confirmed in several studies)
Cycloserine	None
D (vitamin)	None; follow up infant's serum calcium level if mother receives pharmacologic doses
Danthron	Increased bowel activity
Dapsone	None; sulfonamide detected in infant's urine
Dexbrompheniramine maleate with *d*-isoephedrine	Crying, poor sleeping patterns, irritability
Digoxin	None
Diltiazem	None
Dipyrone	None
Disopyramide	None
Domperidone	None
Dyphylline†	None
Enalapril	—
Erythromycin†	None
Estradiol	Withdrawal, vaginal bleeding
Ethambutol	None
Ethanol (cf. alcohol)	—
Ethosuximide	None, drug appears in infant serum
Fentanyl	—
Flecainide	—

Continued

TABLE E-6
Maternal Medication Usually Compatible
with Breast-Feeding—cont'd

Drug	Reported sign or symptom in infant or effect on lactation
Flufenamic acid	None
Fluorescein	—
Folic acid	None
Gold salts	None
Halothane	None
Hydralazine	None
Hydrochlorothiazide	—
Hydroxychloroquine†	None
Ibuprofen	None
Indomethacin	Seizure (1 case)
Iodides	May affect thyroid activity; see iodine
Iodine (providone-iodine/ vaginal douche)	Elevated iodine levels in breast milk, odor of iodine on infant's skin
Iodine	Goiter
Iopanoic acid	None
Isoniazid	None; acetyl metabolite also secreted; ? hepatotoxic
K$_1$ (vitamin)	None
Kanamycin	None
Ketorolac	—
Labetalol	None
Levonorgestrel	—
Lidocaine	None
Loperamide	—
Magnesium sulfate	None
Medroxyprogesterone	None
Mefenamic acid	None
Methadone	None if mother receiving ≤20 mg/24 hr
Methimazole (active metabolite of carbimazole)	None
Methocarbamol	None
Methyldopa	None
Methyprylon	Drowsiness
Metoprolol†	None
Metrizamide	None
Mexiletine	None

Continued

TABLE E-6
Maternal Medication Usually Compatible
with Breast-Feeding—cont'd

Drug	Reported sign or symptom in infant or effect on lactation
Minoxidil	None
Morphine	None; infant may have significant blood concentration
Moxalactam	None
Nadolol†	None
Nalidixic acid	Hemolysis in infant with glucose-6-phosphate dehydrogenase (G6PD) deficiency
Naproxen	—
Nefopam	None
Nifedipine	—
Nitrofurantoin	Hemolysis in infant with G6PD deficiency
Norethynodrel	None
Norsteroids	None
Noscapine	None
Oxprenolol	None
Phenylbutazone	None
Phenytoin	Methemoglobinemia (1 case)
Piroxicam	None
Prednisone	None
Procainamide	None
Progesterone	None
Propoxyphene	None
Propranolol	None
Propylthiouracil	None
Pseudoephedrine†	None
Pyridostigmine	None
Pyrimethamine	None
Quinidine	None
Quinine	None
Riboflavin	None
Rifampin	None
Scopolamine	—
Secobarbital	None
Senna	None
Sotalol	—

TABLE E-7
Food and Environmental Agents: Effect on Breast-Feeding

Agent	Reported sign or symptom in infant or effect on lactation
Aflatoxin	None
Aspartame	Caution if mother or infant has phenylketonuria
Bromide (photographic laboratory)	Potential absorption and bromide transfer into milk; see Table E-6
Cadmium	None reported
Chlordane	None reported
Chocolate (theobromine)	Irritability or increased bowel activity if excess amounts (16 oz/ day) consumed by mother
DDT, benzenehexachlorides, dieldrin, aldrin, hepatachlorepoxide	None
Fava beans	Hemolysis in patient with glucose-6-phosphate dehydrogenase (G6PD) deficiency
Fluorides	None
Hexachlorobenzene	Skin rash, diarrhea, vomiting, dark urine, neurotoxicity, death
Hexachlorophene	None; possible contamination of milk from nipple washing
Lead	Possible neurotoxicity
Methyl mercury, mercury	May affect neurodevelopment
Monosodium glutamate	None
Polychlorinated biphenyls and polybrominated biphenyls	Lack of endurance, hypotonia, sullen expressionless facies
Tetrachlorethylene cleaning fluid (perchloroethylene)	Obstructive jaundice, dark urine
Vegetarian diet	Signs of B_{12} deficiency

Physicians who encounter adverse effects in infants fed drug-contaminated human milk are urged to document these effects in a communication to the American Academy of Pediatrics (AAP) Committee on Drugs and the U.S. Food and Drug Administration. Such communication should include the generic and brand names of the drug, the maternal dose and mode of administration, the concentrations of the drug in milk and maternal and infant blood in relation to time of ingestion, the age of the infant, and the method used for laboratory identification. Such reports may significantly increase the pediatric community's knowledge regarding drug transfer into human milk and the potential or actual risk to the infant.

Acknowledgment

We thank Linda Wilson for her work in reference identification, document retrieval, and manuscript preparation.

Committee on drugs, 1992-1993

- Robert E. Kauffman, MD, PhD, Chairman
- William Banner, Jr., MD, PhD
- Chester M. Berlin, Jr., MD
- Jeffrey L. Blumer, MD, PhD
- Richard L. Gorman, MD
- George H. Lambert, MD
- Geraldine S. Wilson, MD

Liaison representatives

- Donald R. Bennett, MD, PhD, American Medical Association
- Jose F. Cordero, MD, MPH, Centers for Disease Control and Prevention
- Paul Kaufman, MD, Pharmaceutical Manufacturers' Association
- Sam A. Licata, MD, National Health and Welfare, Health Protection Branch, Canada
- Paul Tomich, MD, American College of Obstetricians and Gynecologists
- Gloria Troendle, MD, U.S. Food and Drug Administration
- Sumner J. Yaffe, MD, National Institute of Child Health and Human Development

AAP section liaison

- Charles J. Cote, MD, Section on Anesthesiology

Consultant

- Anthony R. Temple, MD

APPENDIX F

Composition of Nutritional Products

TABLE F-1
Common Caloric Supplements

Component	Calories
Protein	
Casec	1gm = 3.7 kcal, 0.9 gm protein
	1 tbsp = 17 kcal, 4 gm protein
Carbohydrate	
Polycose	Powder: 3.8 kcal/gm
	8 kcal/tsp
	Liquid: 2.0 kcal/mL
	10 kcal/tsp
Fat	
MCT oil	7.7 kcal/mL
Vegetable oil	8.3 kcal/mL

From Siberry G, Iannone R (editors): *The Harriet Lane handbook,* ed 15, St. Louis, 2000, Mosby.

TABLE F-2
Infant Formula Analysis (per liter)

Formula	kcal/mL (kcal/oz)	Protein gm (% kcal)	Carbohydrate gm (% kcal)	Fat gm (% kcal)	Na (mEq)	K (mEq)	Ca (mg)	P (mg)	Fe (mg)	Osmolality (mOsm/kg water)	Suggested uses
Enfamil AR (Mead Johnson)	0.67 (20)	16.7 (10) Nonfat milk Demineralized whey	73 (44) Lactose (57%) Rice starch (30%) Maltodextrins (13%)	34 (46) Palm olein (45%) Soy oil (20%) Coconut oil (20%) HO sun oil (15%)	11	18	520	353	12	230	When a thickened feeding is desired
Enfamil 24 [w/Fe] (Mead Johnson)	0.8 (20)	17 (9) Nonfat milk Whey	88 (43) Lactose	43 (48) Palm olein (45%) Soy oil (20%) HO Sun oil (15%)	10	22	630	430	6 [15]	360	Infants with normal GI tract requiring additional calories
Enfamil Premature Formula 20 [w/Fe] (Mead Johnson)	0.67 (20)	20 (12) Demineralized whey Nonfat milk	75 (44) Corn syrup solids Lactose	35 (44) MCT oil (40%) Soy oil Coconut oil	11	18	1120	560	1.7 [12]	260	Preterm infants

From Siberry G, Iannone R (editors): *The Harriet Lane handbook*, ed 15, St. Louis, 2000, Mosby.

Continued

TABLE F-2
Infant Formula Analysis (per liter)—cont'd

Formula	kcal/mL (kcal/oz)	Protein gm (% kcal)	Carbohydrate gm (% kcal)	Fat gm (% kcal)	Na (mEq)	K (mEq)	Ca (mg)	P (mg)	Fe (mg)	Osmolality (mOsm/kg water)	Suggested uses
Enfamil Premature Formula 24 [w/Fe] (Mead Johnson)	0.8 (24)	24 (12) Demineralized whey Nonfat milk	9 (44) Corn syrup solids Lactose	41 (44) MCT oil (40%) Soy oil Coconut oil	14	21	1340	670	2 [15]	310	Preterm infants
Enfamil 22 with iron (Mead Johnson)	0.73 (22)	20.6 (11) Nonfat milk Demineralized whey	79 (43) Corn syrup solids Lactose	39 (48) HO sun oil Soy oil MCT oil Coconut oil	11	20	890	490	13	—	Preterm infants after hospital discharge until good catch-up growth
Evaporated milk formula[a]	0.69 (21)	28 (16) Cow's milk	75 (43) Lactose Corn syrup	33 (43) Butterfat	20	33	1130	870	2	—	Infants with normal GI tract; need vitamin C and iron supplement
Follow-up (Carnation)	0.67 (20)	18 (10) Nonfat milk	89 (53) Corn syrup (43%) Lactose (37%)	28 (37) Palm olein (47%) Soy oil (26%) Coconut oil (21%) HO saff oil (6%)	11	23	912	608	13	328	Infants 4-12 months with normal GI tract

Follow-up Soy (Carnation)	0.67 (20)	21 (12) Soy isolate Methionine	81 (48) Maltodextrin Sucrose	29 (40) Palm olein (47%) Soy oil (26%) Coconut oil (21%) HO saff oil (6%)	12	20	912	608	12	200	Infants 4-12 months with allergy to cow's milk, lactose malabsorption, galactosemia
Good Start (Carnation)	0.67 (20)	16 (10) Hydrolyzed whey	74 (44) Lactose Maltodextrins	3.5 (46) Palm olein (47%) Soy oil (26%) Coconut oil (21%) HO saff oil (6%)	7	17	432	243	10	265	Infants with normal GI tract
Isomil (Ross)	0.67 (20)	17 (10) Soy isolate Methionine	70 (41) Corn syrup Sucrose	37 (49) Soy oil Coconut oil	13	19	709	507	12	230	Infants with allergy to cow's milk, lactose malabsorption, galactosemia
Isomil DF (Ross)	0.67 (20)	18 (11) Soy isolate Methionine	68 (40) Corn syrup Sucrose Soy fiber	37 (49) Soy oil Coconut oil	13	19	709	507	12	240	Short-term management of diarrhea; contains fiber
Lactofree (Mead Johnson)	0.67 (20)	14 (9) Milk protein isolate	7 (43) Corn syrup solids	36 (48) Palm olein (45%) Soy oil (20%) Coconut oil (20%) HO Sun oil (15%)	9	19	550	370	12	200	Infants with lactose malabsorption

From Siberry G, Iannone R (editors): *The Harriet Lane handbook*, ed 15, St. Louis, 2000, Mosby.
a 13 oz evaporated whole milk, 119 oz water, 12 tbsp corn syrup.

Continued

TABLE F-2
Infant Formula Analysis (per liter)—cont'd

Formula	kcal/mL (kcal/oz)	Protein gm (% kcal)	Carbohydrate gm (% kcal)	Fat gm (% kcal)	Na (mEq)	K (mEq)	Ca (mg)	P (mg)	Fe (mg)	Osmolality (mOsm/kg water)	Suggested uses
MJ3232A (Mead Johnson)	0.42 (12.6)	19 (17) Casein hydrolysate Cystine, Tyr, Trp	28 (25) Tapioca starch CHO selected by physician	28 (57) MCT oil (85%) Corn oil (15%)	13	19	630	420	13	250	Infants with severe CHO intolerance (CHO must be added)
Neocate (Scientific Hospital Supply)	0.69 (21)	20 (12) Free amino acids	78 (47) Corn syrup solids	32 (41) Safflower oil Coconut oil Soy oil	8	16	826	620	10	342	Infants with severe food allergies
Nutramigen (Mead Johnson)	0.67 (20)	19 (11) Casein hydrolysate Cystine, Tyr, Trp	74 (44) Corn syrup solids Modified cornstarch	34 (45) Palm olein (45%) Soy oil (20%) Coconut oil (20%) HO Sun oil (15%)	14	19	640	430	13	320	Infants with food allergies
Portagen (Mead Johnson)	0.67 (20)	24 (14) Na caseinate	78 (46) Corn syrup solids Sucrose	32 (40) MCT oil (85%) Corn oil (15%)	16	22	640	470	13	230	Infants with fat malabsorption

	kcal/mL (kcal/L)	Protein g (%)	Protein source	CHO g (%)	CHO source	Fat g (%)	Fat source							Osmolality	Indications
Pregestimil (Mead Johnson)	0.67 (20)	19 (11)	Casein hydrolysate Cystine, Tyr, Trp	69 (41)	Corn syrup solids (60%) Modified corn-starch (20%) Dextrose (20%)	38 (48)	MCT oil (55%) Corn oil (20%) Soy oil (12.5%) HO Saff oil (12.5%)	11	19	640	430	13		320	Infants with food allergies, protein or fat malabsorption
ProSobee (Mead Johnson)	0.67 (20)	20 (12)	Soy isolate Methionine	73 (42)	Corn syrup solids	37 (48)	Palm olein (45%) Soy oil (20%) Coconut oil (20%) HO Sun oil (15%)	10	21	710	560	12		200	Infants with allergy to cow's milk, lactose malabsorption, galactosemia
RCFa (Ross) [w/Fe]	0.4 (12)	20 (20)	Soy isolate	—	Selected by physician	36 (80)	Soy oil Coconut oil	13	19	709	507	12		—[a]	Infants with severe CHO intolerance (CHO must be added) Modified for ketogenic diet
Similac [w/Fe] (Ross)	0.67 (20)	14 (8)	Nonfat milk Whey protein	73 (43)	Lactose	36 (49)	Soy oil Coconut oil HO saff oil	7	18	527	284	1.5	[12]	300	Infants with normal GI tract
Similac 24 [w/Fe] (Ross)	0.8 (24)	22 (11)	Nonfat milk	85 (42)	Lactose	43 (47)	Soy oil Coconut oil	12	27	726	565	1.8	[15]	380	Infants with normal GI tract requiring additional calories

From Siberry G, Iannone R (editors): *The Harriet Lane handbook*, ed 15, St. Louis, 2000, Mosby.
[a]Available as concentrated liquid. Nutrient values vary depending on amount of added carbohydrate (CHO) and water. A total of 12 fl oz of concentrated liquid with 15 gm CHO and 12 fl oz water yields 20 kcal/fl oz formula with 68 gm CHO/L.

Continued

TABLE F-2
Infant Formula Analysis (per liter)—cont'd

Formula	kcal/mL (kcal/oz)	Protein gm (% kcal)	Carbohydrate gm (% kcal)	Fat gm (% kcal)	Na (mEq)	K (mEq)	Ca (mg)	P (mg)	Fe (mg)	Osmolality (mOsm/kg water)	Suggested uses
Similac Lactose Free (Ross)	0.67 (20)	14.5 (9) Milk isolate	72.3 (43) Corn syrup solids Sucrose	36.5 (49) Soy oil Coconut oil	9	18.5	568	378	12	230	Infants with lactose malabsorption
Similac Neosure (Ross)	0.75 (22)	19 (10) Nonfat milk Whey	77 (41) Corn syrup solids 50% Lactose (50%)	41 (49) MCT oil Soy oil Coconut oil HO saff oil	11	27	784	463	13	250	Preterm infants, after hospital discharge, until good catch-up growth

Similac PM 60/40 (Ross)	0.67 (20)	15 (9) Whey Na caseinate	69 (41) Lactose	38 (50) Soy oil Coconut oil Corn oil	7	15	378	189	1.5	280	Infants who require lowered calcium and phosphorus levels
Similac Special Care 20 [w/Fe] (Ross)	0.67 (20)	18 (11) Nonfat milk Whey	72 (42) Corn syrup solids Lactose	37 (49) MCT oil Soy oil Coconut oil	13	22	1216	676	2.5 (12)	235	Preterm infants
Similac Special Care 24 [w/Fe] (Ross)	0.8 (24)	22 (11) Nonfat milk Whey	86 (42) Corn syrup solids Lactose	44 (49) MCT oil Soy oil Coconut oil	15	27	1452	806	3 [15]	280	Preterm infants

From Siberry G, Iannone R (editors): *The Harriet Lane handbook*, ed 15, St. Louis, 2000, Mosby.

TABLE F-3
Human Milk and Fortifiers Analysis (per liter)

Formula	kcal/mL (kcal/oz)	Protein gm (% kcal)	Carbohydrate gm (% kcal)	Fat gm (% kcal)	Na (mEq)	K (mEq)	Ca (mg)	P (mg)	Fe (mg)	Osmolality (mOsm/kg water)	Suggested uses
Human milk (mature)	0.69 (20)	9 (5) Human milk protein	73 (42) Lactose	42 (54) Human milk fat	8	13	280	147	0.4	286	Infants
Preterm human milk[a]	0.67 (20)	14 (8) Human milk protein	66 (40) Lactose	39 (52) Human milk fat	11	15	248	128	1.2	290	Preterm infants
Enfamil Human Milk Fortifier (per packet) (Mead Johnson)	3.5 —	0.15 (20) Whey protein concentrate Na caseinate	0.68 (76) Corn syrup solids Lactose	0.02 (3.9) From caseinate	0.08	0.1	23	11	0	—	Fortifier for preterm human milk
Similac Natural Care Human Milk Fortifier (Ross)	0.8 (24)	22 (11) Nonfat milk Whey protein concentrate	86 (42) Corn syrup solids Lactose	44 (47) MCT oil Soy oil Coconut oil	15	26.6	1694	935	3	280	Fortifier for preterm human milk

Preterm Human Milk + Similac Natural Care 50:50 ratio	0.74 (22)	18 (10) Human milk protein Nonfat milk Whey protein concentrate	71 (40) Lactose Corn syrup solids	41 (50) Human milk fat MCT oil Soy oil Coconut oil	13	21	971	531	2.1	285	Preterm infants
Preterm Human Milk + Enfamil Human Milk Fortifier (1 pkt/50mL)	0.73 (22)	17.3 (9) Human milk protein Whey protein concentrate Na caseinate	79 (43) Lactose Corn syrup solids	39 (48) Human milk fat	12	16	688	348	1.2	350	Preterm infants

From Siberry G, Iannone R (editors): *The Harriet Lane handbook*, ed 15, St. Louis, 2000, Mosby.
From Ross Products Division, Abbott Laboratories, Inc.
[a]Composition of human milk varies with maternal diet, stage of lactation, within feedings, diurnally, and among mothers.

TABLE F-4
Enteral Feeding Formula Analysis (per liter)

Formula	kcal per oz	gm	PROTEIN %cal	PROTEIN Type	gm	CARBOHYDRATE %cal	CARBOHYDRATE Type	gm	FAT %cal	FAT Type	NA mEq	K mEq	CA mg	P mg	FE mg	GI solute load, mOsm/kg H$_2$O
Enrich	32.5	39.2	15	Na and Ca caseinates, soy protein isolate	160	55	Hydrolyzed corn starch, sucrose, soy fiber	37	30	Corn oil	36.2	42.6	708	708	12.8	480
Ensure	31.3	36.7	14	Na and Ca caseinates, soy protein isolate	143	55	Corn syrup, sucrose	47	31	Corn oil	36.2	37	521	521	9.4	470
Ensure Plus	44.4	54.2	15	Na and Ca caseinates, soy protein isolate	197	53	Corn syrup, sucrose	53	32	Corn oil	48.9	53.3	696	696	12.5	690
Isocal	32	34.0	13	Na and Ca caseinates, soy protein	133	50	Maltodextrins	44	37	Soy oil MCT oil	23.0	34.0	630	630	0.5	300

Jevity	31.3	43.8	Na and Ca caseinate	17	150	Hydrolyzed corn starch, soy fiber	53	36	MCT—50% corn oil, soy oil	30	39.9	39.4	896	746	13.4	310
Osmolite	31.3	36.6	Casein, soy protein isolate	14	143	Hydrolyzed corn starch	55	38	MCT—50% corn oil, soy oil	31	27.2	25.6	521	521	9.4	300
Pediasure	30	29.6	Na caseinate, whey protein concentrate	12	110	Hydrolyzed corn starch, sucrose	44	50	High oleic safflower oil—50% soy oil—30% MCT—20%	44	16.5	33.0	970	800	14.0	325
Pulmocare	45	63.0	Na and Ca caseinates	17	106	Sucrose hydrolyzed corn starch	28	92	Corn oil	55	57.0	49.0	1057	1057	19.0	520
Sustacal	30	61.0	Na and Ca caseinates, soy protein isolate	24	140	Sucrose, corn syrup solids	55	23	Partially, hydrolyzed soy oil	21	41.0	54.0	1010	930	16.9	620
Sustacal HC	44.4	61.0	Na and Ca caseinates	16	190	Corn syrup solids, sucrose	50	58	Corn oil	34	36.0	38.0	850	850	15.0	650

From Johnson KB, editor: *The Harriet Lane handbook*, ed 13, St. Louis, 1993, Mosby.

Continued

TABLE F-4
Enteral Feeding Formula Analysis (per liter)—cont'd

Formula	kcal per oz	PROTEIN			CARBOHYDRATE			FAT			NA	K	CA	P	FE	GI solute load, mOsm/kg H₂O
		%cal	gm	Type	%cal	gm	Type	%cal	gm	Type	mEq	mEq	mgm	mgm	mgm	
Travasorb MCT	30	20	49.2	Lactalbumin K Caseinate	50	123	Corn syrup solids	33	30	Sunflower oil—20% MCT—80%	15.2	25.6	500	500	9.0	250
Vital HN	30	17	41.7	Partially hydrolyzed whey, meat soy, amino acids	74	185	Hydrolyzed corn starch, sucrose	11	9	Safflower oil MCT—45%	20.3	34.1	120	667	667	500
Vivonex TEN	30	15	38.0	Free amino acids	82	206	Maltodextrins	3	3	Safflower oil	20.0	20.0	500	500	9.0	630

From Johnson KB, editor: *The Harriet Lane Handbook*, ed 13, St. Louis, 1993, Mosby.

TABLE F-5
Estimated Daily Requirements of Premature Infants:* Growth and Nongrowth

	BODY WEIGHT INTERVALS (GM)†								
	750-1000	1000-1250	1250-1500	1500-1750	1750-2000	2000-2250	2250-2500	2500-2750	2750-3000
Energy									
Growth (kcal)	21	46	68	79	92	104	114	111	108
Nongrowth (kcal)	71	94	117	133	156	180	204	215	239
Total (kcal/kg)	105	124	127	130	133	133	134	124	121
Protein									
Growth (g)	1.78	3.45	4.44	4.79	4.85	4.90	4.68	4.27	3.77
Nongrowth (g)	0.87	1.12	1.37	1.62	1.87	2.12	2.37	2.62	2.87
Total (g/kg)†	3.02	4.06	4.22	3.94	3.58	3.30	2.96	2.62	2.30
Sodium									
Growth (mEq)	0.95	1.68	2.10	2.21	2.21	2.21	2.10	1.89	1.57
Nongrowth (mEq)	0.18	0.23	0.28	0.34	0.38	0.44	0.49	0.55	0.60
Total (mEq/kg)	1.29	1.69	1.73	1.56	1.38	1.24	1.09	0.92	0.75

From Taeusch HW, Ballard RA, Avery ME (editors): *Diseases of the newborn*, ed 7, Philadelphia, 1998, WB Saunders, p 1362.
*Assuming extent of intestinal absorption as follows: energy: 75% absorption for infants weighing 750-1500 gm, 80% for those weighing 1500-2500 gm, and 85% for those weighing more than 2500 gm; protein: 75% absorption at 750-1250 gm, 77% at 1250-1500 gm, 80% at 1500-2250 gm, 83% at 2250-2500 gm, and 85% above 2500 gm; sodium and potassium, 95% absorption throughout; calcium, 40%; phosphorus, 80%; and magnesium, 20% throughout.
†Based on arithmetic mean weight for the weight interval. (Data from O'Donnell AM, Ziegler EE, Fomon SJ, reproduced with permission of Dr. Fomon.)
Continued

TABLE F-5
Estimated Daily Requirements of Premature Infants:* Growth and Nongrowth

	BODY WEIGHT INTERVALS (GM)†								
	750-1000	1000-1250	1250-1500	1500-1750	1750-2000	2000-2250	2250-2500	2500-2750	2750-3000
Potassium									
Growth (mEq)	0.31	0.73	1.05	1.15	1.26	1.36	1.36	1.36	1.15
Nongrowth (mEq)	0.20	0.26	0.32	0.38	0.43	0.49	0.55	0.61	0.66
Total (mEq/kg)	0.58	0.88	0.99	0.94	0.90	0.87	0.80	0.75	0.63
Calcium									
Growth (mg)	148	317	442	530	592	632	660	627	592
Nongrowth (mg)	—	—	—	—	—	—	—	—	—
Total (mg/kg)	169	282	321	326	316	300	278	239	206
Phosphorus									
Growth (mg)	49	110	148	172	188	197	202	194	177
Nongrowth (mg)	12	27	37	43	47	49	50	49	44
Total (mg/kg)	70	121	135	132	125	116	106	93	77
Magnesium									
Growth (mg)	9.0	18.5	25.5	30.0	33.5	35.5	37.0	35.5	32.5
Nongrowth (mg)	—	—	—	—	—	—	—	—	—
Total (mg/kg)	10.3	16.4	18.6	18.5	17.8	16.7	15.6	13.5	11.3

From Taeusch HW, Ballard RA, Avery ME (editors): *Diseases of the newborn*, ed 7, Philadelphia, 1998, WB Saunders, p 1362.

APPENDIX G

Physical Observations

NEUTRAL THERMAL ENVIRONMENTAL TEMPERATURES

For healthy naked infant in incubator of moderate humidity (50% saturation). Range shown is that needed to maintain normal body temperature without increasing heat production or evaporation loss by more than 25% (Fig. G-1).

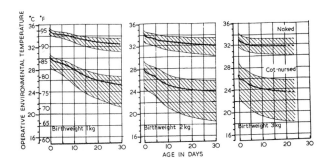

FIG. G-1 Range of temperature to provide neutral environmental conditions for baby lying either dressed in cot or naked on warm mattress in draft-free surroundings of moderate humidity (50% saturation) when mean radiant temperature is same as air temperature. Hatched area shows neutral temperature range for healthy babies weighing 1 kg, 2 kg, or 3 kg at birth. Approximately 1° C should be added to these operative temperatures to derive appropriate neutral air temperature for a single-walled incubator when room temperature is less than 27° C (80° F) and more if room temperature is much less than this. (From Hey F, Katz G: *Arch Dis Child* 45:328, 1970.)

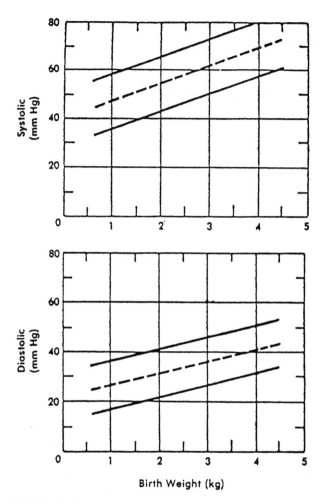

FIG. G-2 Linear regression *(broken lines)* and 95% confidence limits *(solid lines)* of systolic *(top)* and diastolic *(bottom)* aortic blood pressures and birth weight in 61 healthy newborn infants during the first 12 hours after birth. For systolic pressure, $y = 7.13x + 40.45$; $r = 0.79$. For diastolic pressure, $y = 4.81x + 22.18$; $r = 0.71$. For both, $n = 413$ and $P < 0.001$. (From Versmold HT, et al: *Pediatrics* 67:607, 1981.)

TABLE G-1
Time of First Void and First Stool in 500 Infants

Hours	395 Full-Term Infants		80 Preterm Infants		25 Postterm Infants	
	No. of infants	Cumulative %	No. of infants	Cumulative %	No. of infants	Cumulative %
First void						
In delivery room	51	12.9	17	21.2	3	12
1-8	151	51.1	50	83.7	4	38
9-16	158	91.1	12	98.7	14	84
17-24	35	100	1	100	4	100
>24	0	—	0	—	0	—
First stool						
In delivery room	66	16.7	4	5	8	32
1-8	169	59.5	22	32.5	9	68
9-16	125	91.1	25	63.8	5	88
17-24	29	98.5	10	76.3	3	100
24-48	6*	100	18†	98.8	0	—
>48	0	—	1‡	100	0	—

From Clark DA: *Pediatrics* 60:457, 1977.
*At 25, 26, 27, 28, 33, and 37 hours.
†Five stooled more than 36 hours after birth at 38, 39, 40, 42, and 47 hours.
‡At 59 hours.

TABLE G-2
Endotracheal Tube Size

	ENDOTRACHEAL TUBE DIAMETER	
Infant weight (gm)	Inside	Outside
Less than 1000	2.5 mm	12F
1000-1500	3.0 mm	14F
1500-2200	3.5 mm	16F
2200 and over	4.0 mm	18F

From Avery GB, Fletcher MA, MacDonald MG, editors: *Neonatology,* ed 4, Philadelphia, 1994, Lippincott.

TABLE G-3
Depth of Insertion of an Orotracheal Tube From the Lips of a Premature Infant

Infant weight (kg)	Depth of insertion (cm)
1.0	7
2.0	8
3.0	9
4.0	10

From Avery GB, Fletcher MA, MacDonald MG, editors: *Neonatology,* ed 4, Philadelphia, 1994, Lippincott.

APPENDIX H

Neonatal Pharmacology

The differences in drug disposition for newborns when compared with adults are due to the underdevelopment of those organ systems affecting drug absorption, distribution, metabolism, and excretion (Table H-1). For these reasons, a neonate cannot be considered a small adult. There is considerable immaturity.

DRUG DOSES FOR NEONATES

Abbreviations
GI, gastrointestinal
ALT, alanine aminotransferase
AST, aspartate aminotransferase
bid, twice a day
BUN, blood urea nitrogen
CBC, complete blood count
CNS, central nervous system
CSF, cerebrospinal fluid
ECG, electrocardiogram
ET, endotracheal
Hct, hematocrit
HIV, human immunodeficiency virus
IHSS, idiopathic hypertrophic subaortic stenosis
IM, intramuscular
IT, intratracheal
IV, intravenous
LFT, liver function test
PCA (postconceptional age in weeks) = gestational age (weeks) + postnatal age (weeks)
PNA, Postnatal age (days)
PO, by mouth
PR, by rectum
PRN, as needed
PSVT, paroxysmal supraventricular tachycardia
PTT, partial thromboplastin time
PVC, premature ventricular contraction
qd, every day
qid, four times a day

qod, every other day
RDA, recommended dietary allowance
RDS, respiratory distress syndrome
RSV, respiratory syncytial virus
SC, subcutaneous
SGOT, serum glutamic-oxaloacetic transaminase
TIBC, total iron binding content
TSH, thyroid-stimulating hormone

Table H-2, prepared in large part by Dr. Carlton K.K. Lee, contains both generic and trade names, information on how drugs are supplied, and their usual dose and route of administration. Brief remarks regarding side effects, drug interactions, precautions, effect on breast-feeding, and other relevant factors are included.

Note in the How Supplied column that the unit quantity in which a drug is supplied is listed in parentheses after the drug concentration. Suspension formulations marked by an asterisk are not commercially available and must be extemporaneously compounded by a pharmacist. References for these formulations and for the contents of the formulary are provided at the end of this section of the appendix. Drug dilutions may be necessary to enhance the accuracy of dose delivery for certain drugs. Check with your respective pharmacy for specific dosage forms and concentrations available at your institution.

REFERENCES

American Academy of Pediatrics Committee on Infectious Diseases: *1997 Redbook,* Elk Grove, Ill, 1997, the Academy.

American Society of Hospital Pharmacists Committee on Extemporaneous Formulation, SIG on Pediatric Practice: *Handbook on extemporaneous formulations,* Bethesda, Md, 1987, the Society.

Dupuis LL (editor): *1993 Formulary of drugs,* ed 12, Toronto, 1993, The Hospital for Sick Children.

McEveyt G, McQuarrie GM (editors): *Drug information 99,* Bethesda, Md, 1999, American Hospital Formulary Service.

Nelson JD: *Pocketbook of pediatric antimicrobial therapy,* ed 13, Baltimore, 1998-1999, Williams & Wilkins.

Pagliaro LA, Pagliaro AM (editors): *Problems in pediatric drug therapy,* ed 3, Hamilton, Ill, 1995, Drug Intelligence Publications Inc.

Roberts RJ: *Drug therapy in infants,* Philadelphia, 1984, WB Saunders.

Siberry GK, Iannone R: *The Harriet Lane handbook,* ed 15, St. Louis, 2000, Mosby.

Taketomo CK, Hodding JH, Kraus DM (editors): *Pediatric dosage handbook,* ed 6, Hudson, Ohio, 1999-2000, Lexicomp.

Yaffe S, Aranda J: *Pediatric pharmacology,* ed 2, Philadelphia, 1992, WB Saunders.

Young TE, Mangum OB: *Neofax '99: a manual of drugs used in neonatal care,* ed 12, Columbus, Ohio, 1999, Acorn Publishing Inc.

TABLE H-1
General Characteristics of the Pharmacokinetic Process in Neonates as Compared With Adults

Characteristic	Relative to adult	Age until adult level reached	Pharmacokinetic effect	Example drug
ABSORPTION				
Peroral				
PH	Lower acid output	3 mo	↓ Bioavailability of acid drug	Phenobarbitol
GI motility	Gastric emptying time is 6-8 hr at birth	6-8 mo	Unpredictable biovailability	Digoxin
GI contents	Decreased amounts of bile acid pools and pancreatic enzymes; underdeveloped bacterial flora	About 1 year	↓ Bioavailability of fat-soluble drug	Vitamin E
Intramuscular	Low vascular perfusion, delay	?		
Percutaneous	Increased, especially in preterm infants	Months	↑ Absorption	Lindane/Kwell (contraindicated—have caused seizures)

Modified from Pelkon O: *Curr Opin Pediatr* 2:220, 1990; Misap RL, Hill MR, Szefler SL: In Evans WE (editor): *Applied pharmacokinetics*, ed 3, Spokane, Wash, 1992, Applied Therapeutics.

Continued

TABLE H-1
General Characteristics of the Pharmacokinetic Process in Neonates as Compared With Adults—cont'd

Characteristic	Relative to adult	Age until adult level reached	Pharmacokinetic effect	Example drug
DISTRIBUTION				
% Body water	High extracellular and total body water rapidly changes in first year	About 12 years	↑ Volume of distribution	Aminoglycosides
% Fat	Full-term birth at 12%-16%; increases from 5-10 years of age followed by a decrease	About 17 years		
Plasma proteins	Lower total protein, albumin, and α-1 acid glycoprotein	Gradual changes over first year	↑ Volume of distribution and free drug concentration	Phenytoin, lidocaine
	Higher unconjugated bilirubin and free fatty acids	Gradual changes over first year		
Blood-brain barrier	Immature barrier caused by incomplete myelination	?	↑ CSF penetration	Aminoglycosides

METABOLISM

P-450 enzyme	Lower at birth, isoenzyme specific	2 wk-6 mo	↑ Elimination T$_{1/2}$	Phenobarbitol
Glucuronidation	Lower at birth	3-4 yr	Minor metabolite	Acetaminophen
Sulphation	At adult level		Major metabolite	Acetaminophen
Glycine conjugation	At adult level			
Overall capacity	Further impaired by prematurity or disease			

ELIMINATION

Glomerular filtration	Lower, especially in premature infants	About 6 mo	↑ Elimination T$_{1/2}$	Aminoglycosides
Tubular secretion	Lower	About 6 mo	↑ Elimination T$_{1/2}$	Penicillins

Modified from Pelkon O: *Curr Opin Pediatr* 2:220, 1990; Misap RL, Hill MR, Szefler SL: In Evans WE (editor): *Applied pharmacokinetics*, ed 3, Spokane, Wash, 1992, Applied Therapeutics.

TABLE H-2
Drug Doses for Neonates

Drug	How supplied	Dose and route	Remarks
Acetaminophen (Tylenol, Tempra, Panadol, and others)	Infant drops: 80 mg/0.8 ml Elixir: 80 mg/5ml, 120 mg/5 ml, or 160 mg/5 ml Child solution/suspension: 160 mg/5 ml Suppository: 80, 120, 125 mg	5-10 mg/kg/dose q4-6h PO/PR (**maximum** 5 doses per day)	Delayed hepatotoxicity occurs in overdose. Avoid use in suspected G6PD deficiency. Some preparations contain alcohol and/or phenylalanine. Breast-feeding: Compatible.
Acetazolamide (Diamox)	Suspension:* 25, 30, or 50 mg/ml Injection: 500 mg/5 ml Contains 2.05 mEq Na$^+$ per 500 mg drug	IV/PO: 5 mg/kg/24 hr ÷ q8h, increase as required to 25 mg/kg/24 hr *For hydrocephalus (IV/PO):* Day 1: 25 mg/kg/24 hr ÷ q8h Day 2: 50 mg/kg/24 hr ÷ q8h Day 3: 75 mg/kg/24 hr ÷ q8h Day 4 and greater: 100 mg/kg/24 hr ÷ q8h	Contraindicated in hepatic failure, severe renal failure and hypersensitivity to sulfonamides. Paresthesias, polyuria, drowsiness, GI irritation, transient hypokalemia, reduced urate excretion, and metabolic acidosis may occur with long-term therapy. Avoid IM administration because injectable product has a high pH. Bicarbonate replacement therapy may be required, especially during long-term use (see citrate or sodium bicarbonate). Breast-feeding: Compatible.
Acyclovir (Zovirax)	Suspension: 200 mg/5 ml Injection: 500 mg/10 ml Ointment: 5% (15 g) Contains 4.2 mEq Na$^+$ per 1 gm drug	*Herpes simplex virus:* IV: 30-45 mg/kg/24 hr ÷ q8h for 14-21 days Topical use, apply ointment 5-6 times per day for 7 days	Can cause renal impairment. Adequate hydration is essential to prevent renal tubular crystallization. Encephalopathic reactions have been reported. May cause nausea, vomiting, diarrhea, headache, dizziness, arthralgia, fatigue, rash, insomnia, fever. Infuse

	Varicella zoster: Immunocompromised host IV: 1500 mg/m²/24 hr ÷ q8h for 7-10 days Immunocompetent host PO: 80 mg/kg/24 hr ÷ qid for 5 days; begin immediately after signs or symptoms	dose over 1 hr at a concentration ≤7 mg/ml. Adjust dose in renal impairment. Breast-feeding: Compatible.
Adenosine (Adenocard) Injection: 3 mg/ml (2 ml)	*For PSVT:* 0.05 mg/kg IV push; if not effective within 2 minutes, increase dose by 0.05 mg/kg increments every 2 min to a **maximum** of 0.25 mg/kg/dose	$T_{1/2}$ <10 seconds; may precipitate bronchoconstriction. Side effects include facial flushing, headache, shortness of breath, dyspnea, nausea, and chest pain. **Contraindicated** in second- and third-degree AV block. Theophylline and caffeine may antagonize its effect. Breast-feeding: Safety not established.
Albumin, human (Normal serum albumin) Injection: 5% (50 mg/ml), 25% (250 mg/ml); both contain 130-160 mEq Na⁺/L	*Hypoproteinemia:* IV, 0.5-1 gm/kg/dose over 2-4 hr; repeat every 1-2 days or as calculated to replace ongoing losses *Hypovolemia:* IV, 0.5 gm/kg/dose, repeated prn; usually infused over 0.5-1hr (faster rates may be clinically necessary) **(maximum** dose: 6 gm/kg/24 hr)	Fever, chills, rash, tachycardia, and hypervolemia may occur. **Contraindicated** in severe CHF or anemia. Use with **caution** in hypervolemia. 5% concentration generally used; 25% concentration is generally reserved for fluid- and sodium-restricted patients. Dilutions of the 25% product should be made with D5W or NS. Breast-feeding: Safety not established.

*Indicates suspensions not commercially available; must be extemporaneously compounded by a pharmacist. See references.   *Continued*

TABLE H-2
Drug Doses for Neonates—cont'd

Drug	How supplied	Dose and route				Remarks

Alprostadil (PGE₁, Prostaglandin E₁, Prostin VR)

How supplied: Injection: 500 µg/ml

Dose and route: Initial: 0.05-0.1 µg/kg/min; advance to 0.2 µg/kg/min if necessary
Maintenance: When increase in PO_2 is noted, decrease immediately to lowest effective dose; doses >0.4 µg/kg/min not likely to produce additional benefit

Remarks: For palliation only. Continuous vital sign monitoring is essential. May cause apnea, fever, seizures, flushing, bradycardia, hypotension, and diarrhea. Decreases platelet aggregation. Breast-feeding: Safety not established.

Amikacin sulfate (Amikin)

How supplied: Injection: 50 or 250 mg/ml

Dose and route:

PCA	PNA	Dose (mg/kg/dose)	Interval (hr)
≤29 or significant asphyxia	0-28	7.5	24
	>28	10	24
30-36	0-14	10	24
	>14	7.5	12
≥37	0-7	7.5	12
	>7	7.5	8

Remarks: Ototoxicity, nephrotoxicity, rash, fever, eosinophilia, and headache may occur. Monitor levels. **Therapeutic levels: peak, 20-30 mg/L; trough, 5-10 mg/L.** Recommended serum sampling time at steady-state: trough within 30 minutes before the third consecutive dose and peak 30-60 minutes after the administration of the third consecutive dose. Adjust dose with renal impairment. Ototoxic effects are synergistic with furosemide. Administer dose at least 2 hr before or after penicillins and cephalosporins (may blunt serum concentration). Breast-feeding: Safety not established.

Aminophylline
(Somophyllin and various other brand names)

Injection (IV): 25 mg/ml (79% theophylline)
Oral liquid: 105 mg/5 ml (240 ml) (86% theophylline)

IV loading: 6 mg/kg IV over 20 min (each 1.2-mg/kg dose raises the serum theophylline concentration 2 mg/L) IV maintenance (continuous IV drip): Neonates, 0.2 mg/kg/hr *Neonatal apnea:* Loading dose IV or PO, 5-6 mg/kg; maintenance dose IV or PO, 1-2 mg/kg/dose q6-8h

Monitoring serum levels is essential, especially in infants. Side effects: restlessness, GI upset, seizures, arrhythmias.
Therapeutic level: For neonatal apnea, 6-13 mg/L; for bronchospasm 10-20 mg/L.
Recommended guidelines for obtaining levels:
IV bolus: 30 min after infusion IV continuous; 12-24 hr after initiation of infusion
PO liquid (peak): 1 hr after dose
PO liquid (trough): Just before dose. Ideally, obtain levels after achievement of steady-state (1-6 days). However, levels may be obtained before steady-state to assess safety. *Drug interactions:* Increased levels with erythromycin, cimetidine; decreased levels with phenobarbital, rifampin, phenytoin. NOTE: Several oral liquid preparations are dye free. Consult with pharmacist if it is an issue. Breast-feeding: Compatible.

Amoxicillin
(Amoxil, Larotid, Trimox, and others)

Drops: 50 mg/ml (15, 30 ml)
Suspension: 125, 250, mg/5ml (80, 100, 125, 150, 200 ml)

PO: 20-40 mg/kg/24 hr ÷ q8h

Similar to ampicillin. May cause abdominal cramps, cutaneous reactions, diarrhea, hypersensitivity reactions, interstitial nephritis, pancytopenia, pseudomembranous colitis, and urticaria. Adjust dose in renal failure. Breast-feeding: Compatible.

Continued

TABLE H-2
Drug Doses for Neonates—cont'd

Drug	How supplied	Dose and route	Remarks
Amoxicillin-clavulanic acid (Augmentin)	Suspension: 125, 250, mg/5ml (31.25 and 62.5 mg clavulanate/5 ml) (75, 100, 150 ml); or 200, 400 mg/5 ml (28.5 and 57 mg clavulanate/5 ml) (50, 75, 100 ml) Contains 0.63 mEq K⁺ per 125 mg clavulanate	Dosage based on amoxicillin component *Children <3 mo:* 30 mg/kg/24 hr ÷ bid PO (recommended dosage form is 125 mg/5 ml suspension)	See amoxicillin for side effects. Diarrhea primarily caused by clavulanic acid. Reduce dose in renal failure. 200, 400 mg/5 ml concentrations contain phenylalanine and should not be used by phenylketonurics. Breast-feeding: Compatible.
Amphotericin B (Fungizone)	Injection: 50 mg Cream: 3% (20 gm) Lotion: 3% (30 ml) Ointment: 3% (20 gm) Oral suspension: 100 mg/ml (24 ml)	Topical: Apply to affected areas bid-qid IV: Mix with D₅W to a concentration of 0.1 mg/ml, pH >4.2; infuse over 4-6 hr Test dose: 0.1 mg/kg/dose IV up to a **maximum** of 1 mg infused over 2 hr (followed by remaining initial dose) Initial dose: 0.25 mg/kg/24 hr	Fever, chills, nausea, and vomiting are common side effects. Monitor renal, hepatic, electrolytes, and hematologic status *closely*. Hypokalemia (may cause digoxin toxicity—if receiving both drugs), hypomagnesemia, renal tubular acidosis, renal failure, acute hepatic failure, and phlebitis may occur. Drug is incompatible in normal saline. A more-concentrated solution of 0.2 mg/ml can be used for fluid-restricted patients but must be administered only through a central line. Breast-feeding: Safety not established.

Ampicillin
(Omnipen, Polycillin, Principen)

Drops: 100 mg/ml (20 ml)
Suspension: 125, 250 mg/ 5 ml (80, 100, 150, 200 ml)
Injection: 125, 250, 500 mg, 1 gm, 2 gm
Contains 3 mEq Na^+/gm drug

Increment: Increase as tolerated by 0.125-0.25 mg/kg/24 hr qd or qod
Maximum dose: 1.5 mg/kg/ 24 hr
Oral candidiasis: 100 mg PO qid
IV or IM: 50 mg/kg/dose

PCA	PNA	Interval (hr)
≤29	≤28	12
≤29	>28	8
30-36	≤14	12
30-36	>14	8
37-44	≤7	12
37-44	>7	8
≥45	All	6

For meningitis and group B streptococcal sepsis use 100 mg/kg/dose with the same guidelines as above

Same side effects as penicillin, with cross-reactivity. Rash is commonly seen at 5-10 days. May cause interstitial nephritis. Adjust dose in renal failure. Breast-feeding: Use with caution (adverse effects are rare, three potential problems exist for nursing infant: bowel flora modification, allergic response, and interference of culture results for fever work-up).

Atropine sulfate

Injection: 0.05, 0.1, 0.3, 0.4, 0.5, 0.8, 1 mg/ml

Cardiopulmonary resuscitation: IV, IM, SC: 0.01-0.03 mg/kg/dose; repeat q10-15 min prn (may give via ET tube at 2-3 times the above doses)
Minimum dose 0.1 mg
Maximum dose 0.5 mg

Hyperthermia, tachycardia, urinary retention, constipation, and dry mouth may occur. **Caution** with patients sensitive to sulfate. Breast-feeding: Compatible.

Continued

TABLE H-2
Drug Doses for Neonates—cont'd

Drug	How supplied	Dose and route	Remarks
Aztreonam (Azactam)	Injection: 0.5, 1, 2 gm Contains approximately 780 mg L-Arginine per 1 gm of drug	Neonates (IV/IM): 30 mg/kg/dose: <1.2 kg and 0-4 wk age: q12 hr 1.2-2 kg and 0-7 days: q12 hr 1.2-2 kg and >7 days: q8 hr >2 kg and 0-7 days: q8 hr >2 kg and >7 days: q6 hr	Low cross-allergenicity between aztreonam and other beta-lactams. May cause thrombophlebitis, eosinophilia, and liver enzyme elevation. Good CNS penetration. Adjust dose in renal failure. Breast-feeding: Compatible.
Bacitracin (Ak-Tracin)	Ophthalmic ointment: 1% or 500 U/gm (3.5, 3.75 gm)	*Ophthalmic:* Apply a ¼- to ½-inch ribbon to the conjunctival sac qid	Ophthalmic ointment may cause blurred vision. Rash and allergic reactions may occur. Patients sensitive to neomycin may also be sensitive to bacitracin. Breast-feeding: Safety not established.
Beractant (Pulmonary surfactant, bovine lung surfactant, natural lung surfactant) (Survanta)	Suspension: 25 mg/ml (4, 8 ml)	*Prophylactic therapy:* 4 ml/kg/dose intratracheally as soon as possible; up to four doses may be given at intervals no shorter than q6h during the first 48 hr of life *Rescue therapy:* 4 ml/kg/dose intratracheally, immediately after the diagnosis of RDS; may repeat dose as needed q6hr to maximum of 4 total doses	All doses are administered intratracheally. If the suspension settles during storage, gently swirl the contents—**do not shake.** Each dose is divided into four 1 ml/kg aliquots; administer 1 ml/kg in each of four different positions (slight downward inclination with head turned to the right, head turned to the left; slight upward inclination with head turned to the right, head turned to the left). Transient bradycardia, O_2 desaturation, pallor, vasoconstriction, hypotension, endotracheal tube blockage, hypercarbia, hypercapnea, apnea, and hypertension.

Caffeine citrate	Injection: 20 mg/ml (citrate salt) = 10 mg/ml (caffeine base) (3ml) Oral liquid: 20 mg/ml (citrate salt) = 10 mg/ml (caffeine base)	**Doses based on caffeine citrate salt:** *Neonatal apnea:* Loading dose (IV, PO), 20 mg/kg/dose × 1; maintenance dose (IV, PO), 5-10 mg/kg/dose qd, first dose 24 hr after load	**Therapeutic levels for apnea: 5-25 mg/L.** Cardiovascular, neurologic, or GI toxicities occur when levels are >50 mg/L. **Avoid caffeine benzoate, may cause kernicterus.** Breast-feeding: Compatible.
Calcium carbonate (40% calcium)	Suspension: 400 mg/5 ml, 1000 mg/5 ml, 1250 mg/5 ml; each gm of salt contains 20 mEq = 400 mg of elemental calcium	**Doses based on calcium carbonate salt:** *Neonatal hypocalcemia:* 125-375 mg/kg/24 hr PO ÷ q4-6h **Maximum dose** 2500 mg/24 hr	Administer each dose with meals or with lots of fluid. May cause constipation, hypophosphatemia, hypomagnesemia, and vomiting. May reduce absorption of iron. Some products may contain a trace amount of sodium. Breast-feeding: Safety not established.
Calcium chloride (27% calcium)	Injection: 100 mg/ml 10% (1.36 mEq Ca⁺⁺/ml); each gm of salt contains 13.6 mEq = 270 mg of elemental calcium	**Doses based on calcium chloride salt:** *Maintenance/hypocalcemia:* 200-300 mg/kg/24 hr PO as 2% solution ÷ q6h *For cardiac arrest:* IV, 20 mg/kg/dose (0.2 ml/kg/dose) q10min	May cause GI irritation, phlebitis. Use intravenously with **extreme caution.** Acidifying effect; give only 2-3 days, then change to another Ca⁺⁺ salt. Treat IV infiltrate with hyaluronidase. **Maximum IV administration rates:** IV Push: DO NOT EXCEED 100 mg/min IV Infusion: DO NOT EXCEED 45-90 mg/kg/hr with a maximum concentration of 20 mg/ml. Breast-feeding: Safety not established.

Continued

TABLE H-2
Drug Doses for Neonates—cont'd

Drug	How supplied	Dose and route	Remarks
Calcium glubionate (Neocalglucon) (6.4% calcium)	Syrup: 1.8 gm/ml; each 5 ml contains 5.8 mEq = 115 mg of elemental calcium	**Doses based on calcium glubionate salt:** Neonatal hypocalcemia: 1200 mg/kg/24 hr PO ÷ q4-6h Maintenance: 600-2000 mg/kg/24 hr PO ÷ qid (**maximum dose 9 gm/24 h**)	Administer before feeding for best absorption. Absorption inhibited by phosphate load. High osmotic load of syrup (20% sucrose) may cause diarrhea. Breast-feeding: Safety not established.
Calcium gluconate (9% calcium)	Injection: 100 mg/ml (10%); each gm of salt contains 4.8 mEq = 90 mg of elemental calcium	**Dose based on calcium gluconate salt:** Maintenance/hypocalcemia: IV, 200-800 mg/kg/24 hr ÷ q6h; PO, 400-800 mg/kg/24 hr ÷ q6h For cardiac arrest: IV, 100 mg/kg/dose (= 1 ml/kg/dose) q10min	If given by IV route, administer slowly and watch for bradycardia, hypotension, and extravasation. May produce arrhythmias in digitalized patients. Precipitates with bicarbonates. Tissue necrosis may result from infiltrates. **Do not use scalp vein.** **Maximum IV administration rates:** IV push: DO NOT EXCEED 100 mg/min IV infusion: DO NOT EXCEED 150-300 mg/kg/hr with maximum concentration of 55 mg/ml. Breast-feeding: Safety not established.

Calfactant
(Infasurf)

Intratracheal suspension: 6 ml; each ml contains 35 mg phospholipids and 0.26 mg of surfactant protein B.

Prophylactic therapy: 3 ml/kg/dose intratracheally as soon as possible; up to a total of three doses may be given q12h

Rescue therapy: 3 ml/kg/dose intratracheally immediately after the diagnosis of RDS. May repeat doses as needed q12h to a maximum of three total doses

All doses administered intratracheally. If suspension settles during storage, gently swirl the contents—**do not shake.** Manufacturer recommends administration through a side-port adapter into the endotracheal tube with two attendants (one to instill drug and another to monitor and position patient). Each dose is divided into two 1.5 ml/kg aliquots; give 1.5 ml/kg in each of two different positions (infant positioned to the right or left-side dependent). Administration is made while ventilation is continued over 20-30 breaths for each aliquot, with small bursts timed only during the inspiratory cycles. A pause followed by evaluation of the respiratory status and repositioning should separate the two aliquots. Common adverse effects include cyanosis, airway obstruction, bradycardia, reflux of surfactant into the ET tube, requirement for manual ventilation, and reintubation.

Captopril
(Capoten)

Suspension:* 1 mg/ml
Tablets: 12.5, 25, 50, 100 mg

0.1-0.4 mg/kg/24 hr PO ÷ q6-8h
Maximum: 6 mg/kg/24 hr

Adjust with renal failure. May cause rash, coughing, proteinuria, neutropenia, and hypotension. Known to decrease aldosterone and increase renin production. Breast-feeding: Compatible.

Continued

TABLE H-2
Drug Doses for Neonates—cont'd

Drug	How supplied	Dose and route	Remarks
Cefazolin (Ancef, Kefzol) (first generation)	Injection: 0.25, 0.5, 1, 5, 10 gm (contains 2.1 mEq Na$^+$ per 1 gm of drug)	<7 days (IV or IM): 40 mg/kg/ 24 hr ÷ q12h ≥7 days (IM or IV): ≤2 kg, 40 mg/kg/24 hr ÷ q12h > 2 kg, 60 mg/kg/24 hr ÷ q8h	Use caution in penicillin-allergic patients and reduce dose in renal failure. May cause phlebitis, leukopenia, thrombocytopenia, elevated liver enzymes, false-positive urine reducing substance. Breast-feeding: Compatible.
Cefotaxime (Claforan) (third generation)	Injection: 0.5, 1, 2, 10 gm (contains 2.2 mEq Na$^+$ per 1 gm of drug)	<1 wk (IV or IM): 100 mg/kg/ 24 hr ÷ q12h 1-4 wk (IV or IM): 150 mg/kg/ 24 hr ÷ q8h	Use with **caution** in penicillin-allergic patients and reduce dose in renal failure. Toxicities similar to other cephalosporins: allergy, neutropenia, thrombocytopenia, eosinophilia, positive Coombs' test, elevated BUN, creatinine, and liver enzymes. Breast-feeding: Compatible.
Ceftazidime (Fortaz, Tazidime, Tazicef, Ceptaz [arginine salt]) (third generation)	Injection: 0.5, 1, 2 gm (contains 2.3 mEq Na$^+$ per 1 gm of drug) (Ceptaz contains 349 mg L-arginine per 1 gm of drug)	IM or IV (<2 kg): <7 days, 100 mg/kg/24 hr ÷ q12h ≥7 days, 150 mg/kg/24 hr ÷ q8h IM or IV (≥2 kg): <7 days, 100-150 mg/kg/24 hr ÷ q8-12h ≥7 days, 150 mg/kg/24 hr ÷ q8h	Use with **caution** in penicillin-allergic patients and reduce dose in renal failure. Good Pseudomonas coverage and CSF penetration. Breast-feeding: Compatible.

Ceftizoxime (Cefizox)	Injection: 0.5, 1, 2 gm (contains 2.6 mEq Na^+ per 1 gm drug)	150-200 mg/kg/24hr IV/IM ÷ q6-8 hr	Use with caution in penicillin-allergic patients. May cause transient elevation of liver enzymes and diarrhea. Good CNS penetration. Reduce dose in renal failure. Breast-feeding: Compatible.
Ceftriaxone (Rocephin) (third generation)	Injection: 0.25, 0.5, 1, 2, 10 gm (contains 3.6 mEq Na^+ per 1 gm drug)	IV or IM (<2 kg): 50 mg/kg/dose q24h IV or IM (≥2 kg): <7 days, 50 mg/kg/dose q24h ≥7 days, 75 mg/kg/dose q24h *Uncomplicated gonococcal ophthalmia:* 50 mg/kg × 1 **Maximum dose** 125 mg/dose	Use with caution in penicillin-allergic patients. May cause diarrhea, increased hepatic enzymes, reversible cholelithiasis, sludging in gallbladder. Use with caution in neonates at risk for hyperbilirubinemia. Breast-feeding: Compatible.
Cefuroxime (Zinacef, Kefurox) (second generation)	Injection: 0.75, 1.5, 7.5 gm (contains 2.4 mEq Na^+ per 1 gm drug)	IM or IV: 20-60 mg/kg/24 hr ÷ q12h	Use with caution in penicillin-allergic patients and reduce dose in renal failure. May cause thrombophlebitis at infusion site. Other toxicities are those of other cephalosporins. Not recommended for meningitis. Breast-feeding: Compatible.
Chloral hydrate (Noctec, Aquachloral supprettes)	Syrup: 250 mg/5 ml, 500 mg/5 ml Suppository: 324 mg	PO or PR: *Sedative:* 25-50 mg/kg/24 hr ÷ q6-8h *Hypnotic:* 50 mg/kg as a single dose	Gastric irritation (dilute PO doses); caution with hepatic, renal, cardiac, or pulmonary disease. Caution when using with furosemide and anticoagulants. Accumulation of major metabolites may occur with chronic administration. Breast-feeding: Compatible.

Continued

TABLE H-2
Drug Doses for Neonates—cont'd

Drug	How supplied	Dose and route	Remarks
Chloramphenicol (Chloromycetin)	Injection (as sodium succinate): 1 gm (contains 2.25 mEq Na⁺ per 1 gm drug) Otic solution: 0.5% Ophthalmic ointment: 1% (3.5 gm) Topical cream: 1% (30 gm)	Loading dose (all ages): IV 20 mg/kg Neonates: <2 kg: IV 25 mg/kg/24 hr qd ≥2 kg, <7 days: IV 25 mg/kg/24 hr qd ≥7 days: IV 50 mg/kg/24 hr ÷ q12h **Note:** Initiate maintenance therapy for neonates <7 days old beginning **24 hr after** loading dose	Dose recommendations are only guidelines for therapy; monitoring of blood levels is essential in neonates and infants. Drug is poorly absorbed by IM route. Follow hematologic status for dose-related or idiosyncratic marrow suppression. Gray baby syndrome may be seen with levels >50 mg/L. Concomitant use of rifampin may lower serum levels. Chloramphenicol may increase phenytoin levels. **Therapeutic levels: 15-25 mg/L.** IV route preferred because of the lack of an oral liquid dosage form and wide variations in plasma levels with PO route. Breast-feeding: Unknown with concerns.
Chlorothiazide (Diuril)	Suspension: 250 mg/5 ml (237 ml) or 50* mg/ml Injection: 500 mg (20 ml) (contains 5 mEq Na⁺ per 1 gm of drug)	PO/IV: 10-20 mg/kg/dose q12h	Use with caution in liver and severe renal disease. May cause hyperbilirubinemia, hypokalemia, alkalosis, hyperglycemia, hyperuricemia, hypomagnesemia, blood dyscrasias, pancreatitis. Avoid IM administration. Breast-feeding: Compatible.
Cimetidine (Tagamet)	Syrup: 300 mg/5 ml: contains 2.8% alcohol Injection: 150 mg/ml	5-20 mg/kg/24hr IM/PO/IV ÷ q6-12h	May cause diarrhea, rash, and elevated liver function tests. Inhibits cytochrome P450 oxidative system to increase serum levels of theophylline, phenytoin, lidocaine, and diazepam. Reduce dose in renal failure. Breast-feeding: Compatible.

Cisapride
(Propulsid)

Suspension: 1 mg/ml
(450 ml)

Gastroesophageal reflux: 0.2-0.3
mg/kg/dose PO tid-qid

Contraindicated in patients taking medications that
inhibit cytochrome p-450 3A4 and electrolyte disorders; potentially resulting in fatal cardiac arrhythmias. These medications include ketoconazole,
erythromycin, and clarithromycin. Do not use in
patients with cardiac disease (especially, torsades
de pointes, long QT syndrome, sinus node dysfunction and second or third degree atrioventricular
block). Use in premature infants is controversial
because of concerns of immature drug metabolism.
A 12-lead ECG should be obtained before therapy
is initiated. Drug should not be used if QT_c value is
>450 milliseconds. May cause diarrhea and rhinitis.
Breast-feeding: Compatible.

**Citrate: Sodium citrate
and citric acid**
(Bicitra, Cytra-2)

Each ml contains 1 mEq
Na^+ and 1 mEq HCO_3^-
equivalent

Dosing based on citrate: PO:
3-5 mEq/kg/24 hr ÷ tid-qid

Adjust dose to maintain urine pH. 1 mEq of citrate is
equivalent to 1 mEq HCO_3^- provided patient has
normal liver function. Bicitra is preferred over
Polycitra (1 ml = 1 mEq Na and K and 2 mEq citrate) and Polycitra-K (1 ml = 2 mEq K and citrate)
because of hidden amounts of potassium. Breast-
feeding: Safety not established.

Continued

TABLE H-2
Drug Doses for Neonates—cont'd

Drug	How supplied	Dose and route	Remarks
Clindamycin (Cleocin)	Oral liquid (as palmitate): 75 mg/5 ml (100 ml) Injection: 150 mg/ml (contains 9.45 mg/ml benzyl alcohol)	<2 kg (IV, IM): <7 days: 10 mg/kg/24 hr ÷ q12h ≥7 days: 15 mg/kg/24 hr ÷ q8h ≥2 kg (IV, IM): <7 days, 15 mg/kg/24 hr ÷ q8h; ≥7days, 20 mg/kg/24 hr ÷ q6h Full term (IV, IM): 20-30 mg/kg/24 hr ÷ q6h	Not indicated in meningitis. Use with caution in hepatic insufficiency. Pseudomembranous colitis may occur up to several weeks after cessation of therapy but generally is uncommon in pediatric patients. May cause diarrhea, rash, Stevens-Johnson syndrome, granulocytopenia, thrombocytopenia, or sterile abscess at injection site. Breast-feeding: Compatible.
Clotrimazole (Lotrimin, Mycelex)	Cream: 1%, (15, 30, 45, 90 gm) Topical Solution: 1% (10, 30 ml) Lotion: 1% (30 ml)	Topical: Apply to affected skin area bid	May cause erythema, blistering, or urticaria where applied. Avoid contact with eyes. Breast-feeding: Safety not established.

Colfosceril palmitate (pulmonary surfactant, dipalmitoylphosphatidylcholine [DPPC], synthetic lung surfactant) (Exosurf)	Intratracheal suspension: 108 mg (10 ml)	*Prophylactic therapy:* 5 ml/kg intratracheally as soon as possible; two additional doses (12 and 24 hr) after the initial dose for infants remaining on ventilators *Rescue therapy:* 5 ml/kg intratracheally as soon as the diagnosis of RDS is made; a second 5 ml/kg-dose should be administered 12 hr later as two 2.5-ml/kg aliquots	**For intratracheal use only.** Pulmonary hemorrhage, apnea, mucous plugging, and decrease in transcutaneous O_2 of >20% may occur. Drug must be reconstituted with preservative-free sterile water for injection. Suction infant before administration. Monitor O_2 saturation, ECG, and blood pressure during dose administration, and arterial blood gases for post-dose hyperoxia and hypocarbia after administration.
Cortisone			See hydrocortisone, dexamethasone, methylprednisolone, prednisone.
Cyclopentolate (Cyclogel)	Ophthalmic solution: 0.5%, 1%, 2% (2, 5, 15 ml)	1 drop of 0.5% solution in each eyes 5-10 min before examination; apply pressure over nasolacrimal sac for at least 2 min to minimize absorption	Do not use in narrow-angle glaucoma. Onset of action: 15-60 min. May cause burning sensation, tachycardia, loss of visual accommodation. Breast-feeding: Safety not established.

Continued

TABLE H-2
Drug Doses for Neonates—cont'd

Drug	How supplied	Dose and route	Remarks
Dexamethasone (Decadron, Hexadrol)	Elixir: 0.5 mg/5 ml (100 ml) (some preparations contain 5% alcohol) Oral solution: 0.1, 1 mg/ml (30 ml) (some preparations contain 30% alcohol) Injection: 4, 10, 20, 24 mg/ml	*Bronchopulmonary dysplasia:* PO or IV 0.25 mg/kg/dose q12h for 3-7 days, then taper slowly; or 42-day regimen: 0.5 mg/kg/24 hr × 3 days, 0.3 mg/kg/24 hr × 3 days, decrease by 10% every 3 days until 0.1 mg/kg/24 hr (day 34), then 0.1 mg/kg/24 hr × 3 days followed by 0.1 mg/kg/24 hr qod × 7 days	See hydrocortisone. 42-day regimen based on Cummings et al: *N Engl J Med* 320:1505, 1989. Dexamethasone acetate salt for injection is used in IM in adults. Breast-feeding: Safety not established.
Diazepam (Valium)	Oral solution: 1, 5 mg/ml Injection: 5 mg/ml contains 40% propylene glycol, 10% alcohol, and 1.5% benzyl alcohol, Emulsified injections (Diazac, Diazemuls): 5 mg/ml	PO, IV, IM: *Sedative:* 0.02-0.3 mg/kg/dose q6-8h *Seizure:* 0.3-0.75 mg/kg/dose slow IV push	Diluted injection may precipitate. IM absorption is poor. Respiratory depression and hypotension may occur. *IV administration rate:* No faster than 2 mg/min. Currently, no neonatal dosing guidelines available for emulsified injection product. Breast-feeding: Unknown with concerns.

Diazoxide
(Hyperstat,
Proglycem)

Suspension: 50 mg/ml
(30 ml); contains 7.25%
alcohol

Hyperinsulinemic hypoglycemia:
8-15 mg/kg/24 hr PO ÷
q8-12h

Hypoglycemia should be treated initially with IV glucose; diazoxide should be used only if refractory to
glucose infusion. May cause sodium and fluid retention, rash, hyperuricemia, and arrhythmias.
Hyperglycemic effect with PO administration occurs
within 1 hr with a duration of 8 hr. Breast-feeding:
Safety not established.

Didanosine
(ddI, Videx)

Oral pediatric powder (for
10 mg/ml solution); 2,
4 gm

Neonates and infants
<3 months: 100 mg/m²/24 hr
PO ÷ q12h

May cause diarrhea, abdominal pain, peripheral neuropathy (dose related), electrolyte abnormalities,
hyperuricemia, increased liver enzymes, rash, and
pancreatitis. Administer all doses on an empty
stomach. Impairs absorption of drugs requiring an
acidic environment (e.g., ketoconazole). Breast-
feeding: Unknown with concerns.

Continued

TABLE H-2
Drug Doses for Neonates—cont'd

Drug	How supplied	Dose and route	Remarks
Digoxin (Lanoxin)	Pediatric injection: 100 µg/ml (1 ml) Injection: 250 µg/ml (2 ml) (both injection products may contain propylene glycol and alcohol) Elixir: 50 µg/ml (60 ml); (may contain 10% alcohol)	Total digitalizing dose, PO: Preterm: 10 µg/kg × 1 followed by 5 µg/kg q8-18h × 2 Term: 15 µg/kg q8-18h × 1, followed by 7.5 µg/kg q8-18h × 2; IV preterm:7.5 µg/kg × 1, followed by 3.75 µg/kg q8-18h × 1 Term: 10 µg/kg × 1, followed by 5 µg/kg q8-18h × 2 Daily maintenance doses (begin 12 hours after last digitalizing dose), PO: Preterm: 5 µg/kg/24 hr divided bid Term: 8-10 µg/kg/24 hr divided bid IV: Preterm: 3-4 µg/kg/24 hr divided bid; Term: 6-8 µg/kg/24 hr divided bid	*IV route for acute digitalization:* administer IV over 5-10 min. **NOTE:** Two different IV strengths. Adverse effects include arrhythmias, bradycardia, nausea, and vomiting. Should not be given in conjunction with calcium because this may potentiate bradycardia. Therapeutic levels are generally 0.5-2 ng/ml. However, neonates may require higher levels because of the serum assay's inability to differentiate maternal digoxin-like substances. Antiarrhythmic doses may be higher than these (for CHF). IV dose is about 75% of PO dose. Digoxin toxicity may occur when taking amphotericin B (because of hypokalemia). **Antidote:** Digoxin Immune Fab. Breast-feeding: Compatible.

Digoxin immune FAB (Ovine) (Digibind)	Injection: 38 mg/vial	First, determine total body digoxin load (TBL): TBL (mg) = serum digoxin level (ng/ml) × 5.6 × wt (kg) ÷ 1000, or TBL (mg) = mg digoxin ingested × 0.8 Then calculate digoxin immune Fab dose Dose in number of digoxin immune Fab vials: # vials = TBL ÷ 0.5 Infuse IV over 15-30 min (through 0.22 micron filter)	Contraindicated if hypersensitivity to sheep products, or if renal or cardiac failure. May cause severe hypokalemia, decreased cardiac output, rash, edema. Breast-feeding: Safety not established.
Dihydrotachysterol (DHT, Hytakerol, DHT Intensol)	Solution: 0.2 mg/ml (20 ml) (20% alcohol) Solution (in oil): 0.25 mg/ml (15 ml) 1 mg = 120,000 IU of vitamin D_2	*Hypoparathyroidism:* PO: 0.05-0.1 mg/dose qd	Monitor serum Ca^{++} and PO_4. Toxicities include hypercalcemia and hypervitaminosis D. More potent than vitamin D_2, but more rapidly inactivated (half-life is hours vs weeks). Titrate dose with patient response. Oral Ca^{++} supplementation may be required. Activated by 25-hydroxylation in liver, does not require 1-hydroxylation in kidney. Breast-feeding: Safety not established.

Continued

TABLE H-2
Drug Doses for Neonates—cont'd

Drug	How supplied	Dose and route	Remarks
Diphenhydramine (Benadryl)	Elixir/syrup: 12.5 mg/5 ml (120 ml) (elixir may contain 14% alcohol and syrup may contain 5% alcohol) Liquid: 6.25 mg/5ml Injection: 10, 50 mg/ml	PO or IV: 5 mg/kg/24 hr ÷ q6h *For anaphylaxis:* 1-2 mg/kg IV slowly	Sedation, hypotension, paradoxic excitement, nausea, vomiting, dry mucous membranes may occur. Breast-feeding: Safety not established.
Dobutamine (Dobutrex)	Injection: 12.5 mg/ml (contains sulfites)	IV: 2.5-15 µg/kg/min **Maximum recommended dose** 40 µg/kg/min To prepare infusion: 6 × wt (kg) × desired dose (µg/kg/min) ÷ IV infusion rate (ml/hr) = mg of drug to be added to 100 ml compatible IV fluid	Monitor blood pressure and vital signs. Contraindicated in IHSS. Tachycardia, arrhythmias (PVCs), and hypertension may occasionally occur (especially at higher infusion rates). Correct hypovolemic states before use. **Avoid extravasation (phentolamine is the antidote).** Breast-feeding: Safety not established.

Dopamine
(Intropin)

Injection: 40, 80, 160 mg/ml

Low-dose IV: 2-5 µg/kg/min increases renal blood flow with minimal effect on heart rate and cardiac output

Intermediate-dose IV:
5-15 µg/kg/min increases renal blood flow, heart rate, cardiac contractility, cardiac output

High-dose IV: >20 µg/kg/min alpha-adrenergic effects prominent; decreases renal perfusion

Maximum recommended dose 20-50 µg/kg/min

To prepare infusion: Same as for dobutamine

Extravasation may lead to necrosis (phentolamine is the antidote). High dose may constrict renal arteries. Tachyarrhythmias, ectopic beats, hypertension, vasoconstriction, and vomiting may occur. Do not use in pheochromocytoma, tachyarrhythmias, or hypovolemia. Breast-feeding: Safety not established.

Doxapram
(Dopram)

Injection: 20 mg/ml (20 ml) (contains 0.9% benzyl alcohol)

Methylxanthine refractory neonatal apnea: Load with 2.5-3 mg/kg over 15-30 min followed by a continuous infusion of 1 mg/kg/hr titrated to the lowest responsive dose

Maximum dose 2.5 mg/kg/hr

Hypertension occurs with higher doses (> 1.5 mg/kg/hr). May also cause tachycardia, arrhythmias, seizures, hyperreflexia, hyponatremia, abdominal distention, and sweating. Avoid extravasation. Breast-feeding: Safety not established.

Continued

TABLE H-2
Drug Doses for Neonates—cont'd

Drug	How supplied	Dose and route	Remarks
EMLA (eutectic mixture of lidocaine and prilocaine)	Cream: Lidocaine 2.5% + procaine 2.5%; 5-gm kit (with dressings); 30-gm tube Topical anesthetic disc: Lidocaine 2.5% + prilocaine 2.5%; 1 gm (box of 2s or 10s)	*Circumcision:* 1gm/dose × 1. Apply one third of dose to lower abdomen, then extend penis upward and gently press against abdomen. Apply remainder of dose to Tegaderm dressing and place over the penis. Tape dressing over abdomen so the cream surrounds the penis. Leave in place for 60-80 minutes, remove dressing and wipe-off cream. (Based on Taddio, et al: *N Eng J Med* 336:1197, 1997.)	Use with caution in patients with G6PD deficiency and in patients with renal and hepatic impairment. Prilocaine has been associated with methemoglobinemia. Breast-feeding: Safety not established.
Enalaprilat (*Vasotec* IV)	Injection: 1.25 mg/ml (contains 0.9% benzyl alcohol)	IV: 5-10 µg/kg/dose over 5 min q8-24h (intervals determined by blood pressure measurements)	Enalapril is its oral dosage form and is a pro-drug that must be converted to the active Enalaprilat. Side effects include nausea, coughing, diarrhea, headache, hypotension, and hypersensitivity. Reduce dosage in patients with renal impairment. Breast-feeding: Compatible.

Epinephrine
(Adrenaline)

Injection: 1:1000 (aqueous)
as 1 mg/ml (1, 30 ml)
1:10,000 (aqueous) prefilled
syringes as 0.1 mg/ml
(3, 10 ml)

Resuscitation (IV, ET, IM):
1:10,000, 0.1-0.3 ml/kg
(0.01-0.03 mg/kg) q3-5 min
Hypotension (IV drip):
0.1-1 µg/kg/min
To prepare infusion: Same as for
dobutamine

May produce tachycardia, arrhythmias, hypertension,
vomiting. Necrosis may occur at site of repeated
local injections. ET doses should be diluted with
normal saline to a total volume of 1-2 ml before
administration. Follow with several positive pressure
ventilations. Breast-feeding: Safety not established.

Ergocalciferol
(Calciferol, Drisdol,
Vitamin D$_2$)

Oral solution: 8000 IU/ml
(60 ml)
Injection: 500,000 IU/ml
40 IU = 1 µg

Dietary supplementation (PO):
400 IU qd

Monitor serum Ca^{++}, PO$_4$, and alkaline phosphate.
Serum Ca^{++} and PO$_4$ product should be <70
mg/dl. Vitamin D$_2$ must be activated by hydroxyla-
tion in liver and kidney. Breast-feeding: Safety not
established.

Erythromycin
(Erythrocin,
Pediamycin,
and others)

Ophthalmic ointment: 0.5%
(3.5, 3.75 gm)
Suspension: Erythromycin
estolate, 100 mg/ml
(10-ml drops), 125 mg/
5 ml, 250 mg/5 ml;
erythromycin succinate,
100 mg/2.5 ml (50-ml
drops), 200 mg/5 ml,
400 mg/5 ml

Ophthalmic: Apply ½-inch ribbon
to affected eye bid-qid
PO: Weight <2000 gm, 0-7
days: 20 mg/kg/24 hr ÷ q12h
>7 days: 30 mg/kg/24 hr ÷
q8h
Weight ≥2000 gm, 0-7 days:
20 mg/kg/24 hr ÷ q12h
>7 days: 40 mg/kg/24 hr ÷
q8h

Candidiasis (oral, perianal), stomatitis, irritability
caused by esophageal irritation, and epigastric discomfort may occur. Allergic reaction is rare. To prevent cross-infection and ensure sterility, never share
the use of an ophthalmic ointment tube among
multiple patients (all tubes must be individualized).
Interacts with theophylline (aminophylline) by
increasing theophylline levels. Breast-feeding:
Compatible.

Continued

TABLE H-2
Drug Doses for Neonates—cont'd

Drug	How supplied	Dose and route	Remarks
Erythropoietin (Epoetin Alfa, Epogen, Procrit)	Injection: 2,000, 3,000, 4000, 10,000, 20,000 U/ml; multidose vials contain 1% benzyl alcohol	*Anemia of prematurity:* 25-100 U/kg/dose SC 3 × per week; alternatively, 200 U/kg/dose IV/SC qd-qod for 2-6 wk may be used	Evaluate serum iron, ferritin, TIBC before therapy. Iron supplementation recommended during therapy unless iron stores are already in excess. Monitor Hct, blood pressure, clotting times, platelets, BUN, serum creatinine. Peak effect in 2-3 weeks. Reduce dose when target Hct is reached, or when Hct increases >4 points in any 2-week period. May cause hypertension, seizures, hypersensitivity reactions, edema. Breast-feeding: Safety not established.
Fentanyl (Sublimaze)	Injection: 50 µg/ml	IM or IV: 1-2 µg/kg/dose q30-60min prn; may be used as a continuous IV infusion; start with 1 µg/kg/hr, then titrate to effect (usual range 1-3 µg/kg/hr)	Onset of action 1-2 min with a peak action of about 10 min. As with other opiates, respiratory depression occurs and may persist beyond the period of analgesia. Give IV dose over 3-5 min; rapid infusion may cause respiratory depression via severe muscular rigidity. Naloxone is the antagonist. Reduce dose in renal impairment. Breast-feeding: Compatible.
Ferrous gluconate (Fergon, Ferralet, Simron, iron preparations)	Ferrous gluconate (12% elemental Fe); elixir, 300 mg (34 mg Fe)/5 ml (7% alcohol)	As for ferrous sulfate	See ferrous sulfate. Breast-feeding: Safety not established.

Ferrous sulfate (Feosol, Fer-In-Sol, iron preparations, others)	Ferrous sulfate (20% elemental Fe) Drops (Fer-In-Sol): 75 mg (15 mg Fe)/0.6 ml (50 ml) Syrup (Fer-In-Sol): 90 mg (18 mg Fe)/ 5 ml Elixir (Feosol): 220 mg (44 mg Fe)/5 ml (5% alcohol)	*Prophylaxis:* 1-2 mg elemental Fe/kg/24 hr ÷ qd-bid PO *Iron deficiency anemia:* 3-6 mg elemental Fe/kg/24 hr ÷ qd-bid PO	Iron preparations are variably absorbed. Vitamin C enhances absorption, whereas antacids decrease absorption. May cause nausea, constipation, black tarry stool, lethargy, hypotension, and GI upset. Breast-feeding: Safety not established.
Flucytosine (Ancobon, 5-FC, 5-Fluorocytosine)	Oral liquid:* 10 mg/ml	PO: 20-40 mg/kg/dose q6h	Common side effects include nausea, vomiting, diarrhea, rash, CNS disturbance, anemia, leukopenia, and thrombocytopenia. Monitor CBC, BUN, serum creatinine, alkaline phosphatase, AST, and ALT. Reduce dose in renal impairment. **Therapeutic levels: 25-100 mg/L.** Breast-feeding: Unknown with concerns.
Folic acid (Folvite and others)	Oral solution:* 1 mg/ml Injection: 5 mg/ml; contains 1.5% benzyl alcohol	*Folic acid deficiency:* 15 µg/kg/dose qd PO, IM, IV, SC **Maximum dose** 50 µg/24 hr *RDA:* Neonates-6 mo, 25-35 µg qd PO, IM, IV, SC	Normal levels: Serum >3 ng/ml, RBC 153-605 ng/ml. May mask hematologic effects of vitamin B_{12} deficiency but not prevent progression of neurologic abnormalities. Breast-feeding: Compatible.

Continued

TABLE H-2
Drug Doses for Neonates—cont'd

Drug	How supplied	Dose and route	Remarks
Fosphenytoin (Cerebyx)	Injection: 50 mg phenytoin equivalent (PE) (75 mg fosphenytoin)/1 ml (2, 10 ml; each 1 mg PE provides 0.0037 mmol of phosphate)	**All doses are expressed as phenytoin sodium equivalents (PE):** See phenytoin and use the conversion of 1 mg phenytoin = 1 mg PE	**All doses should be prescribed and dispensed in terms of mg phenytoin sodium equivalents (PE) to avoid medication errors.** Fosphenytoin is a prodrug of phenytoin and needs to be metabolized to the active phenytoin. Pharmacokinetics and safety in pediatrics have not been fully established. Use with **caution** in patients with porphyria. Consider amounts of formaldehyde (metabolic by-product in trace amounts) and phosphates delivered by fosphenytoin. May cause hypokalemia (with rapid IV administration), dizziness, ataxia, rash, exfoliative dermatitis, nystagmus, diplopia, and tinnitus. Avoid abrupt withdrawal of drug. Monitor blood pressure and ECG during IV loading dose administration. Maximum IV infusion rate: 3 mg PE/kg/min. IM administration may be given via one or two separate sites. **Therapeutic levels:** 10-20 mg/L (free and bound phenytoin) OR 1-2 mg/L (free only). Recommended peak serum sampling times in adults (may be different for newborns): 4 hours after IM dose or 2 hours after IV dose. See phenytoin for drug interactions. Breast-feeding: Compatible.

Furosemide (Lasix and others)	Injection: 10 mg/ml Oral liquid: 10 mg/ml, 8 mg/ml (60 ml)	IM, IV: 0.5-2 mg/kg/dose q12-24h **IV maximum** 2 mg/kg/dose PO: 1-4 mg/kg/dose q12-24h, **maximum** 6 mg/kg/dose	Half-life is prolonged in premature infants. Can cause alkalosis, hypocalcemia, hypochloremia, hyponatremia, hypokalemia, and increased calcium excretion. Potential ototoxicity with aminoglycosides. Breast-feeding: Safety not established.
Gentamicin (Garamycin and others)	Injection: 10, 40 mg/ml Ophthalmic ointment: 0.3% (3.5 gm) Ophthalmic drops: 0.3% (5 ml) Topical ointment: 0.1% (15 gm) Topical cream: 0.1% (15 gm)	Parenteral (IM or IV): ≤29 wk PCA or significant asphyxia, 0-28 days: 2.5 mg/kg/dose q24h >28 days: 3 mg/kg/dose q24h 30-36 wk PCA, 0-14 days: 3 mg/kg/dose q24h >14 days: 2.5 mg/kg/dose q12h >37 wk PCA, 0-7 days: 2.5 mg/kg/dose q12h >7 days: 2.5 mg/kg/dose q8h	Monitor levels (peak and trough). Monitor renal status; may cause proximal tubule dysfunction. Watch for ototoxicity. **Therapeutic levels: 5-10 mg/L (peak); <2 mg/L (trough).** Peak levels of 8-10 mg/L have been recommended in pulmonary infections, neutropenia, and sepsis. Recommended serum sampling time at steady-state: trough within 30 minutes before the third consecutive dose and peak 30-60 minutes after the third dose. Eliminated more quickly in patients with cystic fibrosis, burns, or neutropenia. Neonatal doses are the same for gentamicin and tobramycin, but amikacin dose is about three times higher. Avoid physical contact with penicillin and cephalosporins (may blunt serum concentration). Breast-feeding: Safety not established.
Glucagon HCl (Glucagon)	Injection: 1, 10 mg/vial (1 U = 1 mg)	*For hypoglycemia:* <10 kg (IM, SC, IV), 0.025-0.3 mg/kg up to 1 mg q30min	Onset of action: 15-30 min. Noted to have cardiostimulatory effect at high doses even in the presence of beta-blockade. Do **not** delay starting glucose infusion while awaiting effect of glucagon. May cause nausea, vomiting, and tachycardia. Breast-feeding: Safety not established.

Continued

TABLE H-2
Drug Doses for Neonates

Drug	How supplied	Dose and route	Remarks
Heparin sodium	Injection: 10, 100, 1000, 2000, 2500, 5000, 7500, 10,000, 15,000, 20,000, 40,000 U/ml; 120 U = approximately 1 mg	Initial: IV 50 U/kg bolus Maintenance IV: 10-25 U/kg/hr as constant infusion, or 50-100 U/kg/dose q4h Heparin flush: Peripheral IV, 1-2 ml of 10 U/ml solution q4h; central lines, 2-3 ml of 100 U/ml solution q24h	Adjust dose to give clotting time of 20-30 min or PTT of 1.5-2.5 times control value before dose. PTT is best measured 6-8 hr after initiation or change in dose. **Toxicities:** bleeding, allergy, alopecia, and thrombocytopenia. **Antidote:** Protamine sulfate (1 mg per 100 U heparin in previous 4 hr). **NOTE:** Central line heparin flush dosage may be heparinizing; if so, use less heparin. A preservative-free flush product is preferred. Breast-feeding: Compatible.
Hepatitis B immune globulin (Bayhep-B, HBIG, Hep-B-Gammagee, HyperHep, Nabi-HB)	Injection: 1, 4, 5 ml Injection (prefilled syringe): 0.5 ml Some preparations may contain thimerosal.	*Positive maternal HBsAg:* IM, 0.5 ml within 12 hours after birth *Percutaneous inoculation:* IM, 0.06 ml/kg/dose × 1 within 24 hours of exposure	Local pain at injection site, urticaria, angioedema. Anaphylaxis is rare. Breast-feeding: Safety not established.

Hepatitis B vaccine (Recombivax HB, Engerix-B)	Injection: Engerix-B, 20 µg/ml (0.5-, 1-, 10-ml vials and 0.5-, 1-ml pre-filled syringes); Recombivax HB, 10 µg/ml (0.5-, 1-, 3-ml vials and 0.5-, 1-ml pre-filled syringes); 40 µg/ml (1-ml vials) Some preparations may contain thimerosal.	*Positive maternal HBsAg:* IM, Engerix-B 10 µg (0.5 ml) or Recombivax HB 5 µg (0.5 ml) at birth (within 12 hours), 1 month, and 6 months of age (total 3 doses) **NOTE:** HBIG × 1 should also be administered at birth *Negative maternal HBsAg:* IM, Engerix-B 10 µg (0.5 ml) or Recombivax HB 2.5 µg (0.25 ml) or 0.5 ml of Recombivax HB pediatric formulation (2.5 µg/0.5 ml) at 0-2 days, 1-2 mo after first dose, and 6-18 mo of age (total three doses)	Local reactions at the injection site, allergic reactions, or neuropathic effects may occur. **NOTE:** Recombivax HB is available in two different concentrations (10 and 40 µg/ml). Breast-feeding: Safety not established.
Hyaluronidase (Wydase)	Injection: 150 U/ml Powder for injection: 150, 1500 U (Pharmacy can make a 15 U/ml dilution)	*Extravasation:* Dilute drug to 15 U/ml; give 1 ml (15 U) by injecting five separate injections of 0.2 ml (3 U) at borders of extravasation site SC or ID using 25- or 26- gauge needle	**Contraindicated** in dopamine and alpha-agonist extravasation. May cause urticaria. Administer as early as possible (minutes to 1 hour) after IV extravasation.

Continued

TABLE H-2
Drug Doses for Neonates—cont'd

Drug	How supplied	Dose and route	Remarks
Hydralazine (Apresoline)	Oral liquid:* 1.25, 2, 4, mg/ml Injection: 20 mg/ml	PO: 0.25-1 mg/kg/dose q6-8h IM/IV: 0.15 mg/kg/dose q6h; increase as needed in 0.1 mg/kg increments up to a **maximum** of 2 mg/kg/dose q6h	Use with caution in severe renal disease (reduce dose in renal impairment) and cardiac disease. May cause lupuslike syndrome (reversible), cardiovascular, GI, neurologic, hematologic, and dermatologic reactions. May cause reflex tachycardia. Breast-feeding: Compatible.
Hydrochlorothiazide (Esidrix, Hydro-T, Thiuretic, Hydrodiuril)	Oral solution: 50 mg/5 ml	PO: 1-2 mg/kg/dose q12h	See chlorothiazide. May cause fluid and electrolyte imbalances, hyperuricemia. Administration with feeding seems to improve absorption. Do not use in patients with renal or hepatic failure. Breast-feeding: Compatible.
Hydrocortisone (Solu-cortef)	Oral suspension (cypionate salt): 10 mg/5 ml (120 ml) Injection (sodium succinate): 100, 250, 500, 1000 mg Injection (sodium phosphate): 50 mg/ml	*Adrenal crisis* (IM, IV): 1-2 mg/kg dose bolus, followed by 25-150 mg/24 hr ÷ q6-8hr *Physiologic replacement* (PO): 15-25 mg/m²/24 hr or 1 mg/kg/24 hr ÷ tid *Congenital adrenal hyperplasia (maintenance therapy):* 15-24 mg/m²/24hr PO ÷ tid	Treatment of more than 7-10 days requires gradual dosage reduction to avoid adrenal insufficiency, immunosuppression, hyperglycemia, growth delay, leukocytosis, and gastric irritation. Breast-feeding: Safety not established.

Drug		Dosage
Imipenem-Cilastatin (Primaxin)	Injection: 250, 500, 750 mg; contains 3.2 mEq Na per 1 gm drug	<1 wk: 40-50 mg/kg/24 hr IV ÷ q12h 1- 4 wk: 60-75 mg/kg/24 hr IV ÷ q8h 4 wk-3 mo: 100 mg/kg/24 hr IV ÷ q6h	Administer IV over 30-60 minutes. May cause pruritus, GI symptoms, seizures, hypotension, elevated LFTs, blood dyscrasias, and penicillin allergy. Reduce dose in renal impairment. Breast-feeding: Safety not established.
Immune globulin	Gammar-IM: 165 ± 15 mg/ml IM Gamastan: 165 ± 5 mg/ml IM Gammagard, Iveegam, Sandoglobulin, Polygam, Venoglobulin-1: 0.5, 1, 2.5, 5, 6, 10 gm per vial IV Gamimune-N: 50 mg/ml IV	*Primary immunodeficiency:* 300-400 mg/kg/dose IV every month or more frequently *Idiopathic thrombocytopenic purpura:* 1 gm/kg/dose IV qd for 1-2 days IV administration guidelines vary among products; check respective package inserts for initial and **maximum** infusion rates	May cause tenderness, erythema, and induration at injection site. Rare hypersensitivity reaction, especially when given rapidly. Gamimune-N contains maltose and may cause an osmotic diuresis. **Contraindicated** in IgA deficiency except Gammagard or Polygam. **Note:** Gamastan and Gammar are IM preparations; Gammagard, Iveegam, Sandoglobulin, Polygam, Venoglobulin-1, and Gamimune-N are IV preparations. Breast-feeding: Safety not established.

Continued

TABLE H-2
Drug Doses for Neonates—cont'd

Drug	How supplied	Dose and route	Remarks
Indomethacin (Indocin)	Injection: 1 mg	*Closure of ductus arteriosus:* Infuse intravenously over 20-30 min Dose (mg/kg, q12-24h) | Age	#1	#2	#3 | |-----|----|----|----| | <48hr | 0.2 | 0.1 | 0.1 | | 2-7 | 0.2 | 0.2 | 0.2 | | >7 | 0.2 | 0.25 | 0.25 | Infant <1500 gm 0.1-0.2 mg/kg q24h may be given for an additional 3-5 days	Maintenance dose regimens have been recommended to improve overall efficacy of PDA closure. In neonates, monitor renal and hepatic function before and during use. **Contraindicated** in neonates with BUN ≥30 mg/dl, creatinine ≥1.8 ml/dl, active bleeding, coagulation defects, and necrotizing enterocolitis. Keep urine output >0.6 ml/kg/hr. IV is the preferred route of administration for treatment of PDA. Reductions in cerebral blood flow have been associated with rapid infusions (<5 min). May decrease platelet aggregation and cause GI distress (ulcer, nausea, diarrhea), headache, and blood dyscrasias. Breast-feeding: Compatible.
Insulin (regular)	Injection: Many preparations at concentrations of 40, 100, 500 U/ml	*Hyperglycemia:* IV infusion, 0.01-0.1 U/kg/hr; SC (intermittent doses), 0.1-0.2 U/kg/dose q6-12h	Only regular insulin for injection may be administered intravenously. For hyperkalemia, administer glucose 0.5 gm/kg with 0.3 U insulin/per gm of glucose over 2 hr. Lower dosage may be required for patients in renal compromise. Breast-feeding: Compatible.

Isoniazid
(INH, Nydrazid,
Laniazid)

Syrup: 50 mg/5 ml
Injection: 100 mg/ml

Tuberculosis (prophylaxis): PO,
10 mg/kg/24 hr qd or 20-40
mg/kg/dose PO twice weekly
(after 1 mo of daily therapy)
for total of 12 mo

Tuberculosis (treatment): PO,
10-15 mg/kg/24 hr qd or 20-
30 mg/kg dose twice weekly
(after 1 month of daily therapy)
for 9 months with rifampin

Should not be used alone for treatment. Peripheral
neuropathy, optic neuritis, seizures, encephalopathy,
psychosis, and hepatic side effects may occur with
higher doses and in combination with rifampin.
Follow LFTs monthly. Diarrhea has been associated
with use of syrup dosage form. Supplemental pyridoxine (1-2 mg/kg/24 hr) is recommended. Inhibits
hepatic microsomal enzymes to increase serum levels of diazepam, phenytoin. May be given IM when
oral therapy is not possible. Breast-feeding:
Compatible.

Isoproterenol
(Isuprel)

Injection: 200 µg/ml (1,
5 ml)

Initial: 0.05-0.1 µg/kg/min;
increase by 0.1 µg/kg/min
q5-10min until desired effect
or when heart rate >180-200
beats/min

Maximum dose 2 µg/kg/min
Prepare infusion as for dobutamine

Use with care in CHF, ischemia, or aortic stenosis.
May precipitate arrhythmias when used in combination with epinephrine. Patients should be monitored
for arrhythmias, hypertension, and myocardial
ischemia. Tachycardia, nervousness, restlessness,
flushing of the face or skin, nausea, vomiting, and
hypoglycemia may occur. Breast-feeding: Safety
not established.

Lamivudine
(3TC, Epivir)

Oral solution: 10 mg/ml
(**Note:** Epivir-HBV is
another oral liquid dosage
form indicated for hepatitis B and comes in a
5-mg/ml concentration)

Neonates: 2 mg/kg/dose PO bid

May be administered with food. May cause fatigue,
nausea, diarrhea, skin rash, pancreatitis, and
abdominal pain. Concomitant use with co-trimoxa-
zole may result in the increase of lamivudine levels.
Adjust dose in renal impairment. Breast-feeding:
Unknown with concerns.

Continued

TABLE H-2
Drug Doses for Neonates—cont'd

Drug	How supplied	Dose and route	Remarks
Lidocaine (Xylocaine)	Injection: 0.5, 1, 1.5, 2, 4, 10, 20% (1% sol = 10 mg/ml) Some preparations may be combined with epinephrine Prefilled syringes: 10 mg/ml (1%) 100 mg/5ml (2%)	*Antiarrhythmic:* IV, 1 mg/kg infused over 5-10 min; may be repeated q10min five times prn; infusion dose 10-50 μg/kg/min (see dobutamine for infusion preparation)	May cause hypotension, seizures, asystole, and respiratory arrest. Decrease dose in presence of hepatic or renal failure. **Contraindicated** in Stokes-Adams attacks, sinoatrial, atrioventricular, or intraventricular block. **Monitor blood levels (therapeutic range 1.5-5 mg/L). Toxicity may occur at levels >5 mg/L for neonates.** Breast-feeding: Compatible.
Lorazepam (Ativan)	Injection: 2, 4 mg/ml (each contains 2% benzyl alcohol)	IV: 0.05-0.1 mg/kg infused over 2-5 min	Limited data in newborns. May cause respiratory depression, especially in combination with other sedatives. Onset of action: 1-5 minutes. Duration of action: 3-24 hours. Breast-feeding: Unknown with concerns.
Magnesium sulfate (9.9% magnesium)	Injection: 100 mg/ml (0.8 mEq/ml), 125 mg/ml (1 mEq/ml), 250 mg/ml (2 mEq/ml), 500 mg/ml (4 mEq/ml)	*Hypomagnesemia:* IV, 50-100 mg/kg/dose q8-12h as needed **Maximum dose** 1 gm/24 hr	When given IV, beware of hypotension, respiratory depression, and hypermagnesemia. Calcium gluconate (IV) should be available as antidote. Use with caution in patients with renal insufficiency. Breast-feeding: Compatible.

Methylene blue	Injection: 10 mg/ml (1%)	*Methemoglobinemia:* IV, 1-2 mg/kg/dose over 5 min; may be repeated in 1 hr if necessary	Use **cautiously** in patients with G6PD deficiency or renal insufficiency. May cause nausea, vomiting, diaphoresis, and abdominal pain. Causes blue-green discoloration of urine. Breast-feeding: Safety not established.
Methylprednisolone (Medrol, Solu-Medrol, Depo-Medrol)	Injection: sodium succinate (Solu-Medrol) 40, 125, 500, 1000, 2000 mg; dilutions may be required to ensure accuracy of dose delivery; consult pharmacist	*Antiinflammatory/immunosuppressive* (IV, IM): 0.5-1.7 mg/kg/24 hr or 5-25 mg/m²/24 hr ÷ q6-12h	Hydrocortisone preferred for physiologic replacement. Less mineralocorticoid effect than hydrocortisone. Intravenous product may contain benzyl alcohol. Dose of methylprednisolone: 1/6 dose of cortisone. Acetate salt form of the drug is used for intramuscular, intraarticular, and intralesional injection in adults. Breast-feeding: Safety not established.
Metoclopramide (Reglan)	Syrup: 1 mg/ml Concentrated solution: 10 mg/ml Injection: 5 mg/ml	*Gastroesophageal reflux* (PO, IV): 0.05-0.1 mg/kg/dose tid-qid	May cause extrapyramidal symptoms, especially at higher doses (give diphenhydramine as remedy). Use with caution in patients with history of seizures. Reduce dosage in renal-compromised patients. Breast-feeding: Unknown with concerns.

Continued

TABLE H-2
Drug Doses for Neonates—cont'd

Drug	How supplied	Dose and route	Remarks
Metronidazole (Flagyl)	Suspension:* 100 mg/5 ml or 50 mg/ml Injection: 500 mg or 5 mg/ml ready to use (contains 28 mEq Na per 1 gm of drug)	*Anaerobic infection:* Loading dose (IV) 15 mg/kg; maintenance dose 7.5 mg/kg (initiate one dosing interval after load): <table><tr><td>PCA</td><td>PNA</td><td>Interval (hr)</td></tr><tr><td>≤29</td><td>0-28</td><td>48</td></tr><tr><td>≤29</td><td>>28</td><td>24</td></tr><tr><td>30-36</td><td>0-14</td><td>24</td></tr><tr><td>30-36</td><td>>14</td><td>12</td></tr><tr><td>37-44</td><td>0-7</td><td>24</td></tr><tr><td>37-44</td><td>>7</td><td>12</td></tr><tr><td>≥45</td><td>All</td><td>8</td></tr></table>	Nausea, diarrhea, urticaria, dry mouth, leukopenia, vertigo. Candidiasis may worsen. Potentiates anticoagulants. IV infusion must be given slowly over 1 hr. Initial drug of choice for antibiotic-associated pseudomembranous colitis over oral vancomycin. Adjust dosage for liver and renal compromise. Breast-feeding: Unknown with concerns.
Mezlocillin (Mezlin)	Injection: 1, 2, 3, 4 gm (contains 1.85 mEq sodium per 1 gm of drug)	IV: 75 mg/kg/dose <table><tr><td>PNA</td><td>Weight (kg)</td><td>Interval (hr)</td></tr><tr><td>≤7</td><td>All</td><td>12</td></tr><tr><td>>7</td><td><2</td><td>8</td></tr><tr><td>>7</td><td>≥2</td><td>6</td></tr></table>	May cause allergic reactions, seizures, nausea, vomiting, hematologic abnormalities (eosinophilia, leukopenia, neutropenia, anemia), and elevated BUN, creatinine, and liver enzymes. Reduce dose in renal impairment. Breast-feeding: Use with caution.
Morphine sulfate (various)	Injection: 0.5, 1, 2, 3, 4, 5, 8, 10, 15, 25 mg/ml Oral solution: 2, 4, 20 mg/ml	*Analgesia/tetralogy spells:* IV, IM, SC, 0.05-0.2 mg/kg/dose q4h prn Continuous IV: 0.01-0.02 mg/kg/hr; begin with lower dose and titrate to effect	PO dose is approximately six times IV/IM dose. Respiratory depression reversible with naloxone. May cause nausea, vomiting, constipation, hypotension, bradycardia, increased intracranial pressure, miosis, and biliary or urinary tract spasm. Breast-feeding: Use with caution.

Morphine sulfate— cont'd

Nafcillin
(Unipen, Nafcil, Nallpen)

Oral solution: 250 mg/5 ml
Injection: 0.5, 1, 2, 4 gm (contains 2.9 mEq Na$^+$ per 1 gm of drug)

Opiate withdrawal: PO, 0.08-0.2 mg/dose q3-4h prn
IV: 25 mg/kg/dose

Weight (kg)	PNA	Interval (hr)
<2	≤7	12
<2	>7	8
≥2	≤7	8
≥2	>7	6

Severe infections:
≤7 days, 100 mg/kg/24 hr ÷ q8-12h
>7 days, 150-200 mg/kg/24 hr ÷ q6-8h

Allergic cross-sensitivity with penicillin. Oral route not recommended because of poor absorption. High incidence of phlebitis with IV route of administration. Reduce dose in renal insufficiency. Breast-feeding: Use with caution.

Naloxone
(Narcan)

Injection: 0.4 mg/ml (1 ml); 1 mg/ml (2 ml)
Neonatal injection: 0.02 mg/ml (2 ml)

Opiate intoxication: IV, IM, SC, 0.1-0.2 mg/kg/dose; may repeat every 2-3 min prn
Continuous infusion: 0.01 mg/kg/hr

Does not cause respiratory depression. Short duration of action may necessitate multiple doses. Use with **caution** in patients with cardiac disease.
Tachycardia, hypertension, tremors, and seizures are possible. Administration to an infant of a drug-addicted mother may result in seizures and withdrawal symptoms. Breast-feeding: Safety not established.

Continued

TABLE H-2
Drug Doses for Neonates—cont'd

Drug	How supplied	Dose and route	Remarks
Neomycin sulfate (Mycifradin)	Oral suspension: 125 mg/ 5 ml	Premature and full-term infants: PO, 50 mg/kg/24 hr ÷ q6h	Follow for renal toxicity or ototoxicity. **Contraindicated** in ulcerative bowel disease or intestinal obstruction. Oral absorption is limited, but levels may accumulate. Consider dosage reduction in renal failure. Breast-feeding: Safety not established.
Neostigmine (Prostigmin)	Injection: 0.25, 0.5, 1 mg/ml (methylsulfate)	*Myasthenia gravis:* Diagnosis, 0.04 mg/kg × 1 IM; treatment, 0.01-0.04 mg/kg/dose q2-3h prn IM/IV/SC *For reversal of nondepolarizing neuromuscular blockade:* IV, 0.025-0.1 mg/kg/dose with atropine or glycopyrrolate to prevent severe vagal reaction	Titrate for each patient, but avoid excessive cholinergic effects. **Caution** in asthmatics. **Contraindicated** in patients with GI and urinary obstruction. May cause cholinergic crisis, bronchospasm, salivation, nausea, vomiting, diarrhea, miosis, diaphoresis, lacrimation, bradycardia, hypotension, fatigue, confusion, respiratory depression, and seizures. Reduce dose in renal impairment. **Antidote:** Atropine 0.01-0.04 mg/kg/dose IV. Breast-feeding: Safety not established.

Nevirapine (NVP, Viramune)	Suspension: 10 mg/ml (240 ml)	*Prevention of HIV perinatal transmission:* Maternal antenatal dose: 200 mg × 1 at the onset of labor Neonatal postpartum dose: 2 mg/kg/dose × 1 within 72 hours of birth	May be administered with food. Use with caution in hepatic or renal dysfunction. May cause skin rash (may be life threatening), sedation, headache, and GI discomfort. **Discontinue** therapy if a severe rash or rash with fever, blistering, oral lesions, conjunctivitis, and muscle aches occurs. Drug induces the CYP 450 3A4 drug metabolizing isoenzyme to cause an autoinduction of its own metabolism within the first 2-4 weeks of therapy. Cimetidine, erythromycin, ketoconazole can increase serum levels of nevirapine. Breast-feeding: Unknown with concerns.
Nystatin (Mycostatin, Nilstat)	Suspension: 100,000 U/ml Topical powder, ointment, cream: 100,000 U/gm (15, 30 gm)	Oral: Preterm infants, 0.5 ml (50,000 U) to each side of mouth qid; term infants: 1 ml (100,000 U) to each side of mouth qid Topical: Apply bid-qid	May produce local irritation, diarrhea, and GI symptoms. Treat until 48-72 hr after resolution of symptoms. Systemic absorption is poor through mucous membranes, intact skin, and GI tract. Breast-feeding: Compatible.

Continued

TABLE H-2
Drug Doses for Neonates—cont'd

Drug	How supplied	Dose and route			Remarks

Oxacillin
(Bactocill, Prostaphlin)

Oral solution: 250 mg/5 ml
Injection: 0.25, 0.5, 1, 2, 4 gm (contains 2.8-3.1 mEq Na/gm)

IV or IM: 25-50 mg/kg/dose

PCA	PNA	Interval (hr)
≤29	0-28	12
≤29	>28	8
30-36	0-14	12
30-36	>14	8
37-44	0-7	12
37-44	>7	8
≥45	All	6

Rash, diarrhea, nausea, vomiting, epigastric discomfort or fullness, and SGOT elevation may occur. PO administration is not recommended. Use higher dosage for meningitis. Reduce dose in renal failure. Breast-feeding: Safety not established.

Palivizumab
(Synagis)

Injection: 100 mg

RSV prophylaxis: ≤2 yr with chronic lung disease, or premature infants (<35 wks gestation) <12 mo of age: 15 mg/kg/dose IM monthly during RSV season

RSV season is typically November through April in the northern hemisphere but may begin earlier or persist later in certain communities. Use with caution in patients with thrombocytopenia or any coagulation disorder because of IM route. May cause rhinitis, rash, pain, increased liver enzymes, pharyngitis, cough, wheeze, diarrhea, vomiting, conjunctivitis, and anemia.

Drug	Preparation	Dose	Comments
Pancuronium bromide (Pavulon)	Injection: 1, 2 mg/ml (contains 1% benzyl alcohol)	Initial: 0.02 mg/kg/dose IV Maintenance: 0.05-0.1 mg/kg/dose IV q0.5-4h prn	Must be prepared to intubate within 2 min of induction. Drug effect accentuated by hypothermia, acidosis, neonatal age, decreased renal function, halothane, succinylcholine, hypokalemia, and aminoglycoside antibiotics. May cause tachycardia, mild salivation, and rash. Reduce dose in severe renal failure. **Antidote:** neostigmine (with atropine or glycopyrrolate). Breast-feeding: Safety not established.
Paregoric (camphorated opium tincture)	Camphorated tincture: 2 mg/5 ml (0.4 mg morphine/ml) (some preparations contain up to 45% alcohol)	*Opiate withdrawal:* Initial, 0.2-0.3 ml/dose q3-4h; increment, 0.05 ml/dose until symptoms abate (rare to exceed 0.7 ml/dose) **Maximum dose** 1-2 ml/kg/24 hr	Same side effects as morphine (e.g., constipation, lethargy). After symptoms are controlled for several days, dose is gradually decreased over 2-4 wk (e.g., by 10% every 2-3 days). **NOTE: Deodorized opium tincture contains 10 mg morphine/ml and is 25 times stronger than the camphorated product.** Breast-feeding: Use with caution.
Penicillin G preparations—benzathine (Permapen, Bicillin L-A)	Injection: 300,000; 600,000 U/ml (may contain parabens and povidone)	*Congenital syphilis* (asymptomatic infants born to mothers with syphilis): IM, 50,000 U/kg × 1	Provides sustained levels for 2-4 weeks. Do **not** administer IV. Use with caution in patients with renal or cardiac impairment and seizure disorders. Breast-feeding: Safety not established.

Continued

TABLE H-2
Drug Doses for Neonates—cont'd

Drug	How supplied	Dose and route	Remarks
Penicillin G preparations— potassium and sodium	Potassium: Injection, 1, 5, 10, 20 million units (contains 1.7 mEq of K^+ and 0.3 mEq of Na^+ per 1 million units of drug) Sodium: Injection, 5 million units (contains 2 mEq of Na^+ per 1 million units of drug)	IV or IM: ≤7 days, <2 kg, 50,000-100,000 U/kg/24 hr ÷ q12h ≥2 kg, 75,000-225,000 U/kg/24 hr ÷ q8h >7 days, < 2 kg, 75,000-150,000 U/kg/24 hr ÷ q8h ≤2 kg, 100,000-200,000 U/kg/24 hr ÷ q6h	1 mg = approximately 1600 units. Side effects: ana-phylaxis, hemolytic anemia, interstitial nephritis. Half-life may be prolonged by concurrent use of probenecid. Reduce dose in renal impairment. For meningitis, use higher daily dose at shorter dosing intervals. Use for 10-14 days in congenital syphilis. Breast-feeding: Safety not established.
Penicillin G preparations— procaine (Duracillin, Wycillin)	Injection: 300,000; 500,000; 600,000 U/ml (contains 120 mg procaine per 300,000 U) (may con-tain parabens, phenol, povidone and formalde-hyde)	*Congenital syphilis:* IM, 50,000 U/kg/dose q24h × 10-14 days	Provides sustained levels for 2-4 days. May cause sterile abscess at injection site. Contains 120 mg procaine per 300,000 U; this may cause allergic reactions, CNS stimulation, or seizures. Use with **caution** in neonates. Do **not** use IV. Breast-feed-ing: Safety not established.

Phenobarbital
(Luminal)

Elixir: 15, 20 mg/5 ml (contains 13.5% alcohol)
Injection: 30, 60, 65, 130 mg/ml (some products may contain benzyl alcohol and propylene glycol)

For withdrawal: IV, IM, PO, 5-12 mg/kg/24 hr ÷ qid
For seizures: Loading dose, IV, 20 mg/kg over 10 min; up to an additional 5 mg/kg until seizure control up to total dose of 40 mg/kg is reached; maintenance, 4-5 mg/kg/24 hr ÷ q12h IV, IM, PO
Chronic anticonvulsant: Initial, 2-4 mg/kg/24 hr ÷ qd-bid × 2 weeks, followed by maintenance, 5 mg/kg/24 hr ÷ qd-bid

IV administration may cause respiratory arrest or hypotension. **Contraindicated** in patients with hepatic or renal disease and porphyria.
Therapeutic levels: 15-40 mg/L. Recommended serum sampling time at steady-state: trough level obtained within 30 minutes before the next scheduled dose after 10-14 days of continuous dosing. However, levels may be obtained before steady-state to assess safety. Induces liver enzymes, thus decreases blood levels of many drugs (e.g., warfarin). Reduce dose in renal failure. **IV push not to exceed 1 mg/kg/min.** Breast-feeding: Use with caution.

Continued

TABLE H-2
Drug Doses for Neonates—cont'd

Drug	How supplied	Dose and route	Remarks
Phenytoin (Dilantin)	Injection: 50 mg/ml (2, 5 ml) Oral suspension: 125 mg/5 ml (240 ml)	Status epilepticus: IV, loading dose, 15-20 mg/kg, infused at a rate <0.5 mg/kg/min; PO, IV, maintenance, 4-8 mg/kg/24 hr qd-bid; flush IV with saline before and after dose Antiarrhythmic: IV, 2-5 mg/kg over 5-10 min (or <0.5 mg/kg/min), repeat up to 20 mg/kg	**Therapeutic blood level monitoring: 10-20 mg/L of free and bound phenytoin (probably lower at 6-14 mg/L because of reduced protein binding in neonates).** Recommended serum sampling times: trough levels (PO/IV) within 30 minutes before next scheduled dose; peak or post load level (IV) 1 hr after end of IV infusion. For routine monitoring, measure trough. Do not administer intramuscularly. Oral absorption is reduced in neonates. Intravenous infusion requires sufficient dilution (<5 mg/ml) with 0.9% NaCl solution. Start IV administration soon after dilution so that precipitation of the drug is avoided. An experienced person should supervise. Breast-feeding: Compatible.

Phosphorous supplements (sodium and potassium = Neutra-Phos); (potassium phosphate = Neutra-Phos-K); sodium phosphate; potassium phosphate	Oral dosage forms (to be reconstituted in 75 ml H_2O per capsule or packet); Na^+ and K^+ phosphate (Neutra-Phos), caps, powder, 7 mEq Na, 7 mEq K, 250 mg (8 mM) P; K phosphate (NeutraPhos-K), caps, powder, 14.25 mEq K, 250 mg (8 mM) P Injection: Na, 94 mg (3 mM) P + 4 mEq Na/ml; K, 94 mg (3 mM) P + 4.4 mEq K/ml Conversion: 31 mg P= 1mM P	PO: 31-46.5 mg (1-1.5 mM) phosphorus/kg/24 hr ÷ bid; consider the additional cations (Na^+ or K^+) in each dosage form	May cause tetany, hyperphosphatemia, hyperkalemia, hypocalcemia. PO dosing may cause nausea, vomiting, abdominal pain, or diarrhea. Use with **caution** in patients with renal impairment. Breast-feeding: Safety not established.
Phytonadione	See Vitamin K_1		

Continued

TABLE H-2
Drug Doses for Neonates—cont'd

Drug	How supplied	Dose and route		Remarks

Piperacillin (Pipracil)

How supplied: Injection: 2, 3, 4 gm (contains 1.85 mEq Na per 1 gm of drug)

Dose and route: IM or IV: 50-100 mg/kg/dose

PCA	PNA	Interval (hr)
≤29	0-28	12
≤29	>28	8
30-36	0-14	12
30-36	>14	8
37-44	0-7	12
37-44	>7	8
≥45	All	6

Remarks: Similar to penicillin. Adjust dosage in renal impairment. May falsely lower aminoglycoside serum level results if the drugs are infused close to one another; allow a minimum of 2 hr between infusions to prevent this interaction. Breast-feeding: Safety not established.

Prednisone (various)

How supplied: Solution: 5 mg/5 ml (may contain alcohol)

Dose and route: *Antiinflammatory or immunosuppressive:* 0.5-2 mg/kg/24 hr ÷ q6-12h

Remarks: See Hydrocortisone. Prednisone must be converted in the liver to methylprednisolone. Breast-feeding: Compatible.

Procainamide (Pronestyl)

How supplied: Injection: 100, 500 mg/ml Suspension:* 5, 50, 100 mg/ml

Dose and route: IV: Initial, 1 mg/kg infused over 5 minutes q5-10min prn to a **maximum** of 15 mg/kg (100 mg total **maximum**); maintenance, 20-50 µg/kg/min (see dobutamine for infusion preparation/calculations)

Remarks: Contraindicated in myasthenia gravis, complete heart block, systemic lupus erythematosus, torsade de pointes. Asystole, myocardial depression, anorexia, vomiting, nausea; rash and lupuslike syndrome may occur. Blood level monitoring is helpful. **Therapeutic range: procainamide, 3-10 mg/L; N-acetyl procainamide (NAPA), 5-30 mg/L.** Monitor IV use closely, along with blood pressure and ECG readings. Administer at a rate of <20 mg/min to avoid severe hypotension. Adjust dose in renal failure. Breast-feeding: Compatible.

Propranolol
(Inderal)

Injection: 1 mg/ml
Solution: 4, 8 mg/ml
Concentrated solution: 80 mg/ml
Suspension:* 1 mg/ml

Arrhythmias: Initial dose, IV, 0.01-0.2 mg/kg infused over 10 min to a **maximum** of 1 mg/dose (may repeat in 10 min); maintenance/non-emergent dose, PO, 0.05-2 mg/kg/dose q6h

Tetralogy spells: Acute, IV, 0.15-0.25 mg/kg/dose over 10 min (may repeat in 15 min × 1); maintenance dose, PO, 1-2 mg/kg/dose q6h

Contraindicated in asthma and heart block. Use with caution in presence of obstructive lung disease, heart failure, or renal or hepatic disease. May cause hypoglycemia, hypotension, nausea, vomiting, depression, weakness, bronchospasm, and heart block. Concurrent use with barbiturates, indomethacin, or rifampin may cause decreased activity of propranolol. Concurrent use with cimetidine, hydralazine, chlorpromazine, or verapamil may lead to increased activity of propranolol. IV and PO doses are not bioequivalent. Administer IV doses over 10 min. Breast-feeding: Compatible.

Propylthiouracil
(PTU)

Tablets: 50 mg
100 mg PTU = 10 mg methimazole

PO: 5-10 mg/kg/24hr ÷ q8h; increase to **maximum** of 10 mg/kg/dose as required; onset of action may be delayed days to weeks

May cause blood dyscrasia, fever, liver disease, dermatitis, urticaria, malaise, and CNS stimulation or depression. Dosage must be adjusted to maintain normal T_3, T_4, and TSH levels. Falsely elevates prothrombin time. Reduce dose in renal impairment. Breast-feeding: Compatible.

Prostaglandin E_1

See Alprostadil

Continued

TABLE H-2
Drug Doses for Neonates—cont'd

Drug	How supplied	Dose and route	Remarks
Protamine sulfate	Injection: 10 mg/ml (5, 10, 25 ml)	*Heparin antidote:* 1 mg will neutralize approximately 100 U of heparin; for IV heparin, base dose on amount received in previous 2 hr; <30 min (IV, 1 mg/100 U heparin; 30-60 min (IV), 0.5- 0.75 mg/100 U heparin; >120 min (IV), 0.25-0.375 mg/100 U heparin **Maximum dose** IV, 50 mg with rate not to exceed 5 mg/min	Dosage depends on route of administration and time elapsed since heparin dose. Can cause hypotension, bradycardia, dyspnea, and anaphylaxis. Rarely, heparin rebound has occurred. Breast-feeding: Safety not established.
Pyridoxine (Vitamin B₆)	Injection: 100 mg/ml Tablets: 10, 25, 50, 100 mg	*Pyridoxine-dependent seizures:* Diagnostic dose, IV/IM, 50-100 mg × 1; maintenance dose, PO, 50-100 mg qd	May be given IV, IM, or SC when oral administration is not feasible. Sedation may occur. Breast-feeding: Compatible.
Pyrimethamine (Daraprim)	Tablets: 25 mg Suspension:* 1, 2 mg/ml	*Congenital toxoplasmosis* (administer with sulfadiazine): PO, loading dose, 2mg/kg/24hr ÷ q12h × 2 days	Blood dyscrasias, glossitis, leukopenia, folic acid deficiency, rash, or seizures may occur. Folinic acid supplementation (5 mg every 3 days) is recommended so that hematologic complications are avoided. For additional information on congenital toxoplasmosis see *Clin Infect Dis* 18:38-72, 1994. Breast-feeding: Compatible.

Pyrimethamine—cont'd		Maintenance 1 mg/kg/24hr PO-qd × 2-6 months, then 1 mg/kg/24 hr three times per week to complete 12 months of therapy	
Ranitidine (Zantac)	Injection: 25 mg/ml Syrup: 15 mg/ml	PO: 2-4 mg/kg/24hr ÷ q8-12h IV: 2 mg/kg/24hr ÷ q6-8h IV continuous infusion: Administer daily IV dosages over 24 hours (may be added to parenteral nutrition solutions)	GI disturbance, malaise, sedation, arthralgia, and hepatotoxicity may occur. Data limited in neonates. Adjust dose in renal failure. Breast-feeding: Compatible.
Respiratory Syncytial Virus Immune Globulin (RSVIG, Respigam)	Injection: 50 mg/ml (20, 50 ml)	*RSV prophylaxis:* <2 yrs: 750 mg/kg/dose IV monthly during RSV season (typically November through April in the northern hemisphere but may begin earlier or persist later in certain communities). Start infusion at 1.5 mg/kg/hr for 15 minutes, if tolerated, gradually increase rate to 3 ml/kg/hr for the next 15 minutes then to 6 ml/kg/hr to the end of infusion	Although this product has a broad indication for use in children <2 yr old with bronchopulmonary dysplasia or history of prematurity (<35 wk gestation), see latest version of the *AAP Redbook* for specific recommendations. **Contraindicated** in IgA deficiency. Should not be used in patients with cyanotic heart disease. May cause fever, respiratory distress, vomiting, and wheezing. Monitor heart rate, blood pressure, temperature, respiratory rate. Injectable live virus vaccines (i.e, MMR, measles, varicella) should be deferred for 9-10 months after the last dose of RSVIG.
			Continued

*Indicates suspensions not commercially available; must be extemporaneously compounded by a pharmacist. See references.

TABLE H-2
Drug Doses for Neonates—cont'd

Drug	How supplied	Dose and route	Remarks
Rifampin (Rimactane, Rifadin)	Oral suspension:* 15 mg/ml Injection: 600 mg	*Tuberculosis* (use with isoniazid): IV/PO, 10-20 mg/kg/24hr ÷ q12-24h or 10-20 mg/kg/dose twice weekly (CDC recommendations) *Meningitis prophylaxis* (<1 month): *Neisseria meningitidis*, PO, 10 mg/kg/24 hr ÷ q12h × 2 days; *Haemophilus influenzae*, PO, 10 mg/kg/24 hr qd × 4 days	Causes red discoloration of body secretions (urine, saliva, and tears). Induces hepatic microsomal enzymes; may need increased doses of digoxin, phenytoin, theophylline, etc. Use with caution in liver disease. May cause GI irritation, allergy, headache, fatigue, ataxia, confusion, fever, hepatitis, blood dyscrasia, and elevated BUN and uric acid. Reduce dose in renal failure. Food ingestion delays absorption. IV dose is similar to PO dose. Breast-feeding: Compatible.
Silver nitrate	Ophthalmic drops: 1% (single-use wax ampules)	*Prophylaxis:* 2 drops into the lower conjunctival sack of each eye no later than 1 hr after delivery	Chemical conjunctivitis, cauterization of the cornea, and staining of the skin may occur. Breast-feeding: Safety not established.

Sodium bicarbonate	Injection: 8.4% (1 mEq/ml) 50 ml Prefilled syringes: 4.2% (0.5 mEq/ml), 8.4% (1 mEq/ml), 10 ml (1 mEq bicarbonate provides 1 mEq Na^+)	*Resuscitation:* IV, 1-2 mEq/kg/dose (using 4.2% strength) infuse slowly only if infant is ventilated adequately *Correction of metabolic acidosis:* HCO_3 (mEq) = $0.3 \times$ wt (kg) $\times$ base deficit (mEq/L)	$NaHCO_3$ comes in 8.4% and 4.2% strengths. Use 4.2% for peripheral line administration because of a lower osmolarity of 900 mOsm/L. The 8.4% strength (1800 mOsm/L) is hyperosmolar and may cause tissue necrosis. The 8.4% solution should be diluted 1:1 with preservative-free sterile water. Metabolic alkalosis, hypernatremia, hypokalemia, hypocalcemia, edema, and tissue necrosis (during extravasation) may occur. Breast-feeding: Safety not established.
Sodium polystyrene sulfonate (Kayexalate, SPS)	Powder: 454 gm (1 tsp = 3.5 gm) Suspension: 15 g/60 ml (contains 21.5 ml sorbitol and 65 mEq Na per 60 ml) Contains 4.1 mEq NA^+ per 1 gm of drug	*Practical exchange ratio:* 1 mEq K per 1 gm resin Calculate dose according to desired exchange; usual dose: 1 g/kg/dose PO q6h or q2-6h rectally **NOTE:** Suspension may be given PO or PR	1 mEq Na is delivered for each mEq K removed. Use cautiously in presence of renal failure. Do not administer with antacids or laxatives containing magnesium or aluminum. May cause hypokalemia, hypomagnesemia, hypocalcemia, and systemic alkalosis. Breast-feeding: Safety not established.
Spironolactone (Aldactone)	Suspension:* 1, 2, 5 mg/ml	PO: 1-3 mg/kg/24 hr ÷ bid	Contraindicated in patients with acute renal failure. May potentiate ganglionic blocking agents and other antihypertensives. May cause GI distress, rash, and hyperkalemia. Breast-feeding: Compatible.

Continued

TABLE H-2
Drug Doses for Neonates—cont'd

Drug	How supplied	Dose and route	Remarks
Streptomycin sulfate	Injection: 400 mg/ml (2.5 ml)	Administer by IM route only: Newborns, 10-20 mg/kg/dose q24h; infants, 20-30 mg/kg/24 hr ÷ q12h	Adjust dose in presence of renal insufficiency. Follow auditory status. May cause CNS depression or other neurologic problems, myocarditis, serum sickness, nephrotoxicity, and ototoxicity. **Therapeutic levels: peak 20-30 mg/L, trough <5 mg/L.** Recommended serum sampling time at steady-state: trough within 30 minutes before the third consecutive dose and peak 30-60 minutes after the third dose. Therapeutic levels are not achieved in CSF. For tuberculosis, use in conjunction with other antituberculosis drugs. Breast-feeding: Compatible.
Sulfadiazine	Suspension:* 100 mg/ml	*Congenital toxoplasmosis:* (Administer with pyrimethamine and folinic acid) PO, 85 mg/kg/24 hr ÷ q6h	Contraindicated in porphyria and hypersensitivity to sulfonamides. Use caution in infants <2 mo because of risk of hyperbilirubinemia, and in hepatic or renal dysfunction. May cause crystalluria (keep output high and alkaline), fever, rash, hepatitis, lupuslike syndrome, vasculitis, or bone marrow depression. For additional information on congenital toxoplasmosis, see *Clin Infec Dis* 18:38-72, 1994. Breast-feeding: Use with caution.

Surfactant, pulmonary See Beractant (Survanta), calfactant (Infasurf), or colfosceril palmitate (Exosurf)

Theophylline See Aminophylline

Ticarcillin Injection: 1, 3, 6, 20, 30 gm (Ticar) (contains 5.2–6.5 mEq Na⁺ per 1 gm of drug)

IV: 75 mg/kg/dose

Weight (kg)	PNA	Interval (hr)
<2	0–7	12
<2	>7	8
≥2	0–7	8
≤2	>7	6

May cause inhibition of platelet aggregation, bleeding diathesis, hypernatremia, hypocalcemia, allergy, rash, or increased SGOT. **Do not mix** with aminoglycoside in same solution. Reduce dosage in renal failure. Breast-feeding: Compatible.

Tobramycin Injection: 10, 40 mg/ml (Nebcin, Tobrex) Ophthalmic ointment: 0.3% (3.5 g) Ophthalmic solution: 0.3% (5 ml)

Neonates (IV or IM): See gentamicin
Ophthalmic: Apply thin ribbon of ointment to affected eye bid-tid or 1–2 drops of solution to affected eye q4h

Therapeutic levels: peak 5–10 mg/L, trough:
<2 mg/L. Recommended serum sampling times at steady-state: trough within 30 minutes before the third consecutive dose and peak 30–60 minutes after the third dose. Ototoxicity, nephrotoxicity, myelotoxicity, and allergic reaction may occur. Ototoxic effects are synergistic with furosemide. Higher doses may be needed in patients with cystic fibrosis, burns, or neutropenia. Adjust dose in renal impairment. Breast-feeding: Safety not established.

Continued

TABLE H-2
Drug Doses for Neonates—cont'd

Drug	How supplied	Dose and route	Remarks
Tolazoline (Priscoline)	Injection: 25 mg/ml (4 ml)	Pulmonary hypertension: Test dose (IV): 1-2 mg/kg over 10 min; maintenance dose: (IV) 1-2 mg/kg/hr To prepare infusions: 50 mg/kg × wt (kg) in 50 ml D₅W, so that 1 ml/hr = 1 mg/kg/hr Acute vasospasm: 0.25/mg/kg/hr	For pulmonary hypertension infuse via a vein in an upper extremity or scalp. Hypotension, gastrointestinal and pulmonary bleeding, and renal dysfunction may occur. Monitor vital signs continuously and renal status (renally eliminated; decrease dose 50% if urinary output is <0.9 ml/kg/hr). Volume expanders or dopamine may be needed at bedside.
Tolnaftate (Tinactin, Aftate)	Topical aerosol liquid: 1% (113 gm) Aerosol powder: 1% (100, 150 gm) Cream: 1% (15, 30, 45 gm) Gel: 1% (15 gm) Powder: 1% (45, 90 gm) Topical solution: 1% (10, 60 ml)	Apply 1-2 drops of solution or small amount of gel, liquid, cream, or powder bid for 2-6 weeks	May cause mild irritation and sensitivity. Avoid eye contact. Do not use for nail or scalp infections.

Vancomycin
(Vancocin)

Injection: 500, 1000 mg
Oral solution: 1, 10 gm (reconstitute to 500 mg/6 ml)

IV: 10-15 mg/kg/dose

PNA	Weight (kg)	Interval (hr)
<7	<1	24
<7	1-2	18
<7	>2	12
≥7	<1	18
≥7	1-2	12
≥7	>2	8

Give 15 mg/kg/dose if CNS is involved
For colitis: PO, 10 mg/kg/dose q6h

Ototoxicity, nephrotoxicity, allergy may occur. "Red man" syndrome associated with rapid IV infusion. Infuse over 60 min, may be infused over 120 min if 60 min not tolerated. Adjust dose in renal failure. **Note:** Diphenhydramine is used to treat "red man" syndrome. **Therapeutic levels: peak 25-40 mg/L, trough 5-10 mg/L.** Recommended serum sampling time at steady-state: trough within 30 minutes before the third to fifth consecutive dose and peak 60 minutes after the third to fifth dose. The intravenous dosage form may be given orally as a more cost-effective alternative. Metronidazole (PO) is the drug of choice for colitis caused by *Clostridium difficile*. Breast-feeding: Safety not established.

Varicella-zoster immune globulin
(VZIG)

1 vial: 125 U (volume in each vial varies but is typically ≤2.5 ml)

Weight 10 kg or less: 125 U IM
10.1-20 kg: 250 U IM; administer dose within 96 hr postexposure

Contraindicated in severe thrombocytopenia because of IM injection. May induce anaphylactic reactions in IgA-deficient individuals. Interferes with immune response to live virus vaccines such as measles, mumps, and rubella; defer administration of live vaccines 5 months after VZIG dose. Local discomfort at injection site may occur. Do not administer intravenously because serious systemic reactions could occur. Breast-feeding: Safety not established.

Continued

TABLE H-2
Drug Doses for Neonates—cont'd

Drug	How supplied	Dose and route	Remarks
Verapamil (Isoptin, Calan)	Injection: 2.5 mg/ml	IV: 0.1-0.2 mg/kg (**maximum dose** 5 mg) infused over 2 min; if response is inadequate repeat in 30 min × 1	**Contraindicated** in cardiogenic shock, severe CHF, sick sinus syndrome, or third-degree atrioventricular block and during treatment with beta blockers. Monitor ECG during infusion. Bradycardia, atrioventricular block, asystole, hypotension, and apnea may occur. Have calcium and isoproterenol ready to reverse hypotension and bradycardia. Breast-feeding: Compatible.
Vitamin A (Aquasol A)	Drops: 50,000 IU/ml (30 ml) Injection: 50,000 IU/ml (2 ml)	*Prophylactic therapy for children at risk for deficiency:* 100,000 IU q4-6mo PO *Daily dietary supplement:* Infants up to 1 yr (PO), 1250 IU qd	Avoid toxicity. Adverse effects seen with high doses include irritability, drowsiness, increased intracranial pressure, erythema, vomiting, diarrhea, papilledema, and visual disturbances. May increase adverse effects of warfarin. Breast-feeding: Safety not established.
Vitamin D₂ **Vitamin E** (Aquasol E)	See Ergocalciferol Oral drops: 50 IU/ml (12 ml) 1 IU = 1 mg of dl-alphatocopherol acetate	*Vitamin E deficiency:* PO, 25-50 IU/24 hr *Prevention of RBC hemolysis:* PO, 25 IU/24 hr	Nausea, diarrhea, and intestinal cramps may occur. Breast-feeding: Safety not established.

Vitamin E—cont'd		
Vitamin K₁ (Aqua-Mephyton, Konakion, Phyto- nadione, Mephyton)	Tablets: 5 mg Injection: 2, 10 mg/ml (contains benzyl alcohol)	RDA: Premature infant (<3 mo): 25 IU/24 hr Infant (<6 mo): 3 IU/24 hr Infant (6-12 mo), 4 IU/24 hr *Neonatal hemorrhagic disease:* Prophylaxis, 0.5-1 mg/dose IM, SC, or IV × 1; treatment, 1-2 mg/dose/24 hr IM, SC, or IV *Oral anticoagulant overdose:* Infants (IM, SC, or IV), 1-2 mg/dose q4-8h *Vitamin K deficiency:* Infants (IM or IV), 1-2 mg/dose × 1; PO: 2.5-5 mg/24 hr	Follow PT/PTT. Use with **caution** in presence of severe hepatic disease. Large doses (>25 mg) in newborn may cause hyperbilirubinemia. **IV injection rate not to exceed 3 mg/m²/min or 1 mg/min.** IV doses may cause flushing, dizziness, hypotension, or anaphylaxis. **IV administration is indicated only when other routes of administration are not feasible.** Breast-feeding: Compatible.
Zidovudine (AZT, Azidothymidine, Retrovir)	Syrup: 50 mg/5 ml Injection: 10 mg/ml	*Prevention of HIV maternal transfer:* PO, 2 mg/kg/dose q6h × 6 wk; IV, 1.5 mg/kg/dose q6h × 6 wk; initiate first dose (PO or IV) within 8-12 hr after birth; IV administration over 1 hr with a concentration ≤ 4 mg/ml	Side effects include anemia, granulocytopenia, nausea, and headache. Use with caution in renal or hepatic impairment. Drug interactions: acyclovir, ganciclovir, and drugs inhibiting glucuronidation enhance toxic effects of AZT. **Do not administer IM.** See *N Engl J Med* 331(18):1173, 1994, for entire dosing protocol (antenatal and postnatal). Breast-feeding: Unknown with concerns.

APPENDIX I

Newborn Nursery Policy Statements*

I. ONGOING CARE OF THE NEWBORN

A. Indications.

1. All newborns who meet the criteria for admission to a full-term nursery.
2. All newborns who meet the criteria for Combined Care/Mother-Baby Care. The infant may return to the nursery anytime as desired by the mother.

B. Responsibility.

1. The pediatrician should be notified before all deliveries regarding maternal/fetal criteria listed below.
2. The pediatrician/practitioner will assess the newborn after delivery and determine whether the infant may remain with the mother or must be admitted to a setting in which consistent professional observation is available.
3. Infants on Combined Care will be cared for by the registered nurse (RN) who is assigned to care for the mother. The Combined Care RN will provide nursing care for the infant for the duration of the hospital stay except when the infant is returned to Nursery Care.
4. The RN assigned to care for the infant is responsible for instructing the mother and/or her significant other on infant care.

C. Pediatrician notification.

1. Assess maternal/fetal status continuously for the presence of risk factors before delivery. Collaboration with the pediatric staff should occur before delivery to determine whether they should be called for delivery.
2. Maternal/fetal criteria for mandated pediatrician's attendance at a delivery. Contact the pediatrician for mandatory attendance at a delivery for the following:
   a. All cesarean sections.

*Modified in large part from policies developed for the Nelson 2 Nursery at The Johns Hopkins Hospital in Baltimore, Maryland. The gracious cooperation of Diann L. Snyder and Angella Olden of the Department of Gynecology and Obstetrics is gratefully acknowledged.

    b. Meconium-stained amniotic fluid at any time during labor or delivery (moderate, thick, particulate, pea soup).

    c. Prematurity (gestation of <37 weeks).

    d. Fetal distress.

    e. Multiple gestation.

    f. Any situation requiring double set-up procedures.

    g. Hydrops fetalis.

    h. Mid-pelvis delivery by forceps.

    i. Suspected placental previa or abruption.

    j. Intrauterine growth retardation (IUGR).

    k. Suspected fetal anomaly (at discretion of the obstetrician).

3. Maternal/fetal criteria for mandatory notification of pediatrician within 1 hour after delivery. The RN caring for the infant will notify the pediatrician regarding any of the following:

    a. Rupture of membranes >18 hours.

    b. Chorioamnionitis.

    c. Maternal fever >38° C.

    d. Positive test for human immunodeficiency virus (HIV).

    e. Intrapartum treatment with magnesium sulfate.

    f. Hepatitis B positive or surface antigen positive.

    g. Infant weight <2500 gm.

4. Notify the pediatrician/pediatric nurse practitioner (PNP) whenever any of the following are present:

    a. Respiratory distress.

    b. Abnormal skin color (e.g., jaundice in first 24 hours, ruddy, central cyanosis, pallor).

    c. Hypertonic/hypotonic.

    d. Suspected neonatal fractures.

    e. Blood glucose <40 mg/dl (see Section G).

    f. Rectal temperature <36.5° or >37.5° C (see Section G).

    g. Apical pulse <110 or >170.

    h. Respiration rate <30 or >70.

    i. Systolic blood pressure <60 or >80 mmHg.

    j. Projectile vomiting; abdominal distention, green-stained vomitus.

    k. Excessive irritability or tremors.

    l. Hemoglobin <15 or >22 mg/dl.

D. Newborn assessment: transitional period.

1. Assess umbilical cord immediately after placing cord clamp for the number of vessels and absence of active bleeding.

2. Assess axillary temperature, apical pulse, respirations, color, tone, respiratory effort and activity within 30 minutes after birth, every 30 minutes thereafter for three times, then every hour for 2 hours or until stable.

3. Perform physical examination, including measurement of head circumference, length, and weight, and assessment of gestational age by 4 hours of age. **Note:** Assess infant in well-lighted area. Use overhead bed light or warmer light.

4. Obtain blood glucose level at 1 hour of age for the following maternal or neonatal conditions AND continue to monitor before

feedings until blood glucose is greater than or equal to 40 mg/dl for 12 hours:

    a. Gestational or insulin-dependent diabetes.

    b. Apgar score <5 at 5 minutes.

    c. Hypotonia or hypertonia.

    d. Changes in levels of consciousness.

    e. Excessive tremors.

    f. Hypothermia (rectal temperature <36.5° C).

5. Obtain blood glucose level at 2 hours of age for the following maternal or neonatal conditions AND continue to monitor before feedings until blood glucose is greater than or equal to 40 mg/dl for 12 hours:

    a. Birth outside of the hospital or department.

    b. Respiratory distress at delivery.

    c. Intrapartum meconium-stained amniotic fluid.

    d. Weight <2500 gm.

    e. Small for gestational age (SGA).

    f. Postmature by examination or >42 0/7 weeks gestation.

    g. Large for gestational age (LGA) or weight >3800 gm.

    h. Premature delivery (<37 weeks).

    i. Premature rupture of membranes (PROM) >18 hours.

    j. No prenatal care.

    k. Maternal morbid obesity.

6. Obtain blood glucose level whenever any of the following maternal or neonatal conditions are present:

    a. Excessive irritability or tremors.

    b. Feeding problem (>40 minutes to feed, <30 cc q4h, unable to latch on to breast >8 hours, and lethargic, weak suck and swallow).

    c. Polycythemia (hemoglobin >22 mg/dl).

    d. Respiratory distress.

    e. Hypotonia.

    f. Hypothermia (temperature <36.5° C).

7. Obtain hemoglobin level after 4 hours of age for the following maternal or neonatal conditions:

    a. Birth outside hospital or department.

    b. Maternal hemorrhage (placenta previa, accreta, abruption).

    c. Weight <2500 gm or SGA.

    d. Nuchal cord requiring transection before delivery.

    e. Premature delivery (<37 weeks).

    f. Respiratory distress, tachypnea, apnea, 5-minute Apgar score <5.

    g. Ruddy color.

    h. Rh sensitization.

8. Obtain a urine toxicology for the following maternal or neonatal conditions:

    a. Positive toxicology screen on mother this admission.

    b. Maternal history of positive toxicology screen during current pregnancy.

    c. Mother with significant history of drug abuse within the past year.

    d. No toxicology screen obtained from mother on admission to labor and delivery.

E. Ongoing care (period after transitional care).

1. Routine vital signs.

    a. All infants will have their vital signs taken every 4 hours until they are 24 hours old. If the infant's condition is stable after 24 hours of age, vital signs will be taken every 8 hours until discharge.

    b. Infants on Nursery Care will continue to have their vital signs taken every 3 to 4 hours or per pediatrician/PNP order (e.g., prematurity, respiratory distress, phototherapy, isolette care, drug withdrawal, sepsis, polycythemia).

    c. Infants on Nursery Care because of the mother's inability to care for the infant will have vital signs taken every 8 hours after 24 hours of age.

2. Perform physical assessment.

    a. For infants on Combined Care, assess at least every 24 hours.

    b. For infants on Nursery Care, assess at least every 12 hours. Abnormal assessments should be reassessed every 8 hours and as needed.

    c. Assessment should be completed in a well lighted area (e.g., use the overhead bed light in patient's room or radiant warmer).

3. Assess and document voiding, stools amount, frequency, and tolerance of feeding every 2 to 5 hours.

4. Assess and document bonding behaviors and mother's ability to provide infant care every shift.

F. Nursing interventions.

1. Establish and maintain a patent airway.

    a. Suction the nasooropharynx after delivery and as needed.

       (1) Suctioning may be accomplished by use of a bulb syringe, Delee suction device, or wall suction device set on low (<100 mmHg).

       (2) Limit suctioning to 5 to 10 seconds and provide blow-by oxygen every 5 seconds until airway is opened.

       (3) Keep bulb syringe within reach at all times.

    b. Position newborn with head slightly lower than chest to facilitate drainage of secretions.

2. Maintain stable body temperature:

    a. Dry infant thoroughly and keep it away from drafts and direct contact with cold surfaces.

    b. Swaddle infant in a blanket and cover the head with a hat when infant is not under a radiant warmer.

    c. Place nude infant under radiant warmer or directly next to mother's skin. A skin probe is required when infant is under the radiant warmer. The skin probe is placed on the right upper quadrant of the abdomen. **Note:** The probe should be moved to the infant's back if it is medically necessary for the infant to be in the prone position.

d. Bathe infant under radiant warmer when medically stable (e.g., axillary temperature >36.5° C for two readings, normal respiratory effort). **Note:** Parents may choose not to have infant bathed before discharge.

   (1) A radiant warmer, and suction must be set up and available during the bath. The equipment should be brought to the mother's room if the infant is bathed at the mother's bedside.

   (2) Vernix in the folds does not need to be removed unless it is mixed with blood.

   (3) Parents may hold the infant immediately after the bath. Minimize heat loss by dressing and wrapping the infant in two blankets and covering its head with a hat.

   (4) Repeat axillary temperature reading in 30 to 60 minutes. The infant may go to an open bassinet if its weight is >2500 gm and its axillary temperature is >36.5° C.

3. Promote infant-parent attachment:

  a. Provide parents with information about infant's status.

  b. Encourage parents to touch, hold, and interact with infant as much as possible.

4. Obtain and label cord blood in Labor and Delivery department. If mother is Rh negative, send cord blood to laboratory for ABO, Rh, and direct Coombs' test. Inform pediatrician/PNP if you are unable to obtain cord blood.

5. Identify infant and mother with matching bands.

6. Provide adequate nutrition.

  a. Put infant to the mother's breast within the first hour after birth when possible if mother has decided to breast-feed, then every 2 to 3 hours on demand thereafter.

  b. Offer bottle-fed infants 15 ml of formula with iron (20 kcal/oz). If infant tolerates formula, feed every 2 to 5 hours on demand as prescribed. Position on right side or back after feeding.

7. Protect the infant from infection and trauma.

  a. Wash hands. Use gloves and gown when handling the infant.

  b. Apply Betadine (Prepodyne) scrub to scalp electrode site immediately after delivery. (Do not rinse the site.) Cover the infant's head with stockinet cap after scalp scrub.

  c. Instill a thin line (1 to 2 cm) of erythromycin 0.5% into the conjunctiva sac of each eye, from inner canthus outward, soon after birth; remove excess after 1 minute. (Eyelids should be cleaned of blood and vernix before application of ointment).

  d. Administer Phytonadione (Aquamephyton) 1 mg (0.5 ml) intramuscularly soon after birth; using the vastus lateralis muscle as the injection site. (Clean site thoroughly two times with alcohol swabs to remove all blood and vernix before administering intramuscular medication).

    e. Apply triple dye to umbilical cord and skin area around the base of the cord after the bath.

    f. Remove cord clamp after 24 hours when the cord is dry. Begin applying alcohol to the cord every 4 hours or with each diaper change after 24 hours.

    g. Clean skin with mild soap after each diaper change.

8. Administer hepatitis B vaccine per physician order.

9. Assess readiness of mother and infant for Combined Care. Exclusion criteria for Combined Care include the following:

    a. Respiratory distress symptoms.

    b. Gestational age <37 weeks.

    c. Isolette care.

    d. Signs and symptoms of drug withdrawal.

    e. Polycythemia (hemoglobin >22 mg/dl).

    f. SGA or weight <2500 gm.

    g. Hypoglycemia (blood glucose level <40 mg/dl on two measurements).

    h. Maternal mental and/or physical limitations that precludes care of infant.

    i. Maternal tuberculosis.

    j. Maternal group B streptococcus, possible chorioamnionitis, PROM >18 hours and infant receiving antibiotics.*

    k. Phototherapy care.*

10. Provide infant care instructions to mother and her significant other.

11. Review infant safety and security guidelines with mother and her significant other.

12. Stock infant's bassinet according to nursery standard.

13. Give a verbal report to the Combined Care nurse including pertinent delivery information and infant's status.

14. Follow established policy for guidelines related to infant's discharge.

G. Newborn conditions.

1. Hypoglycemia (blood glucose <40 mg/dl).

    a. Feed infant immediately. Supplementation must be considered if infant is breast-feeding and cannot latch on to the breast.

    b. Repeat blood glucose measurement in 45 to 60 minutes and report abnormal value to pediatrician/PNP.

2. Hypothermia (rectal temperature <36.5° C).

    a. If axillary temperature is <36.5° C, obtain rectal reading. If rectal temperature is <36.5° C, double wrap infant in warm blankets and cover head with hat. If infant is in an isolette, follow policies regarding infant in isolette.

    b. Check blood glucose level. If blood glucose is <40 mg/dl, see above.

    c. Repeat assessment of rectal temperature, respirations, and heart rate in 1 hour. If temperature is <36.5° C, place infant (nude)

---

*The decision to place an infant on Combined Care will be made at the discretion of the pediatrician/PNP and by a written medical order.

under radiant warmer and report abnormal vital signs to pediatrician/PNP.

3. Hyperthermia (rectal temperature >37.5° C). Unwrap infant and recheck temperature in 1 hour. If rectal temperature remains >37.5° C, notify pediatrician/PNP.

H. Documentation.

1. Indicate pediatrician's attendance and criteria on the following:
   a. Delivery/cesarean section note.
   b. Labor and delivery data record.
2. Admission note, assessments, interventions, response to interventions, and reportable conditions on Nursing Flow Sheet.
3. Application of vitamin K and erythromycin ointment.
4. Hepatitis B vaccine.
5. Teaching/learning activity provided.
6. Situations that occur that are listed on the multidisciplinary problem list.
7. Maternal-infant bonding behaviors and maternal ability to care for infant.

II. MANAGEMENT OF THE INFANT IN THE ISOLETTE AND WEANING THE INFANT FROM THE ISOLETTE

A. Indications for use of an isolette.

1. Weight <2500 gm.
2. <37 weeks gestation.
3. Respirations >70 at rest, or persistent tachypnea.
4. Rectal temperature 36.5° C or less after 2 hours.
5. At the discretion of the nurse caring for the infant.
6. A medical order is needed to wean the infant from the isolette. A nursing order is sufficient to initiate placing the infant in an isolette.

B. Responsibility for the isolette belongs to the RN/licensed practical nurse (LPN) caring for the infant.

C. Assessment.

1. Maintaining the isolette includes obtaining the infant's vital signs and monitoring the isolette temperature before feedings.
2. Weaning from isolette includes the following:
   a. Obtaining the infant's vital signs before the weaning process and then every 4 hours.
   b. Monitoring the isolette temperature every 4 hours until a temperature of 27° C is obtained.
   c. After weaning, assess vital signs every 4 hours for 24 hours, then every 8 hours thereafter.

D. Interventions.

1. Adjust isolette temperature as needed.
2. Infant may be removed for 30 minutes for every feeding.
3. For weaning, dress infant in shirt, hat, diaper, and one blanket. Lower temperature of isolette 1 to 2° C every 4 hours. As room temperature is approached (27° C), wrap infant in two blankets.

4. Wean infant from isolette to bassinet when the isolette has been at room temperature for 2 hours and the infant's axillary temperature >36.5° C for 2 hours.
5. After weaning, repeat axillary temperature measurement every 4 hours for 24 hours and then every 8 hours thereafter.

E. Reportable conditions.
1. Rectal temperature <36.5° C or >37.2° C.
2. Respirations >70 at rest.
3. Any respiratory distress (e.g., tachypnea, grunting, flaring, retractions).

F. Safety.
1. Ensure that thermostat is in place and operating properly.
2. Ensure that temperature dial is set on air.
3. Ensure that isolette portholes are properly closed.
4. Ensure that plug is secure in outlet.
5. Isolette should be thoroughly reconditioned after each patient use.

G. Documentation.
1. All vital signs and isolette temperatures should be recorded on a daily infant flow sheet.
2. Record infant's response to weaning process on daily infant flow sheet.
3. Record completion of weaning process on daily flow sheet.

III. INFANT GAVAGE FEEDING—INTERMITTENT

All infants requiring gavage feeding must have a written order specifying need and details. This procedure may be performed by an RN, nursing graduate, or LPN.

A. Equipment.
1. Feeding tube: 5F or 8F sterile.
2. 20-ml sterile syringe (new one for each feeding); 3-ml sterile syringe (to inject air).
3. ½-inch tape.
4. Stethoscope.
5. Suction equipment.
6. Formula or breast milk; sterile water.

B. Procedure.
1. Wash hands and put on gloves.
2. Ensure that suction equipment is operable.
3. Insert nasogastric tube (start with step 4; to feed through existing tube, start with step 10).
4. Use 5F tube if the infant is <1500 gm; use 8F tube if the infant is >1500 gm.
5. Measure feeding tube from tip of nose to earlobe to a point just past xiphoid process. Mark length of tube with a piece of tape.
6. Place infant in supine position, head slightly hyperflexed or nose pointed toward the ceiling.
7. Lubricate tube with sterile water with one hand and stabilize head with the other.
8. Insert tube through mouth, directing it toward the back of the throat, holding the infant's head in a slightly hyperextended posi-

tion until the premeasured length of tube is reached; using the nose, slip the tube along the base and direct it straight back toward the occiput.

9. If the tube is to be left in place, tape it securely to the infant's cheek using 1 to 1½ inches of tape.

N.B.: Cap tube and leave in place if gavaging all feedings by order. Change the indwelling feeding tube every 72 hours. Note that infants are obligatory nose breathers; insertion through the mouth is more comfortable and contributes to sucking.

10. Place infant in right lateral oblique position by placing rolled blanket behind its back.

11. Place a stethoscope over the stomach area. Inject 0.5 to 1.0 ml of air into the tube and listen for a whispering sound to confirm proper placement of the tube in the stomach. Aspirate air before feeding.

12. Place a 20-ml syringe on the end of the tube. Aspirate gastric contents. If aspirate measures >2 ml, the exact amount should be refed and that amount substracted from this feeding.

13. Slowly administer the feeding at the rate of 3 ml per minute using a 20-ml syringe. The plunger may be used to gently initiate flow of formula but should not be used again after flow is started except to instill air after formula is gavaged. A usual feeding may take from 15 to 30 minutes to complete.

14. If the infant begins to cough, gag, or regurgitate, stop the feeding until the episode passes. Aspirate immediately if there is any question about respiratory distress.

15. Assess quality of suck and encourage muscular development by offering a nipple or pacifier during gavage feeding.

N.B.: During insertion, watch for choking or cyanosis, signs that the tube has entered the trachea. If there is any suspicion of this, remove the tube, pause for a moment, and start over. Watch for signs of vagal stimulation, bradycardia, and apnea.

16. Pinch the tube off quickly before air enters the stomach; withdraw tube quickly and smoothly.

17. Burp infant to decrease abdominal distention.

18. Leave infant in right lateral oblique position for 1 hour (facilitates gastric emptying, forestalls aspiration in event of regurgitation).

19. Remove gloves and wash hands.

C. **Documentation.** Record the following information on the infant flow sheet:

1. Volume of any aspirate in stomach before feeding.
2. Volume of fluid instilled and how tolerated by infant.
3. Comment on quality of suck, gag, and swallow reflex.
4. Date and time tube was changed.

IV. MANAGEMENT OF INFANT RECEIVING PHOTOTHERAPY

The responsible practitioner must leave a written order based on clinical decision regarding the course of the infant's hyperbilirubinemia.

A. Responsibility. The registered nurse providing direct care carries out the order.

B. Assessment.

1. Obtain vital signs every 4 hours.
2. Inspect the skin for appearance of and increase in jaundice at least every 4 hours.
   a. Observe in daylight (preferably) or white fluorescent light.
   b. Blanche the skin over a bony prominence (remove capillary coloration).
3. Observe for behavior or feeding changes. Note any lethargy, change in suck quality, vomiting, or dehydration.
4. Obtain a urine specimen for reducing substances at the beginning of phototherapy per physician order (if necessary, infant may be placed under phototherapy before obtaining urine specimen).

C. Procedure. Administer phototherapy with overhead bili lights and blanket or per physician order.

1. Undress the infant to expose entire skin surface. Distance between infant and lights should be 16 inches.
2. Place illuminator on hard, flat surface, no more than 3 feet from where the infant will be lying or held.
3. Insert the panel into the end of the disposable vest and secure the vest around the cable with the tape tabs provided.
4. Lay the vest-covered panel flat in the bassinet. Ensure that the light-emitting side is face up. Place the infant on its back or chest directly on the panel. The fiberoptic panel cord should be at the infant's feet and secured in place to the bassinet.
5. Secure the vest to the infant.
   a. Wrap the side without the tape tab around the midsection of the infant.
   b. Wrap the side with the tape tab over the infant.
   c. Peel off the protective cover on the tab and secure it.
   d. Ensure that the vest is wrapped securely, but not too tightly.
6. Ensure that the irradiance level selector switch is on the highest level or as ordered by the practitioner.
7. Protect the infant's eyes with an opaque mask placed securely to prevent retinal injury.
8. Change eye pads and perform eye care every 12 hours.
9. Turn infant every 2 hours to expose all surfaces.
10. Maintain thermoregulations of isolette or bassinet depending on infant's temperature stability.
11. Remove infant from lights one half hour out of every 4 hours for feeding, stimulation, and human contact.
    a. Turn off overhead bili lights and remove eye mask.
    b. Leave bili blanket in place. Infant may be swaddled in blanket, picked up, rocked, and cuddled with blanket in place.
12. Prevent skin breakdown, especially diaper area. Cleanse diaper area at least every 3 hours and prn.
13. Foster parent-infant relationship.
    a. Encourage parent to visit infant as much as possible.

    b. Allow parents to cuddle, hold, and feed infant; provide privacy.
    c. Support the breast-feeding mother, especially if breast-feeding is temporarily discontinued. Encourage mother to pump and store milk.
14. Maintain adequate hydration of infant per physician's order.

D. Report the following conditions.
1. Increasing jaundice (judged by inspection, preferably in daylight).
2. Lethargy.
3. Poor feeding.
4. Significant weight loss.
5. Temperature <36.5° C.

E. Documentation (on nursing flow sheets).
1. All assessments and reportable conditions.
2. Presence of eye pads every 3 hours.
3. Intake and output.
4. Parent-infant interactions.

V. INFECTION CONTROL (NEWBORN NURSERY)

All nursing personnel in the newborn nursery will observe and enforce the following infection control guidelines. To prevent cross-contamination in the newborn nursery, everyone will observe the following guidelines:

A. All personnel will prepare their hands and arms before touching the newborn infant according to the following procedure:
1. Equipment.
    a. Antiseptic soap impregnated scrub sponge with nail cleaner.
    b. Paper towels.
2. Procedure.
    a. Remove all jewelry, including watch and rings.
    b. Initial preparation required before any contact with newborn or at the beginning of a shift includes the following:
      (1) Prescrub.
        (a) Open scrub packet.
        (b) Retain the packet as a clean surface on which to set the brush and nail cleaner.
        (c) Adjust water temperature. (Very hot water will cause skin irritation).
        (d) Wet hands.
        (e) Remove nail cleaner from brush.
        (f) Clean under each nail with the nail cleaner.
        (g) Rinse nail cleaner as necessary.
        (h) Discard nail cleaner.
        (i) Rinse hands.
      (2) Two-minute scrub.
        (a) During scrub, keep fingers higher than elbows at all times.
        (b) Lather with sponge side of brush.
        (c) Never rescrub an area.

(d) With the brush, begin scrubbing fingers one side at a time until all surfaces have been scrubbed.

(e) Scrub the fronts and backs of hands.

(f) Scrub the first half of the forearm.

(g) Scrub up to the elbow.

(3) Rinse.

(a) During rinse, keep fingertips higher than elbows at all times.

(b) Allow water to flow from fingertips toward elbows. Be careful not to touch the faucet.

(c) Rinse thoroughly to remove all soap.

(d) Dry hands with a paper towel from fingertips toward elbows.

(e) Turn off water using a paper towel to protect the hand from contamination.

(f) Discard paper towel.

c. Hand washing after the initial scrub.

(1) Between infants, wash hands for 15 seconds with approved liquid hand soap.

(2) Wash hands for 15 seconds with approved antimicrobial soap after eating, breaks, going to the bathroom, blowing the nose, adjusting hair, and wiping eyes or face.

N.B.: A small individual vial of lotion may be brought to work by personnel. If lotion is applied during the shift, it must be followed by the full 2-minute scrub before resuming patient care.

B. Personnel with skin, gastrointestinal, or respiratory infections are not allowed inside the nursery.

C. Articles dropped on the floor are considered contaminated.

D. There will be no exchange of clean linen or equipment between bassinets.

E. Bassinets should be placed at least 2 feet apart.

F. Babies with presumed or diagnosed communicable diseases will be isolated according to control procedures appropriate for the particular disease.

G. Care of equipment.

1. Wipe examining equipment with Wescodyne 150 ppm or equivalent after each use.

2. Place soiled linen in laundry bag. Replace bag at least once each shift, and place soiled bag in laundry chute.

3. Wipe circumcision boards with Wescodyne 150 ppm or equivalent after each use.

4. Clean bassinets and warmers with Wescodyne or its equivalent daily and after each infant's discharge.

VI. TOXIC SUBSTANCE: SCREENING AND MANAGEMENT

The urine of all infants meeting the following criteria will be collected by the nurse admitting the infant. The urine will be sent for a screen to detect heroin, cocaine, marijuana, and barbiturates.

A. Criteria for urine screening.

1. Maternal conditions.
   a. History or suspicion of substance abuse.
   b. Unregistered for prenatal care.
   c. Late registrants (>28 weeks).
   d. Premature deliveries (<37 weeks).
   e. Precipitous deliveries.
   f. Born outside of asepsis (BOA).
   g. Placental abruptions.
   h. History of hepatitis, syphilis, or other sexually transmitted diseases.
   i. History of more than two abortions (spontaneous or elective).
2. Infant status.
   a. SGA/IUGR.
   b. Excessive irritability, difficult to console.
   c. Jitteriness; tremors, hypertonic, myoclonic jerks.
   d. Loose, watery stools.
   e. Stuffy nose.
   f. Increased sweating.
   g. Disorganized suck, poor feeding.
   h. Wakefulness after feeding.
   i. Projectile vomiting.

B. Procedure.

1. Consult prenatal chart or admission date for maternal history.
2. Bag infants with symptoms or maternal criteria on admission to the nursery.
3. Wash vernix from genital area to ensure a tight seal on the urine collection bag.
4. Stimulate Perez reflex to induce voiding.
   a. Hold infant prone in one hand.
   b. Press gently with the thumb sliding along the spine from the sacrum to the neck.
5. Remove collection bag and send specimen for toxicology screening.

N.B.: If the toxicology screen is positive, continue with the following assessment.

C. Assessment.

1. Take vital signs every 4 hours.
2. Note the presence of tachypnea, fever, or tachycardia.
3. Observe for infant signs and symptoms listed under Infant status above.

D. Interventions.

1. Reduce noise.
2. Dim lights.
3. Swaddle infant.
4. Hold close, rock, offer pacifier.
5. Provide small, frequent feedings per medical order. Feed in the upright position to facilitate sucking.
6. Provide opportunity for mother and infant to interact. Encourage parents to actively participate in infant's care.

7. The pediatrician/PNP will inform the mother about her and the infant's toxicology screen results.
8. The pediatrician/PNP will discuss with the mother the need for observation, estimated length of stay, and symptoms of withdrawal.
9. A social worker will meet with the mother before baby's discharge.

E. Reportable conditions.
1. Respiratory rate >70; heart rate >160.
2. Temperature >37.5°C (rectal).
3. Projectile vomiting.
4. Lack of sleep (sleeps less than 1 hour after feeding).
5. Myoclonic jerks or seizure activity.

F. Documentation.
1. Presence of withdrawal symptoms and behavioral states.
2. Infant's response to interventions.
3. Maternal-infant interactions and conversations with mother regarding infant's behavior, weight, feedings, and sleep pattern.
4. Other assessments such as feeding, elimination, activity, vital signs on nursing flow sheet.
5. Reportable conditions, interventions, and outcomes.

VII. CIRCUMCISION
All male infants whose parents decide on circumcision will have the procedure performed when possible before discharge from the hospital according to the following criteria and procedure:

A. Criteria for circumcision.
1. The infant has stabilized and has been transferred to a bassinet.
2. The infant has been examined by the pediatrician, physician's assistant, or nurse practitioner, has been determined to be healthy, and has voided.
3. The infant has had nothing by mouth (NPO) for at least 30 minutes before the procedure.
4. The physician performing the procedure explains the major risks of the operation and the alternatives to the parents.
5. The parent signs the informed consent in the presence of the practitioner.

B. Equipment.
1. Circumcision instrument set and board.
2. Circumcision gauze (Vaseline).
3. Postcircumcision care instructions.
4. Petroleum jelly packets.
5. Surgical scrub.
6. Sterile water.
7. Equipment and medications, including EMLA cream for local anesthesia as instructed by physician.
8. Gown and gloves.

C. Procedure.
1. Apply EMLA cream to penis approximately 1 hour before procedure or per physician's order. Cover with an occlusive dressing.
2. Place the infant on the circumcision board.

N.B.: *Never* leave the infant unattended on the circumcision board. The door of the treatment room will remain closed when in use for circumcisions. RN or designee is to be in attendance throughout the procedure.

3. Secure the arms and legs into position on the board.
4. Prepare the penis with surgical scrub and sterile water.
5. Comfort infant as needed.
6. Remove the infant from the board after circumcision, put on diaper, and place infant on his side in the bassinet.
7. Clean the circumcision board with antimicrobial cleaning solution.
8. Rinse the circumcision instruments with water before placing them in the nursery soiled utility room. Change straps on circumcision board.
9. Stock the bassinet with circumcision gauze (Vaseline) packets.
10. Return the infant to the mother and review the postcircumcision care instructions with the mother. Instruct her to leave original gauze in place for 24 hours unless it is soiled.

D. Postcircumcision.

1. Babies circumcised immediately before discharge must remain 1 hour to be observed for bleeding.
2. Assess site for bleeding within and no later than 1 hour after circumcision.
3. Assess site every shift thereafter for swelling, bleeding, and exudate until time of discharge to home.
4. Interventions.
   a. Apply cloth diaper after circumcision.
   b. Apply petroleum jelly gauze strip if original strip becomes soiled or falls off before 24 hours.
   c. Apply petroleum jelly to penis after gauze strip is removed.
   d. Cuddle infant liberally and as necessary.
5. Reportable conditions.
   a. Bleeding.
   b. Swelling.
   c. Exudate.
   d. Denuding.
   e. Inability to void within 12 hours.
6. Documentation. Record observation on infant flow sheet: time, date, prep, operator, and assessment of the site after the procedure.

VIII. BREAST-FEEDING
A. Contraindications.

1. Mother
   a. HIV seropositive if tested.
   b. Positive hepatitis B surface antigen. (If positive, infant may breast-feed after receiving HBIG and initial dose of hepatitis B vaccine).
   c. Active tuberculosis.
   d. Taking medication, including lithium.
   e. Positive drug screen during this pregnancy (e.g., cocaine, heroin).
   f. Breast cancer.
2. Infant diagnosed with galactosemia.

B. Responsibilities.

1. The RN caring for the infant is responsible for supporting and teaching the mother who is breast-feeding.
2. The RN caring for the infant is responsible for assessing the infant's latch every 8 hours and prn.
3. The RN may delegate observation of a breast-feeding session to her designee.
4. This protocol should be initiated as soon as possible in the Labor and Delivery area by the primary nurse/designee unless infant's or mother's condition is unstable (e.g. mother is heavily sedated, infant's 5-minute Apgar score is low, infant is transferred to nursery immediately after delivery, infant has choanal atresia).

C. Assessment.

1. Perform a breast examination on mother before the initiation of breast-feeding. Check for the presence of any surgical scars, flat or inverted nipples, and normal glandular development.
2. Assess proper placement of mother's hand on breast during breast-feeding.
3. Assess mother and infant's body position for proper alignment during feeding.
4. Observe the quality of the breast-feeding session every 8 hours using the LATCH Charting System (Table I-1). If the nurse/designee is unable to observe the breast-feeding session, the LATCH score is obtained by asking the patient to give a verbal report of the breast-feeding session.
5. Assess for nutritive sucking at each breast-feeding session.
   a. Movement of jaw (wide jaw excursions).
   b. Sustained audible swallowing. If difficult to hear, place a stethoscope at the base of the infant's chin as he swallows.
   c. Cheeks rounded (no smacking sounds or dimpling in the cheeks).
   d. Mother does not report nipple pain after infant has latched onto breast.

D. Interventions.

1. Encourage rooming-in whenever possible to provide opportunity for short, frequent feedings as often as every 2 to 3 hours and no longer than 15 minutes on each side before mother's milk comes in.
   a. Short, frequent feedings are the most beneficial means of establishing the mother's milk supply.
   b. Watch for signs that the infant may be ready to nurse (e.g., sucking on fingers or blanket, rooting, awake and alert). If the infant is in the nursery, take the infant to the mother when baby is awake. If the infant is crying and frantic, calm before beginning a feeding.
   c. If the baby is sleepy, rouse for feeding by talking and playing and massaging chest and back.
2. Help the mother find a comfortable position. Use lots of pillows to support her back and arms.
3. Help the mother to position the infant for feeding. Infant should be nursed in different positions (cradle, football, lying down). The in-

TABLE I-1
LATCH Charting System*

	0	1	2
L (latch)	Too sleepy or reluctant; no latch achieved	Repeated attempts, holds nipple in mouth; stimulated to suck	Grasps breast; tongue down; lips flanged; rhythmical sucking
A (audible swallowing)	None	Few swallows with stimulation	Spontaneous and intermittent at <24 hr old; spontaneous and frequent at >24 hr old
T (type of nipple)	Inverted	Flat	Everted (after stimulation)
C (comfort: breast/nipple)	Breast engorged; nipples cracked, bleeding; large blisters or bruises; severe discomfort	Breast filling; nipples reddened; small blisters or bruises; mild to moderate discomfort	Breast soft and nontender
H (hold positioning)	Full assist (staff holds)	Minimal assist (i.e., pillows, raise or lower head of bed); teach one side, mom does other; staff holds then mom takes over	No assist from staff; mom able to position and hold baby

From Jensen D, Wallace S, Kelsay P: *JOGNN* 23(1):27-31, 1994.
*Assess each dimension on a scale of 0-1-2; the higher the result, the better.

fant's body should be held so that the ventral (front) surface of the infant faces the mother.

4. Help the mother to correctly hold her breast for her infant. Have the mother tickle the infant's lower lip with her breast or nipple, then draw the infant in close to the breast as soon as the mouth is open wide.
   a. Never push the infant's head toward the breast because the infant may push back, often arching away from the breast.
   b. Timing should be casual and not with stopwatch rigidity. Usually infants nurse about 5 to 15 minutes at one or both breasts per feeding in the first days after birth.

5. When the mother is producing milk, follow the infant's cues in determining when the infant is finished nursing.

6. If the infant falls asleep without releasing the breast, instruct the mother to gently remove the infant from her breast. To remove the infant from the breast, gently insert a finger into the corner of the infant's mouth between the gums, releasing the suction.

7. Gently burp the infant. Help the mother reposition the infant on the second breast if the infant is still interested (awake) after releasing the first side. The mother may need to wait a little, wake the infant, and move to the second side.

8. Obtain a blood glucose level immediately after feeding for the following conditions:
   a. Infant is lethargic.
   b. Infant has not latched on to the breast and nursed over an 8-hour period.
   c. Risk factors such as respiratory distress, maternal history of insulin-dependent or gestational diabetes, temperature instability.

9. Supplementation must be considered if any of the following conditions are present:
   a. The infant cannot latch on to the breast AND blood glucose is <40 mg/dl.
   b. The infant is premature (<37 weeks gestation) and unable to latch onto the breast.
   c. The mother's nipples are severely inverted and latching on has failed.

10. Supplementation should be provided with a medical order.
    a. Obtain a medical order for supplementation.
    b. Supplement the full-term infant (<37 weeks gestation) with the use of a 5-ml syringe, by finger feeding with gavage tubing, or use of an orthodontic nipple (NUK) to minimize the risk of nipple confusion.
    c. Premature infants (<37 weeks gestation) must have a medical order for mode and type of supplementation.

11. Do not routinely give pacifiers to breast-feeding infants before successful breast-feeding has been established.

12. Initiate regular milk expression with breast pump when infant and mother are separated. Mother should begin pumping within 6 to 12 hours after delivery or when she is physically able to use a breast pump.

13. Provide breast-feeding counseling.
    a. Engorgement.
        (1) Encourage frequent nursing (every 2 to 3 hours). It is the most effective mechanism for removal of milk and prevention of engorgement. Do not skip feedings during the night.
        (2) Apply warm soaks or advise the mother to take a warm shower just before a feeding to facilitate manual expression and latching on to the breast.
        (3) Manually express or pump breasts to soften the areola before nursing.
        (4) Compress and hold onto areola between two fingers to make it easier for the infant to grasp.
        (5) Offer pain medication if needed. Offer medication immediately after nursing so that the least amount possible reaches mother's milk and the baby (most medications take 30 minutes to get into the milk).
        (6) Advise the mother to wear a well-fitted brassiere.
        (7) Apply ice packs to breast between feedings to relieve discomfort.
    b. Sore, painful, or cracked nipples (best prevented by proper latch-on and positioning).
        (1) Use relaxation and massage to facilitate milk let-down before nursing.
        (2) Nurse on the least affected or sore side first. Rotate infant's position at each feeding (cradle, lying down, football hold).
        (3) Let expressed breast milk dry on nipples and areola after feeding.
        (4) Apply dry heat to nipples with a hair dryer, held at arm's length, on low setting after feedings.
        (5) Provide pain medication immediately after nursing if needed.
        (6) Avoid routine use of ointments, creams, and lotions on nipple, areola, or breast.
        (7) Avoid nipple shields.
    c. Flat or inverted nipples.
        (1) Assist mother with positioning and latch-on.
        (2) Plastic breast shells may be worn inside the mother's bra between feedings. Instruct the mother to remove the breast shells during sleep.
        (3) Discard milk that accumulates in the shells.
        (4) Shells may be washed with mild soap and water.
    d. Review patient teaching on nutrition, breast pump rental, pumping and storage, and breast and nipple care.

E. Reportable conditions.
1. Refer to pediatrician, lactation consultant, or PNP if any of the following conditions occur:
    a. Infant has not latched on and nursed by 8 hours of age.
    b. Premature infant (<37 weeks).
    c. IUGR.
    d. Multiple gestation.

    e. Severe or persistent nipple soreness; inverted nipples.

    f. Infant has excessive weight loss (greater than 10% of birth weight).

    g. Mother requests consult.

    h. Persistent maternal anxiety about breast-feeding.

    i. Mother being discharged before infant's discharge.

    j. Maternal medical-surgical history (e.g., history of breast surgery, diabetes mellitus, multiple sclerosis, cystic fibrosis).

2. Refer to pediatrician or PNP if the infant has any of the following conditions:

    a. Hypoglycemia (blood glucose <40 mg/dl).

    b. Lethargy.

    c. Infant is breast-feeding poorly (has not latched on to the breast for >8 hours).

3. Refer to obstetrician or certified nurse manager (CNM) if the following conditions occur:

    a. Maternal breasts are hot, red, swollen, and painful.

    b. Maternal fever (temperature >38° C).

F. Documentation.

1. Medical order to supplement infant.

2. Breast-feeding education on multidisciplinary patient education flow sheet.

3. Reportable condition on nursing flow sheet.

4. Document the total LATCH on the infant's flow sheet.

IX. RISKY SITUATIONS (Table I-2)

A. Indications of risk and predisposing factors for infants.

1. Respiratory rate >60 or <30.

2. Heart rate >180 or <60.

3. Respiratory distress (stridor, grunting, nasal flaring, retractions, audible wheezing).

4. Cyanosis, pallor.

5. Diminishing level of consciousness, lethargy.

6. Seizures, hypertonicity.

7. Fever or sepsis.

B. Assessment.

1. Assess for predisposing factors listed above.

2. Assess the following ABCs:

    a. **A**irway patency.

    b. **B**reathing (breath sounds, lung expansion, respiratory effort).

    c. **C**irculation (heart rate, blood pressure, color, muscle tone).

C. Interventions.

1. Respiratory distress (stridor, grunting, nasal flaring, retractions, audible wheezing).

    a. Observe and evaluate infant respirations; help to keep airway patent.

2. Notify pediatrician.

3. Provide free-flowing oxygen if central cyanosis is present.

4. Respiratory arrest (infant not breathing spontaneously after opening airway).

TABLE I-2
Risk Factors and Associated Laboratory Tests
in the Newborn Nursery

Risk factors	Urine toxicology	Hemoglobin	Glucose
Abortion (≥2 therapeutic or spontaneous abortions)	X		
Apgar score ≤5 at 5 minutes		X	XX
Born outside the hospital or department	X	X	X
Changes in level of consciousness			XXO
Excessive irritability	X		XO
Excessive tremors			XXO
Feeding problems			O
Hypertonia	X		XX
Hypothermia (rectal temperature <36.5° C)			XXO
Hypotonia (lethargic)			XXO
Late registrant after 28 weeks or fewer than three visits	X		
LGA (Dubowitz) or weight >3800 gm			X
Maternal history of ≥2 sexually transmitted diseases (e.g., gonorrhea, syphilis, trichomonas, chlamydia, herpes, human papilloma virus)	X		
Maternal history of hepatitis B infection	X		
Maternal history of substance abuse in this or other pregnancies	X		
Maternal positive toxicology screen at this admission or during this pregnancy	X		

XX, Measure glucose by 1 hour of age; *X,* by 2 hours of age; *O,* whenever.

TABLE I-2
**Risk Factors and Associated Laboratory Tests
in the Newborn Nursery—cont'd**

Risk factors	Urine toxicology	Hemoglobin	Glucose
Maternal diabetes mellitus (gestational or insulin dependent), large amounts of IV glucose			XX
Maternal morbid obesity			X
Meconium-stained amniotic fluid (intrapartum)			X
Multiple births			X
No prenatal care	X		X
Nuchal cord requiring transection before delivery		X	
Placenta previa or accreta		X	
Placenta abruption	X	X	
Polycythemia (hemoglobin >22 mg/dl)			XO
Postterm by examination (>42 0/7 weeks)			X
Precipitous delivery (<3 hours from the onset of labor)	X		
Premature delivery (<37 weeks)	X	X	X
Prolonged rupture of membranes ≥18 hr			X
Respiratory distress (tachypnea, apnea, cyanosis, stridor, grunting, retractions, nasal flaring)		X	XO
Rh sensitization		X	
Ruddy color		X	
SGA (Dubowitz) or weight <2500 gm	X	X	X

a. **Call for help.**
b. Give positive-pressure ventilation with bag and mask to infants who are apneic or having gasping respirations after stimulation.
c. If unable to get a good "seal" for effective ventilation, reposition infant, check equipment, suction oropharynx, and attempt to reventilate.

5. Cardiac arrest (heart rate <60, with respiratory arrest requiring positive pressure ventilations).
   a. Place infant on backboard under a warmer and begin cardiopulmonary resuscitation (CPR).
   b. **Call for help.**
   c. Continue CPR until help arrives.
   d. Assist physician as needed.

6. Role delineation of team members during a cardiopulmonary arrest.
   a. Patient's nurse.
      (1) Remains at bedside initiating CPR while calling for help.
      (2) Assists the Pediatric department arrest team by doing the following:
         (a) Provides a report of the patient medical history and status before the arrest.
         (b) Retrieves medications.
         (c) Retrieves supplies for special procedures.
         (d) Obtains the infant's blood glucose level.
         (e) Communicates with recording and charge nurses the infant's status and response to interventions.
         (f) Ensures completeness and accuracy of nursing documentation of arrest activities after the episodes.
   b. Pediatrician. The most senior medical staff will manage the code.
   c. Charge nurse.
      (1) Responsible for delegation of or checking emergency equipment at the start of the shift.
      (2) Responsible for assignment and reassignment of nursing roles during an emergency.
      (3) Ensures that the arrest team members are present and carrying out assigned roles.
      (4) Ensures crowd control, insisting that personnel who are not needed leave the area.
      (5) Ensures that all patients in the unit are being adequately cared for by utilizing resource people such as a clinical nurse specialist, nurse educator, or case manager.
   d. Recorder nurse.
      (1) Responsible for documentation of drugs given and time of administration, and procedures.
      (2) Documents highlights of resuscitation effort (i.e., patient's response to medication or intervention).
   e. Ancillary support staff.
      (1) Places call to the pediatric arrest team.
      (2) Retrieves additional supplies from clean utility room.

    (3) Assists in attending to other patients' needs.

    (4) Should not leave the floor when an arrest is taking place.

D. The following documentation should be made on the pediatric arrest flow sheet.

1. Resuscitation efforts.
2. Patient's response.
3. Medications and time of administration.
4. Procedures performed.
5. Disposition of the infant.

REFERENCES

Wong D: *Whaley and Wong's nursing care of infants and children,* ed 5, St. Louis, 1995, Mosby.

Cultural Considerations

TABLE J-1
Some Religious Beliefs That Affect Newborn Care

Religion		Beliefs about birth	Beliefs regarding medical care
Adventist (Seventh Day Adventist; Church of God)	**Birth:**	Opposed to infant baptism Baptism in adulthood	Some believe in divine healing and practice anointing with oil and use of prayer May desire communion or baptism when ill Believe in man's choice and God's sovereignty
Baptist (27 groups)	**Birth:**	Opposed to infant baptism Believers baptized by immersion as adults	"Laying on of hands" (some) May encounter some resistance to some therapies, such as abortion
	Death:	Counsel and prayer with clergy, family, patient	Believe God functions through physician Some believe in predestination; may respond passively to care
Buddhist Churches of America	**Birth:**	No infant baptism Infant presentation	Illness believed to be a trial to aid development of soul; illness is due to karmic causes May be reluctant to have surgery or certain treatments on holy days
	Death:	Last rites chanting often practiced at bedside soon after death Priest should be contacted	Cleanliness believed to be of great importance Family may require Buddhist priest for counseling

Modified from Seidel HM, Ball JW, et al: Mosby's guide to physical examination, ed 3, St Louis, 1995, Mosby.

Continued

TABLE J-1
Some Religious Beliefs That Affect Newborn Care—cont'd

Religion	Beliefs about birth		Beliefs regarding medical care
Church of Christ Scientist (Christian Science)	**Birth:**	No baptism	Deny the existence of health crisis; see sickness and sin as errors of mind that can be altered by prayer
	Death:	No last rites	Oppose human intervention with drugs or other therapies; however, most accept legally required immunizations
			Many adhere to belief that disease is a human mental concept that can be dispelled by "spiritual truth" to extent that they refuse all medical treatment
Church of Jesus Christ of Latter Day Saints (Mormon)	**Birth:**	No baptism at birth	Devout adherents believe in divine healing through anointment with oil and "laying on of hands" by church official (elder)
		Infant is "blessed" by church official at first opportunity after birth (in church)	Medical therapy not prohibited
		Baptism by immersion at 8 years	
	Death:	No special rites	
Eastern Orthodox (e.g., Turkey, Egypt, Syria, Romania, Bulgaria, Cyprus, Albania)	**Birth:**	Most believe in infant baptism by immersion 8 to 40 days after birth	Anointment of the sick
	Death:	Last rites obligatory for impending death	No conflict with medical science

Episcopal (Anglican)	**Birth:** Infant baptism mandatory; urgent if poor prognosis **Death:** Last rites available but not mandatory	Some believe in spiritual healing Rite for anointing sick available but not mandatory
Friends (Quakers)	**Birth:** No baptism Infant's name recorded in official book	No special rites or restrictions
Greek Orthodox	**Birth:** Baptism considered important Performed 40 days after birth If not possible to baptize by sprinkling or immersion, Church allows child baptism "in the air" by moving the child in the form of a cross as appropriate words are said **Death:** Last rites, administration of Sacrament of Holy Communion; should be performed while dying person is still conscious	Each health crisis handled by ordained priest; deacon may also serve in some cases Holy Communion administered in hospital Some may desire Sacrament of the Holy Unction performed by priest

Continued

Modified from Seidel HM, Ball JW, et al: *Mosby's guide to physical examination*, ed 3, St Louis, 1995, Mosby.

TABLE J-1
Some Religious Beliefs That Affect Newborn Care—cont'd

Religion	Beliefs about birth	Beliefs regarding medical care
Hindu	**Birth:** No ritual **Death:** Special prescribed rites Priest pours water into the mouth of dead child, ties a thread around neck or wrist to signify blessing (should not be removed) Family washes body and is particular about who touches body	Illness or injury believed to represent sins committed in previous life Accept most modern medical practices
Islam (Muslim/Moslem)	**Birth:** No baptism **Death:** Family should be present Family washes and prepares body, then turns it to face Mecca Only relatives and friends may touch body	Faith healing not acceptable unless psychologic condition of patient is deteriorating; performed for morale Ritual washing after prayer; prayer takes place five times daily (on rising, midday, afternoon, early-evening, and before bed); during prayer, face Mecca and kneel on prayer rug
Jehovah's Witness	**Birth:** No baptism **Death:** No last rites	Adherents are generally absolutely opposed to blood transfusions, including banking of own blood; individuals can sometimes be persuaded in emergencies

Judaism (Orthodox and Conservative)	**Birth:**	No baptism Ritual circumcision of male infants on eighth day; performed by Mohel (ritual circumciser familiar with Jewish law and aseptic technique) Reform Jews favor ritual circumcision, but not as a religious imperative	May resist surgical procedures during Sabbath, which extends from sundown Friday until sundown Saturday
	Death:	Remains are ritually washed by members of the Ritual Burial Society Burial should take place as soon as possible	
Lutheran	**Birth:**	Baptism only for living infants shortly after birth	If grave prognosis, family may request anointing and blessing of sick or visit by church official
	Death:	Last rites optional	
Mennonite (similar to Amish)	**Birth:**	No baptism in infancy	No illness rituals
Methodist	**Birth:**	No baptism at birth	Communion may be requested before surgery or similar crisis
	Death:	No ritual	

Modified from Seidel HM, Ball JW, et al: *Mosby's guide to physical examination,* ed 3, St Louis, 1995, Mosby.

Continued

TABLE J-1
Some Religious Beliefs That Affect Newborn Care—cont'd

Religion	Beliefs about birth		Beliefs regarding medical care
Nazarene	**Birth:**	Baptism optional	Church official administers communion and laying on of hands
	Death:	No last rites	Adherents believe in divine healing but not exclusive of medical treatment
Pentecostal (Assembly of God, Foursquare)	**Birth:**	No baptism at birth	No restrictions regarding medical care
	Death:	No last rites	Deliverance from sickness is provided for in atonement; may pray for divine intervention in health matters and seek God in prayer for themselves and others when ill
Orthodox Presbyterian	**Birth:**	Infant baptism by sprinkling	Communion administered when appropriate and convenient
	Death:	Last rites not a sacramental procedure; scripture reading and prayer	Blood transfusion accepted when advisable
			Pastor or elder should be called for ill person
			Believe science should be used for relief of suffering

Roman Catholics	**Birth:**	Infant baptism mandatory; especially urgent in poor prognosis, when it may be performed by anyone
	Death:	Rites for anointing of the sick are mandatory Family or patient may request anointing if prognosis is grave	Encourage anointing of the sick, although this may be interpreted by older members of church as equivalent to the old terminology, "extreme unction" or "last rites"; they may require a careful explanation if their reluctance is associated with fear of imminent death
Russian Orthodox	**Birth:**	Baptism by priest only
	Death:	Traditionally after death, arms are crossed, fingers set in a cross	Cross necklace is important and should be removed only when necessary and replaced as soon as possible Adherent believe in divine healing, but not exclusive of medical treatment
Unitarian Universalist	**Birth:**	Some practice infant baptism; most consider it unnecessary	Believe God helps those who help themselves Some may prefer not to have clergy visit them in hospital
	Death:	No ritual

Continued

Modified from Seidel HM, Ball JW, et al: *Mosby's guide to physical examination*, ed 3, St Louis, 1995, Mosby.

TABLE J-2
Cultural Characteristics Related to Newborn Care—cont'd

Cultural group	Health beliefs	Health and diet practices	Family relationships	Communication	Comments
Asian Americans Chinese	A healthy body is viewed as a gift from parents and ancestors and must be cared for Health is one of the results of balance between the forces of *yin* (cold) and *yang* (hot), energy forces that rule the world Illness is caused by imbalance Believe blood is source of life and is not regenerated *Chi* is innate energy	Goal of therapy is to restore balance of *yin* and *yang* Wide use of medicinal herbs procured and applied in prescribed ways Folk healers are herbalist, spiritual healer, temple healer, fortune healer Milk intolerance relatively common	Extended family pattern common Strong concept of loyalty of young to old Family and individual honor and "face" important Self-reliance and self-restraint highly valued; self-expression repressed Males valued more highly than females; women submissive to men in family	Open expression of emotions unacceptable Often smile when do not comprehend	Are especially upset by drawing of blood Deep respect for their bodies and believe it best to die with bodies intact; therefore may refuse surgery May believe in reincarnation Children sometimes breast-fed for up to 4 or 5 years*

Japanese	Lack of *chi* and blood result in deficiency that produces poor constitution and long illness Three major belief systems: *Shinto*—religious influence, human inherently good, evil caused by contact with polluting agents (e.g., blood, corpses, skin disease; *Chinese and Korean influence*—health achieved through harmony and balance between self and	Believe evil removed by purification *Kampo* medicine—use of natural herbs Believe in removal of diseased parts Trend is to use both Western and Eastern healing methods Care for disabled viewed as family's responsibility Take pride in child's good health	Close intergenerational relationships Family provides anchor Family tends to keep problems to self Value self-control and self-sufficiency Many adopt practices of contemporary middle class Co-sleeping of infants with parents is common	*Issei*—born in Japan; usually speak Japanese only *Nisei, Sansei,* and *Yonsei* have few language difficulties New immigrants able to read and write English better than to speak or understand it	Generational categories: *Issei*—first generation to live in United States *Nisei*—second generation *Sansei*—third generation *Yonsei*—fourth generation Cleanliness highly valued

Modified from Wong DL: *Whaley & Wong's nursing care of infants and children,* ed 3, St Louis, 1995, Mosby.
*Most Asian cultures consider the child 1 year old at the time of birth. Traditional Chinese custom adds 1 year on January 1 regardless of the birthday—a child born in December is 2 years old the next January.

Continued

TABLE J-2
Cultural Characteristics Related to Newborn Care—cont'd

Cultural group	Health beliefs	Health and diet practices	Family relationships	Communication	Comments
Japanese—cont'd	society, disease caused by disharmony with society and not caring for body; *Portuguese influence*—upholds germ theory of disease	Seek preventive care, medical care for illness		Make significant use of nonverbal communication with subtle gestures and facial expressions Tend to suppress emotions Will often wait silently	Time considered valuable, to be used wisely Tendency to practice emotional control may make assessment of situation more difficult
Vietnamese	Good health considered to be balance between *yin* (cold) and *yang* (hot) Believe person's life has been predisposed toward certain phenomena by cosmic forces Health believed to be result of harmony	Fortune-tellers determine disturbance that caused disturbance May visit temple to procure divine instruction Regard health as family responsibility; outside aid sought when resources run out	Family is revered institution Multigenerational families Family is chief social network Children highly valued Individual needs and interests are subordinate to those of family group	Many immigrants are not proficient in speaking and understanding English May hesitate to ask questions Questioning authority is sign of disrespect; asking questions	Consider status more important than money Time concept more relaxed—consider punctuality less significant than other values (e.g., propriety) Place high value on social harmony

	with existing universal order, harmony attained by pleasing good spirits and avoiding evil ones Belief in *am duc*, the amount of good deeds accumulated by ancestors Many use rituals to prevent illness Practice some restrictions to prevent illness by incurring wrath of evil spirits	Certain illnesses considered only temporary (such as pustules, open wounds) and ignored Seek generalist health healers Lactose intolerance prevalent	Father is main decision maker Women taught submission to men	considered impolite Use indirectness rather than forthrightness in expressing disagreement May avoid eye contact with health professionals as a sign of respect	
Filipino	Believe God's will and supernatural forces govern universe Illness, accidents, and other misfortunes are God's punishment for violations of his will	Some use amulets as a shield from witchcraft or as good luck pieces Catholics substitute religious medals and other items	Family is highly valued, with strong family ties Multigenerational family structure common, often with collateral members as well	Immigrants and older persons may not be able to speak or understand English	Tend to have a fatalistic outlook on life Believe time and Providence will solve all

Modified from Wong DL: *Whaley & Wong's nursing care of infants and children*, ed 3, St Louis, 1995, Mosby.

Continued

TABLE J-2
Cultural Characteristics Related to Newborn Care—cont'd

Cultural group	Health beliefs	Health and diet practices	Family relationships	Communication	Comments
Filipino—cont'd	Widely accept "hot" and "cold" balance and imbalance as cause of health and illness		Personal interests are subordinated to family interests and needs Members avoid any behavior that would bring shame on the family		
African American	Illness classified as *natural*—affected by forces of nature without adequate protection (e.g., cold air, pollution, food, and water); *unnatural*—evil influences (e.g., witchcraft, voodoo, hoodoo, hex, fix, rootwork); symp-	Self-care and folk medicine prevalent Folk therapies usually religious in origin Attempt home remedies first; poorer people do not seek help until illness is serious Prayer is common means for prevention and treatment	Strong kinship bonds in extended family; members come to aid others in crisis Less likely to view illness as a burden Sex-role sharing among parents	Alert to any evidence of discrimination Place importance on nonverbal behavior May use nonstandard English or "Black English" Use "testing" behaviors to assess person-	High level of caution and distrust of majority group Social anxiety related to tradition of humiliation, oppression, and loss of dignity Will elect to retain dignity rather than seek care if values are compromised

	Health/Illness beliefs	Health practices	Family/social organization	Communication	Health care
(African American)	...toms often associated with eating Believe serious illness sent by God as punishment (e.g., parents punished by illness or death of child) Believe serious illness can be avoided May resist health care because illness is "will of God"			nel in health care situations before seeking active care	Strong sense of peoplehood Minister a strong influence in African American community Visits by family minister are sought, expected, and valued in helping to cope with illness and suffering
Haitian	Illness has supernatural or natural origin Supernatural illnesses are caused by angry voodoo spirits, enemies, or the dead, especially ancestors	Health is a personal responsibility Food has properties of "hot"/"cold" and "light"/"heavy" and must be in harmony with one's life cycle and bodily states	Maintenance of family reputation is paramount Lineal authority supreme; children in a subordinate position in family hierarchy	Recent immigrants and older persons may speak only Haitian Creole May prefer family/friends to act as translators and confidants	Will use biomedical and ethnomedical (folk) systems simultaneously Adherence to prescribed treatments directly related to perceived severity of illness

Continued

Modified from Wong DL: *Whaley & Wong's nursing care of infants and children*, ed 3, St Louis, 1995, Mosby.

TABLE J-2
Cultural Characteristics Related to Newborn Care—cont'd

Cultural group	Health beliefs	Health and diet practices	Family relationships	Communication	Comments
Haitian—cont'd	Natural illnesses based on concep- tions of natural causes: Irregularities in blood Movement and consistency of mother's milk Hot/cold imbalance in the body Health is maintained by good dietary and hygienic habits	Natural illnesses are treated by home remedies first Supernatural illnesses are treated by heal- ers: voodoo priest (houngan) or priest- ess (mambo), mid- wife (fam saj), and herbalist or leaf doctor (dokte fey) Amulets and prayer used to protect against illness caused by curses or willed by evil people	Children valued for parental social security in old age and expected to contribute to family welfare at an early age Children viewed as "gifts from god" and treated with indul- gence and affection	Often smile and nod in agree- ment when do not understand Quiet and gentle communication style and lack of assertiveness may lead health care providers to believe wrongly that they com- prehend health teaching and are compliant Will not ask ques- tions if health care provider is busy or rushed	

Hispanic American Mexican-American (Latino, Chicano, Raza-Latino)	Health beliefs have strong religious association Believe in body imbalance as a cause of illness, especially imbalance between *caliente* (hot) and *frio* (cold) or "wet" and "dry" Some maintain good health is a result of "good luck"—a reward for good behavior Illness is a punishment from God for wrongdoing, forces of nature, and the supernatural	Treatments involve use of herbs, rituals, and religious artifacts; visit shrines, offer medals and candles, offer prayers Adhere to "hot" and "cold" food prescriptions and prohibitions for prevention and treatment of illness	Traditionally men considered breadwinners, women homemakers Males are considered big and strong *(macho)* Strong kinship; extended families include compadres (godparents) established by ritual kinship Children valued highly and desired	May use nonstandard English Most bilingual; may speak only Spanish May have a strong preference for native language and revert to it in times of stress	High degree of modesty—often a deterrent to seeking medical care Magicoreligious practices common

Continued

Modified from Wong DL: *Whaley & Wong's nursing care of infants and children*, ed 3, St Louis, 1995, Mosby.

TABLE J-2
Cultural Characteristics Related to Newborn Care—cont'd

Cultural group	Health beliefs	Health and diet practices	Family relationships	Communication	Comments
Puerto Rican	Subscribe to the "hot-cold" theory of causation of illness Believe some illness caused by evil spirits and forces	Infrequent use of health care systems Seek folk healers—use of herbs, rituals Treatment classified as "hot" or "cold"	Family usually large and home centered—the core of existence Father has complete authority in family—family provider and decision maker Wife and children subordinate to father Children valued—seen as a gift from God	May use nonstandard English Spanish speaking or bilingual Strong sense of family privacy—may view questions regarding family as impudent	Relaxed sense of time Pay little attention to exact time of day Suspicious and fearful of hospital
Cuban American	Prevention and good nutrition are related to good health	Diligent users of the medical model Eclectic health-seeking practices, including preventive measures and, in some instances,	Strong family ties with mother and father kinship	Most are bilingual (English/Spanish) except for segments of the senior population	In less than 30 years Cubans have been able to obtain a higher standard of living than other Hispanic groups in United States

folk medicine of both religious and nonreligious origins; home remedies; in many instances seek assistance of *santeros* (Afro-Cuban healers) and spiritualists to complement medical treatment Nutrition is important; parents show overconcern with eating habits of their children	Have been able to retain many of their former social institutions Many do not feel discriminated against or harbor feelings of inferiority with respect to Anglo-Americans or "mainstream" population

Continued

Modified from Wong DL: *Whaley & Wong's nursing care of infants and children*, ed 3, St Louis, 1995, Mosby.

TABLE J-2
Cultural Characteristics Related to Newborn Care—cont'd

Cultural group	Health beliefs	Health and diet practices	Family relationships	Communication	Comments
Native American (numerous tribes)	Believe health is state of harmony with nature and universe Respect of bodies through proper management All disorders believed to have aspects of supernatural Violation of a restriction or prohibition thought to cause illness	Medicine persons: altruistic persons who must use powers in purely positive ways Persons capable of both good and evil—perform negative acts against enemies	Extended family structure—usually includes relatives from both sides of family Elder members assume leadership roles	Most speak both their own language and English Nonverbal communication important	Time orientation—present Respect for age Going to hospital associated with illness or disease; therefore may not seek prenatal care because pregnancy viewed as natural process

Fear of witchcraft
May carry objects
 believed to guard
 against witchcraft
Theology and medi-
 cine strongly
 interwoven

Diviner-diagnosti-
 cians—diagnose
 but do not have
 powers or skill to
 implement medical
 treatment
Specialist—use herbs
 and curative but
 nonsacred medical
 procedures
Medicine persons—
 use herbs and ritual
Singers—cure by the
 power of their song
 obtained from
 supernatural
 beings, effect cures
 by laying on of
 hands

Modified from Wong DL: *Whaley & Wong's nursing care of infants and children*, ed 3, St Louis, 1995, Mosby.
*Most Asian cultures consider the child 1 year old at the time of birth. Traditional Chinese custom adds 1 year on January 1 regardless of the birth-
day—a child born in December is 2 years old the next January.

Index

Note: Page numbers in *italics* indicate illustrations and boxed material. Page numbers followed by *t* indicate tables.